Hematology and Oncology:
An Evidence-Based Approach

Hematology and Oncology: An Evidence-Based Approach

Edited by Dylan Hill

hayle
medical

New York

Hayle Medical,
750 Third Avenue, 9th Floor,
New York, NY 10017, USA

Visit us on the World Wide Web at:
www.haylemedical.com

ISBN: 978-1-63241-894-4

Cataloging-in-Publication Data

Hematology and oncology : an evidence-based approach / edited by Dylan Hill.
    p. cm.
Includes bibliographical references and index.
ISBN 978-1-63241-894-4
1. Hematology. 2. Oncology. 3. Blood--Diseases. 4. Cancer. 5. Leukemia. I. Hill, Dylan.
RC636 .H46 2020
616.15--dc23

Table of Contents

Preface

Blood is a body fluid which delivers nutrients and oxygen to the cells. It also transports metabolic wastes away from the cells. Any anomaly in the production of blood and its components, such as hemoglobin, bone marrow, platelets, spleen, blood proteins, the mechanism of coagulation, etc. is expressed as a blood disorder. Leukemia, myelodysplastic syndrome, thrombocytosis, polycythemia vera, etc. are some of the disorders of cell proliferation. Coagulation disorders include hemophilia, thrombophilia and coagulopathy. Hematological malignancies are malignant neoplasms affecting the blood, lymph, bone marrow and lymphatic system. These may derive from either the myeloid or lymphoid cell lines. All such disorders are treated in the domain of hematology and oncology. This book contains some path-breaking studies in the fields of hematology and oncology. The topics included herein are of utmost significance and bound to provide incredible insights to readers. This book aims to serve as a resource guide for students and experts alike and contribute to the growth of these disciplines.

All of the data presented henceforth, was collaborated in the wake of recent advancements in the field. The aim of this book is to present the diversified developments from across the globe in a comprehensible manner. The opinions expressed in each chapter belong solely to the contributing authors. Their interpretations of the topics are the integral part of this book, which I have carefully compiled for a better understanding of the readers.

At the end, I would like to thank all those who dedicated their time and efforts for the successful completion of this book. I also wish to convey my gratitude towards my friends and family who supported me at every step.

Editor

NF-κB signaling and its relevance to the treatment of mantle cell lymphoma

Swathi Balaji, Makhdum Ahmed, Elizabeth Lorence, Fangfang Yan, Krystle Nomie and Michael Wang[*]

Abstract

Mantle cell lymphoma is an aggressive subtype of non-Hodgkin B cell lymphoma that is characterized by a poor prognosis determined by Ki67 and Mantle Cell International Prognostic Index scores, but it is becoming increasingly treatable. The majority of patients, especially if young, achieve a progression-free survival of at least 5 years. Mantle cell lymphoma can initially be treated with an anti-CD20 antibody in combination with a chemotherapy backbone, such as VR-CAP (the anti-CD20 monoclonal antibody rituximab administered with cyclophosphamide, doxorubicin, and prednisone) or R-CHOP (the anti-CD20 monoclonal antibody rituximab administered with cyclophosphamide, doxorubicin, vincristine, and prednisone). While initial treatment can facilitate recovery and complete remission in a few patients, many patients experience relapsed or refractory mantle cell lymphoma within 2 to 3 years after initial treatment. Targeted agents such as ibrutinib, an inhibitor of Bruton's tyrosine kinase, which has been approved only in the relapsed setting, can be used to treat patients with relapsed or refractory mantle cell lymphoma. However, mantle cell lymphoma cells often acquire resistance to such targeted agents and continue to survive by activating alternate signaling pathways such as the PI3K-Akt pathway or the NF-κB pathways.

NF-κB is a transcription factor family that regulates the growth and survival of B cells; mantle cell lymphoma cells depend on NF-κB signaling for continued growth and proliferation. The NF-κB signaling pathways are categorized into canonical and non-canonical types, wherein the canonical pathway prompts inflammatory responses, immune regulation, and cell proliferation, while the non-canonical leads to B cell maturation and lymphoid organogenesis. Since these pathways upregulate survival genes and tumor-promoting cytokines, they can be activated to overcome the inhibitory effects of targeted agents, thereby having profound effects on tumorigenesis. The NF-κB pathways are also highly targetable in that they are interconnected with numerous other pathways, including B cell receptor signaling, PI3K/Akt/mTOR signaling, and toll-like receptor signaling pathways. Additionally, elements of the non-canonical NF-κB pathway, such as NF-κB-inducing kinase, can be targeted to overcome resistance to targeting of the canonical NF-κB pathway.

Targeting the molecular mechanisms of the NF-κB pathways can facilitate the development of novel agents to treat malignancies and overcome drug resistance in patients with relapsed or refractory mantle cell lymphoma.

Keywords: NF-κB, Mantle cell lymphoma, Canonical pathway, Non-canonical pathway

Background

Mantle cell lymphoma (MCL) is an aggressive B cell lymphoma with one of the worst prognoses of all non-Hodgkin lymphomas. MCL cells are marked by a t(11;14) chromosomal translocation and overexpression of cyclin D1. Although MCL is incurable to date, impressive response rates have been achieved via targeted agents, such as ibrutinib, a Bruton's tyrosine kinase (BTK) inhibitor. Unfortunately, MCL cells inevitably develop resistance to ibrutinib, making it difficult to treat. While some MCL cell lines are highly sensitive to the B cell receptor (BCR) signaling inhibitors ibrutinib and sotrastaurin, other MCL cell lines, including Z-138 and Maver-1, are insensitive and demonstrate activation of the non-canonical NF-κB pathway, instead of the canonical pathway [1]. This finding suggests that patients with drug-resistant MCL may benefit from alternate treatment approaches, particularly those that are independent of the BCR signaling pathway.

* Correspondence: miwang@mdanderson.org
Department of Lymphoma/Myeloma, University of Texas MD Anderson Cancer Center, 1515 Holcombe Blvd. Unit 0429, Houston, TX 77030-4009, USA

The nuclear factor kappa-light-chain enhancer of activated B cells (NF-κB) is a transcription factor family that regulates the expression of growth factors, cytokines, chemokines, adhesion molecules, and apoptosis inhibitors [2]. NF-κB is known for its regulatory role in inflammatory responses and other pathological processes, including cell differentiation and survival. The NF-κB family has five monomers: RelA, RelB, c-Rel, p50, and 52, which combine to form up to 15 different NF-κB complexes, of which p50–p65 (canonical) and p52-RelB (non-canonical) are paradigmatic.

There are several pathways for NF-κB activation, but the two primary pathways are the canonical and non-canonical pathways. The canonical pathway is triggered by toll-like microbial pattern recognition receptors (TLRs) and pro-inflammatory cytokines such as tumor necrosis factor alpha (TNFα) and interleukin-1 (IL-1), which leads to the activation of RelA- or cRel-containing complexes [3]. The non-canonical pathway is activated by TNF (tumor necrosis factor) family cytokines, including lymphotoxin β (TNFSF3), CD40 ligand (CD40L and TNFSF5), and B cell-activating factor (BAFF and TNFSF13B). The canonical pathway has downstream effects including inflammatory responses, immune regulation, and cell proliferation, while the non-canonical pathway's downstream effects lead to B cell maturation and lymphoid organogenesis. An understanding of NF-κB pathway mechanisms in MCL tumorigenesis will facilitate the development of more effective therapeutic agents that suit different patient populations (Table 1).

Main text
The canonical pathway

The p50–p65 heterodimer is a transcription factor of the NF-kB family that is bound to and inhibited by IκB. Activation of the canonical pathway leads to proteasomal degradation of IκB, leading to downstream gene expression.

The p50–p65 heterodimer is initially bound to IκB, which prevents the heterodimer from entering the nucleus and enabling gene expression. Lipopolysaccharides (LPSs), tumor necrosis factor alpha (TNF-α), and interleukin-1 (IL-1) activate toll-like receptors (TLR), tumor necrosis factor receptors (TNFR), and interleukin-1 receptors (IL-1R), respectively. Activation of these receptors initiates adapter protein and signaling kinase responses, leading to activation of the IκB kinase (IKK) complex. The IKK complex consists of IKKα, IKKβ, and two IKKγ (NEMO) kinases, which phosphorylate IκB on the serine residues S32 and S36, leading to the poly-ubiquitination and proteasomal degradation of IκB [4]. This allows the p50 and p65-RelA heterodimer (a complex from the NF-κB family) to be released into the nucleus to induce gene expression.

Interactions with signaling pathways that coordinate with the NF-κB canonical pathway

BCR signaling The downstream effects of antigen-mediated BCR signaling lead to activation of BTK and eventually the IKK complex, which leads to gene expression via the canonical pathway. The BCR signaling pathway is mediated by receptor tyrosine kinase-mediated signal transduction. The B cell receptor consists of the immunoglobulins IgM, IgD, Ig-alpha, and Ig-beta, which are expressed by B cells and bound to CD79a/CD79b. When antigens bind to these immunoglobulins, tyrosine kinases including LYN, FYN, and B lymphocyte tyrosine kinase (BLK) phosphorylate the dual-tyrosine containing immunoreceptor tyrosine-based activation motifs (ITAMs) in the cytoplasmic tails of Ig-alpha and Ig-beta [5]. Spleen tyrosine kinase (SYK) binds to the phosphorylated ITAMs and becomes activated, then mediating tyrosine phosphorylation of proteins including B cell linker (BLNK) and B cell adaptor for phosphoinositide 3-kinase (BCAP) (Fig. 1) [6]. Upstream Src family kinases including BLK and LYN, which phosphorylates CD19, activate Bruton's tyrosine kinase (BTK) [7]. BTK phosphorylates and activates 1-phosphatidylinositol-4,5-bisphosphate phosphodiesterase gamma-2 (PLCγ2), which leads to downstream signaling involving Ca^{2+} release and phosphorylation of CARMA/CARD11 by protein kinase C beta (PKCβ) [8]. CARMA/CARD11 associates with B cell lymphoma/leukemia 10 protein (BCL10) and mucosa-associated lymphoid tissue lymphoma translocation protein 1 (MALT1), forming the CARD11-BCL10-MALT1 (CBM) signalosome complex [9]. Once the CBM complex is formed, the IKK complex is activated, leading to p50 and p65-RelA translocation to the nucleus via the canonical NF-κB pathway.

Molecular mechanisms involved in canonical BCR-driven signaling have profound effects on tumorigenesis. For instance, the dysregulation of NF-κB in chronic lymphocytic leukemia (CLL) cells causes overexpression of anti-apoptotic genes; CLL cells have elevated SYK, LYN, and BTK expression and elevated PI3K activity. Ligation of the B cell receptor in vitro has been shown to induce more NF-κB DNA-binding activity in the nucleus of CLL cells, thereby increasing cellular survival [10]. Survival of diffuse large B cell lymphoma (DLBCL) cells and other lymphoma cells similarly depends on CARMA1/CARD11 and NF-κB signaling [11, 12]. Two cell lines of activated B cell-like diffuse large B cell lymphoma (ABC-DLBCL) had high levels of NF-κB DNA-binding activity in the nucleus, constitutive IKK activity, and rapid IκB degradation that were not observed in germinal center B cell-like diffuse large B cell lymphoma (GCB-DLBCL) [11], demonstrating the

Table 1 Various agents targeting the NF-κB pathway

Agent name	Agent mechanism	Relevant target pathway	Tested in MCL cells/patients?
Ibrutinib	Bruton's tyrosine kinase (BTK) inhibitor	Canonical NF-κB pathway; BCR signaling	Yes—tested in vitro, in vivo, in clinical trials; approved by the FDA; 68% overall response rate in MCL patients [54]
Acalabrutinib	Second-generation Bruton's tyrosine kinase (BTK) inhibitor	Canonical NF-κB pathway; BCR signaling	Yes—tested in relapsed or refractory mantle cell lymphoma in a single-arm, multicenter, phase 2 trial; 81% overall response and 40% complete response for 124 patients at a median follow-up of 15.2 months [55]
Bortezomib	Proteasome inhibitor → prevents degradation of ubiquitinated IκB; induces cell death via oxidative and ER stress → NOXA upregulation (NF-κB independent)	Canonical NF-κB pathway	Yes—tested in vitro, in vivo, and in clinical trials; approved by the FDA; 33% overall response rate in R/R MCL patients [56]
Rituximab	Chimeric anti-CD20 antibody; downregulates Bcl-x(L) expression; decreases the phosphorylation of NF-κB-inducing kinase, IκB kinase, and IκBα; diminishes IKK kinase activity; and decreases NF-κB DNA-binding activity	Canonical and non-canonical NF-κB pathways	Yes—widely used in clinical treatment of patients with non-Hodgkin lymphoma (NHL); also tested in vitro in CD20(+) drug-resistant cell lines Ramos (Bcl-2(−)/Bcl-x(L)(+)) and Daudi (Bcl-2(+)/Bcl-x(L)(+)) [57]
Lenalidomide	Downregulates pro-inflammatory cytokines, such as TNF-α, IL-1, and IL-6	Canonical NF-κB pathway	Yes—approved for the treatment of patients with MCL whose disease has relapsed or progressed after two prior therapies, one of which included bortezomib
Idelalisib	PI3Kδ inhibitor	Cross-talk between NF-κB and PI3K/Akt pathways	Yes—phase I study in 2014 for treatment of relapsed/refractory MCL patients, overall response rate of 40% (16/40 patients) [58]; phase I study in 2014 for treatment of patients with indolent non-Hodgkin lymphoma (NHL), overall response rate of 47% (30/64 patients) [44]
Auranofin	Inhibits homodimerization of toll-like receptor 4 (TLR4), thereby suppressing TLR-mediated activation of NF-κB [59]	Canonical NF-κB pathway; TLR signaling	Phase I/II clinical trial at University of Kansas Medical Center to evaluate safety and efficacy of auranofin in chronic lymphocytic leukemia (CLL), small lymphocytic lymphoma (SLL), and/or prolymphocytic lymphoma (PLL) patients (clinicaltrials.gov)
Duvelisib	PI3K inhibitor	Cross-talk between NF-κB and PI3K/Akt pathways	Yes—tested in vitro and in patient-derived xenograft studies; inhibited MCL growth in vitro and in PDX mice [45]
ACP-319	PI3K inhibitor	Cross-talk between NF-κB and PI3K/Akt pathways	Yes—undergoing phase 1/2 clinical trial in combination with ACP-196 in subjects with B cell malignancies, including MCL (no study results posted yet—clinicaltrials.gov)
AM-0216 and AM-0561	NIK inhibitors	Non-canonical NF-κB pathway	Tested in vitro in multiple myeloma cells; was not possible to do in vivo studies due to poor pharmacokinetic properties, but drug combination may be more promising [35]
ASN002	Syk/jak inhibitor	Canonical NF-κB pathway; BCR signaling	Showed anti-proliferative activity in many cell lines and inhibited tumor growth in a multiple myeloma xenograft model; phase I/II ongoing clinical study [60]
CUDC-907	PI3K/histone deacetylase (HDAC) inhibitor	Canonical NF-κB pathway; BCR and TCR signaling	Yes—inhibits tumor growth of ibrutinib-resistant MCL in vitro and in PDX model [61]; phase I/II trial for relapsed or refractory lymphoma or multiple myeloma (clinicaltrials.gov)
Emetine	IκBα phosphorylation inhibitor	Canonical NF-κB pathway	Tested in vitro and in vivo in diffuse large B cell lymphoma cells; induced cell death and demonstrated significant inhibition of tumor growth [62]
Lestaurtinib	IκBα phosphorylation inhibitor	Canonical NF-κB pathway	Showed biological and clinical activity in phase 1/2 trial for patients with relapsed or refractory acute myeloid leukemia [63]
Mesalamine	Blocks p65-dependent transactivation	Canonical NF-κB pathway	Not tested in MCL cells; first line agent for treating ulcerative colitis; maintains remission in mild to moderate UC [64]
Fenofibrate	Inhibits the TNF-α/NF-κB axis to induce apoptosis; modulates the expression of anti-apoptotic genes associated with MCL; decreases DNA binding of NF-κB	Canonical NF-κB pathway, cross-talk with TNF signaling	Tested in vitro—decreases growth of Mino, SP53, and Jeko-1 cell lines; induces apoptosis in MCL cell lines Mino and Jeko-1 in vitro; decreases cyclin D1 expression in Mino and SP53 [65]

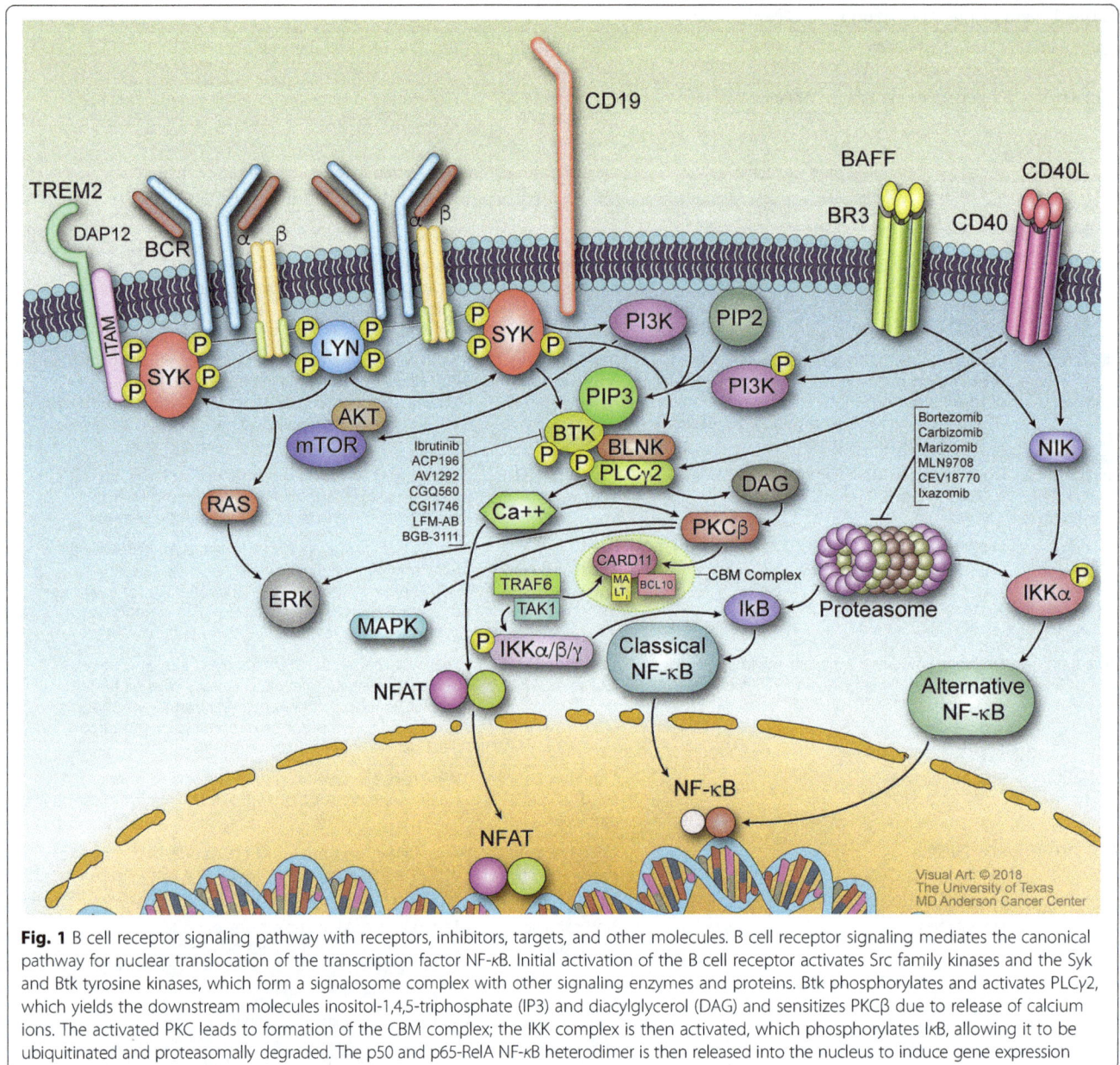

Fig. 1 B cell receptor signaling pathway with receptors, inhibitors, targets, and other molecules. B cell receptor signaling mediates the canonical pathway for nuclear translocation of the transcription factor NF-κB. Initial activation of the B cell receptor activates Src family kinases and the Syk and Btk tyrosine kinases, which form a signalosome complex with other signaling enzymes and proteins. Btk phosphorylates and activates PLCγ2, which yields the downstream molecules inositol-1,4,5-triphosphate (IP3) and diacylglycerol (DAG) and sensitizes PKCβ due to release of calcium ions. The activated PKC leads to formation of the CBM complex; the IKK complex is then activated, which phosphorylates IκB, allowing it to be ubiquitinated and proteasomally degraded. The p50 and p65-RelA NF-κB heterodimer is then released into the nucleus to induce gene expression

key role of NF-κB activity in the proliferation of various subtypes of lymphoma cells.

BTK is a major player in initiating the canonical pathway involving BCR signaling. Inhibition of BTK can cause apoptosis in lymphoma cells, which makes BTK a critical therapeutic target [13]. Ibrutinib (PCI-32765) and acalabrutinib, a second-generation BTK inhibitor, effectively block downstream signaling, subsequently inhibiting B cell activation (Table 1) [14–16]. In ABC-DLBCL and Waldenström macroglobulinemia, ibrutinib is highly effective due to the activation of BTK via mutations in CD79B or the myeloid differentiation primary response gene 88 (MyD88), but in mantle cell lymphoma, these mutations are rare [17–19].

To identify what confers ibrutinib sensitivity in mantle cell lymphoma with respect to NF-κB signaling, Saba et al. [17] analyzed the gene expression profiles of 55 tumor samples from 43 previously untreated patients with MCL that were about to undergo therapy. MCL cells of the lymph node demonstrated activation of canonical NF-κB signaling and BCR signaling [17]. Gene expression differed between MCL cells in peripheral blood and lymph nodes because of activation of signaling pathways in the lymph nodes [17]. The ability of tumor cells to proliferate corresponded with the degree of BCR activation.

Saba et al. found that the canonical NF-κB signature with 18 genes dependent on IKKβ activation was on average

2.1-fold more highly expressed in lymph node biopsies than in purified MCL cells ($p < .0001$) [17]. One set of tumors demonstrated dependence on the lymph node environment for BCR and NF-κB activation, whereas another set indicated that BCR and NF-κB genes were not as independent on the lymph node microenvironment [17]. NF-κB-inducing kinase (NIK) signature genes, as markers of the non-canonical NF-κB pathway, were less expressed than the canonical NF-κB signature genes [17]. In MCL cells from the lymph nodes, SYK and p65 were highly phosphorylated, reflecting BCR-dependent activation of the canonical NF-κB pathway [17]. When ibrutinib was administered to inhibit BTK, ibrutinib reduced phosphorylation of p65 and killed 35 to 50% of the tumor cells within 48 h of administration [17]. BCR signaling is activated in the lymph node microenvironment in vivo and appears to promote tumor proliferation and survival, making the canonical pathway a viable target.

TLR signaling Toll-like receptor (TLR) signaling is of particular relevance in mantle cell lymphoma, as TLRs are important proteins involved in the innate immune system. Specifically, increased TLR4 expression in MCL cells can contribute to tumor progression [20]. TLRs recognize pathogen-associated microbial patterns (PAMPs) and danger-associated molecular patterns (DAMPs) to help cells recognize foreign invaders and trigger inflammatory responses. TLR4 activation in patients with recurrent bacterial infections promotes tumor growth and shields MCL cells from surveillance by the immune system [20]. Toll-like receptor signaling is twofold: one pathway involving TLR4 depends on MyD88, mediating early NF-κB activation, and the other pathway depends on TIR-domain-containing adapter-inducing interferon-β (TRIF), mediating late activation of NF-κB.

Both TLR pathways begin with lipopolysaccharide (LPS) binding to LPS-binding protein and forming a complex that binds CD14 to the cell membrane. LPS is then transferred to MD-2 and TLR-4 [21]. TLR-4 subsequently activates the MyD88-dependent pathway with Mal/TIRAP and the TRIF-dependent pathway with TRAM. Unlike IL-1R signaling, MyD88 interacts with Mal for recruitment to the receptor complex [22]; complexes I, II, and III otherwise form in the same manner as that for IL-1R signaling. MyD88 additionally recruits TNF receptor-associated factor 6 (TRAF6) and members of the interleukin-1 receptor-associated kinase (IRAK) family, i.e., IRAK-1, which interact with BCL10 in complex I. BCL10 then binds to Pellino2 and MALT1 (in complexes II and III, respectively), facilitating the activation of TRAF6 [23]. TRAF6, along with Ubc13 and Uev1A, which are ubiquitin-conjugating proteins, activates the TAK1 complex [24]. The TAK1 complex can then activate IKK, triggering the usual cascade of events

in the canonical pathway. Targeting TLR-mediated NF-κB signaling may increase the susceptibility of MCL cells to immune surveillance and subsequently minimize tumor progression.

Stimulation of TLR4 signaling via LPS has been found by Wang et al. to increase proliferation of the following MCL cell lines: SP53, Jeko-1, Mino, and Granta-519 [20]. MCL cells expressed many different TLRs, of which TLR4 was one of the most highly expressed [20]. LPS-induced TLR4 signaling also increased NF-κB phosphorylation and activated expression of important cytokines, including interleukin-1 and the vascular endothelial growth factor (VEGF) in MCL cell lines and primary patient cells with TLR4 and MyD88 expression [20]. LPS-mediated TLR4 signaling in MCL cells also facilitated immune evasion by inhibiting T cell proliferation. Cells without TLR4 had a much weaker ability to inhibit T cell proliferation, confirming the key pro-tumor role of TLR4 in MCL cell survival [20].

TLR1/2 and TLR5 have also been found to be expressed in MCL cell lines and primary MCL cells [25]. The activation of TLR2 and TLR5 further activates Akt and MAPK signaling, leading to overexpression of cyclin D1 and D3 and increased proliferation of MCL cells. TLR1/2 and TLR5 activation also affects the canonical NF-κB pathway and enhances the survival and migration of MCL cells [25]. Primary MCL cells have also shown an intermediate response to stimulation with CpG oligodeoxynucleotides, which are detected by TLR9 [26]. TLR9 upregulates the expression of CD20 upon binding with the CpG motif and interacts with BTK to induce B cell proliferation [26, 27].

TLR signaling interplays with BCR signaling mechanisms, affecting the overall survival of MCL patients. Akhter et al. used the NanoString nCounter technology to digitally quantify BCR and TLR signaling molecules in a cohort of 81 MCL patients [27]. This cohort was split into two subsets: those with high BCR activation and those with low BCR activation (> 1.5-fold change in expression, $p < 0.05$) [27]. There was a significant difference in expression of TLR6, TLR7, and TLR9 between the subsets of patients, with fold changes of 2.2, 1.9, and 2.4, respectively ($p < 0.05$ for all) [27]. Overexpression of TLR6 and TLR9 was associated with a poor clinical outcome and worse overall survival in patients with hyperreactive BCR signaling [27]. TLR4 expression was not significantly different between the two subsets of patients, which failed to validate the findings of Wang et al. [20] that MCL cells have high expression of TLR4 [27]. TLR9, on the other hand, was overexpressed in the subset with high BCR activation, in sync with the overexpression of key mediators in the BCR signaling pathway, including BTK, BLNK, and SYK, suggesting that BCR may be activated in a tonic, antigen-independent, or restricted antigen manner [27]. Targeting MCL through TLR inhibitors in combination with other agents targeting NF-κB pathways may be a promising therapeutic choice.

TNF-R signaling NF-κB activation can lead to apoptosis or survival, depending on the apoptotic stimulus. Interestingly, TNF-α signaling causes NF-κB to have anti-apoptotic effects, protecting the proliferating tumor cells; inhibition of NF-κB sensitizes tumor cells to TNF-α-induced apoptosis [28].

Upon activation, a TNF receptor uses its death domain, tumor necrosis factor receptor type 1-associated death domain (TRADD), to bind to RIP1 and TRAF2 [29]. Once the TNF receptor is endocytosed, TRADD detaches from the receptor and associates with another protein: Fas-associated protein with death domain (FADD). The interaction of FADD with caspase-8 activates a caspase cascade, which leads to apoptosis [30]. Meanwhile, TRAF2 ubiquitinates itself and RIP1, bound to TAB2 and NEMO/ IKKγ, prompting recruitment of TAK1 (which regulates MAP3K3 activity) and IKKβ. TNF stimulation causes RIP1 to recruit MEKK3/MAP3K3, which phosphorylates IKKβ [31]. The IKK complex is then activated, leading to the poly-ubiquitination and proteasomal degradation of IκB, allowing the p50–p65 heterodimer to enter the nucleus. RIP1 can also act independently of TAK1 by interacting with p62, which leads to activation of atypical protein kinase C (aPKC) and subsequent activation of the IKK complex [32].

2′-Deoxy-2′-β-fluoro-4′-azidocytidine (FNC) is a cytidine analogue that inhibits proliferation of mantle cell lymphoma cells in vitro and in vivo by inducing apoptosis. Zhang et al. found that administration of FNC to Jeko-1 cells induces apoptosis through the signaling of death receptors, which are members of the TNF superfamily [33]. FNC treatment increased expression of TNF-α, Fas, and the Fas ligand [33]. Upregulation of TNF-α in combination with inhibition of NF-κB activation can increase apoptosis in mantle cell lymphoma cells, presenting a route by which MCL tumors can be targeted.

The non-canonical pathway

The non-canonical pathway is activated by initiation of B cell activation factor (BAFFR), CD40, lymphotoxin β-receptor (LTβR), or receptor activator for nuclear factor kappa B (RANK) signaling. The non-canonical NF-κB pathway involves the processing of p100, where p100 is phosphorylated by IKKα on the serine residues S866 and S870 and then poly-ubiquitinated (Fig. 2) [34]. This leads to the activation of RelB-p52 complexes, which are heterodimeric subunits of NF-κB. IKKα is activated by the upstream kinase NF-κB-inducing kinase (NIK), which promotes the processing of p100 into the active p52 isoform. NIK is downregulated by the expression of

TRAF2 and TRAF3, which are negative regulators of non-canonical NF-κB signaling that interact with BIRC2 and BIRC3 [1]. Unlike the canonical pathway, the non-canonical pathway does not rely on IKKβ or IKKγ (NEMO); it only needs IKKα to phosphorylate the p52 precursor, p100. Targeting non-canonical signaling mechanisms can overcome resistance to therapies that only target canonical NF-κB signaling.

Interactions with signaling pathways that coordinate with the NF-κB non-canonical pathway

CD40 signaling When a CD40 ligand binds to the CD40 receptor on the cell membrane, TRAF proteins are recruited to and directly bind to the CD40 receptor. TRAF proteins negatively regulate NIK. When the NF-κB pathway is inactive, NIK is constantly degraded via ubiquitination by TRAF3. NIK activity is also suppressed by expression of cellular inhibitor of apoptosis 1 (cIAP1) and cellular inhibitor of apoptosis 2 (cIAP2) [35]. However, when the pathway is activated via CD40 ligation, TRAF2 and cIAP 1/2 cause TRAF3 to be proteasomally degraded [36]. NIK can then accumulate with increased stability and phosphorylate IKKα, which is required for the phosphorylation and processing of p100 to form p52.

CD40 is expressed in mature B cells, including mantle cell lymphoma cells. While some MCL cells are sensitive to BCR signaling inhibition by ibrutinib, many patients still demonstrate resistance to inhibition of the canonical NF-κB pathway [37]. Culturing the MCL Rec-1 cell line with the CD40 ligand weakened the ability of ibrutinib to inhibit proliferation of Rec-1 cells. The effectiveness of ibrutinib, a BTK inhibitor, was undermined due to how CD40 signaling activates the NF-κB p52 isoform via the non-canonical pathway, which promotes cell survival in opposition to ibrutinib's inhibitory effects on the canonical pathway [38]. Targeting CD40-mediated NF-κB signaling, in addition to targeting canonical BCR signaling, may help overcome ibrutinib resistance in patient populations with activated CD40-CD40L pathways [38].

BAFFR signaling B cell-activating factor receptor (BAFFR) signaling mechanisms are similar to those of CD40 signaling. BAFFR is a member of the TNFR family, and it predominantly activates the non-canonical NF-κB pathway [39]. BAFFR can interact with TRAF3 but not TRAF2, which is why BAFFR cannot trigger the canonical pathway. Degradation of TRAF3 triggers non-canonical NF-κB signaling [40]. This leads to p100 processing via NIK activation and the same downstream molecular interactions as with CD40 signaling. BAFFR may be a key biomarker of both normal and abnormal B cells, especially due to its role in activating the non-canonical NF-κB

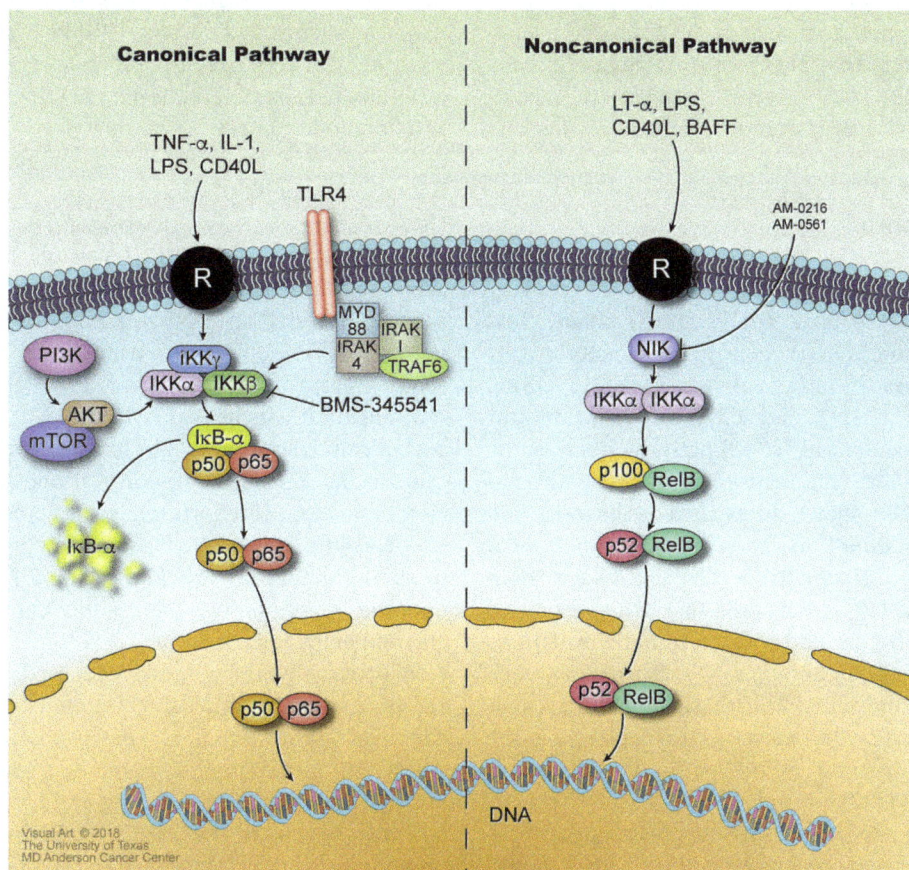

Fig. 2 NF-κB signaling pathways with receptors, inhibitors, targets, and other molecules The canonical and non-canonical pathways for NF-κB signaling are mediated by various receptors and signaling molecules, including toll-like receptors (TLR), tumor necrosis factor receptors (TNFR), interleukin-1 receptor (IL-1R), CD40, initiation of B cell activation factor (BAFFR), lymphotoxin β- receptor (LTβR), and receptor activator for nuclear factor kappa B (RANK). The canonical NF-κB pathway involves the inhibition of NF-κB by IκB, which binds to the p50–p65 heterodimer in the cytoplasm and prevents it from entering the nucleus. Activation of BCR, TNFR, and IL-1R receptors initiates adapter protein and signaling kinase responses, leading to activation of the IκB kinase (IKK) complex. Kinases in the IKK complex phosphorylate IκB and lead to its poly-ubiquitination and proteasomal degradation. This allows the p50 and p65-RelA heterodimer (a complex from the NF-κB family) to be released into the nucleus to induce gene expression. In the non-canonical pathway, IKKα is activated by the upstream kinase NF-κB-inducing kinase (NIK), which promotes the processing of p100 into the active RelB-p52 isoform of NF-κB. NIK is downregulated by the expression of TRAF2 and TRAF3, which are negative regulators of non-canonical NF-κB signaling that interact with BIRC2 and BIRC3 [1]. Unlike the canonical pathway, the non-canonical pathway does not rely on IKKβ or IKKγ (NEMO); it only needs IKKα to phosphorylate the p52 precursor, p100

pathway. Targeting BAFFR-mediated NF-κB signaling may offer a novel approach in suppressing neoplastic B cell maturation and proliferation.

Interaction with the PI3K/AKT pathway

NF-κB signaling is also mediated through interactions with other pathways, such as the PI3K/Akt pathway. In Burkitt's lymphoma, an aggressive form of non-Hodgkin lymphoma, NF-κB activation and STAT3 activation depend on upstream signaling of phosphatidylinositol 3-kinase (PI3K), which plays a key role in survival signaling [41]. Inhibition of PI3K blocks interleukin-1 signaling (IL-1), preventing eventual translocation of the p65-RelA heterodimer to the nucleus. Lipid products of PI3K

activate the serine/threonine kinase Akt/PKB, which mediates cell survival and proliferation [42]. While Akt does not directly phosphorylate NF-κB, it affects the canonical NF-κB signaling pathway by phosphorylating IKKα, which targets the IκB inhibitor protein and allows NF-κB to translocate to the nucleus [42]. Overexpression of IκB conversely interferes with the ability of PI3K and Akt to induce oncogenic transformation, indicating that the PI3K/Akt and NF-κB pathways depend on one another.

Through gene expression profiling, several genes in mantle cell lymphoma cells have been identified that relate to the PI3K/Akt pathway; the following genes were found to be altered or upregulated: PIK3CA, PDK2, PDPK1, AKT1, RPS6KB2, FOXO3A, PPP2R2C, and PDK1 [43].

The PI3K/Akt pathway may confer resistance to apoptosis in MCL cells. PI3K inhibitors such as duvelisib and idelalisib have been found to have anti-tumor activity in relapsed MCL [44, 45]. PI3K/Akt survival signaling is supplemented by the survival signaling of NF-κB, suggesting that targeting both pathways in a joint manner may be highly effective in limiting MCL cell proliferation and preventing tumor growth in patients.

Relevance of NF-κB pathways for the treatment of MCL

Mantle cell lymphoma does not have any single clear oncogenic driver and is heterogeneous, characterized by mutations in genes including ATM, CCND1, UBR5, TP53, BIRC3, NOTCH1/2, and TRAF2 [46]. Mutations in elements of the canonical NF-κB pathway, such as the CBM complex or IKK-beta, cause activation of the canonical pathway. This allows drugs such as ibrutinib and acalabrutinib, BTK inhibitors, to effectively inhibit BCR signaling and suppress growth in cells sensitive to BCR signaling inhibition [47]. MCL cells that are resistant to BCR signaling inhibition tend to have somatic mutations in inhibitors of the non-canonical NF-κB pathway, such as cIAP1, cIAP2, and TRAF2/3; these mutations cause resistant cell lines (Z-138, Maver-1) to depend on the deregulated non-canonical NF-κB pathway for survival and proliferation (Fig. 2).

When PKC-B, an important kinase upstream of the CBM complex in BCR signaling, was depleted via sh-RNA, proliferation of the ibrutinib-sensitive MCL cell line Jeko-1 was suppressed, while the insensitive cell line Granta-519 was left unaffected. This indicates that a subset of cell lines strongly depends on canonical NF-κB signaling. Treatment with sotrastaurin (STN) was also found to selectively modulate IκBα phosphorylation and reduce RelB cleavage, which is a marker of CBM complex activity, in STN-sensitive MCL cell lines [48]. In addition, the CBM complex component CARD11 appeared to be highly expressed in sensitive MCL lines, suggesting that BCR pathway components can be deregulated to treat cells that are sensitive to inhibition of the canonical NF-κB pathway [49].

MCL tumors can also be targeted via other pathways that interact with NF-κB signaling, for instance, through the PI3K /Akt pathway, CD40 signaling, BAFFR signaling, or transglutaminase (TG2) signaling. The expression of transglutaminase (TG2), a calcium-dependent protein encoded by the TGM2 gene associated with tumor cell proliferation, metastasis, and drug resistance, is closely linked with constitutive activation of NF-κB [50]. Upregulation of TG2 expression increased IL6 expression 1.8- to 2.9-fold and stimulated autophagy formation, a protective mechanism for tumor cells [50]. In comparison with normal B cells, patients with a blastoid type of MCL, an aggressive variant with a worse overall survival, displayed elevated TGM2 levels with up to 150-fold increases; these blastoid MCL subtypes also had higher TGM2 levels than classical MCL [50]. By silencing TG2 via CRISPR/Cas9, Zhang et al. observed that p53, p21, and p27 levels increased and cyclin gene levels decreased, indicating cell cycle arrest, levels of anti-apoptotic genes including BCL-XL and BCL-2 decreased, and levels of pro-apoptopic genes including BAX, BAK, and NOXA increased [50]. NF-κB p50 and p65 DNA-binding activity, downstream activation of IL8, p-STAT3 expression, and IL6 levels were significantly decreased in TG2 knockout MCL cells whereas signaling activity increased in TG2 overexpression cells [50]. TG2 silencing also conferred sensitivity to chemotherapeutic drugs whereas cells overexpressing TG2 exhibited drug resistance with higher IC50 values [50]. In patients with bortezomib resistance, TG2 signaling can be inhibited by a calcium blocker such as perillyl alcohol and administered in combination with bortezomib to suppress NF-κB expression and improve MCL cell sensitivity to bortezomib [51]. Inhibiting autophagy in MCL cells via TG2 silencing may thus be a promising therapeutic choice to overcome chemotherapy resistance.

Many targeted therapies have focused on targeting B cell receptor signaling in MCL cells, which indirectly reduces canonical NF-κB signaling. Direct inhibitors of NF-κB are scarce, but more targeted therapies are focusing on inhibition of non-canonical signaling and cross-talk with other pathways, such as the PI3K/Akt pathway to overcome resistance to inhibitors of the canonical pathway. For instance, the combination of TGR-1202, a PI3K delta inhibitor, with ibrutinib had an overall response rate of 67% with six out of nine patients achieving a partial response in a phase I/Ib multicenter trial for patients with relapsed/refractory MCL [52]. Other combination therapies that target both canonical and non-canonical pathways have also been effective in inhibiting MCL cell growth and proliferation (Table 2). For instance, the combination of CC-292 with NIK inhibitors, AM-0216 and AM-0561, in Z138 and MAVER-1, cell lines resistant to CC-292 and ibrutinib, resulted in a significant decrease in p52 levels, via inhibition of the non-canonical pathway, and a complete lack of IκB phosphorylation, indicating total inhibition of the NF-κB pathway [53]. This combination was also effective in primary MCL cells with BIRC3 inactivation and is a promising therapeutic choice for further investigation in vivo and in the clinical setting [53].

Conclusions

Overall, the NF-κB pathways have numerous molecular mechanisms that lead to the eventual expression of NF-κB target genes. These genes prompt inflammatory responses, immune regulation, and cell proliferation via the canonical pathway and B cell maturation and lymphoid organogenesis via the non-canonical pathway. The multifaceted NF-κB pathways play a crucial role in the growth and proliferation

Table 2 Combination therapies targeting the NF-κB pathway

Combination therapy	Target pathway and mechanism	Tested in MCL cells/patients?
Ibrutinib with rituximab	Canonical and non-canonical NF-κB pathways; inhibits BTK; rituximab decreases phosphorylation of NIK, IκB kinase, and IκBα; diminishes IKK kinase activity; and decreases NF-κB DNA-binding activity	Yes; ongoing phase II trial at the MD Anderson Cancer Center of rituximab in combination with ibrutinib in relapsed/refractory MCL (clinicaltrials.gov)
Thalidomide with rituximab	Canonical and non-canonical NF-κB pathway; thalidomide inhibits IKK and reduces TNF-α production, along with effects of rituximab	Yes—thalidomide combined with rituximab has antitumor activity in relapsed/refractory MCL; 81% overall response rate to rituximab plus thalidomide [66]
Lenalidomide with rituximab	Canonical and non-canonical NF-κB pathway; downregulates pro-inflammatory cytokines, such as TNF-α, IL-1, and IL-6, along with effects of rituximab	Yes—overall response rate of 87% when combined with rituximab in MCL patients [67]
TGR-1202 with ibrutinib	Cross-talk between NF-κB and PI3K/Akt pathways; TGR-1202 inhibits PI3K Delta	Yes—tested in relapsed or refractory MCL and CLL patients in combination with ibrutinib in a phase 1/1b study; overall response rate of 85% in combination with ibrutinib (11/13) [52]
Perillyl alcohol (calcium blocker) with bortezomib	Cross-talk between NF-κB and TG2 signaling; inhibition of autophagy to improve sensitivity to bortezomib	Not tested in patients but tested in MCL cells; was found to suppress NF-κB signaling and improve cytotoxicity of bortezomib [51]
CC-292 with lenalidomide and NIK inhibitors, AM-0216 and AM-0561	Canonical and non-canonical NF-κB pathway; CC-292 inhibits BTK in a highly selective manner; lenalidomide downregulates pro-inflammatory cytokines, such as TNF-α, IL-1, and IL-6; NIK inhibitors inhibit alternative NF-κB signaling	Not tested in patients, but tested in MCL cell lines and primary cells; CC-292 significantly reduced BTK phosphorylation and its activity was enhanced by lenalidomide co-treatment; combination of CC-292 with NIK inhibitors had a significant cooperative effect that inhibited cell growth and induced apoptosis in Z138 and MAVER-1 [53]

of mantle cell lymphoma cells. Drugs that target various components of the NF-κB pathway have the potential to treat MCL, depending on the pathway to which the cells are sensitive. Targeting NF-κB mechanisms may prove to be a valuable tool in the development of targeted agents to overcome drug resistance and can lead to effective therapies for mantle cell lymphoma.

Abbreviations

ABC-DLBCL: Activated B cell-like diffuse large B cell lymphoma; BAFF/TNFSF13B: B cell-activating factor; BAFFR: B cell-activating factor receptor; BCAP: B cell adaptor for phosphoinositide 3-kinase; BCL10: B cell lymphoma/leukemia 10 protein; BCR: B cell receptor; BLK: B lymphocyte tyrosine kinase; BLNK: B cell linker protein; BTK: Bruton's tyrosine kinase; C40L/TNFS5: CD40 ligand; CBM: CARD11-BCL10-MALT1 signalosome complex; cIAP1: Cellular inhibitor of apoptosis 1; cIAP2: Cellular inhibitor of apoptosis 2; CLL: Chronic lymphocytic leukemia; DAG: Diacylglycerol; DAMP: Danger-associated molecular patterns; DLBCL: Diffuse large B cell lymphoma; ER: Endoplasmic reticulum; FADD: Fas-associated protein with death domain; FNC: 2'-Deoxy-2'-β-fluoro-4'-azidocytidine; GCB-DLBCL: Germinal center B cell-like diffuse large B cell lymphoma; HDAC: Histone deacetylase; IKK: IκB kinase; IKKα: IκB kinase; IKKβ: IκB kinase; IKKγ: IκB kinase; IL-1: Interleukin-1; IL-1R: Interleukin-1 receptor; IP3: Inositol-1,4,5-triphosphate; IRAK: Interleukin-1 receptor-associated kinase; ITAM: Immunoreceptor tyrosine-based activation motifs; LPS: Lipopolysaccharide; LTβR: Lymphotoxin β-receptor; MALT1: Mucosa-associated lymphoid tissue lymphoma translocation protein 1; MCL: Mantle cell lymphoma; MyD88: Myeloid differentiation primary response gene 88; NF-κB: Nuclear factor kappa-light-chain enhancer of activated B cells; NIK: NF-κB-inducing kinase; PAMP: Pathogen-associated molecular patterns; PCI-32765: Ibrutinib, an inhibitor of Bruton's tyrosine kinase; PI3K: Phosphatidylinositol 3-kinase; PKCβ: Protein kinase C beta; PLCγ2: 1-Phosphatidylinositol-4,5-bisphosphate phosphodiesterase gamma-2; RANK: Receptor activator for nuclear factor kappa B; STN: Sotrastaurin; SYK: Spleen tyrosine kinase; TG2: Transglutaminase; TLR: Toll-like microbial pattern recognition receptors; TLR1: Toll-like receptor 1; TLR2: Toll-like receptor 2; TLR4: Toll-like receptor 4; TLR5: Toll-like receptor 5; TLR9: Toll-like receptor 9; TNFR: Tumor necrosis factor receptor; TNFSF3: Lymphotoxin β; TNFα: Tumor necrosis factor alpha; TRADD: Tumor necrosis factor receptor type 1-associated death domain protein; TRAF: TNF receptor-associated factor; TRIF: TIR-domain-containing adapter-inducing interferon-β; VEGF: Vascular endothelial growth factor

Funding

This work was supported by the generous contributions made to the B-cell Lymphoma Moon Shot Program at MD Anderson Cancer Center.

Authors' contributions

SB was the major contributor in compiling research for and writing the manuscript. MA and EL made equal contributions in revising the manuscript. FY helped prepare the figures and revise the manuscript. KN and MW made final revisions to the manuscript and oversaw its completion. All authors have read and approved this manuscript.

Competing interests

The authors declare that they have no competing interests.

References

1. Rahal R, Frick M, Romero R, Korn JM, Kridel R, Chan FC, Meissner B, Bhang HE, Ruddy D, Kauffmann A, et al. Pharmacological and genomic profiling identifies NF-kappaB-targeted treatment strategies for mantle cell lymphoma. Nat Med. 2014;20:87–92.
2. Broide DH, Lawrence T, Doherty T, Cho JY, Miller M, McElwain K, McElwain S, Karin M. Allergen-induced peribronchial fibrosis and mucus production mediated by IkappaB kinase beta-dependent genes in airway epithelium. Proc Natl Acad Sci U S A. 2005;102:17723–8.
3. Lawrence T, Gilroy DW, Colville-Nash PR, Willoughby DA. Possible new role for NF-kappaB in the resolution of inflammation. Nat Med. 2001;7:1291–7.

4. Taylor JA, Bren GD, Pennington KN, Trushin SA, Asin S, Paya CV. Serine 32 and serine 36 of IkappaBalpha are directly phosphorylated by protein kinase CKII in vitro. J Mol Biol. 1999;290:839–50.

5. Gauld SB, Cambier JC. Src-family kinases in B-cell development and signaling. Oncogene. 2004;23:8001–6.

6. Fu C, Turck CW, Kurosaki T, Chan AC. BLNK: a central linker protein in B cell activation. Immunity. 1998;9:93–103.

7. Marcotte DJ, Liu YT, Arduini RM, Hession CA, Miatkowski K, Wildes CP, Cullen PF, Hong V, Hopkins BT, Mertsching E, et al. Structures of human Bruton's tyrosine kinase in active and inactive conformations suggest a mechanism of activation for TEC family kinases. Protein Sci. 2010;19:429–39.

8. Rohacs T. Regulation of transient receptor potential channels by the phospholipase C pathway. Adv Biol Regul. 2013;53:341–55.

9. Blonska M, Lin X. NF-kappaB signaling pathways regulated by CARMA family of scaffold proteins. Cell Res. 2011;21:55–70.

10. Hewamana S, Alghazal S, Lin TT, Clement M, Jenkins C, Guzman ML, Jordan CT, Neelakantan S, Crooks PA, Burnett AK, et al. The NF-kappaB subunit Rel A is associated with in vitro survival and clinical disease progression in chronic lymphocytic leukemia and represents a promising therapeutic target. Blood. 2008;111:4681–9.

11. Davis RE, Brown KD, Siebenlist U, Staudt LM. Constitutive nuclear factor kappaB activity is required for survival of activated B cell-like diffuse large B cell lymphoma cells. J Exp Med. 2001;194:1861–74.

12. Bognar MK, Vincendeau M, Erdmann T, Seeholzer T, Grau M, Linnemann JR, Ruland J, Scheel CH, Lenz P, Ott G, et al. Oncogenic CARMA1 couples NF-kappaB and beta-catenin signaling in diffuse large B-cell lymphomas. Oncogene. 2016;35:4269–81.

13. Seda V, Mraz M. B-cell receptor signalling and its crosstalk with other pathways in normal and malignant cells. Eur J Haematol. 2015;94:193–205.

14. Honigberg LA, Smith AM, Sirisawad M, Verner E, Loury D, Chang B, Li S, Pan Z, Thamm DH, Miller RA, Buggy JJ. The Bruton tyrosine kinase inhibitor PCI-32765 blocks B-cell activation and is efficacious in models of autoimmune disease and B-cell malignancy. Proc Natl Acad Sci U S A. 2010;107:13075–80.

15. Wu J, Zhang M, Liu D. Acalabrutinib (ACP-196): a selective second-generation BTK inhibitor. J Hematol Oncol. 2016;9:21.

16. Wu J, Liu C, Tsui ST, Liu D. Second-generation inhibitors of Bruton tyrosine kinase. J Hematol Oncol. 2016;9:80.

17. Saba NS, Liu D, Herman SE, Underbayev C, Tian X, Behrend D, Weniger MA, Skarzynski M, Gyamfi J, Fontan L, et al. Pathogenic role of B-cell receptor signaling and canonical NF-kappaB activation in mantle cell lymphoma. Blood. 2016;128:82–92.

18. Davis RE, Ngo VN, Lenz G, Tolar P, Young RM, Romesser PB, Kohlhammer H, Lamy L, Zhao H, Yang Y, et al. Chronic active B-cell-receptor signalling in diffuse large B-cell lymphoma. Nature. 2010;463:88–92.

19. Treon SP, Tripsas CK, Meid K, Warren D, Varma G, Green R, Argyropoulos KV, Yang G, Cao Y, Xu L, et al. Ibrutinib in previously treated Waldenstrom's macroglobulinemia. N Engl J Med. 2015;372:1430–40.

20. Wang L, Zhao Y, Qian J, Sun L, Lu Y, Li H, Li Y, Yang J, Cai Z, Yi Q. Toll-like receptor-4 signaling in mantle cell lymphoma: effects on tumor growth and immune evasion. Cancer. 2013;119:782–91.

21. Nagai Y, Akashi S, Nagafuku M, Ogata M, Iwakura Y, Akira S, Kitamura T, Kosugi A, Kimoto M, Miyake K. Essential role of MD-2 in LPS responsiveness and TLR4 distribution. Nat Immunol. 2002;3:667–72.

22. Verstak B, Nagpal K, Bottomley SP, Golenbock DT, Hertzog PJ, Mansell A. MyD88 adapter-like (Mal)/TIRAP interaction with TRAF6 is critical for TLR2- and TLR4-mediated NF-kappaB proinflammatory responses. J Biol Chem. 2009;284:24192–203.

23. Liu Y, Dong W, Chen L, Xiang R, Xiao H, De G, Wang Z, Qi Y. BCL10 mediates lipopolysaccharide/toll-like receptor-4 signaling through interaction with Pellino2. J Biol Chem. 2004;279:37436–44.

24. Yamamoto M, Okamoto T, Takeda K, Sato S, Sanjo H, Uematsu S, Saitoh T, Yamamoto N, Sakurai H, Ishii KJ, et al. Key function for the Ubc13 E2 ubiquitin-conjugating enzyme in immune receptor signaling. Nat Immunol. 2006;7:962–70.

25. Mastorci K, Muraro E, Pasini E, Furlan C, Sigalotti L, Cinco M, Dolcetti R, Fratta E. Toll-like receptor 1/2 and 5 ligands enhance the expression of cyclin D1 and D3 and induce proliferation in mantle cell lymphoma. PLoS One. 2016;11:e0153823.

26. Jahrsdorfer B, Muhlenhoff L, Blackwell SE, Wagner M, Poeck H, Hartmann E, Jox R, Giese T, Emmerich B, Endres S, et al. B-cell

27. Akhter A, Street L, Ghosh S, Burns BF, Elyamany G, Shabani-Rad MT, Stewart DA, Mansoor A. Concomitant high expression of toll-like receptor (TLR) and B-cell receptor (BCR) signalling molecules has clinical implications in mantle cell lymphoma. Hematol Oncol. 2017;35:79–86.

28. Wang CY, Cusack JC Jr, Liu R, Baldwin AS Jr. Control of inducible chemoresistance: enhanced anti-tumor therapy through increased apoptosis by inhibition of NF-kappaB. Nat Med. 1999;5:412–7.

29. Hsu H, Huang J, Shu HB, Baichwal V, Goeddel DV. TNF-dependent recruitment of the protein kinase RIP to the TNF receptor-1 signaling complex. Immunity. 1996;4:387–96.

30. Hu WH, Johnson H, Shu HB. Activation of NF-kappaB by FADD, Casper, and caspase-8. J Biol Chem. 2000;275:10838–44.

31. Lee TH, Huang Q, Oikemus S, Shank J, Ventura JJ, Cusson N, Vaillancourt RR, Su B, Davis RJ, Kelliher MA. The death domain kinase RIP1 is essential for tumor necrosis factor alpha signaling to p38 mitogen-activated protein kinase. Mol Cell Biol. 2003;23:8377–85.

32. Sanz L, Sanchez P, Lallena MJ, Diaz-Meco MT, Moscat J. The interaction of p62 with RIP links the atypical PKCs to NF-kappaB activation. EMBO J. 1999;18:3044–53.

33. Zhang Y, Zhang R, Ding X, Peng B, Wang N, Ma F, Peng Y, Wang Q, Chang J. FNC efficiently inhibits mantle cell lymphoma growth. PLoS One. 2017;12:e0174112.

34. Fong A, Sun SC. Genetic evidence for the essential role of beta-transducin repeat-containing protein in the inducible processing of NF-kappa B2/p100. J Biol Chem. 2002;277:22111–4.

35. Demchenko YN, Brents LA, Li Z, Bergsagel LP, McGee LR, Kuehl MW. Novel inhibitors are cytotoxic for myeloma cells with NFkB inducing kinase-dependent activation of NFkB. Oncotarget. 2014;5:4554–64.

36. Liao G, Zhang M, Harhaj EW, Sun SC. Regulation of the NF-kappaB-inducing kinase by tumor necrosis factor receptor-associated factor 3-induced degradation. J Biol Chem. 2004;279:26243–50.

37. Martin P, Maddocks KJ, Noto K, Christian B, Furman RR, Andritsos LA, Flynn JM, Jones JA, Ruan J, Chen-Kiang S, et al. Poor overall survival of patients with ibrutinib-resistant mantle cell lymphoma. Blood. 2014;124:3047.

38. Sun Z, Luo L. Abstract 1298: CD40L-CD40 signaling on B-cell lymphoma response to BTK inhibitors. Cancer Res. 2016;76:1298.

39. Claudio E, Brown K, Park S, Wang H, Siebenlist U. BAFF-induced NEMO-independent processing of NF-kappa B2 in maturing B cells. Nat Immunol. 2002;3:958–65.

40. Morrison MD, Reiley W, Zhang M, Sun SC. An atypical tumor necrosis factor (TNF) receptor-associated factor-binding motif of B cell-activating factor belonging to the TNF family (BAFF) receptor mediates induction of the noncanonical NF-kappaB signaling pathway. J Biol Chem. 2005; 280:10018–24.

41. Han SS, Yun H, Son DJ, Tompkins VS, Peng L, Chung ST, Kim JS, Park ES, Janz S: NF-kappaB/STAT3/PI3K signaling crosstalk in iMyc E mu B lymphoma. Mol Cancer 2010, 9:97.

42. Bai D, Ueno L, Vogt PK. Akt-mediated regulation of NFkappaB and the essentialness of NFkappaB for the oncogenicity of PI3K and Akt. Int J Cancer. 2009;125:2863–70.

43. Rizzatti EG, Falcao RP, Panepucci RA, Proto-Siqueira R, Anselmo-Lima WT, Okamoto OK, Zago MA. Gene expression profiling of mantle cell lymphoma cells reveals aberrant expression of genes from the PI3K-AKT, WNT and TGFbeta signalling pathways. Br J Haematol. 2005;130:516–26.

44. Flinn IW, Kahl BS, Leonard JP, Furman RR, Brown JR, Byrd JC, Wagner-Johnston ND, Coutre SE, Benson DM, Peterman S, et al. Idelalisib, a selective inhibitor of phosphatidylinositol 3-kinase-delta, as therapy for previously treated indolent non-Hodgkin lymphoma. Blood. 2014;123:3406–13.

45. Wang J, Zhang V, Bell T, Liu Y, Guo H, Zhang L. The effects of PI3K-δ/γ inhibitor, duvelisib, in mantle cell lymphoma in vitro and in patient-derived xenograft studies. Blood. 2016;128:3016.

46. Saba N, Wiestner A. Do mantle cell lymphomas have an 'Achilles heel'? Curr Opin Hematol. 2014;21:350–7.

47. Colomer D, Campo E. Unlocking new therapeutic targets and resistance mechanisms in mantle cell lymphoma. Cancer Cell. 2014;25:7–9.

48. Rauert-Wunderlich H, Rudelius M, Ott G, Rosenwald A. Targeting protein kinase C in mantle cell lymphoma. Br J Haematol. 2016;173:394–403.

lymphomas differ in their responsiveness to CpG oligodeoxynucleotides. Clin Cancer Res. 2005;11:1490–9.

49. Knies N, Alankus B, Weilemann A, Tzankov A, Brunner K, Ruff T, Kremer M, Keller UB, Lenz G, Ruland J. Lymphomagenic CARD11/BCL10/MALT1 signaling drives malignant B-cell proliferation via cooperative NF-kappaB and JNK activation. Proc Natl Acad Sci U S A. 2015;112:E7230–8.

50. Zhang H, Chen Z, Miranda RN, Medeiros LJ, McCarty N. TG2 and NF-kappaB signaling coordinates the survival of mantle cell lymphoma cells via IL6-mediated autophagy. Cancer Res. 2016;76:6410–23.

51. Jung HJ, Chen Z, Wang M, Fayad L, Romaguera J, Kwak LW, McCarty N. Calcium blockers decrease the bortezomib resistance in mantle cell lymphoma via manipulation of tissue transglutaminase activities. Blood. 2012;119:2568–78.

52. Davids MS, Kim HT, Nicotra A, Savell A, Francoeur K, Hellman JM, Miskin H, Sportelli P, Bashey A, Stampleman L, et al. Updated results of a multicenter phase I/IB study of TGR-1202 in combination with ibrutinib in patients with relapsed or refractory MCL or CLL. Hematol Oncol. 2017;35:54–5.

53. Vidal-Crespo A, Rodriguez V, Matas-Cespedes A, Lee E, Rivas-Delgado A, Giné E, Navarro A, Beà S, Campo E, López-Guillermo A, et al. The Bruton tyrosine kinase inhibitor CC-292 shows activity in mantle cell lymphoma and synergizes with lenalidomide and NIK inhibitors depending on nuclear factor-κB mutational status. Haematologica. 2017;102:e447.

54. Wang ML, Rule S, Martin P, Goy A, Auer R, Kahl BS, Jurczak W, Advani RH, Romaguera JE, Williams ME, et al. Targeting BTK with ibrutinib in relapsed or refractory mantle-cell lymphoma. N Engl J Med. 2013;369:507–16.

55. Wang M, Rule S, Zinzani PL, Goy A, Casasnovas O, Smith SD, Damaj G, Doorduijn J, Lamy T, Morschhauser F, et al. Acalabrutinib in relapsed or refractory mantle cell lymphoma (ACE-LY-004): a single-arm, multicentre, phase 2 trial. Lancet. 2018;391:659–67.

56. Fisher RI, Bernstein SH, Kahl BS, Djulbegovic B, Robertson MJ, de Vos S, Epner E, Krishnan A, Leonard JP, Lonial S, et al. Multicenter phase II study of bortezomib in patients with relapsed or refractory mantle cell lymphoma. J Clin Oncol. 2006;24:4867–74.

57. Jazirehi AR, Huerta-Yepez S, Cheng G, Bonavida B. Rituximab (chimeric anti-CD20 monoclonal antibody) inhibits the constitutive nuclear factor-{kappa}B signaling pathway in non-Hodgkin's lymphoma B-cell lines: role in sensitization to chemotherapeutic drug-induced apoptosis. Cancer Res. 2005;65:264–76.

58. Kahl BS, Spurgeon SE, Furman RR, Flinn IW, Coutre SE, Brown JR, Benson DM, Byrd JC, Peterman S, Cho Y, et al. A phase 1 study of the PI3Kdelta inhibitor idelalisib in patients with relapsed/refractory mantle cell lymphoma (MCL). Blood. 2014;123:3398–405.

59. Youn HS, Lee JY, Saitoh SI, Miyake K, Hwang DH. Auranofin, as an anti-rheumatic gold compound, suppresses LPS-induced homodimerization of TLR4. Biochem Biophys Res Commun. 2006;350:866–71.

60. Reddy S, Damle NK, Venkatesan AM, Thompson SK, Rao N, Smith RA, Gupta S. Abstract 792: ASN002: a novel dual SYK/JAK inhibitor with strong antitumor activity. Cancer Res. 2015;75:792.

61. Boyle JN, Kim CR, Guo H, Bell T, Huang S, Li CJ, Liu Y, Zhang H, Wang J, Zhang V, et al. CUDC-907: an oral HDAC/PI3K dual inhibitor with strong preclinical efficacy in MCL model. Blood. 2016;128:4183.

62. Aoki T, Shimada K, Sakamoto A, Sugimoto K, Morishita T, Kojima Y, Shimada S, Kato S, Iriyama C, Kuno S, et al. Emetine elicits apoptosis of intractable B-cell lymphoma cells with MYC rearrangement through inhibition of glycolytic metabolism. Oncotarget. 2017;8:13085–98.

63. Smith BD, Levis M, Beran M, Giles F, Kantarjian H, Berg K, Murphy KM, Dauses T, Allebach J, Small D. Single-agent CEP-701, a novel FLT3 inhibitor, shows biologic and clinical activity in patients with relapsed or refractory acute myeloid leukemia. Blood. 2004;103:3669–76.

64. Ham M, Moss AC. Mesalamine in the treatment and maintenance of remission of ulcerative colitis. Expert Rev Clin Pharmacol. 2012;5:113–23.

65. Zak Z, Gelebart P, Lai R. Fenofibrate induces effective apoptosis in mantle cell lymphoma by inhibiting the TNFalpha/NF-kappaB signaling axis. Leukemia. 2010;24:1476–86.

66. Kaufmann H, Raderer M, Wohrer S, Puspok A, Bankier A, Zielinski C, Chott A, Drach J. Antitumor activity of rituximab plus thalidomide in patients with relapsed/refractory mantle cell lymphoma. Blood. 2004;104:2269–71.

67. Ruan J, Martin P, Shah B, Schuster SJ, Smith SM, Furman RR, Christos P, Rodriguez A, Svoboda J, Lewis J, et al. Lenalidomide plus rituximab as initial treatment for mantle-cell lymphoma. N Engl J Med. 2015;373:1835–44.

2

Novel antibodies against GPIbα inhibit pulmonary metastasis by affecting vWF-GPIbα interaction

Yingxue Qi[1], Wenchun Chen[2], Xinyu Liang[1], Ke Xu[3*], Xiangyu Gu[1], Fengying Wu[4], Xuemei Fan[5], Shengxiang Ren[4], Junling Liu[5], Jun Zhang[6], Renhao Li[2], Jianwen Liu[1*] and Xin Liang[1*]

Abstract

Background: Platelet glycoprotein Ibα (GPIbα) extracellular domain, which is part of the receptor complex GPIb-IX-V, plays an important role in tumor metastasis. However, the mechanism through which GPIbα participates in the metastatic process remains unclear. In addition, potential bleeding complication remains an obstacle for the clinical use of anti-platelet agents in cancer therapy.

Methods: We established a series of screening models and obtained rat anti-mouse GPIbα monoclonal antibodies (mAb) 1D12 and 2B4 that demonstrated potential value in suppressing cancer metastasis. To validate our findings, we further obtained mouse anti-human GPIbα monoclonal antibody YQ3 through the same approach.

Results: 1D12 and 2B4 affected the von Willebrand factor (vWF)-GPIbα interaction via binding to GPIbα aa 41-50 and aa 277-290 respectively, which markedly inhibited the interaction among platelets, tumor cells, and endothelial cells in vitro, and reduced the mean number of surface nodules in the experimental and spontaneous metastasis models in vivo. As expected, YQ3 inhibited lung cancer adhesion and demonstrated similar value in metastasis. More importantly, for all three mAbs in our study, none of their Fabs induced thrombocytopenia.

Conclusion: Our results therefore supported the hypothesis that GPIbα contributes to tumor metastasis and suggested potential value of using anti-GPIbα mAb to suppress cancer metastasis.

Keywords: GPIbα, vWF, Platelets, Antibody, Metastasis

Background

The association between elevated platelet number and malignant tumors was initially reported in 1872 [1, 2] and has been demonstrated in several common cancers [3–6]. Tumor cells are capable of activating and aggregating platelets to form tumor thrombus—a process referred to as tumor cell-induced platelet aggregation (TCIPA) [7]. Extensive evidence indicates that the formation of tumor thrombus contributes to critical steps in cancer metastasis, including shielding cancer cells from physiological clearance and immune surveillance and facilitating the migration, invasion, and arrestment of tumor cells within the vasculature [2, 8]. It is increasingly recognized that the formation of tumor thrombus involving platelets is the first and one of the most important steps in cancer metastasis.

Two important platelet membrane receptors, glycoprotein Ib-IX-V (GPIb-IX-V) and glycoprotein IIb-IIIa (GPIIb-IIIa, also known as integrin $\alpha_{IIb}\beta_3$), are essential for tumor cell-platelet adhesion and aggregation when tumor cells invade into vasculature [2]. An increasing number of studies have focused on the role of platelet membrane receptors in tumor metastasis [7, 9–11]. Although it is generally believed that the deficiency of GPIIb-IIIa or blockade of GPIIb-IIIa by monoclonal

* Correspondence: xin.liang@ecust.edu.cn; liujian@ecust.edu.cn; cola519@163.com
[1]State Key Laboratory of Bioreactor Engineering & Shanghai Key Laboratory of New Drug Design, School of Pharmacy, East China University of Science and Technology, 130 Meilong Rd, Shanghai 200237, People's Republic of China
[3]Central laboratory, General Surgery, Putuo Hospital, and Interventional Cancer Institute of Chinese Integrative Medicine, Shanghai University of Traditional Chinese Medicine, 164 Lanxi Rd, Shanghai 200062, People's Republic of China
Full list of author information is available at the end of the article

antibodies may lead to severe bleeding complications [11], which is the main reason to limit the clinical use of these anti-GPIIb-IIIa agents in cancer therapy, the anti-metastatic agent anti-GPIIIa49-66 scFv Ab A11 that has a slight effect on platelet count and vein bleeding time was found to have therapeutic potential in metastasis [7, 12]. While the mechanism of GPIIb-IIIa involvement in tumor metastasis is largely clarified, the role of another important adhesion receptor GPIb-IX-V in metastasis remains debatable [13]. Here, we evaluated the role of GPIb-IX-V and its therapeutic potential in metastasis.

The GPIb-IX-V complex consists of four subunits: GPIbα, GPIbβ, GPIX, and GPV. It interacts with many important extracellular ligands. GPIbα is the largest and most important component of the complex. The N-terminal domain of GPIbα contains the binding sites for several molecules, including vWF [14], P-selectin (CD62P) [15], and thrombin [16], which are essential for primary hemostasis and blood coagulation. The interaction between vWF and GPIbα was found to be particularly critical in the formation of thrombus [17]. Although there are studies that showed that knocking out the mouse GPIbα or replacing mouse GPIbα extracellular domain could significantly inhibit tumor cell metastasis [18], the deletion of GPIbα extracellular domain unfortunately induced platelet depletion, leading to severe bleeding complications [18]. In addition, blockage of GPIbα by monoclonal antibody p0p/B did not have the same influence on tumor metastasis as GPIbα knock out models [9], raising the concern if GPIbα truly participates in the metastatic process. To address this question, we screened out three anti-GPIbα mAbs with minimal effect on platelet activation as the tools to dissect the therapeutic value of GPIbα in cancer metastasis.

Methods
Materials and animals
Platelet agonist ADP and collagen (equine tendon) were from HELENA laboratories (USA). Ristocetin was from Sigma (R7752, USA). Anti-human GPIbα monoclonal antibody SZ2, VM16d, and AK2 were from GenTex (GTX28822, USA), YO Proteins (656, USA), and Bio-Rad (MCA740T, USA), respectively. Secondary antibody anti-human/mouse CD62P (P-selectin) APC was from Thermo Fisher scientific (17-0626, USA), and FITC-conjugated anti-human PAC-1 was from Biolegend (362803, USA). Peptides of GPIbα fragments were synthesized by GL Biochen (China) Ltd. Recombinant mouse vWF protein was from Creative BioMart (VWF-1432 M, USA), and human vWF protein was from Sino Biological (10973-H08C, USA). C57BL/6J mice, BCLB/C mice, and Wistar rat were from JSJ laboratories (China) and were bred and housed at Putuo animal care facility. Transgenic mice expressing no mouse but only human GPIbα (hTg) were described previously [19]. Animal experiments were

conducted in mice or rats using protocols approved by the IACUC of Putuo Hospital. Six- to eight-week-old mice or rats were used in the study, and investigators were blinded to group allocation during data collection.

Human blood collection
Written, informed consent was obtained from all participants prior to their inclusion in studies. Venous blood was collected from healthy adult volunteers at East China University of Science and Technology, as well as lung cancer patients at Shanghai Pulmonary Hospital. In addition, the use of donor-derived human platelets was approved by IRB in Shanghai Pulmonary Hospital.

Production and characterization of GPIbα mAbs
Rat anti-mouse GPIbα monoclonal antibodies and mouse anti-human GPIbα monoclonal antibodies were prepared according to the methods described by Koehler and Milstein [20]. Briefly, to develop mouse anti-human antibodies, BALB/C female mouse (6 to 8 weeks) were immunized by four injections of human platelet lysate at a 28-day interval. To develop rat anti-mouse antibodies, Wistar female rats were given an intraperitoneal injection of washed mouse platelets four times at a 20-day interval. Three days after the fourth immunization, mouse or rat splenocytes were fused with Sp2/0-Ag14 myeloma cells and cultured in HAT selection medium. IgGs were purified from hybridoma supernatants using a protein G-Sepharose 4B column (6518-1, Biovision, CA, USA).

The ELISA assay was then used to characterize these antibodies. Ninety-six well microtiter plates were coated overnight at 4 °C with 50 μl of 4 μg/ml anti-human/mouse CD42a Ab (MBS9206081, MyBioSource). After washing three times, the wells were blocked with 2% (w/v) BSA-PBS for 2 h. The wells were then incubated with lysate of human or mouse platelets for 2 h. After that, hybridoma supernatants or purified mAbs were added to the wells and incubated for 60 min. The bound antibodies were detected by HRP-conjugated goat anti-mouse IgG or goat anti-rat IgG. After the background signal had been subtracted, the binding curve was fitted to the eq. $Y = B_{max} \times [ligand]/(K_d + [ligand])$
where Y is the specific binding, [ligand] the ligand concentration, B_{max} the binding maximum, and K_d the equilibrium dissociation constant.

The specificities of the antibodies were also determined by Western blot as previously described [21].

Preparation of Fab fragment
The generation of Fab fragment was following previously described protocol with the modification in incubation time with immobilized papain (20341, Thermo Scientific) [21]. After papain was removed via centrifugation, the

generated Fab fragment was purified using Protein A beads (6501-5, Biovision, CA, USA).

Platelet activation

Washed platelets (1.2×10^7 cells/ml) were treated with hybridoma supernatants or purified mAbs at room temperature (RT) for 20 min and detected with FITC or APC-conjugated antibody. Platelet activation induced by tumor cells was by adding 1×10^5 cells/100 µl tumor cells to 1.2×10^6 cells/100 µl washed platelets. When needed, the antibody was added to the platelets and incubated for at least 20 min before their stimulation by tumor cells. The signal of platelet activation was quantitated by the mean fluorescence intensity for the entire cell population (10,000 cells) on a Becton-Dickinson FACS Canto II instrument (BD Biosciences, San Jose, CA, USA).

Platelet aggregometry

Platelet-rich plasma (PRP) was generated as previously described [21]. The final platelet count in PRP was adjusted to 2.5×10^8 cells/ml. Aggregation was initiated in 300 µl of stirred PRP by the addition of noted agonists or 1×10^5 cells/50 µl MCF-7 cells to form the mixture of platelets and tumor cells. When required, the antibody was added to PRP and incubated for at least 5 min before stimulation with either agonists or tumor cells. Agonist-induced platelet aggregation was monitored in dual-channel Chrono-Log aggregometer (Havertown, PA, USA)

Assay of tumor cells adhesion to platelets, platelet adhesion to endothelial cells, or tumor cell adhesion to endothelial cells

The adhesion between tumor cells, platelets, and endothelial cells was measured as previously described [7].

Animal experiments

Experimental lung metastasis assay

In the Lewis lung carcinoma (LLC) model, 6-week-old C57BL/6J mice were randomly divided into six groups. There were eight mice per group, and half of the mice are male and half are female in each group. Female and male mice were separately cultured to avoid mating. For groups 1–6, mice were injected with LLC tumor cells (2.5×10^5 cells/mouse) with control IgG, control Fab, 2B4, 1D12, 2B4 Fab, or 1D12 Fab, respectively, at the dose of 50 µg/mouse through the lateral tail vain, along with the tumor cells. After 14 days, the lungs were removed, rinsed with PBS, and the number of metastasis foci on the lung surface was counted. The pulmonary lobes were subsequently kept in 4% paraformaldehyde for later paraffin embedding and hematoxylin and eosin staining. The same experiment

was repeated using B16F10 melanoma mouse model (1×10^6 B16F10 cells/mouse).

Spontaneous metastasis assay

For spontaneous metastasis, 6-week-old BCLB/C female mice were subcutaneously injected with 1×10^5 4T1 tumor cells. The mice were treated with 50 µg/mouse 2B4, 2B4 Fab, 1D12, or 1D12 Fab, respectively, when the tumor volume reached 80 mm³. After 3 weeks, the mice were killed, and the surface metastatic nodules on the lung were counted and the volume of primary tumor was recorded.

Determination of mouse platelet count

The platelet number was quantitated by a Becton-Dickinson FACS Canto II instrument equipped with BD Trucount Tubes (340334). The subsequent steps were then carried out by following the manufacturers' instructions.

Bleeding time

The bleeding time was measured as previously described [22]. Briefly, the mouse tail vein was severed 2 mm from its tip and blotted every 30 s on a circular sheet of filter paper to obtain an objective measurement. Bleeding time was calculated when there was absence of blood on the filter paper. Bleeding time differences were recorded by an unbiased observer and confirmed by two other observers blinded to the experimental status of the mice.

Statistical analysis

Statistical analysis was performed using Prism 6 software. All experiments were carried out at least three times, and the results are presented as the mean ± standard deviation. Statistical significance was assessed by using the one-way analysis of variance (ANOVA) followed by Dunnett's post hoc test. P values < 0.05 were considered statistically significant.

Results

Generation and screening of mAbs targeting mouse platelet GPIbα

To generate antibodies that bind to mouse platelet GPIbα, washed mouse platelet lysate was used as the antigen for rat immunization. Obtained hybridoma clones were screened in ELISA for binding affinity to the GPIb-IX complex. Positive clones were further screened for their abilities to inhibit platelet-cancer cell adhesion (Additional file 1: Table S1A). After screening, we obtained six positive clones that could bind to GPIb-IX complex (Fig. 1a) and inhibit platelet-tumor cell adherence to different extents (Additional file 2: Figure S1A). At static condition, two of the six antibodies, 2B4 and 1D12, had virtually no effect on the activation of integrin $\alpha II_b\beta_3$, which is used to indicate platelet activation [21], while the other four could activate

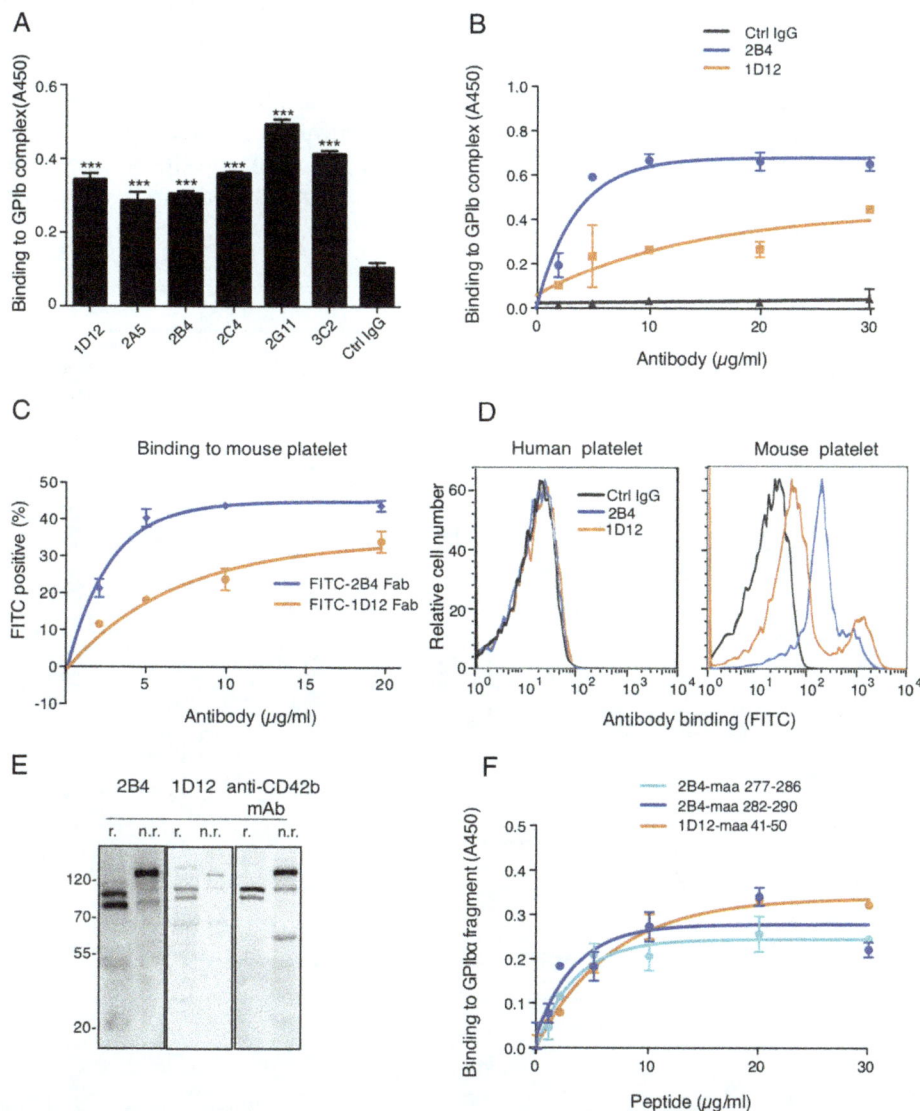

Fig. 1 2B4 and 1D12 specifically bind to mouse glycoprotein (GP)Ibα. **a** Binding of rat anti-mouse antibodies to GPIb-IX complex was detected in ELISA. GPIb-IX was captured by anti-GPIX antibody which complex was immobilized in microtiter plates. Supernatant of hybridoma cells, each identified by the clone name, and the negative control, in the form of RPMI-1640 fetal bovine culture medium with 5 μg/ml rat IgG, were added to the coated wells. The bound Ab was detected with HRP-conjugated rabbit anti-rat IgG. ***$P < 0.001$. **b** Binding of 2B4 and 1D12 to GPIb-IX complex were detected in ELISA. Purified mAbs, colored as indicated, and negative controls, in the form of rat IgG, were added to the GPIb-IX immobilized microtiter plates. The bound Ab was detected with HRP-conjugated rabbit anti-rat IgG. **c** Binding of FITC-conjugated Fab to washed mouse platelets was detected in flow cytometry. Washed mouse platelets were incubated with each Fab at indicated concentration. Binding of Fab was detected by flow cytometry and quantitated by mean fluorescence intensity. **d** 2B4 and 1D12 specifically bound to mouse platelets. Washed human or mouse platelets were incubated with 10 μg/ml FITC-conjugated 2B4 or 1D12, respectively. Binding of Ab was detected by flow cytometry and quantitated by mean fluorescence intensity. **e** 2B4 and 1D12 recognized specifically GPIbα in Western blot under nonreducing (n.r.) and reducing (r.) conditions. Total lysates of mouse platelets were immunoblotted with either 2B4 or 1D12. Molecular weight marker (M) was shown and labeled in kDa on the left. **f** Binding of 5 μg/ml of 2B4 or 1D12 to indicated concentration of GPIbα peptide fragments were detected in ELISA. GPIbα peptide fragment was immobilized in microtiter plates. Indicated concentration antibodies were added to the coated wells. The bound Ab was detected with HRP-conjugated rabbit anti-rat IgG. Each figure or histogram is a representative of three independent experiments

platelet to a certain degree in the same condition (Additional file 2: Figure S1B). Therefore, 2B4 and 1D12 were eventually selected for study.

Purified 2B4 and 1D12 (Additional file 2: Figure S1C) exhibited higher binding affinity to immobilized GPIb-IX

complex than the negative control (Ctrl IgG) (Fig. 1b). The K_d of 2B4 and 1D12 was 2.47 ± 0.28 and 9.62 ± 0.52 μg/ml, respectively. Like 2B4 and 1D12 antibodies, their Fab fragments exhibited strong binding affinity to fresh washed mouse platelets but not human platelets as detected by flow cytometry using FITC-conjugated Fab (Fig. 1c, d). Immunoblotting of platelet lysate with 2B4 and 1D12 produced almost the same protein bands as those blotted with a commercialized well-documented anti-mouse GPIbα antibody (Fig. 1e). These results illustrated that 2B4 and 1D12 specifically recognize mouse GPIbα.

By using synthetic peptides, we obtained 20 purified recombinant GPIbα fragment (Additional file 3: Table S2B) to characterize the binding sites of 2B4 and 1D12. In ELISA, aa 277-290 showed the highest binding with 2B4; meanwhile, 1D12 bound to aa 41-50 (Additional file 4: Figure S2A and B), and the binding of the antibody to the peptide fragment was in a concentration-dependent

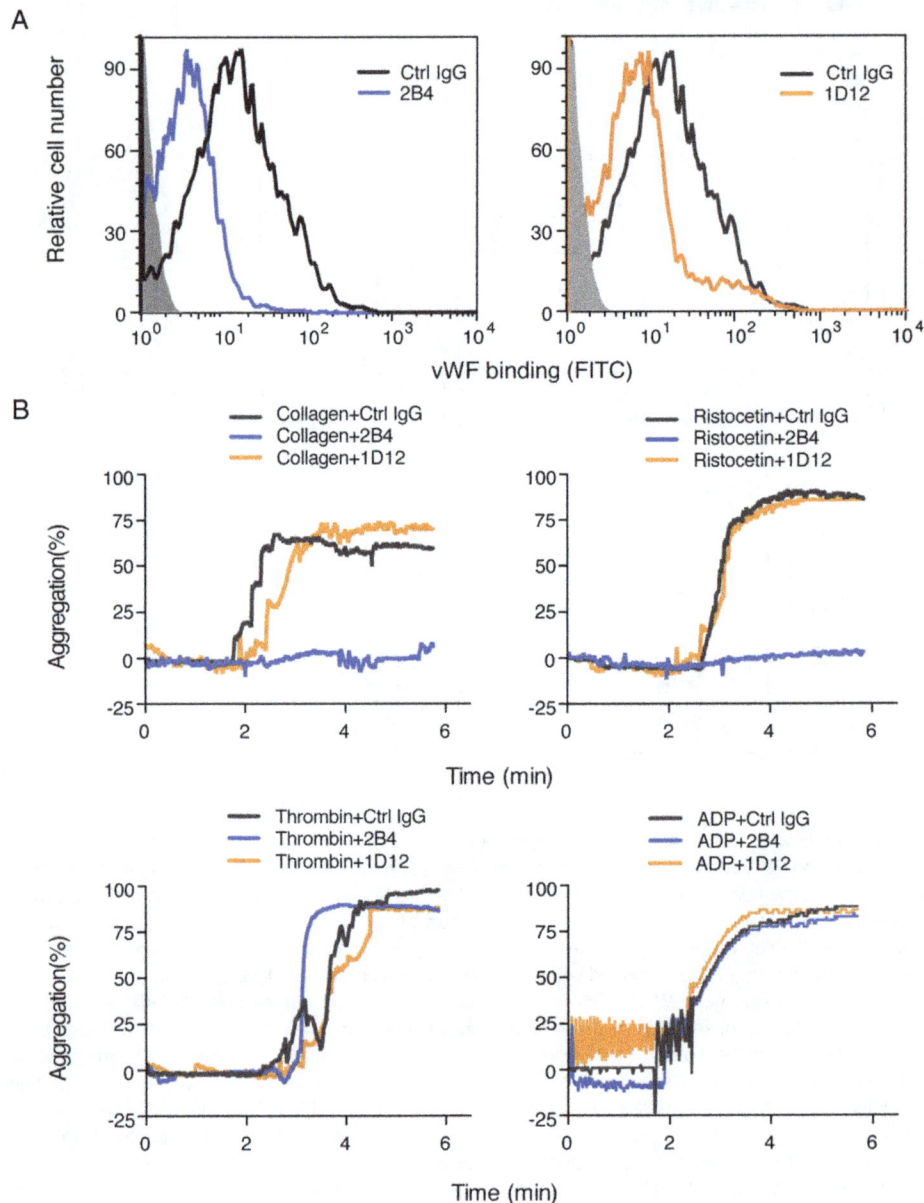

Fig. 2 2B4 and 1D12 inhibit vWF binding. **a** The vWF binding was inhibited by 2B4 and 1D12 and detected by flow cytometry. Washed mouse platelets were incubated with 10 µg/ml 2B4 or 10 µg/ml 1D12 for 20 min, and then 2 µg/ml recombind mouse vWF was added in the presence of 1 mg/ml ristocetin. Binding of vWF was detected with FITC-conjugated mouse vWF IgG by flow cytometry and quantitated by mean fluorescence intensity. **b** 2B4 inhibited ristocetin- and collagen-induced platelet aggregation. Different agonist-induced aggregation of PRP that had been pretreated with 10 µg/ml rat IgG (negative control, gray), 10 µg/ml 2B4 (blue), and 10 µg/ml 1D12 (orange) were detected for 6 min. Agonists: ristocetin (1 mg/ml), thrombin (0.05 U/ml), ADP (10 nM), and collagen (2 µg/ml). The histograms are representative of three independent experiments

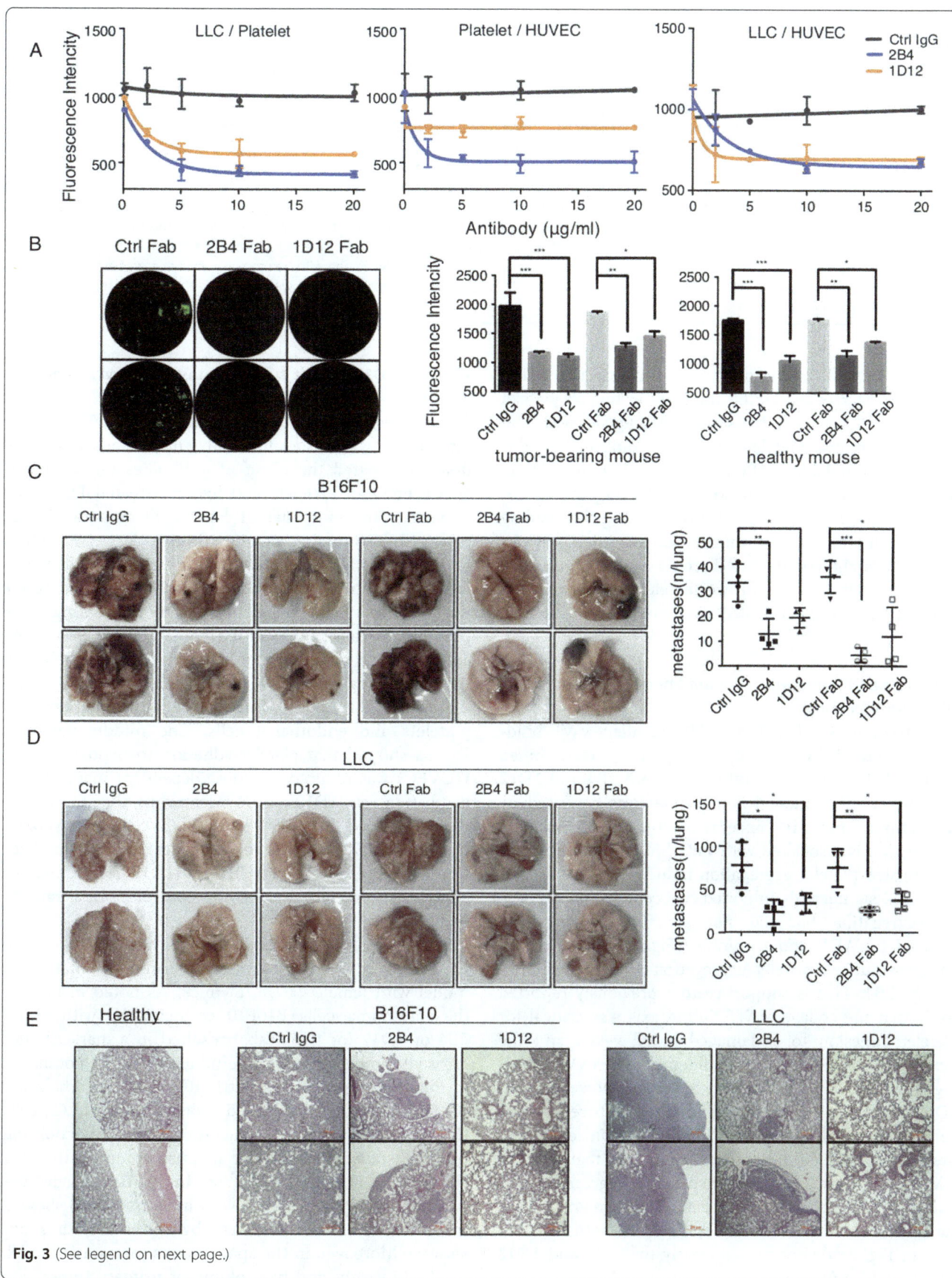

Fig. 3 (See legend on next page.)

(See figure on previous page.)
Fig. 3 2B4 and 1D12 inhibit cancer adhesion in vitro and metastasis in vivo. **a** 2B4 and 1D12 inhibited platelet, LLC cell, and endothelial cell adhesion between each other. Effect of 2B4 (blue) and 1D12 (orange) on the adhesion of LLC with BCECF-labeled platelet (Left panel), mouse BCECF-labeled platelets with HUVECs (middle panel), and BCECF-labeled LLC cells with HUVECs (right panel) in vitro. The negative control was in the form of rat IgG (gray). **b** 2B4 and 1D12 inhibited adhesion of LLC to mouse platelets from mice with pulmonary metastasis. Washed mouse platelets were divided from tumor-bearing mouse blood and healthy mouse blood. The adhesion of LLC with BCECF-labeled platelet was detected with a fluorescence plate reader and observed under a fluorescence microscope. The negative control is in the form of rat IgG or rat Fab. Average fluorescence intensity was shown in right graphs (± SD, P value is indicated; *$P < 0.05$; **$P < 0.01$; ***$P < 0.001$). **c, d** Pulmonary metastasis was assessed after B16F10 and LLC injection with control IgG (50 μg/mouse), 2B4 (50 μg/mouse), 1D12 (50 μg/mouse), control Fab (50 μg/mouse), 2B4 Fab (50 μg/mouse), or 1D12 Fab (50 μg/mouse) through the lateral tail vein ($n = 4$ mice in each group). Metastasis was analyzed 14 days after injection of tumor cells. Representative examples of the lungs (one of each group) with metastatic foci were depicted. Average number of lung metastasis in each of the groups was shown in right graphs (± SD, P value is indicated; *$P < 0.05$; **$P < 0.01$; ***$P < 0.001$). **e** Representative histologic evidence from tumor sections of the different groups. Four percent of paraformaldehyde-embedded lungs of all mice were cut completely, stained with hematoxylin and eosin, and examined histologically. Representative sections of two mice from 2B4 groups, 1D12 groups, and control IgG groups were shown. Each figure is a representative of three independent experiments

manner (Fig. 1f). Interestingly, SZ2 antibody was found binding to aa 268-282 GPIbα fragment in human platelet [23]; it therefore shares the similar binding site with that of 2B4 on mouse platelets (this was confirmed in this study shown in Additional file 4: Figure S2D). In addition, AK2 antibody recognized aa 36-59 GPIbα fragment in human platelet [24], therefore also overlapping the binding site with that of 1D12 on mouse platelet. Since previous experiments showed that vWF could bind to these two binding sites in GPIbα [25], we therefore speculated that 2B4 and 1D12 could also affect vWF binding.

Anti-mouse GPIbα monoclonal antibodies 2B4 and 1D12 inhibit vWF binding

To determine whether 2B4 and 1D12 affect vWF binding, we tested by flow cytometry using recombined mouse vWF. Figure 2a showed that both 2B4 and 1D12 inhibited vWF binding when platelet was activated by ristocetin (1 mg/ml). Since ristocetin-induced platelet aggregation is associated with vWF binding [26], we next investigated platelet aggregation induced by several agonists. 2B4 significantly inhibited ristocetin-induced platelet aggregation but did not affect the aggregation induced by ADP and thrombin (Fig. 2b). In addition, collagen-induced platelet aggregation was totally inhibited by 2B4. This is supportive to a previously reported study that the collagen-vWF-GPIbα axis was critical for platelet adhesion to a damaged blood vessel and the binding to collagen could be influenced when vWF binding is inhibited [27]. It is noteworthy, however, that 1D12 had no influence on neither ristocetin- nor collagen-induced aggregation. This is reminiscent of a previously reported antibody p0p/1-5 [28] that affected vWF binding without influencing the aggregation induced by ristocetin and collagen. These might be because of the different binding epitopes. Nonetheless, our data in Fig. 2a demonstrated clearly that 2B4 and 1D12 could inhibit vWF binding.

2B4 and 1D12 inhibit tumor metastasis in vivo and in vitro

To investigate whether the inhibition of vWF-GPIbα interaction was associated with tumor metastasis, we first investigated the effect of antibodies on the interaction between platelets and hypoxic-treated LCC cells in vitro. The left panel of Fig. 3a demonstrated that platelet-LLC adhesion was significantly decreased with a maximum of approximately 60% inhibition when platelets were pretreated with 2B4 or 1D12. A similar result was observed using platelets from tumor-bearing mice (Fig. 3b). Because vWF-GPIbα and vWF-collagen interactions play a critical role in the adhesion of platelets to the endothelial cells [29], we therefore reasoned that 2B4 and 1D12 could inhibit the adhesion between platelets and endothelial cells. The middle panel in Fig. 3a showed that platelet adhesion to hypoxic-treated HUVECs was reduced in a dose-dependent manner after incubation with 1D12 or 2B4. Meanwhile, the adhesion of BCECF-labeled hypoxic-treated LLC cells to hypoxic-treated HUVECs was also markedly decreased when platelets were pretreated with 2B4 or 1D12 (Fig. 3a, right panel). As expected, the negative control, normal rat IgG had no effect.

We further investigated the inhibitory effect of these antibodies in vivo using an experimental metastasis model with female C57BL/6J mice. As noted in Fig. 3c, the melanoma cells B16F10 co-incubated with either 2B4 or 1D12 (or their Fabs) resulted in a markedly decreased number of surface pulmonary nodules compared to the control group using ctrl IgG or its Fab. The same phenomenon was observed when using LLC cells (Fig. 3d). This finding was again confirmed by counting the metastatic lesions under microscopy using the H-E slides of the lung tissue (Fig. 3e). In addition, in vivo experimental metastasis assay with male mice also showed inhibition of tumor metastasis by antibodies (data not shown). Moreover, in the spontaneous metastasis model, the body weight and the volume of primary tumor was

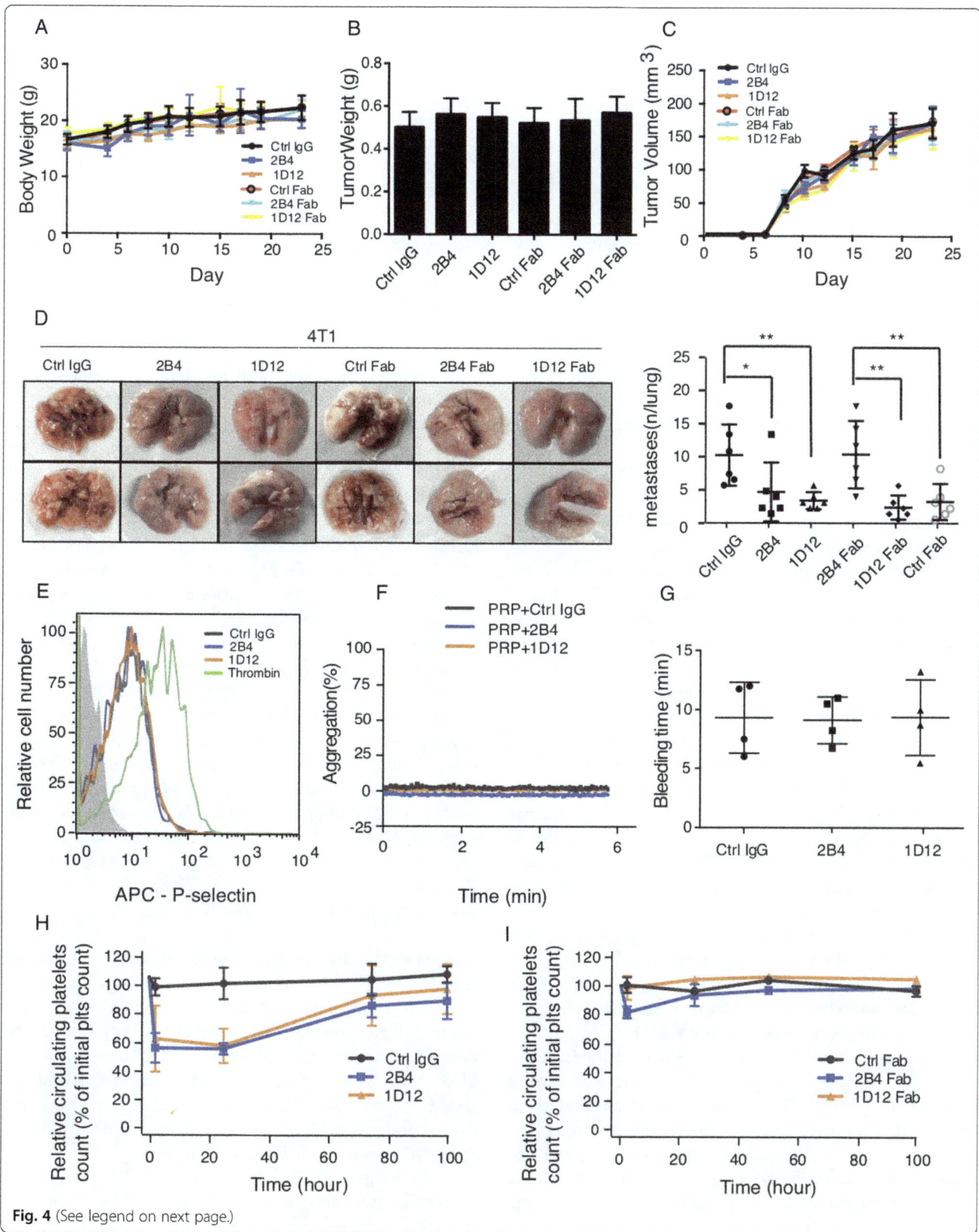

Fig. 4 (See legend on next page.)

(See figure on previous page.)
Fig. 4 2B4 and 1D12 inhibit spontaneous metastasis but have no effect on platelet activation and hemostatic function. Effect of 2B4 (50 µg/mouse), 1D12 (50 µg/mouse), and their Fabs (50 µg/mouse) on (**a**) mice weight, (**b**) tumor weight, (**c**) tumor volume, and (**d**) pulmonary metastasis on spontaneous metastasis of 4T1 ($n = 6$ mice in each group). Metastasis was analyzed 3 weeks after injection of tumor cells. Representative examples of the lungs (one of each group) with metastatic foci were depicted. Average number of lung metastasis in each of the groups was shown in right graphs (± SD, P value is indicated; $*P < 0.05$; $**P < 0.01$; $***P < 0.001$). **e** 2B4 and 1D12 did not affect platelet activation. Increased expression of APC-conjugated P-selectin indicated the degree of platelet activation. Washed platelets were treated with 10 µg/ml purified 2B4 (blue), 1D12 (orange), negative control (rat IgG, gray), or 0.05 U/ml thrombin (green) as positive control, then probed with APC-conjugated anti-P-selectin Ab. The florescence intensity was detected by flow cytometry. **f** 2B4 and 1D12 did not induce platelet aggregation. The aggregation of PRP pretreated with 10 µg/ml 2B4 (blue) and 10 µg/ml 1D12 (orange) was detected. Negative control was in the form of rat IgG. **g** Bleeding time did not prolonged 2 h after the injection of intact 2B4 or 1D12 (50 µg/mouse) ($n = 4$ mice in each group). **h** Platelet survival curves for mice injected with 2B4 (50 µg/mouse), 1D12 (50 µg/mouse), or negative control (normal rat IgG, 50 µg/mouse) ($n = 6$ mice in each group). **i** Platelet survival curves for mice injected with 2B4 Fab (50 µg/mouse), 1D12 Fab (50 µg/mouse), or negative control (normal rat Fab, 50 µg/mouse) ($n = 6$ mice in each group). Blood was drawn from mice at the time of antibody injection (0 h), 2 h after injection, and every 24 h following until 96 h after antibody injection. Platelet count determined by flow cytometry. The histograms are representative of three independent experiments

not be influenced by antibody injection (Fig. 4a–c), but the lung metastasis was obviously suppressed (Fig. 4d). All together, these data suggested 2B4 and 1D12 could potently inhibit the adhesion of cancer cells in vitro and metastasis in vivo.

2B4 and 1D12 have no effect on platelet activation and hemostatic function

Since platelet activation and subsequent clearing induced by antibodies targeting GPIbα limited the clinical application of previous platelet antibodies in suppressing cancer metastasis [18, 30], it is therefore important to investigate whether 2B4 and 1D12 could affect platelet activation and/or induce thrombocytopenia in vivo. Treatment of washed mouse platelets with 2B4 or 1D12 did not induce increased expression of P-selectin (Fig. 4e). Furthermore, the addition of 2B4 or 1D12 to PRP did not induce platelet aggregation (Fig. 4f). Injection of 2B4 or 1D12 at the dose of 50 µg/mouse did not affect tail-bleeding time (Fig. 4g). While the injection of 2B4 or 1D12 decreased almost 40% of the platelet count, that of their respective Fab fragments did not change the platelet count (Fig. 4h, i). Therefore, 2B4 and 1D12 can potentially suppress cancer metastasis without significantly affecting the number and function of platelets.

Generation and characterization of mouse anti-human platelet GPIbα monoclonal antibody YQ3

Based on the above findings, we then decided to use the same approach to generate a series of mouse anti-human platelet GPIbα monoclonal antibodies to explore the role of human GPIbα in cancer metastasis (Additional file 1: Table S1B). After screening, we obtained a potent antibody, YQ3, as the best candidate for the subsequent studies. Our screening results showed that compared to other candidates, YQ3 exhibited the strongest binding affinity to GPIb-IX complex (Fig. 5a) and inhibitory effect on adhesion (Additional file 2: Figure S1D).

Further experiments illustrated that purified YQ3 (Additional file 2: Figure S1E) exhibited strong binding to immobilized GPIb-IX complex in a dose-dependent manner (Fig. 5b, K_d of YQ3 is 2.26 ± 0.37 µg/mL). Meanwhile, it specifically recognized human but not mouse platelet GPIbα (Fig. 5c–e). By using 20 purified human GPIbα fragments (Additional file 3: Table S2A) in ELISA, we found that YQ3 bound to aa 31-56 and aa 277-290 of human GPIbα in a dose-dependent manner. (Fig. 5f left panel, Additional file 4: Figure S2C). These two binding sites overlapped those of the above-mentioned two rat anti-mouse antibodies. In addition, the Fab of YQ3 was found to bind to aa 41-56 and aa 277-286 (Fig. 5f right panel, Additional file 4: Figure S2E). To further verify the accuracy of the binding sites, we conducted a competitive binding assay. Briefly, washed human platelets were pretreated with aa41-55 or aa277-286, or both peptides before adding FITC-conjugated YQ3 Fab. As expected, peptides aa 41-56 and aa 277-286 inhibited 50% binding of YQ3 Fab to platelets. When aa 41-56 or aa 277-286 was used alone, such binding was also impaired, but to a lesser degree (Fig. 5g).

YQ3 inhibits adhesion and cancer cell-induced platelet activation

We next investigated whether YQ3 could affect vWF binding. Figure 6a showed that vWF binding induced by ristocetin in vitro was decreased when incubated with YQ3. Meanwhile, ristocetin- and collagen-induced aggregation were also significantly inhibited by YQ3 and its Fab fragment. However, ADP and thrombin-induced aggregation was not influenced (Fig. 6b).

To investigate inhibitory potential of YQ3 in cancer metastasis, we first tested YQ3 on TCIPA. Figure 6c showed that platelet aggregation induced by breast cancer cells MCF-7 was partially inhibited by the addition of YQ3. We then tested the effect of YQ3 on adhesions between platelet, tumor cells (e.g., colorectal cancer

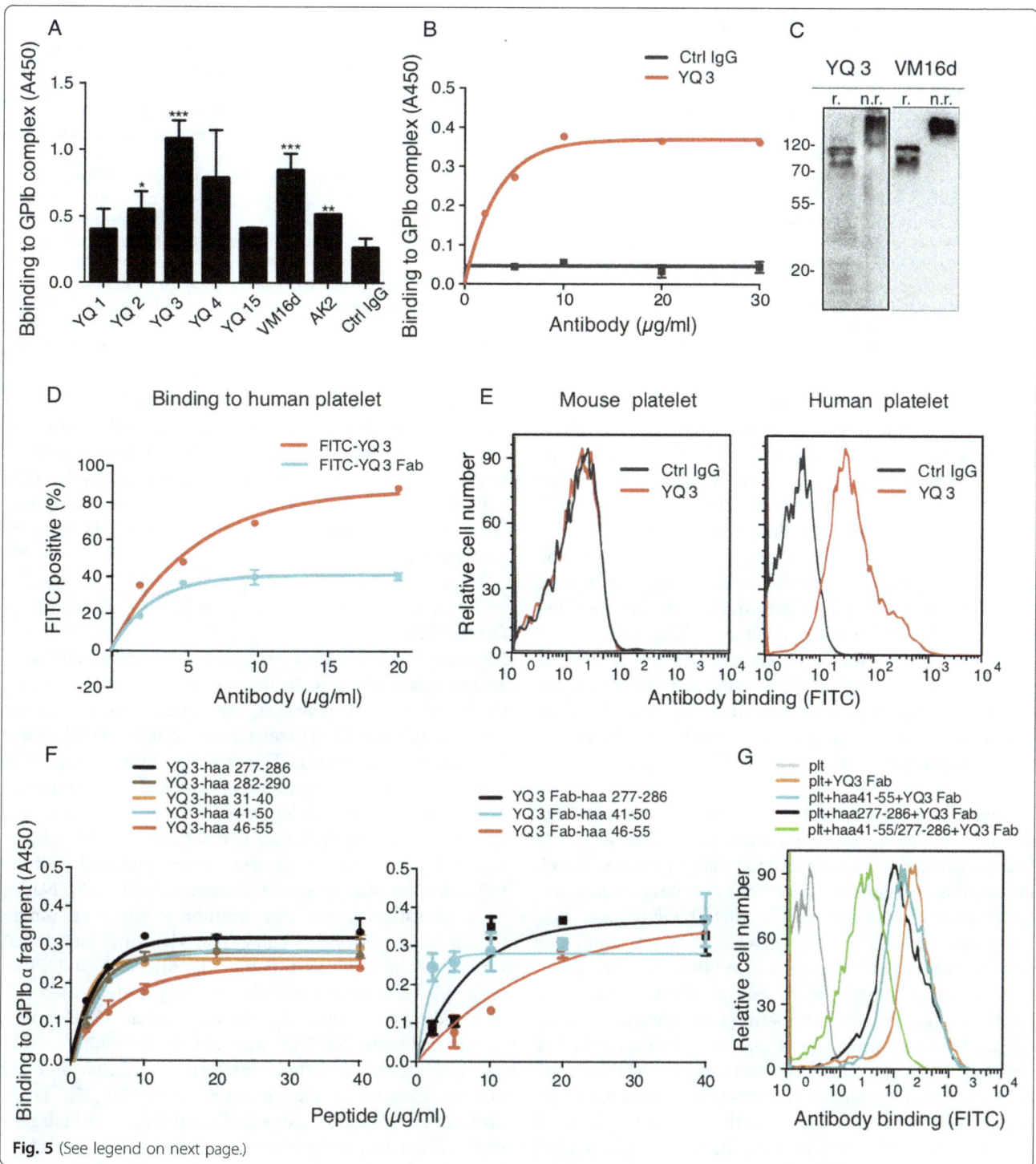

Fig. 5 (See legend on next page.)

HCT116), and HUVECs. Figure 6d showed that YQ3 inhibited cell adhesion between HCT116 cells and platelets, platelets and HUVECs, and HUVECs and HCT116 cells. Similar results were observed when we used other tumor cell lines such as breast cancer MDA-MB-231 and lung cancer A549 cells (data not shown).

We then tested the effect of YQ3 on tumor cell-induced platelet activation. Different types of tumor cells (e.g., HCT116, A549, and MDA-MB-231) were incubated with platelet with or without YQ3. The expression of P-selectin was used to indicate the degree of platelet activation. Again, YQ3 was found able to inhibit tumor cell-induced platelet activation (Fig. 6e). These results together suggested that YQ3 might have the potential to inhibit metastasis.

YQ3 inhibits the adhesion between patients' platelets and tumor cells without accelerating platelet clearance

We next tested the effect of YQ3 using patients' blood. Pre-incubated platelets collected from lung cancer patients (patients II and III had no metastasis; patients IV–VII presented with metastasis) with YQ3 Fab dramatically attenuated their adhesion to A549 cells (Fig. 7a, b). It is therefore supportive to our previous finding that YQ3 inhibited the adhesion between platelets and tumor cells. Moreover, while the expression levels of GPIbα were higher in lung cancer patients than in healthy controls, no difference was found between patients with metastasis and without, suggesting the expression level of GPIbα could not be correlated to the progression of cancer metastasis (Fig. 7c).

We then tested whether in patients' blood, YQ3 could affect platelet activation or platelet count. Figure 7d demonstrated that YQ3 did not induce PRP aggregation. Moreover, treatment of washed human platelets with YQ3 did not induce activation of integrin $\alpha II_b\beta_3$ or increase the expression of P-selectin (Fig. 7e). To explore the effect of YQ3 on platelet count, hTg mice were treated with YQ3 or YQ3 Fab, and platelet count was monitored over a 4-day period after injection. Figure 7f showed that the injection of YQ3 induced severe decrease of platelet count, but its Fab did not. Therefore, mouse anti-human GPIbα monoclonal antibody YQ3 will likely not have concerning bleeding complications, and it is worth a further exploration in humanized models.

Discussion

Multiple studies have shown that the platelet GPIbα is an important receptor in the process of tumor metastasis [9, 18, 31, 32]. However, the biggest obstacle to use GPIbα inhibition for cancer treatment is potential severe bleeding complications. This is even more concerning when conventional chemotherapy is used since it almost universally affects platelet count. However, several antibodies specifically targeting platelet GPIbα and inhibiting vWF binding to platelet were reported not to influence the platelet count dramatically [33–35]. Nancy et al. investigated the anti-thrombotic effect of human GPIbα mAb 6B4 Fab fragment in vivo and found that through inhibition of the binding of vWF to GPIbα, fewer platelets were activated, resulting in decreased risk of bleeding [33]. Similarly, the anti-human vWF monoclonal antibody SZ-123 was found to inhibit vWF-collagen and vWF-platelet interactions in vivo and did not significantly prolong bleeding time [34, 35]. These findings are important considering inhibition of collagen-vWF-GPIbα axis is therefore considered as a new strategy in anti-thrombotic therapy [29]. Nevertheless, contradictory findings were reported that vWF deficiency could promote tumor metastasis instead [36]. It remains debatable whether this was due to enhanced platelet GPIbα availability that promoted metastasis in the absence of vWF. If this is the case, then inhibiting the interactions among collagen, vWF, and GPIbα might be valuable. Indeed, in this study, we have confirmed such strategy is useful with minimal effect on platelet number and function.

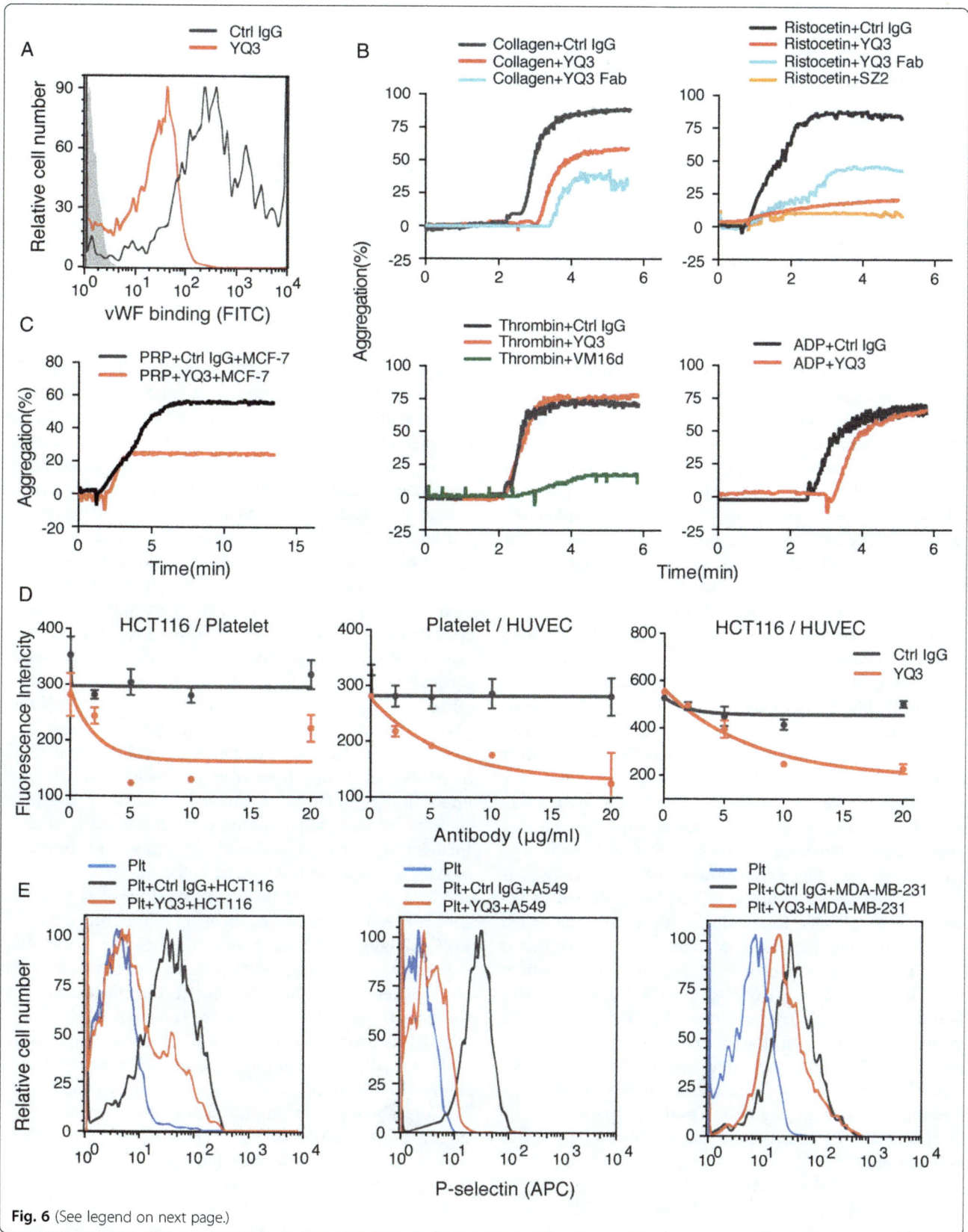

Fig. 6 (See legend on next page.)

(See figure on previous page.)
Fig. 6 YQ3 inhibits adhesion and cancer cell-induced platelet activation. **a** The vWF binding was inhibited by YQ3 detected by flow cytometry. Washed human platelets were incubated with 2 μg/ml recombinant human vWF in the presence of 1 mg/ml ristocetin. Binding of vWF was detected with FITC-conjugated human vWF IgG by flow cytometry and quantitated by mean fluorescence intensity. **b** YQ3 inhibited ristocetin- and collagen-induced platelet aggregation. Different agonist-induced aggregation of PRP that had been pretreated with 10 μg/ml mouse IgG (negative control), 10 μg/ml YQ3, or 10 μg/ml YQ3 Fab was detected for 6 min. **c** YQ3 inhibited MCF-7-induced platelet aggregation. Fifty microliters of MCF-7 cell suspension with 1×10^5 cells/ml was added to PRP. Platelet had previously been incubated with 10 μg/ml YQ3 for 5 min. Aggregation was detected for 13 min. **d** YQ3 inhibited platelet, HCT 116 cell, and endothelial cell adhesion between each other. Left panel, the quantitative analysis of adhesion of HCT116 with BCECF-labeled platelet in the presence of various concentration of YQ3. Middle panel, the effect of YQ3 on the adhesion of BCECF-labeled platelets to HUVECs. Right panel, the effect of YQ3 on platelet-mediated BCECF-labeled HCT116 cells adhesion to HUVECs in vitro. **e** YQ3 inhibited tumor cell-induced platelet activation. Fifty microliters of different tumor cell (HCT116, A549, or MDA-MB-231) suspension with 1×10^5 cells/ml was added to washed platelet. Platelet was pretreated with 10 μg/ml YQ3 or negative control (normal mouse IgG). Platelet activation was detected by APC-conjugated P-selectin Ab. The histograms are representative of three independent experiments

Compared with traditional anti-platelet drugs, which prevent thrombosis by inhibiting normal platelet function, the monoclonal antibodies developed in this study utilize a different mechanism of action. In our report, we developed two novel rat anti-mouse GPIbα monoclonal antibodies, 2B4 and 1D12, and a mouse anti-human GPIbα monoclonal antibody YQ3. These antibodies exhibited inhibitory potential on cancer metastasis by blocking the vWF-GPIbα axis without affecting platelet activation and hemostatic function. Therefore, we proved that it is possible to use antibodies to inhibit metastasis without inducing thrombocytopenia by blocking the vWF-GPIbα interaction.

Several anti-GPIbα monoclonal antibodies which inhibit vWF binding to platelet have already been developed, these include p0p/B [9, 28], SZ2 [23], AK2 [24], and VM16d [37]. Luise et al. [9] investigated the effect of Fab fragment of p0p/B, a mAb directed against the vWF-binding site on mouse GPIbα, on pulmonary metastasis. An unexpected increase in experimental metastasis after blockade of GPIbα was observed. The mechanism of p0p/B promotion on metastasis was thought that the blockade of GPIbα by p0p/B led to the decrease in platelet interaction with P-selectin, which then resulted in increased availability of P-selectin for the direct interaction of cancer cells with endothelium cells. In comparison, in our study, 1D12 and 2B4 were found to inhibit metastasis likely due to their capacity of inhibiting the vWF-GPIbα interaction. Therefore, despite using GPIbα as the same target, using antibodies binding to different sites of GPIbα, hence affecting its binding partners through the resultant spatial conformations, distinct influence on cancer metastasis could be observed.

Interestingly, the binding site of our YQ3 overlaps the previously reported monoclonal antibody SZ2, which binds to vWF-binding site aa 268-282 on mouse GPIbα [23]. Leslie et al. [38] reported previously that MCF-7-induced platelet aggregation was inhibited by 46% when tumor cells were pretreated with SZ2. However, SZ2 failed to affect the extent of platelet-LS174T cell hetero-aggregation [39]. Furthermore, the human GPIbα monoclonal antibody AK2 [24], which has an overlap-binding site aa 41-55 with YQ3, was not reported on its effect on metastasis. Based on the above reports, we tested the effect of SZ2 and AK2 on platelet-tumor cell binding. SZ2 did not affect the adhesion between patients' platelets and tumor cells (Additional file 4: Figure S2F). In addition, AK2 also had no effect on the adhesion of platelet to HCT116 cells (data not shown). As spatial conformation is critical for function, for example, normal thrombus formation was performed primarily through tethering of GPIbα to the A1 domain of immobilized vWF[14], different antibodies may exert different effects despite their binding to similar sites (secondary structure) on GPIbα. We therefore propose that YQ3, SZ2, and AK2 may have distinct spatial conformation upon binding to GPIbα. Meanwhile, our data did suggest such possibility: YQ3 not only inhibited vWF binding (platelet aggregation induced by ristocetin) but also platelet aggregation induced by collagen. Similarly, 1D12 and 2B4 also inhibited the aggregation induced by collagen. Therefore, likely a broader effect on collagen-vWF-GPIbα interaction played the role in promoting metastasis, which is different from the mechanism of the other platelet antibodies used in anti-thrombotic therapy. Certainly, more definitive evidence is warranted.

It is interesting that injection of YQ3 full-length antibody to hTg mice induced severe thrombocytopenia similar to the traditional anti-platelet drugs, but injection of Fab fragment alone did not. Such phenomenon might be explained by a recently proposed theory that anti-GPIbα antibodies harboring bivalent structure may exert a pulling force on platelet GPIbα by crosslinking platelets under shear flow [30]. The bivalent structure of YQ3 full-length antibody could therefore exert pulling force to induce platelet clearing, while the univalent structure of YQ3 Fab will

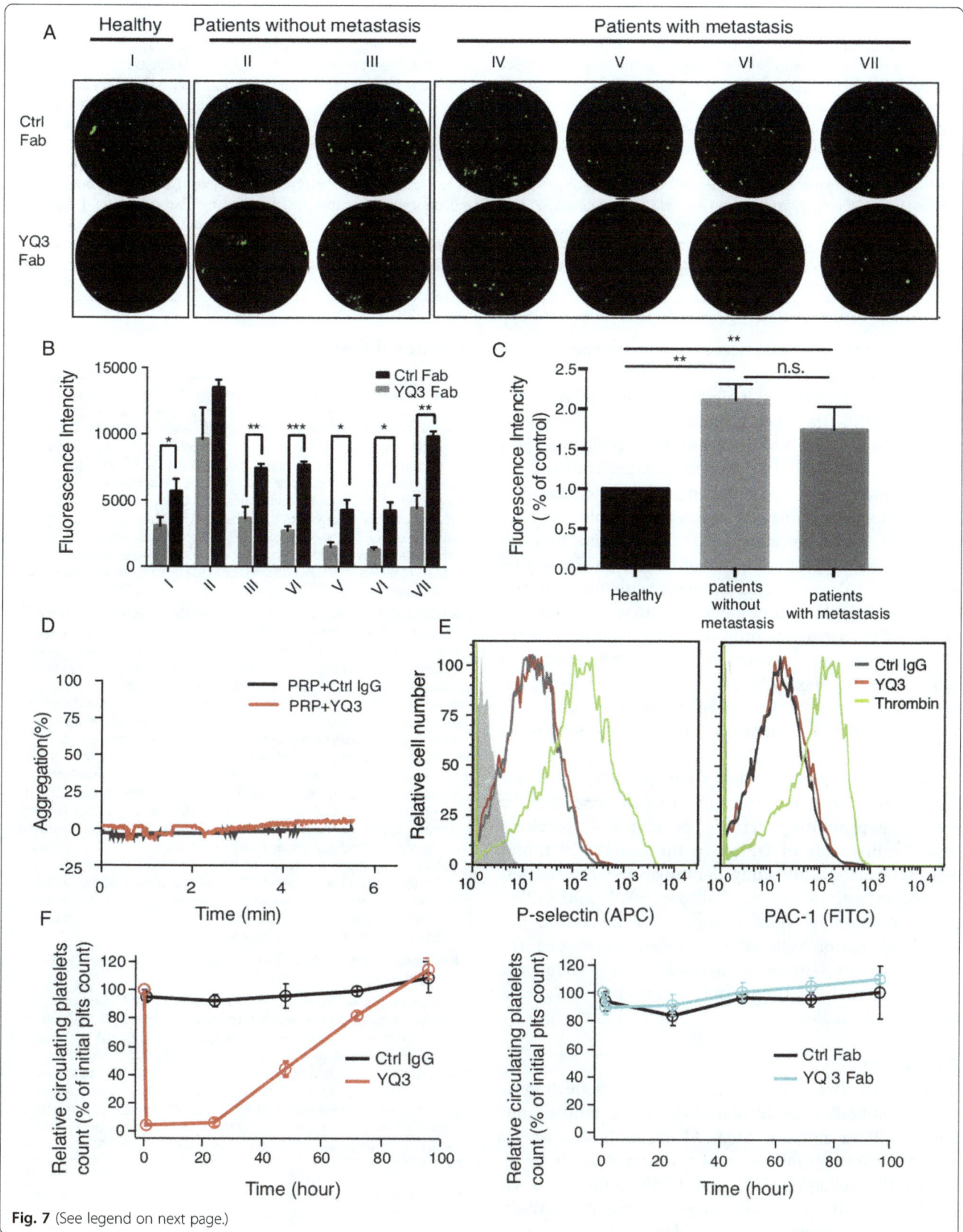

Fig. 7 (See legend on next page.)

(See figure on previous page.)
Fig. 7 YQ3 inhibits the adhesion between patients' platelets and tumor cells without accelerating platelet clearance. **a**, **b** YQ3 inhibited adhesion of A549 lung cancer cells to patients' platelets. **a** The adhesion of A549 to patients' platelets pretreated with 10 μg/ml YQ3 Fab as observed under fluorescence microscope. I: healthy person; II/III: patients without metastasis; IV/V/VI/VII: patients with metastasis. The quantitative analysis of adhesion was shown in **b**, P value is indicated; $*P < 0.05$; $**P < 0.01$; $***P < 0.001$. **c** Expression of GPIbα on platelets that were from healthy controls, patients without metastasis, or patients with metastasis. Fluorescence intensity was detected by flow cytometry. $**P < 0.01$, n.s., no signifance. **d** YQ3 did not induce platelet aggregation. The aggregation of PRP pretreated with 10 μg/ml YQ3 was detected. Negative control was in the form of normal mouse IgG. **e** YQ3 did not affect platelet activation. Increased expression of P-selectin and PAC-1 indicated the degree of platelet activation. Washed human platelets were treated with 10 μg/ml purified YQ3 (red) and negative control (mouse IgG, gray) or 0.05 U/ml thrombin (green) as positive control, then probed with APC-conjugated P-selectin Ab and FITC-conjugated APC-1 Ab. The fluorescence intensity was detected by flow cytometry. **f** Platelet survival curves for hTg mice injected with YQ3 (15 μg/mouse), YQ3 Fab (15 μg/mouse), or negative control (mouse IgG or Fab, 15 μg/mouse) ($n = 6$ mice in each group). Blood was drawn from mice at the time of antibody injection (0 h) and every 24 h following until 96 h after antibody injection. Platelet count determined by flow cytometry. Each figure or histogram is a representative of three independent experiments

not. The YQ3 Fab could serve as a prototype for further exploration.

Currently, metastasis inhibition potential of anti-human GPIIb-IIIa agents including oral antagonist XV454 [10], abciximab, tirofiban, and eptifibatide [40] have been investigated in murine models. However, as the key receptor in the most important and common final pathway of platelet aggregation, blockade of GPIIb-IIIa will likely influence the hemostasis and coagulation. Even though the humanized anti-GPIIIa49-66 scFv Ab A11 demonstrated significant inhibition in metastasis with prolonged bleeding time that could recover in 24 h, the precipitous drop of platelet count by about 70% is concerning [12]. In addition, cancer metastasis still cannot be maximally inhibited because metastasis can be carried out by the adherence between tumor cells and GPIbα. Novel compounds such as YQ3 need to be pursued.

Various ligands of GPIbα, such as vWF, thrombin [16], and P-selectin [15, 41], are all essential for metastasis-promoting activity of platelets, resulting in a complex role of GPIbα in the process of tumor cell metastasis. This study demonstrated that targeting the interaction among collagen, vWF, and GPIbα in cancer therapy could attenuate the metastatic potential of tumor cells. We therefore reinforced the importance of GPIbα in metastasis, as well as the great potential in suppressing metastasis via novel targeting strategies.

Conclusion

In summary, we obtained two novel rat anti-mouse GPIbα antibodies, 1D12 and 2B4, and a mouse anti-human GPIbα antibody YQ3. All of antibodies have a potential effect on inhibition of tumor metastasis by affecting the collagen, vWF, and GPIbα interaction via binding to GPIbα aa 41-50 and aa 277-290, respectively. We therefore demonstrated the role of GPIb in promoting tumor metastasis and found a new target for the inhibition of tumor metastasis.

Additional files

Additional file 1: Table S1. The screening of hybridoma cell clones. (A) Rat anti-mouse platelet clones and (B) mouse anti-human platelet clones. Binding of clones to GPIb-IX complex was detected in ELISA. GPIb-IX complex was captured by anti-GPIX antibody, which was immobilized in microtiter plates. Supernatant of hybridoma cells were added to the coated wells. The bound clone was detected with HRP-conjugated rabbit anti-rat IgG or rabbit anti-mouse IgG. Effect of clones on BCECF-labeled platelets adherence to tumor cells was recorded by fluorescence plate reader. BCECF-labeled platelets pretreated with supernatant of different hybridoma cells were added into tumor cells coated plates. The adherence between platelets and tumor cells was detected by fluorescence plate reader. (XLSX 36 kb)

Additional file 2: Figure S1. Screening of six rat anti-mouse GPIbα antibodies and five mouse anti-human GPIbα antibodies. (A) The quantitative analysis of adhesion of LLC cells with BCECF-labeled mouse platelets in the presence of various antibodies was measured of fluorescent intensity under fluorescence plate reader. (B) Effect of antibodies on platelet activation was detected by flow cytometry. Washed platelets were treated with hybridoma supernatant and negative control (RPMI-1640 fetal bovine culture medium with rat IgG) and then probed with APC-conjugated anti-P-selectin Ab. (C) Purified of 2B4 and 1D12 and its Fab fragments were run in 10% Bis-Tris SDS gel electrophoresis under reducing (r.) and nonreducing (n.r.) conditions. Molecular weight marker (M) was shown and labeled in kDa. (D) The quantitative analysis of adhesion of HCT116 cells with BCECF-labeled human platelets in the presence of various antibodies was measured of fluorescent intensity under fluorescence plate reader. (E) Purified of YQ3 and its Fab fragment were run in 10% Bis-Tris SDS gel electrophoresis under reducing (r.) and nonreducing (n.r.) conditions. Molecular weight marker (M) was shown and labeled in kDa on the left. P value is indicated; $*P < 0.05$; $**P < 0.01$; $***P < 0.001$. Each figure is a representative of three independent experiments. (TIFF 8219 kb)

Additional file 3: Table S2. Mouse (B) and human (A) GPIbα peptides fragment sequences. (XLSX 43 kb)

Additional file 4: Figure S2. Characterization of antibodies' binding sites. Mouse platelet GPIbα fragments bound to (A) 2B4 and (B) 1D12. Human platelet GPIbα fragments bound to (C) YQ3, (D) SZ2 and (E) YQ3 Fab. 20 μg/ml platelet GPIbα fragment was immobilized in microtiter plates. Ten micrograms per milliliter of antibody was added to the coated wells, respectively. (F) SZ2 did not affect adhesion of A549 lung cancer cells to patients' platelets. The adhesion of A549 to patients' platelets pretreated with 10 μg/ml SZ2 as observed under fluorescence microscope. IV/V/VI/VII: patients with metastasis. N.S.: No Significant Difference. (TIFF 8219 kb)

Abbreviations
GPIbα: Platelet glycoprotein Ibα; mAB: Monoclonal antibodies; TCIPA: Tumor cell-induced platelet aggregation; vWF: von Willebrand factor

Acknowledgements
We thank Dr. Zhenghua Wu and Prof. Dawei Li at Shanghai Jiao Tong University School of Pharmacy and Dr. Wei Deng at Emory University for their technical support.

Funding
This work was supported by the National Natural Science Foundation of China (No. 81502540) and Fundamental Research Fund for the Central Universities of China (No. 222201514333). This work was also partially supported by the University of Iowa Start-up Funds (J.Z.), as well as the Grant IRG-15-176-40 from the American Cancer Society, administered through The Holden Comprehensive Cancer Center at The University of Iowa (J.Z.).

Authors' contributions
YQ, KX, JWL, and XL designed the research. YQ, WC, XYL, XG, and XF performed the research and analyzed results. FW, SR, and JLL provided the critical reagents. YQ, KX, and XL wrote the paper. JZ, RL, and JWL edited the manuscript and provided critical comments. All authors read and approved the final manuscript.

Consent for publication
Not applicable

Competing interests
The authors declare that they have no competing interests.

Author details
[1]State Key Laboratory of Bioreactor Engineering & Shanghai Key Laboratory of New Drug Design, School of Pharmacy, East China University of Science and Technology, 130 Meilong Rd, Shanghai 200237, People's Republic of China. [2]Aflac Cancer and Blood Disorders Center, Children's Healthcare of Atlanta, Department of Pediatrics, Emory University School of Medicine, Atlanta, GA 30322, USA. [3]Central laboratory, General Surgery, Putuo Hospital, and Interventional Cancer Institute of Chinese Integrative Medicine, Shanghai University of Traditional Chinese Medicine, 164 Lanxi Rd, Shanghai 200062, People's Republic of China. [4]Department of Medical Oncology, Shanghai Pulmonary Hospital, Thoracic Cancer Institute, Tongji University School of Medicine, Shanghai, People's Republic of China. [5]Department of Biochemistry and Molecular Cell Biology, Shanghai Key Laboratory of Tumor Microenvironment and Inflammation, Shanghai Jiao Tong University School of Medicine, Shanghai 200025, People's Republic of China. [6]Division of Hematology, Oncology and Blood & Marrow Transplantation, Department of Internal Medicine, Holden Comprehensive Cancer Center, University of Iowa Carver College of Medicine, Iowa City, IA 52242, USA.

References
1. Wojtukiewicz MZ, Hempel D, Sierko E, Tucker SC, et al. Antiplatelet agents for cancer treatment: a real perspective or just an echo from the past? Cancer Metastasis Rev. 2017;36:1–25.
2. Bambace NM, Holmes CE. The platelet contribution to cancer progression. J Thromb Haemost. 2011;9:237.
3. Ikeda M, Furukawa H, Imamura H, Shimizu J, et al. Poor prognosis associated with thrombocytosis in patients with gastric cancer. Ann Surg Oncol. 2002; 9:287–91.
4. Monreal M, Fernandezllamazares J, Piñol M, Julian JF, et al. Platelet count and survival in patients with colorectal cancer--a preliminary study. Thromb Haemost. 1998;79:916.
5. Symbas NP, Townsend MF, Elgalley R, Keane TE, et al. Poor prognosis associated with thrombocytosis in patients with renal cell carcinoma. British Journal of Urology International. 2001;87:715–6.
6. Gücer F, Moser F, Tamussino K, Reich O, et al. Thrombocytosis as a prognostic factor in endometrial carcinoma. Gynecol Oncol. 1998;70:210–4.
7. Zhang W, Dang S, Hong T, Tang J, et al. A humanized single-chain antibody against beta 3 integrin inhibits pulmonary metastasis by preferentially fragmenting activated platelets in the tumor microenvironment. Blood. 2012;120:2889–98.
8. Poggi A, Vicenzi E, Cioce V, Wasteson A. Platelet contribution to cancer cell growth and migration: the role of platelet growth factors. Pathophysiol Haemost Thromb. 1988;18:18–28.
9. Erpenbeck L, Nieswandt B, Schön M, Pozgajova M, et al. Inhibition of platelet GPIbα and promotion of melanoma metastasis. J Investig Dermatol. 2010;130:576–86.
10. Amirkhosravi A, Mousa SA, Amaya M, Blaydes S, et al. Inhibition of tumor cell-induced platelet aggregation and lung metastasis by the oral GpIIb/IIIa antagonist XV454. Thromb Haemost. 2003;89:549–54.
11. Trikha M, Zhou Z, Timar J, Raso E, et al. Multiple roles for platelet GPIIb/IIIa and alphavbeta3 integrins in tumor growth, angiogenesis, and metastasis. Cancer Res. 2002;62:2824–33.
12. Nardi M, Feinmark SJ, Hu L, Li Z, et al. Complement-independent Ab-induced peroxide lysis of platelets requires 12-lipoxygenase and a platelet NADPH oxidase pathway. J Clin Invest. 2004;113:973–80.
13. Jain S, Harris J, Ware J. Platelets: linking hemostasis and cancer. Arterioscler Thromb Vasc Biol. 2010;30:2362–7.
14. Terraube V, Marx I, Denis CV. Role of von Willebrand factor in tumor metastasis. Thromb Res. 2007;120 Suppl 2:S64.
15. Chen M, Geng JG. P-selectin mediates adhesion of leukocytes, platelets, and cancer cells in inflammation, thrombosis, and cancer growth and metastasis. Arch Immunol Ther Exp. 2006;54:75–84.
16. Nierodzik ML, Plotkin A, Kajumo F, Karpatkin S. Thrombin stimulates tumor-platelet adhesion in vitro and metastasis in vivo. J Clin Investig. 1991;87:229–36.
17. Löf A, Müller JP, Breehm MA. A biophysical view on von Willebrand factor activation. J Cell Physiol. 2017;233:799–810.
18. Jain S, Zuka M, Liu J, Russell S, et al. Platelet glycoprotein Ib alpha supports experimental lung metastasis. Proc Natl Acad Sci U S A. 2007;104:9024.
19. Ware J, Russell S, Ruggeri ZM. Generation and rescue of a murine model of platelet dysfunction: the Bernard-Soulier syndrome. Proc Natl Acad Sci U S A. 2000;97:2803.
20. Köhler G, Milstein C, Köhler G, Milstein C. Continuous cultures of fused cells secreting antibody of predefined specificity. Biotechnology. 1975;24:524.
21. Liang X, Russell SR, Estelle S, Jones LH, et al. Specific inhibition of ectodomain shedding of glycoprotein Ibα by targeting its juxtamembrane shedding cleavage site. J Thromb Haemost. 2013;11:2155–62.
22. Chen W, Liang X, Syed AK, Jessup P, et al. Inhibiting GPIbalpha shedding preserves post-transfusion recovery and hemostatic function of platelets after prolonged storage. Arterioscler Thromb Vasc Biol. 2016;36:1821–8.
23. Cauwenberghs N, Vanhoorelbeke K, Vauterin S, Westra DF, et al. Epitope mapping of inhibitory antibodies against platelet glycoprotein Ibalpha reveals interaction between the leucine-rich repeat N-terminal and C-terminal flanking domains of glycoprotein Ibalpha. Blood. 2001;98:652.
24. Ward CM, Andrews RK, Smith AI, Berndt MC. Mocarhagin, a novel cobra venom metalloproteinase, cleaves the platelet von Willebrand factor receptor glycoprotein Ibalpha. Identification of the sulfated tyrosine/anionic sequence Tyr-276-Glu-282 of glycoprotein Ibalpha as a binding site for von Willebra. Biochemistry. 1996;35:4929–38.
25. Ruan CG, Du XP, Xi XD, Castaldi PA, et al. A murine antiglycoprotein Ib complex monoclonal antibody, SZ 2, inhibits platelet aggregation induced by both ristocetin and collagen. Blood. 1987;69:570–7.
26. Li C, Piran S, Chen P, Lang S, et al. The maternal immune response to fetal platelet GPIbα causes frequent miscarriage in mice that can be prevented by intravenous IgG and anti-FcRn therapies. The Journal of clinical investigation. 2011;121:4537–47.
27. Wu D, Vanhoorelbeke K, Cauwenberghs N, Meiring M, et al. Inhibition of the von Willebrand (VWF)-collagen interaction by an antihuman VWF monoclonal antibody results in abolition of in vivo arterial platelet thrombus formation in baboons. Blood. 2002;99:3623–8.
28. Bergmeier W, Rackebrandt K, Schröder W, Zirngibl H, et al. Structural and functional characterization of the mouse von Willebrand factor receptor GPIb-IX with novel monoclonal antibodies. Blood. 2000;95:886–93.
29. Vanhoorelbeke K, Ulrichts H, Schoolmeester A, Deckmyn H. Inhibition of platelet adhesion to collagen as a new target for antithrombotic drugs. Curr Drug Targets Cardiovasc Haematol Disord. 2003;3:125–40.

30. Quach ME, Dragovich MA, Chen W, Syed AK, et al. Fc-independent immune thrombocytopenia via mechanomolecular signaling in platelets. Blood. 2017;131:787–96. blood-2017-05-784975

31. Jain S, Russell S, Ware J. Platelet glycoproteinVI facilitates experimental lung metastasis in syngenic mouse models. J Thromb Haemost. 2009;7:1713–7.

32. Karpatkin S, Pearlstein E, Ambrogio C, Coller BS. Role of adhesive proteins in platelet tumor interaction in vitro and metastasis formation in vivo. J Clin Investig. 1988;81:1012–9.

33. Cauwenberghs N, Meiring M, Vauterin S, van Wyk V, et al. Antithrombotic effect of platelet glycoprotein Ib-blocking monoclonal antibody Fab fragments in nonhuman primates. Arterioscler Thromb Vasc Biol. 2000; 20:1347–53.

34. Zhao YM, Jiang M, Ji SD, He Y, et al. Anti-human VWF monoclonal antibody SZ-123 prevents arterial thrombus formation by inhibiting VWF-collagen and VWF-platelet interactions in Rhesus monkeys. Biochem Pharmacol. 2013;85:945–53.

35. Zhao Y, Dong N, Shen F, Xie L, et al. Two novel monoclonal antibodies to VWFA3 inhibit VWF-collagen and VWF-platelet interactions. J Thromb Haemost. 2007;5:1963–70.

36. Terraube V, Pendu R, Baruch D, Gebbink MF, et al. Increased metastatic potential of tumor cells in von Willebrand factor-deficient mice. J Thromb Haemost. 2006;4:519.

37. Mazurov AV, Vinogradov DV, Vlasik TN, Repin VS, et al. Characterization of an antiglycoprotein Ib monoclonal antibody that specifically inhibits platelet-thrombin interaction. Thromb Res. 1991;62:673–84.

38. Oleksowicz L, Mrowiec Z, Schwartz E, Khorshidi M, et al. Characterization of tumor-induced platelet aggregation: the role of immunorelated GPIb and ja: math expression by MCF-7 breast cancer cells. Thromb Res. 1995;79:261.

39. McCarty OJ, Jadhav S, Burdick MM, Bell WR, et al. Fluid shear regulates the kinetics and molecular mechanisms of activation-dependent platelet binding to colon carcinoma cells. Biophys J. 2002;83:836–48.

40. Leclerc JR. Platelet glycoprotein IIb/IIIa antagonists: lessons learned from clinical trials and future directions. Crit Care Med. 2002;30:332–40.

41. Palumbo JS, Kombrinck KW, Drew AF, Grimes TS, et al. Fibrinogen is an important determinant of the metastatic potential of circulating tumor cells. Blood. 2000;96:3302.

3

Function and clinical significance of circRNAs in solid tumors

Yiting Geng[1], Jingting Jiang[2*] and Changping Wu[1,2*]

Abstract

Circular RNA (circRNA) is a new type of endogenous non-coding RNAs (ncRNAs). circRNA regulates gene expression in many biological processes, and it also participates in the initiation and development of various diseases, including tumors, which are the focus of present research. With the development of high-throughput sequencing technique, an increasing number of circRNAs closely related to tumors have been discovered. According to numerous studies, there is a significant difference in the expressions of circRNAs among a variety of tumor tissues and para-carcinoma normal tissues. Some specifically expressed circRNAs may potentially serve as new biomarkers for tumor diagnosis and prognosis. This systemic review briefly introduces the characteristics, biogenesis, and functions of circRNAs, as well as discusses their relationship with cancer in detail. In addition, this article also describes several research strategies for circRNAs.

Keywords: circRNA, microRNA sponge, Solid tumors, Biomarker

Background

More than 70% human genomes are transcribed, and protein-coding genes only account for 1–2%. Most transcripts are non-coding RNAs (ncRNAs) [1]. Circular RNA (circRNA) is a type of new ncRNA different from linear RNA as it is a continuous covalently closed loop without the 5′-cap structure and the 3′-poly A tail. Most circRNAs are universal, stable, and conserved, and they are often specifically expressed in different tissues and developmental stages. In 1979, Hsu and Coca-Prados at Rockefeller University observed that circRNA exists in the cytoplasm of eukaryotic cells [2]. Within decades after the 1970s, circRNA has been considered as an outcome of a splicing error. With the development of RNA sequencing (RNA-seq) technology and bioinformatics in the twenty-first century, a large number of circRNAs have been discovered. There are four types of circRNAs, namely, exonic circRNA (ecircRNA), circRNAs from introns, exon-intron circRNA (EIciRNA), and intergenic circRNA [3]. More than 80% of the circRNAs are ecircRNAs, which are formed by the reverse covalent attachment of the 3′ splice donors and the 5′ splice acceptors

of the precursor mRNA (pre-mRNA). circRNAs from introns are a general term for a class of circRNAs, including circular intronic RNAs (ciRNAs), excised group I introns, excised group II introns, excised tRNA introns, and intron lariats. EIciRNA is a type of circRNAs that are circularized simultaneously by exons and introns, probably similar to ecircRNAs. Intergenic circRNA is another non-exonic circRNA found by circRNA Identifier (CIRI). This integrated circRNA is formed by two intronic circRNA fragments (ICFs) flanked by GT-AG splicing signals acting as the splice donor (SD) and splice acceptor (SA) of the circular junction.

Two basic models of circRNA biogenesis have been proposed as follows: (1) intron-pairing-driven circularization, also known as direct back-splicing (Fig. 1a), is the main form of ecircRNA production, in which the flanking intronic complementary sequences of the pre-mRNA form a lariat by direct base-pairing, forming an ecircRNA when introns are removed, and (2) lariat-driven circularization, also known as exon-skipping (Fig. 1b), in which the pre-mRNA is partially folded during transcription, allowing the 3′-SD of the downstream exon to connect to the 5′-SA of the upstream exon, resulting in exon-skipping and the formation of a RNA lariat containing both exons and introns. With the removal of introns, an ecircRNA is formed. Generally, introns between circular exons will be

* Correspondence: jiangjingting@suda.edu.cn; wcpjjt@163.com
[2]Department of Tumor Biological Treatment, The Third Affiliated Hospital of Soochow University, 185 Juqian Street, Changzhou 213003, Jiangsu, China
[1]Department of Oncology, The Third Affiliated Hospital of Soochow University, 185 Juqian Street, Changzhou 213003, Jiangsu, China

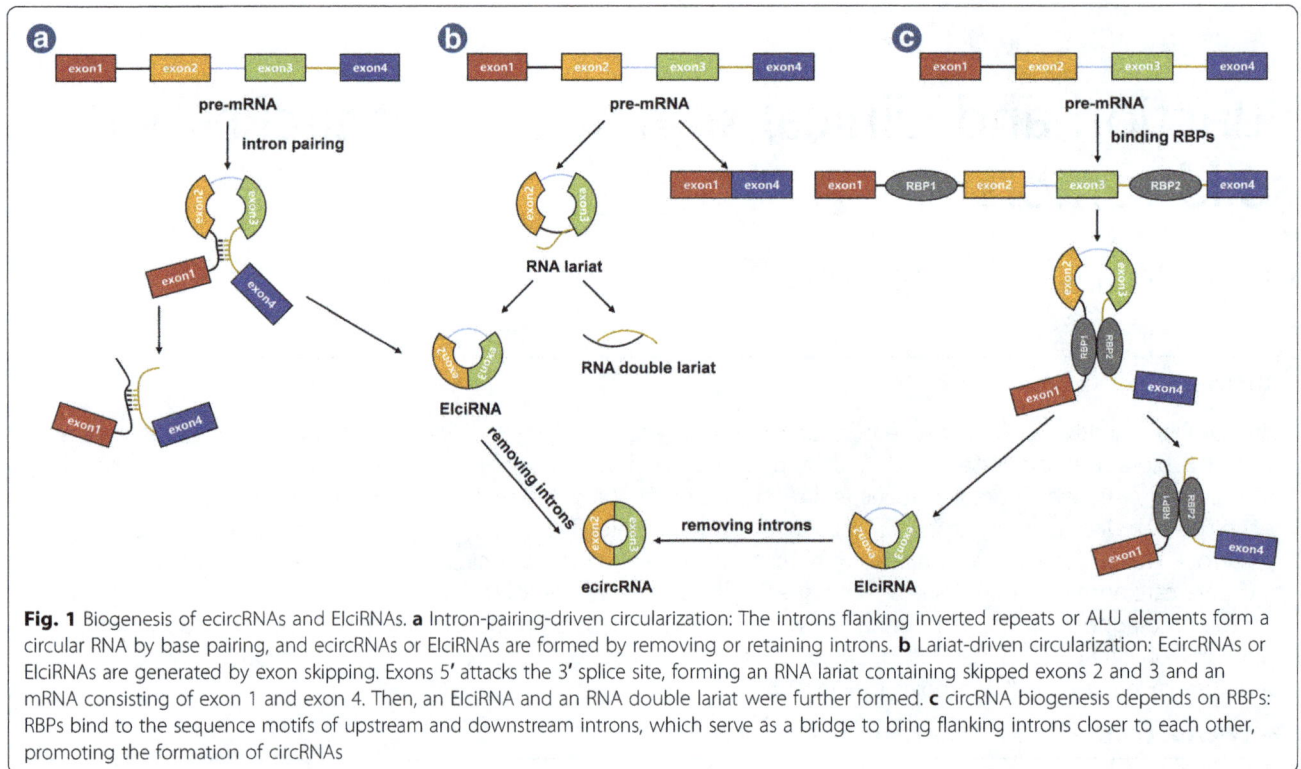

Fig. 1 Biogenesis of ecircRNAs and EIciRNAs. **a** Intron-pairing-driven circularization: The introns flanking inverted repeats or ALU elements form a circular RNA by base pairing, and ecircRNAs or EIciRNAs are formed by removing or retaining introns. **b** Lariat-driven circularization: EcircRNAs or EIciRNAs are generated by exon skipping. Exons 5' attacks the 3' splice site, forming an RNA lariat containing skipped exons 2 and 3 and an mRNA consisting of exon 1 and exon 4. Then, an EIciRNA and an RNA double lariat were further formed. **c** circRNA biogenesis depends on RBPs: RBPs bind to the sequence motifs of upstream and downstream introns, which serve as a bridge to bring flanking introns closer to each other, promoting the formation of circRNAs

excised. However, in some cases, these introns are retained as EIciRNAs. Some introns containing key nucleotide sequences are not decomposed by the debranching enzyme after splicing but instead independently cyclize into ciRNAs, which is called intron cyclization. In addition, there is another pattern of circRNA biogenesis that depends on RNA-binding proteins (RBPs) (Fig. 1c). The formation of circRNAs from introns and intergenic circRNAs is detailed in Fig. 2a-c and d, respectively.

circRNA has several features as follows: (1) abundance and diversity: more than 20,000 different circRNAs have been identified in eukaryotes; (2) stability: the half-life of circRNA is long because circRNA is a covalently closed circular structure without a 5′-cap and 3′-poly A tail, which is not easily degraded by exonuclease, resulting in far superior stability of circRNA than that of linear mRNA; (3) conservation: circRNA is highly conserved among different species, such as humans, mice, nematodes, zebrafish, drosophila, protists, and plants;(4) positioning: ecircRNA accounts for the majority of all circRNA types, which mainly exist in the cytoplasm, and intron-containing circRNAs including ciRNA and EIciRNA, which are mainly located in the nuclei of eukaryotes; and (5) specificity: circRNA is often specifically expressed in different tissues and different developmental stages.

circRNA has abundant biological functions and is involved in various physiological and pathological processes of tumor cells, including proliferation, apoptosis, invasion, and migration. One of the most frequently studied functions of circRNA is the microRNA (miRNA) sponge [4–6], namely, eliminating the miRNA's regulation of a target gene via binding to the miRNA as a competing endogenous RNA (ceRNA) through the base complementary pairing principle. Moreover, circRNAs can also regulate gene expression at the transcriptional and post-transcriptional levels through other mechanisms, and they play a role as RBP sponges and protein scaffolds [7], some of which even have the ability to translate proteins [8, 9]. In addition, circRNAs are involved in RNAP II elongation [10, 11], alternative splicing [12], translation regulation [13], protein localization [14], histone modification [15, 16], and RNA maturation [17]. Recent studies have shown that circRNAs exert their biological functions through various mechanisms (Table 1, Fig. 3).

More and more circRNAs have been reported to be dysregulated in many human malignancies, such as lung cancer, breast cancer, gastric cancer, colorectal cancer, and liver cancer; they may serve as new diagnostic biomarkers and targets for cancer therapy. In this paper, we performed a systematic review of literature to provide information about the expression patterns and roles of circRNAs in solid tumors.

Main text

One hundred eighteen articles that investigated the expressions of circRNAs in various solid tumors were

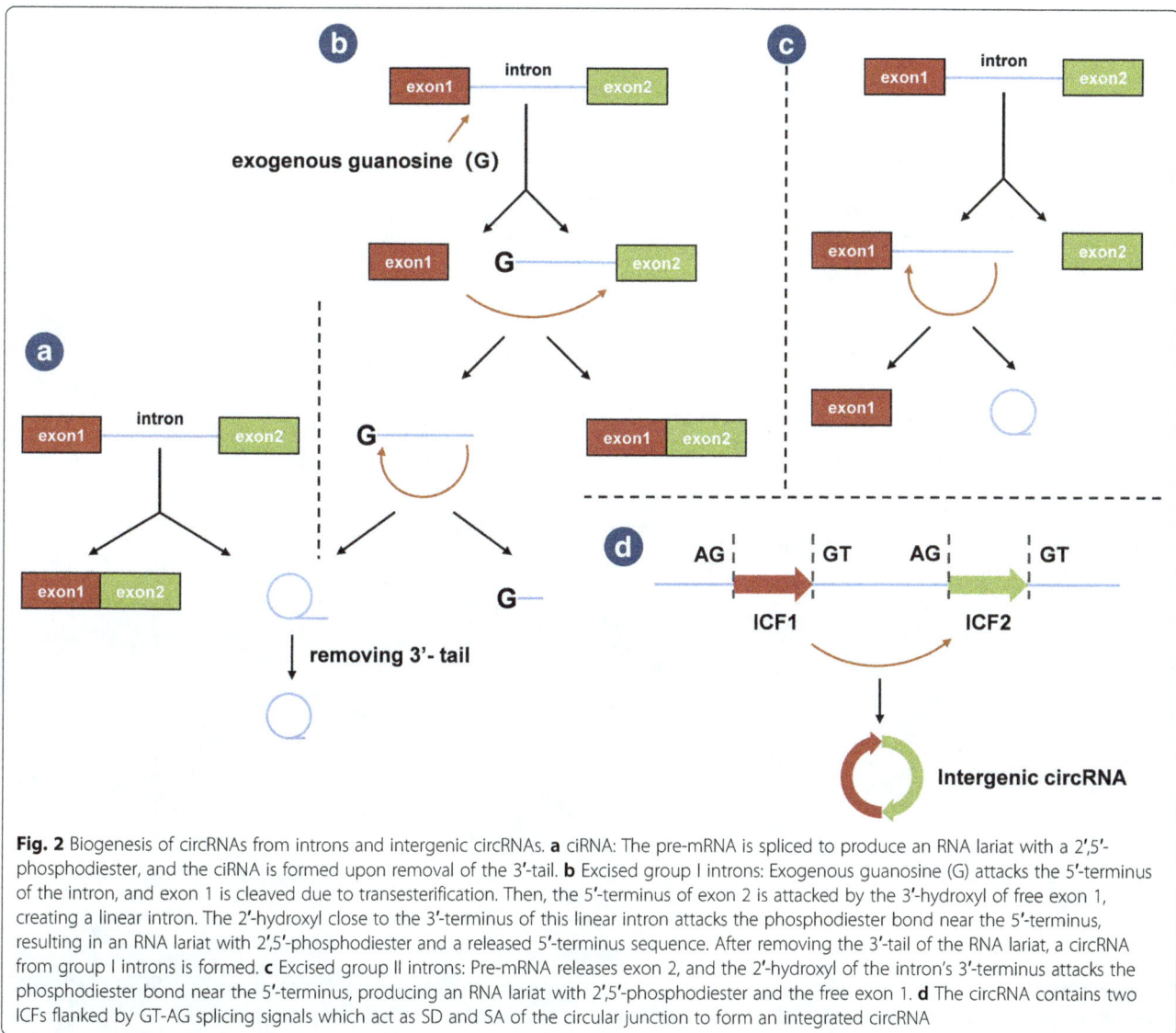

Fig. 2 Biogenesis of circRNAs from introns and intergenic circRNAs. **a** ciRNA: The pre-mRNA is spliced to produce an RNA lariat with a 2',5'-phosphodiester, and the ciRNA is formed upon removal of the 3'-tail. **b** Excised group I introns: Exogenous guanosine (G) attacks the 5'-terminus of the intron, and exon 1 is cleaved due to transesterification. Then, the 5'-terminus of exon 2 is attacked by the 3'-hydroxyl of free exon 1, creating a linear intron. The 2'-hydroxyl close to the 3'-terminus of this linear intron attacks the phosphodiester bond near the 5'-terminus, resulting in an RNA lariat with 2',5'-phosphodiester and a released 5'-terminus sequence. After removing the 3'-tail of the RNA lariat, a circRNA from group I introns is formed. **c** Excised group II introns: Pre-mRNA releases exon 2, and the 2'-hydroxyl of the intron's 3'-terminus attacks the phosphodiester bond near the 5'-terminus, producing an RNA lariat with 2',5'-phosphodiester and the free exon 1. **d** The circRNA contains two ICFs flanked by GT-AG splicing signals which act as SD and SA of the circular junction to form an integrated circRNA

Table 1 Functions of circRNAs

Function	Figure 1	Representative circRNA	Reference
miRNA sponge	a	circHIPK3	[4]
		ciRS-7	[5, 6]
RNAP II elongation	b	ci-ankrd52	[10]
		ElciEIF3j	[11]
Alternative splicing	c	circMbl	[12]
Translation regulation	d	circPABPN1	[13]
Protein scaffold	e	circ-Foxo3	[7]
Protein localization	f	circ-Foxo3	[14]
Translation template	g	circ-ZNF609	[8]
		circMbl	[9]
Histone modification	h	cANRIL	[15, 16]
RNA maturation	i	circANRIL	[17]

selected for the systemic review through searching PubMed, Embase, and Cochrane libraries (as of March 26, 2018), including nine cases of lung cancer, 14 cases of breast cancer, three cases of esophageal squamous cell carcinoma (ESCC), 20 cases of gastric cancer, 17 cases of colorectal carcinoma (CRC), 16 cases of hepatocellular carcinoma (HCC), 10 cases of gliomas, seven cases of bladder cancer, four cases of pancreatic cancer, five cases of osteosarcomas, and 14 cases of other tumors [two cases of ovarian cancer, one case of kidney cancer, one case of thyroid cancer, one case of basal cell carcinoma (BCC), one case of cutaneous squamous cell carcinoma (CSCC), two cases of oral squamous cell carcinoma (OSCC), one case of laryngeal squamous cell cancer (LSCC), one case of hypopharyngeal cancer, two cases of cholangiocarcinoma, one case of cervical cancer, and one case of prostate cancer].

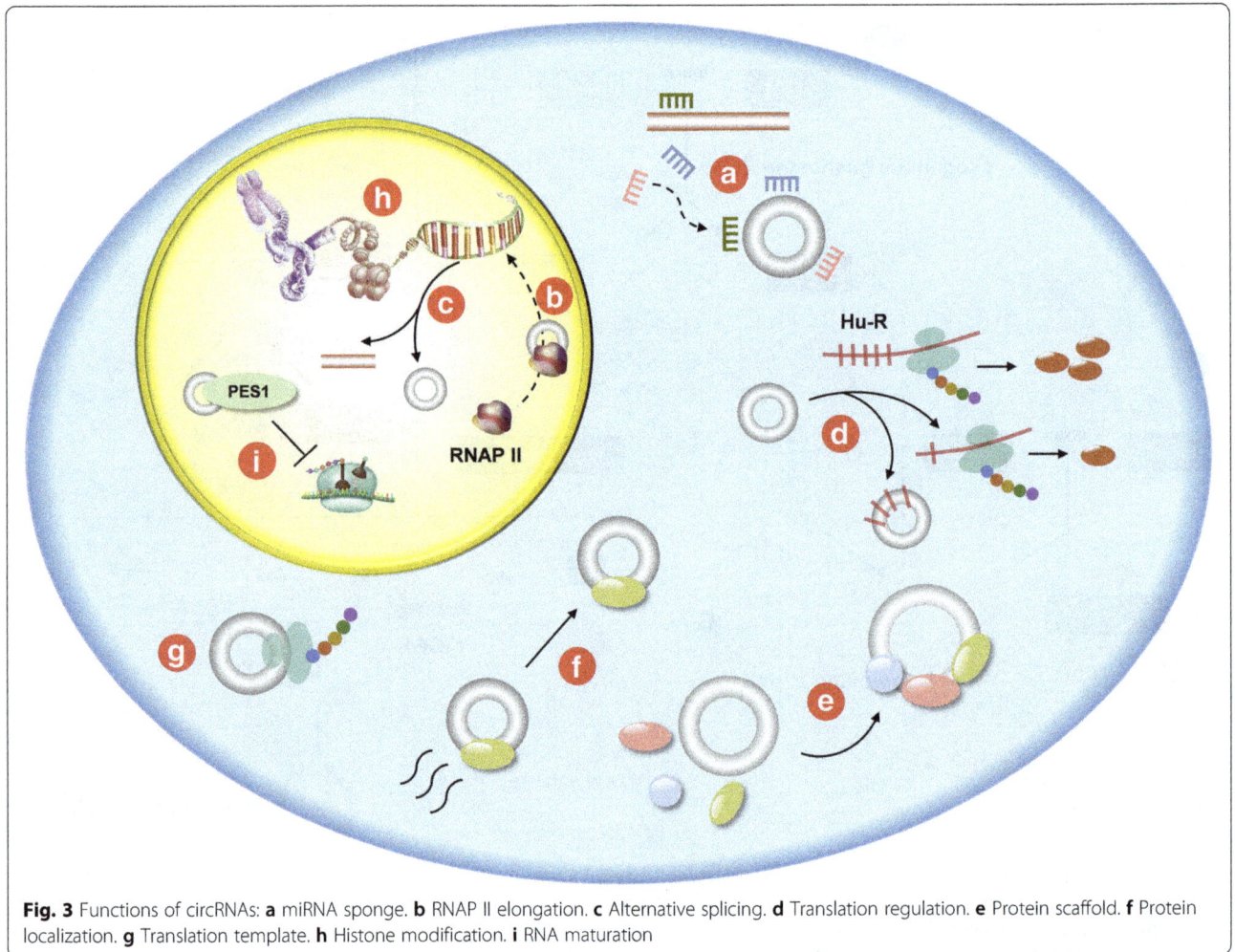

Fig. 3 Functions of circRNAs: **a** miRNA sponge. **b** RNAP II elongation. **c** Alternative splicing. **d** Translation regulation. **e** Protein scaffold. **f** Protein localization. **g** Translation template. **h** Histone modification. **i** RNA maturation

Lung cancer

Zhao et al. screened four pairs of high-throughput circRNA microarrays of lung cancer and para-carcinoma tissues and found that 357 circRNAs are dysregulated [18]. circ-ITCH, a sponge of many oncogenic miRNAs, plays an important inhibitory role in the progression of lung cancer. Wan et al. detected the circ-ITCH levels in cancer tissues and para-carcinoma tissues in 78 lung cancer cases, and they reported that circ-ITCH expression is significantly reduced in approximately 73% of lung cancer tissues. Overexpression of circ-ITCH inhibits the proliferation of lung cancer cells and is associated with the expressions of host genes [19]. Another non-small cell lung cancer (NSCLC) study showed that the expression of circRNA_100876 (circ-CER) is significantly upregulated in cancer tissues. Such high expression of circ-CER is significantly associated with local lymph node invasion and advanced tumor. Patients with high circ-CER expression have significantly worse overall survival (OS) than those with low circ-CER expression [20]. Functional experiments have shown that circ-CER may be involved in the

growth, progression, and metastasis of NSCLC cells [21]. Therefore, circ-CER may serve as a good diagnostic marker of NSCLC, and it is also a potential therapeutic target. In addition, hsa_circ_0013958 from the ACP6 gene is overexpressed in lung adenocarcinoma and correlated with tumor TNM staging [22]. Hsa_circ_0012673 is also upregulated in lung adenocarcinoma tissues and mainly located in the cytoplasm, regulating the proliferation of lung adenocarcinoma cells by adsorbing miR-22 [23]. Hsa_circ_0007385 is overexpressed in both NSCLC tissues and cells. Downregulation of hsa_circ_0007385 significantly inhibits the proliferation and invasion of NSCLC [24]. Hsa_circ_0014130 is highly expressed in NSCLC tissues and is closely related to lymph node metastasis and TNM staging, which can be used for prognostic evaluation [25]. In addition, the overexpression of hsa_circ_0000064 in lung cancer is positively correlated with T and N stage. Knockout of hsa_circ_0000064 significantly inhibits cell proliferation and promotes apoptosis [26]. The expression and function of circRNAs in lung cancer are shown in Table 2.

Table 2 circRNAs in lung cancer

circBase ID (alias)	Host gene	Putative function	Upregulated/downregulated	miRNA sponge	Target gene/pathway	Reference
hsa_circ_0013958	ACP6	miRNA sponge	Upregulated	miR-134	–	[22]
circ-ITCH	ITCH	miRNA sponge	Downregulated	miR-7, miR-214	Wnt/β-Catenin	[19]
circ-CER	CER	miRNA sponge	Upregulated	miR-136	MMP13	[20]
						[21]
hsa_circ_0007385	MEMO1	miRNA sponge	Upregulated	miR-181	–	[24]
hsa_circ_0012673	DHCR24	miRNA sponge	Upregulated	miR-22	ErbB3	[23]
hsa_circ_0014130	PIP5K1A	miRNA sponge*	Upregulated	–	–	[25]
hsa_circ_0000064	B4GALT2	miRNA sponge*	Upregulated	–	MMP-2, MMP-9	[26]

*Not validated experimentally

Breast cancer

Approximately 20% of breast cancers detected by mammography are ductal carcinomas in situ (DCIS) [27]. Some of these highly curative tumors will develop into invasive ductal carcinoma (IDC), which is life-threatening. However, the underlying determinants still remain unclear. A recent study has identified two circRNAs (hsa_circ_0122662 and hsa_circ_0001358) in five patients with DCIS/IDC and the MCF-7 invasive breast cancer cell line. Five miRNAs (miR-200b-3p, miR-200c-3p, miR-376a-3p, miR-376b-3p, and miR-429) have been confirmed to bind to hsa-circ-0001358 [28]. Further study of differentially expressed circRNAs in DCIS/IDC can aid the understanding of the molecular mechanisms underlying the progression from DCIS to IDC.

Nair et al. found 411 tumor-specific circRNAs from 885 breast cancer samples from TCGA in triple-negative (TN) breast cancer, including 256 estrogen receptor-positive (ER+), and 288 HER-2-positive (HER-2+) breast cancer cases [29]. Lu et al. found that 715 out of 1155 differentially expressed circRNAs are upregulated in breast cancer tissues compared to para-carcinoma tissues but that the other 440 circRNAs are downregulated. Validation studies have shown that hsa_circ_103110, hsa_circ_104821, and hsa_circ_104689 are upregulated in breast cancer tissues but that hsa_circ_100219, hsa_circ_006054, and hsa_circ_406697 are downregulated. The combination of hsa_circ_006054, hsa_circ_100219, and hsa_circ_406697 provides valuable insights into the diagnosis of breast cancer [30]. Some scholars believe higher diagnostic value of circRNAs in breast cancer than CEA and CA-153 [31].

circ-Foxo3 is a potential tumor suppressor that is significantly downregulated in breast cancer tissues [32] and may be involved in tumor progression [33]. Overexpression of circ-Foxo3 in the MDA-MB-231 breast cancer cell line significantly reduces cell proliferation in vitro. Subcutaneous injection of MDA-MB-231 cells transfected with circ-Foxo3 into nude mice inhibits tumor growth and promotes apoptosis [32]. A total of 25 binding sites of circ-Foxo3 for eight miRNAs (miR-22, miR-136, miR-138, miR-149, miR-433, miR-762, miR-3614-5p, and miR-3622b-5p) are detected [34], and transfection of these miRNAs into MDA-MB-231 cells can reduce apoptosis.

circ-VRK1 is also one of the downregulated circRNAs in breast cancer, especially in breast cancer stem cells (BCSCs). Upregulation of circ-VRK1 will inhibit the stemness of BCSCs [35]. In addition, circ_000911 is poorly expressed in breast cancer. In vitro experiments have confirmed that upregulation of circ_000911 increases Notch1 expression via binding to miR-449a, thereby suppressing the proliferation, invasion, and metastasis of breast cancer cells [36].

In contrast, hsa_circ_0001982, hsa_circ_0005239, and hsa_circ_0008717 are upregulated in breast cancer, and knockdown of their expressions inhibits cell proliferation and promotes apoptosis [37–39]. circ_0006528 is highly expressed in chemotherapy-resistant breast cancer cell lines, and the sensitivity of these cells to chemotherapy is significantly increased after knocking down circ_0006528 [40]. The expression of circ-DENND4C is increased in breast cancer cell lines under hypoxic conditions, and downregulation of circ-DENND4C inhibits the proliferation of breast cancer cells [41]. The expression and function of circRNAs in breast cancer are shown in Table 3.

ESCC

Several dysregulated circRNAs are found in ESCC, including hsa_circ_000167, hsa_circ_001059, hsa_circ_0067934, and circ-ITCH [42–44]. Similar to lung cancer, downregulation of circ-ITCH is also observed in 684 ESCC tissues and para-carcinoma tissues [42]. circRNAs may be associated with the radio-resistance of ESCC. In a circRNA microarray analysis of radiation-sensitive and radio-resistant cells, researchers have found that 57 significantly upregulated circRNAs and 17 downregulated circRNAs in radio-resistant ESCC cells, excluding circ-ITCH. KEGG analysis has shown that more than 400 differentially expressed target genes of circRNAs are enriched in the Wnt signaling pathway. Su et al. identified more than 3700 human circRNAs, among which hsa_circ_000167 and hsa_circ_001059 in the KYSE-150R

Table 3 circRNAs in breast cancer

circBase ID (alias)	Host gene	Putative function	Upregulated/ downregulated	miRNA sponge	Target gene/pathway	Reference
circ-Foxo3	FOXO3	Protein scaffolding	Downregulated	–	p53	[32]
circ-Foxo3	FOXO3	miRNA sponge	Downregulated	miR-22, miR-136, miR-138, miR-149, miR-433, miR-762, miR-3614-5p, miR-3622b-5p	–	[34]
hsa_circ_0008717	ABCB10	miRNA sponge	Upregulated	miR-1271	–	[37]
hsa_circ_0001358	SEC62	miRNA sponge*	Upregulated	–	ZEB1/2	[28]
hsa_circ_000911	IFNGR2	miRNA sponge	Downregulated	miR-449a	Notch1	[36]
hsa_circ_0001982	RNF111	miRNA sponge	Upregulated	miR-143	–	[38]
hsa_circ_0005239	GFRA1	miRNA sponge	Upregulated	miR-34a	GFRA1	[39]
hsa_circ_0006528	PRELID2	miRNA sponge	Upregulated	miR-7	Raf1	[40]
circ-DENND4C	DENND4C	–	Upregulated	–	HIF1α	[41]

*Not validated experimentally

human radiation-resistant esophageal cancer cell line are significantly different from the KYSE-150 parental cell line. These two circRNAs were confirmed by circRNA-miRNA co-expression analysis to be the most important factors in the potential circRNA/miRNA networks [44]. Xia et al. found that hsa_circ_0067934 encoded by PRKCI is upregulated in 51 cases of ESCC tissues compared to adjacent noncancerous tissues, and they reported that hsa_circ_0067934 is associated with poor tumor differentiation and advanced TNM stage. Silencing hsa_circ_0067934 by siRNA induces cell cycle arrest and inhibits proliferation and migration of ESCC cells [43]. Given that TNM staging is applied to predict patient outcomes, hsa_circ_0067934 may serve as a potential prognostic marker for ESCC. The expression and function of circRNAs in ESCC are shown in Table 4.

Gastric cancer

Several studies have examined the differential expression of circRNAs between gastric cancer and para-carcinoma tissues by circRNA microarrays [45–50]. Chen et al. found 180 circRNAs differentially expressed in gastric cancer and normal tissues using RNA-seq analysis. Among which, circ-PVT1 is upregulated, and the overexpression of circ-PVT1 suggests a better OS and disease-free survival (DFS). A luciferase reporter assay

has confirmed that circ-PVT1 indirectly regulates the expression of the E2F2 transcription factor as a sponge of miR-125 family, promotes the colony formation, and is involved in cell cycle regulation [45].

Hsa_circ_0047905, hsa_circ_0087198, and hsa_circ_0138960 are also highly expressed in gastric cancer tissues. Inhibition of these circRNAs significantly suppresses the proliferation of gastric cancer cells [50]. Sui et al. found that hsa_circRNA_000792 and hsa_circRNA_400071 are upregulated in gastric cancer but that hsa_circRNA_001066, hsa_circRNA_001959, and hsa_circRNA_400066 are downregulated [49].

Hsa_circ_0000096, also known as circ-HIAT1, is downregulated in gastric cancer cells and tissues. Knockdown of hsa_circ_0000096 reduces the expression of cyclin D1, CDK6, matrix metalloproteinase (MPP)-2, and MMP-9, and it significantly inhibits cell proliferation and migration and blocks cell cycle (preventing gastric cancer cells from leaving G0/G1 phase to enter S phase), as well as inhibits tumor growth in a xenograft nude mouse model. The circRNA database shows that hsa_circ_0000096 can interact with 17 different types of miRNAs. Downregulation of hsa_circ_0000096 results in a decrease in miR-224 (a modulator of CD40) and an increase in miR-200a (targeting E-cadherin) [51].

Table 4 circRNAs in ESCC

circBase ID (alias)	Host gene	Putative function	Upregulated/ downregulated	miRNA sponge	Target gene/ pathway	Reference
hsa_circ_0067934	PRKCI	–	Upregulated	–	–	[43]
hsa_circ_0000554	PRB4	miRNA sponge*	Downregulated	miR-30c-1, miR-30c-2, miR-122, miR-139-3p, miR-339-5p, miR-1912	–	[44]
hsa_circ_0000518	RPPH1	miRNA sponge*	Downregulated	miR-181a-2, miR-512-5p, miR-521, miR-556-5p, miR-663b, miR-1204	–	[44]
circ-ITCH	ITCH	miRNA sponge		miR-7, miR-17, miR-214	Wnt/β-catenin	[42]

*Not validated experimentally

Both circ-LPHN2 and circ-LARP4 are lowly expressed in gastric cancer tissues. The former acts as a sponge of miR-630 and inhibits the proliferation of gastric cancer cells [52]. The latter exerts biological functions by adsorbing miR-424, and it acts as an independent prognostic factor for gastric cancer [53]. Hsa_circ_002059 has also been confirmed to be downregulated in gastric cancer tissues. The low expression of hsa_circ_002059 is significantly associated with gender, age, distant metastasis, and TNM staging [54]. In particular, the postoperative level of plasma hsa_circ_002059 in gastric cancer patients is lower than that before surgery. Hsa_circ_0000190 is downregulated in gastric cancer tissues and plasma, and its low expression level is related to tumor size, lymph node and distant metastasis, and TNM staging. Hsa_circ_0000190 is considered to have better sensitivity and specificity compared to CEA and CA19-9 [55]. The low expression of hsa_circ_0001895 in gastric cancer tissues is significantly associated with histological types and grade [56]. Hsa_circ_0014717 is also lowly expressed in gastric cancer, and such downregulation is associated with distant metastasis and clinical staging. Additionally, hsa_circ_0014717 can be stably detected in gastric juice [48]. Hsa_circ_0000181, hsa_circ_0001649, hsa_circ_0000520, hsa_circ_0003159, and hsa_circ_0074362 are also lowly expressed in tissues or plasma of gastric cancer patients, and their expression is negatively correlated with distant metastasis and TNM staging. Therefore, these circRNAs may be used as diagnostic indexes to indicate if there is distant metastasis [57–61]. The plasma levels of hsa_circ_0001017 and hsa_circ_0061276 are also downregulated, making them suitable for the diagnosis and prognosis of gastric cancer [62]. Moreover, hsa_circ_0000745 is expressed at a higher level in gastric cancer tissues than normal tissues, and its expression in plasma of gastric cancer patients is also higher than that of healthy controls. Hsa_circ_0000745 expression in gastric cancer tissues and plasma is associated with tumor differentiation and lymph node metastasis, respectively, and plasma hsa_circ_0000745 combined with CEA has a greater diagnostic value for gastric cancer [63]. The expression of circRNA may be a predictor of early recurrence in patients with radical resection of stage III gastric cancer [64], but the major shortcoming of this previous study was that the follow-up time was too short. The expression and function of circRNAs in gastric cancer are shown in Table 5.

CRC

Bachmayr-Heyda et al. found that 11 circRNAs are upregulated and 28 circRNAs are downregulated in CRC tissues compared to para-carcinoma tissues by RNA-seq analysis [65]. In addition, the ratio of some circRNAs (circ3204/USP3, circ0817/CUL5, circ7374/TNS4, and circ6229/METTL3) to linear RNA is lower in CRC tissues than in normal tissues. Zhang et al. [66] also found that there are more circRNAs downregulated in CRC tissues and that the most significant downregulated circRNA is derived from the PTK2 tumor suppressor gene. This phenomenon can be attributed to the high stability of circRNA as it accumulates in non-proliferating cells and is dispersed in daughter cells of proliferating cells [65].

Similar to lung cancer, circ-ITCH is also significantly downregulated in CRC tissues. circ-ITCH is a sponge of some miRNAs which downregulate many target genes involved in G1/S transition, including miR-7, miR-20a, and miR-214. Overexpression of circ-ITCH reduces the proliferation of SW480 and HCT116 cells. Therefore, circ-ITCH may have anti-proliferative effects in CRC [67].

The downregulation of Hsa_circ_001988 in CRC is significantly related to differentiation and neural invasion of cancer cells. Because nerve invasion is a definite negative prognostic factor in CRC patients, hsa_circ_001988 may be a promising prognostic biomarker of patients with CRC [68]. In addition, hsa_circ_0001649, hsa_circ_0003906, and circRNA derived from ITCH78 are also downregulated in CRC, and the first two circRNAs are related to the pathological differentiation of CRC and may be used as diagnostic indicators of CRC [69, 70].

In contrast, the expression of ciRS-7 is upregulated in CRC, and it is the most significantly upregulated circRNA, deriving from METTL3, a m6A methyltransferase gene [65]. A large study by Weng et al., including 153 trial cohorts and 165 validation cohorts, has also confirmed the upregulation of ciRS-7 in CRC tissues. The high expression of ciRS-7 is positively correlated with tumor size, lymph node metastasis, TNM staging, and OS of patients [71]. Knockdown of ciRS-7 inhibits the activity of miR-7 target genes, such as EGFR and IGF-1R, thereby suppressing the proliferation and invasion of CRC.

As a positive regulator of CRC cell proliferation and invasion, hsa_circ_001569 exhibits higher expression in CRC tissues than noncancerous tissues [65, 72, 73]. Hsa_circ_001569, the sponge of miR-145, increases the number of cells in S and G2/M phase and accelerates the proliferation and invasion of CRC cells by preventing miR-145 from downregulating target genes, such as E2F5, FMNL2, and BAG4 [72]. Knockdown of hsa_circ_001569 in LOVO and SW620 cells reverses the invasive ability [72].

Hsa_circ_0000069 is also overexpressed in CRC tissues. siRNA-mediated knockdown of hsa_circ_0000069 inhibits the proliferation, migration, and invasion of HT-29 cells and induces G0/G1 phase arrest [74]. The expression of circRNAs derived from STIL60 and BANP79 genes in CRC tissues is also higher than that in normal tissues. Knockdown of circ-BANP reduces the proliferation and colony formation of the HCT116 and HT29 cell lines. Moreover, the expression of p-Akt is also decreased, suggesting that the PI3K-Akt pathway may be involved in circ-BANP-induced cell proliferation

Table 5 circRNAs in gastric cancer

circBase ID (alias)	Host gene	Putative function	Upregulated/downregulated	miRNA sponge	Target gene/pathway	Reference
hsa_circ_0001821	PVT1	miRNA sponge	Upregulated	miR-125a/b	–	[45]
hsa_circ_0000190	CNIH4	–	Downregulated	–	–	[55]
hsa_circ_0000096	HIAT1	–	Downregulated	–	CDK6, MMP9, MMP2	[51]
hsa_circ_002059	KIAA0907	–	Downregulated	–	–	[54]
hsa_circ_0014717	CCT3	–	Downregulated	–	–	[48]
hsa_circ_0001895	PRRC2B	–	Downregulated	–	–	[56]
hsa_circ_0003159	CACNA2D1	–	Downregulated	–		
hsa_circ_0000520	RPPH1	miRNA sponge*	Downregulated	–	–	[59]
hsa_circ_0001649	SHPRH	–	Downregulated	–	–	[57]
hsa_circ_0074362	ARHGAP26	–	Downregulated	–	–	[58]
hsa_circ_0061276	NRIP1	–	Downregulated	–	–	[62]
hsa_circ_0001017	XPO1	–	Downregulated	–	–	[62]
hsa_circ_0000181	TATDN3	–	Downregulated	–	–	[60]
hsa_circ_0000745	SPECC1	–	Downregulated	–	–	[63]
hsa_circ_101057	LARP4	miRNA sponge	Downregulated	miR-424	LATS1	[53]
circ-LPHN2	LPHN2	miRNA sponge	Downregulated	miR-630	–	[52]
hsa_circ_0014717	CCT3	–	Downregulated	–	–	[48]
hsa_circ_0047905	SERPINB5	–	Upregulated	–	–	[50]
hsa_circ_0138960	GDA	–	Upregulated	–	–	[50]
hsa_circ_0087198	GDA	–	Upregulated	–	–	[50]

*Not validated experimentally

[75]. Zeng et al. found that circ-HIPK3 is overexpressed in CRC cells and tissues, and they reported that the prognosis of CRC patients with high circ-HIPK3 expression is poor. Knockdown of circ-HIPK3 significantly inhibits the proliferation, invasion, and metastasis of CRC. Additionally, changes in cell function induced by circ-HIPK3 are reversed by miR-7 [76]. The high expression of hsa_circ_0007534 in CRC tissues is associated with lymph node metastasis and tumor staging. Interfering with the expression of hsa_circ_0007534 significantly inhibits the proliferation and promotes the apoptosis of CRC cells [77]. Hsa_circ_000984 is also significantly overexpressed in CRC tissues and cells, and knockdown of hsa_circ_000984 reduces the proliferation, invasion, and metastasis of CRC cells. Moreover, competitively binding to miR-106b as a ceRNA, hsa_circ_000984 effectively upregulates CDK6 expression, thereby affecting the function of CRC cells [78]. Hsa_circ_0020397 is highly expressed in CRC cells, which promotes CRC cell proliferation and invasion. In addition, hsa_circ_000984 upregulates the expression of oncogenic TERT and PD-L1 by binding to miR-106b [79].

Hsiao et al. found that circCDK13, circCCNB, and circCCDC66 are upregulated in CRC tissues. The expression of circ-CCDC66 has been detected in various tumor cell lines. circ-CCDC66 acts as a miRNA sponge to protect MYC mRNA from the miRNA-33b- and miR-93-mediated degradation, and it is involved in cell proliferation, migration, and invasion [80].

Comparison of three syngeneic CRC cell lines with different KRAS mutation status, including DLD-1, DKO-1, and DKs-8, has shown that extracellular circRNAs are more abundant than intracellular circRNAs, and most circRNAs are downregulated in the KRAS-mutated CRC cell lines [81]. circRNA is associated with KRAS mutations, and it is a promising biomarker of CRC, especially for KRAS-mutated CRC. The expression and function of circRNAs in CRC are shown in Table 6.

HCC

Studies have shown that circRNAs are involved in the development of HCC, although the mechanism remains unclear. Shang et al. found 61 circRNAs expressed differentially between HCC and adjacent tissues, including 26 upregulated and 35 downregulated circRNAs [82]. Fu et al. identified 527 circRNAs in HCC and reported that most of them are downregulated in HCC. The two most significantly downregulated circRNAs are hsa_circ_0004018 encoded by SMYD4 and hsa_circ_0003570 encoded by FAM53B, which are associated with the clinicopathological features of HCC [83, 84]. Hsa_circ_0001649 [85], which is derived from the SHPRH gene, and circZKSCAN1 [86], which is derived from the ZKSCAN1 gene, are also significantly downregulated in HCC tissues. Tumor number,

Table 6 circRNAs in CRC

circBase ID (alias)	Host gene	Putative function	Upregulated/downregulated	miRNA sponge	Target gene/pathway	Reference
hsa_circ_0000523	METTL3	–	Downregulated	–	–	[65]
hsa_circ_0001346	RNF13	–	Downregulated	–	–	[65]
hsa_circ_0001793	IKBKB	–	Upregulated	–	–	[65]
hsa_circ_0001946	CDR1	–	Upregulated	–	–	[65]
hsa_circ_0001946	CDR1	miRNA sponge	Upregulated	miR-7	EGFR, RAF1	[71]
hsa_circ_0000069	STIL	–	Upregulated	–	–	[74]
circ-CCDC66	CCDC66	miRNA sponge	Upregulated	miR-33b, miR-93	–	[80]
hsa_circ_001569	ABCC1	miRNA sponge	Upregulated	miR-145	E2F5, BAG4, FMNL2	[72]
circ-ITCH	ITCH	miRNA sponge	Downregulated	miR-7, miR-20a, miR-214	Wnt/β-catenin	[67]
hsa_circ_001988	FBXW7	–	Downregulated	–	–	[68]
circ-BANP	BANP	–	Upregulated	–	p-Akt	[75]
circ-HIPK3	HIPK3	miRNA sponge	Upregulated	miR-7	FAK, IGF1R, EGFR, YY1	[76]
hsa_circ_0001649	SHPRH	–	Downregulated	–	–	[69]
hsa_circ_0007534	DDX42	–	Upregulated	–	–	[77]
hsa_circ_0003906	–	–	Downregulated	–	–	[70]
hsa_circ_000984	CDK6	miRNA sponge	Upregulated	miR-106b	CDK6	[78]
hsa_circ_0020397	DOCK1	miRNA sponge	Upregulated	miR-138	TERT, PD-L1	[79]

cirrhosis, vascular invasion, microvascular infiltration (MVI), and tumor grade are the major factors associated with the circ-ZKSCAN1 expression level. Overexpression of circZKSCAN1 inhibits HCC progression both in vitro and in vivo. The circRNA encoded by the MTO1 gene is also downregulated in HCC tissues. As a sponge of miR-9, circ-MTO1 can inhibit HCC progression by upregulating the expression of p21. Decreased expression of circ-MTO1 is associated with poor outcome in HCC patients, and intratumoral administration of circ-MTO1 siRNA promotes HCC growth in vivo, indicating that circ-MTO1 is a potential prognostic marker and therapeutic target for HCC [87]. The low expression of circ-ITCH in HCC is also associated with a shorter OS [88]. Hsa_circ_0001649 was also lowly expressed in HCC tissues compared to normal tissues, and the expression level of hsa_circ_0001649 is related to tumor size and tumor thrombus. Knockdown of hsa_circ_0001649 increases the levels of MMP9, MMP10, and MMP13, suggesting that it may be a protective factor for HCC metastasis [85] and can be used as a potential diagnostic and prognostic marker. Moreover, hsa_circ_0001445 (cSMARCA5), hsa_circ_0005986, and hsa_circ_0067531 [89] are also downregulated in HCC. CSMARCA5 is regulated by DHX9, and it promotes the expression of TIMP3 and inhibits the proliferation and metastasis of HCC cells by adsorbing miR-17 and miR-181b [90]. HCC patients with cSMARCA5 low expression are usually accompanied by shorter OS and RFS. The expression level of hsa_circ_0005986 in HCC cell lines, including HepG2, Huh7, SMMC7721, HCCLM3, MHCC97H, and MHCC97L, is significantly lower than that in the L02

normal liver cell line. Both hsa_circ_0005986 and Notch1 mRNA can bind to miR-129-5p, and downregulation of hsa_circ_0005986 releases miR-129-5p to decrease the level of Notch1 mRNA, accelerating the cell proliferation by promoting G0/G1 to S phase transition [91].

By using a circRNA chip, Huang et al. identified 189 circRNAs significantly upregulated and 37 circRNAs downregulated in HCC compared to adjacent tissues. circRNA_100338 acts as an endogenous sponge of miR-141-3p in HCC to regulate the invasion function of hepatoma cells, and its high expression is closely related to a poorer OS and PFS of HCC patients [92]. ciRS-7 (hsa_circ_0001946) is significantly upregulated in HCC tissues [93] and is negatively correlated with miR-7 expression [94]. Overexpression of ciRS-7 is a risk factor for MVI in the liver. When ciRS-7 is knocked down, miR-7 is released and proliferation and invasion of HCC cells are also significantly inhibited [93, 94]. However, Xue et al. found that ciRS-7 is downregulated in HCC cells and tissues [95]. Zheng et al. reported that circRNA encoded by exon 2 of HIPK3 is upregulated in HCC tissues. circ-HIPK3 is a highly stable circRNA which can adsorb and inactivate a variety of miRNAs, including miR-124, the well-known tumor suppressor [4]. Therefore, targeting circ-HIPK3 may inhibit the growth of HCC cells in patients. Hsa_circ_0067934, which is highly expressed in HCC tissues and cells, can directly adsorb miR-1324, affect the expression level of FZD5, and regulate the Wnt/β-catenin signaling pathway. Knockdown of has_circ_0067934 significantly inhibits the proliferation, invasion, and metastasis of Hep3B and HuH7 cells and induces apoptosis [96]. Hsa_circ_0005075 is considered to be closely related to cell adhesion, which is an important part of tumor cell proliferation and metastasis. A recent study showed that the expression level of hsa_circ_0005075 is significantly different between HCC and normal liver tissues and is related to HCC tumor size. Larger tumor sizes correlated with higher expression of hsa_circ_0005075. Thus, hsa_circ_0005075 has the potential to become an ideal biomarker for HCC. Hsa_circ_0005075 has binding sites for four miRNAs, namely, miR-23a-5p, miR-23b-5p, miR-93-3p, and miR-581, in which miR-23b-5p is a key factor [82]. The specific molecular mechanism of hsa_circ_0005075 as the miR-23b-5p sponge to regulate the development of HCC remains to be further studied. The combination of circRNAs and traditional biomarkers of HCC will have greater diagnostic value. The expression and function of circRNAs in HCC are shown in Table 7.

Brain glioma

Song et al. selected 476 differentially expressed circRNAs from the RNA-seq data of 46 cases with brain glioma. The expression levels of circ_COL1A2, circ_PTN, circ_VCAN, circ_PLOD2, circ_SMO, circ_CLIP2, circ_GLIS3, and circ_EPHB4 in glioblastoma (GBM) are significantly higher than those in normal tissues. These circRNAs may act as miRNA sponges, which in turn increase the expressions

of certain genes involved in pathological processes. The circRNA derived from the VCAN gene is associated with the development of gliomas, and it is upregulated in oligodendrogliomas and GBM [97]. Barbagallo et al. [98] found that miR-671-5p is overexpressed in GBM cells and tissues, which is associated with downregulation of ciRS-7. Hsa_circ_0046701 is highly expressed in glioma tissues. Silencing hsa_circ_0046701 upregulates miR-142, resulting in a decrease of ITGB8 and inhibition of cell proliferation and invasion. The hsa_circ_0046701/miR-142/ITGB8 axis may contribute significantly to the development of gliomas [99]. circ-SHKBP1 is highly expressed in high-grade gliomas, and knockdown of circ-SHKBP1 significantly inhibits cell proliferation and metastasis. The regulation of cell function by circ-SHKBP1 is achieved by targeted uptake of miR-544a/miR-379 and upregulation of FOXP1/FOXP2 [100].

In addition, the expression levels of circZNF292 [101] and TTBK2 gene-derived circRNAs [102] in gliomas are downregulated and upregulated, respectively. Under hypoxic conditions, cZNF292 is a circRNA expressed in endothelial cells involved in glioma cell proliferation and tube formation. Silencing cZNF292 inactivates the Wnt/β-catenin signaling pathway in U87MG and U251 cells, thereby arresting cell cycle and inhibiting cell proliferation [101]. Hsa_circ_022705 (circ-FBXW7) is lowly expressed in glioma tissues and cells, and it is positively

Table 7 circRNAs in HCC

circBase ID (alias)	Host gene	Putative function	Upregulated/downregulated	miRNA sponge	Target gene/pathway	Reference
hsa_circ_0001649	SHPRH	–	Downregulated	–	–	[85]
hsa_circ_0001727	ZKSCAN1	miRNA sponge*	Downregulated	–	–	[86]
hsa_circ_0005075	EIF4G3	miRNA sponge*	Upregulated	–	–	[82]
hsa_circ_0000284	HIPK3	miRNA sponge*	Upregulated	miR-124, miR-152 miR-193a, miR-29a miR-29b, miR-338 miR-379, miR-584 miR-654	–	[4]
hsa_circ_0007874	MTO1	miRNA sponge	Downregulated	miR-9	p21	[87]
hsa_circ_0004018	SMYD4	miRNA sponge*	Downregulated	–	–	[83]
hsa_circ_0003570	FAM53B	–	Downregulated	–	–	[84]
hsa_circ_0001946	CDR1	miRNA sponge	Upregulated	miR-7	CCNE1, PIK3CD	[93]
hsa_circ_0001946	CDR1	miRNA sponge	Upregulated	miR-7	–	[94]
has_circ_0067934	–	miRNA sponge	Upregulated	miR-1324	FZD5/Wnt/β-catenin	[96]
hsa_circ_0067531	PIK3CB	–	Downregulated	–	–	[89]
hsa_circ_0001445	SMARCA5	miRNA sponge	Downregulated	miR-17, miR-181b	TIMP3	[90]
hsa_circ_0001946	CDR1	miRNA sponge	Downregulated	miR-7	EGFR	[95]
hsa_circRNA_100,338	–	miRNA sponge	Upregulated	miR-141	–	[92]
hsa_circ_0005986	PRDM2	miRNA sponge	Downregulated	miR-129	Notch1	[91]

*Not validated experimentally

correlated with the prognosis of patients with glioma. In addition, hsa_circ_022705 encodes the FBXW7-185aa protein. Upregulation of FBXW7-185aa significantly inhibits the proliferation of tumor cells, while silencing this protein promotes the malignant phenotype [103]. circ-SMARCA5 is significantly downregulated in gliomas and negatively correlated with the histological grade of gliomas. Overexpression of circ-SMARCA5 significantly decreases the metastatic capacity of U87MG cells. circ-SMARCA5 has abundant binding motifs with several RBPs, and it can directly bind to SRSF1 and regulate its expression [104]. circ-SHPRH is abundantly expressed in normal human brain, but it is significantly downregulated in GBM. It has the ability to encode the SHRH-146aa protein with the help of an open reading frame (ORF) driven by an internal ribosome entry site (IRES). Overexpression of SHRH-146aa in U251 and U373 GBM cells reduces the malignant phenotype [105].

The expression of circ-TTBK2 is increased in glioma tissues, which promotes cell proliferation, migration, and invasion but inhibits apoptosis [102]. In addition, circ-BRAF is significantly reduced in glioma patients with a higher pathological grade. The high expression of circ-BRAF is an independent predictive marker for PFS and OS in glioma patients [106]. In the future, more research is needed to reveal the regulatory mechanism of circRNAs in gliomas. The expression and function of circRNAs in gliomas are shown in Table 8.

Bladder cancer

Bladder cancer is a common urinary system malignancy, especially in males [107]. The circRNAs in bladder cancer show an overall upregulation, indicating that there are more upregulated circRNAs than downregulated circRNAs in bladder cancer tissues [108–110]. High-throughput microarray analysis has been used to identify six circRNAs that are differentially expressed in bladder cancer and normal tissues as follows: circPTK2 (hsa_circ_0005273), circTCF25 (hsa_circ_0041103), circBC048201 (hsa_circ_0061265), and circZFR (hsa_circ_0072088) are significantly upregulated and circTRIM24 (hsa_circ_0082582) and circFAM169A (hsa_circ_0007158) are downregulated [108]. The gene expression profiles of the linear transcripts corresponding to the overexpressed circRNAs are favorable for protein modification, binding, and intracellular metabolic processes, while those downregulated circRNAs are favorable for molecular function and catalytic activity [111]. Overexpression of circTCF25 increases CDK6 expression via adsorbing miR-103a-3p and miR-107, and it promotes cell proliferation and migration [108]. Both circRNA-MYLK and vascular endothelial growth factor (VEGF) A are significantly upregulated in bladder cancer. circRNA MYLK directly binds to miR-29a and reduces its ability to target VEGFA, a molecule that activates the VEGFA/VEGFR2 signaling pathway. Functionally, overexpression of circRNA MYLK promotes cell proliferation, migration, tube formation, and rearrangement of cytoskeleton [112].

Several circRNAs are downregulated in bladder cancer. For example, circ-ITCH is downregulated in bladder cancer tissues and cell lines, and patients with low circ-ITCH expression are significantly associated with a shorter OS. Overexpression of circ-ITCH inhibits the malignant biological behavior of bladder cancer cells, such as proliferation, migration, invasion, and metastasis, by upregulating p21 and PTEN through the uptake of miR-17 and miR-224 [113]. The expression of circ-BCRC4 in bladder cancer tissues is also lower than that in adjacent normal tissues. Overexpression of circ-BCRC4 inhibits the level of miR-101, thereby upregulating EZH2 expression, which promotes the apoptosis and inhibits the activity of T24T and UMUC3 cells [114]. circ-HIPK3 is expressed at a low level in bladder cancer cells and tissues, and it is negatively associated with differentiation, infiltration, and lymph node metastasis. Overexpression of circ-HIPK3 effectively inhibits

Table 8 circRNAs in glioma

circBase ID (alias)	Host gene	Putative function	Upregulated/downregulated	miRNA sponge	Target gene/pathway	Reference
circ-VCAN	VCAN	–	Upregulated	–	–	[97]
circ-ZNF292	ZNF292	–	Downregulated	–	Wnt/β-catenin	[101]
hsa_circ_0000594	TTBK2	miRNA sponge	Upregulated	miR-217	HNF1β/Derlin-1	[102]
hsa_circ_0001946	CDR1	miRNA sponge	Downregulated	miR-671	–	[98]
circ-BRAF	BRAF	–	Downregulated	–	–	[106]
hsa_circ_0046701	YES1	miRNA sponge	Upregulated	miR-142	ITGB8	[99]
circ-SHKBP1	SHKBP1	miRNA sponge	Upregulated	miR-544a, miR-379	FOXP1, FOXP2	[100]
circ-FBXW7	FBXW7	Translating protein	Downregulated	–	–	[103]
hsa_circ_0001445	SMARCA5	RNA-binding proteins	Downregulated	–	SRSF1	[104]
circ-SHPRH	SHPRH	Translating protein	Downregulated	–	–	[105]

growth, migration, invasion, and angiogenesis. circ-HIPK3 contains two key binding sites for miR-558, which significantly adsorbs miR-558, thereby inhibiting HPSE expression [110]. The expression and function of circRNAs in bladder cancer are shown in Table 9.

Pancreatic cancer

In pancreatic ductal adenocarcinoma (PDAC), 351 differentially expressed circRNAs (including 209 upregulated and 142 downregulated) between cancer tissues and normal tissues are identified by microarray analysis. Hsa_circ_0000977 is abnormally upregulated in pancreatic cancer tissues, and silencing hsa_circ_0000977 inhibits cell proliferation and induces cell cycle arrest. The interaction of hsa_circ_0000977, hsa-miR-874-3p, and PLK1A has been verified by dual luciferase reporter assay and fluorescence in situ hybridization (FISH) assay, and inhibition of hsa_circ_0000977 can reduce the expression of PLK1. In animal experiments, silencing hsa_circ_0000977 inhibits tumor growth [115]. circ-LDLRAD3 is overexpressed in cells, tissues, and plasma samples of pancreatic cancer patients. High expression of circ-LDLRAD3 is significantly correlated with venous or lymphatic infiltration and metastasis, and it may be used as a diagnostic biomarker for pancreatic cancer [116]. Hsa_circ_0000284 (circRNA_100782) is significantly upregulated in PDAC tissues, which is a sponge of miR-124. Knockdown of circRNA_100782 inhibits the proliferation and colony formation of BxPC3 cells by downregulating the target genes of miR-124, namely, IL6R and STAT3 [117]. In addition, hsa_circ_0005785 has binding sites for miR-181a and miR-181b [118]. Since miR-181a and miR-181b are associated with the growth/migration and gemcitabine resistance of pancreatic cancer cells, respectively, hsa_circ_0005785 may be involved in PDAC progression and gemcitabine resistance. The expression and function of circRNAs in pancreatic cancer are shown in Table 10.

Osteosarcoma

The circRNA encoded by oncogenic KCNH1 is upregulated in osteosarcoma tissues and cells, and it promotes cell proliferation, invasion, and metastasis [119]. The circRNA encoded by UBAP2 is the most prominently upregulated circRNA in osteosarcoma tissues, and patients with high circUBAP2 expression are often associated with a poor OS. In vitro and in vivo experiments have shown that circ-UBAP2 promotes osteosarcoma cell growth and inhibits apoptosis [120]. Hsa_circ_0001564 is significantly overexpressed in osteosarcoma tissues and cells. Knockdown of hsa_circ_001564 significantly inhibits osteosarcoma cell proliferation by inducing G0/G1 cell cycle arrest and promotes apoptosis of HOS and MG-63 cells. Hsa_circ_0001564 mediates tumorigenesis as a sponge of miR-29c-3p, and miR-29c can reverse the oncogenic effects of hsa_circ_001564 [121]. Hsa_circ_0009910 is also overexpressed in osteosarcoma cells. Knockdown of circ_0009910 inhibits the proliferation of osteosarcoma cells, leading to cell cycle arrest and apoptosis. However, inhibition of miR-449a eliminates this effect. As the sponge of miR-449a, circ_0009910 upregulates the functional target gene IL6R and promotes the development of osteosarcoma [122]. In osteosarcoma cells and tissues, hsa_circRNA_103801 is upregulated, while hsa_circRNA_104980 is downregulated. The potential target miRNAs for hsa_circRNA_103801 include hsa-miR-338-3p, hsa-miR-370-3p, and hsa-miR-877-3p, which are involved in the HIF-1, Rap1, PI3K-Akt, VEGF, and angiogenesis pathways. The potential target miRNAs for hsa_circRNA_104980 are hsa-miR-660-3p and hsa-miR-1298-3p, which participate in the tight junction pathway [123]. The expression and function of circRNAs in osteosarcoma are shown in Table 11.

Other tumors

The expression and function of circRNAs in other tumors are shown in Table 12.

Ovarian cancer

Ahmed et al. identified a total of 67,580 candidate circRNAs from primary and metastatic lesions of three patients with stage IIIC ovarian cancer, and they confirmed that the differential expression of circRNAs between primary and metastatic ovarian cancer is more pronounced than corresponding mRNAs [124]. Bachmayr-Heyda et al. found that the levels of circRNAs in immortalized normal ovarian epithelial cells are generally lower than those of ovarian cancer cells [65] because immortalized normal ovarian epidermal cells proliferate faster than ovarian cancer cells, resulting in reduced accumulation of circRNAs.

Table 9 circRNAs in bladder cancer

circBase ID (alias)	Host gene	Putative function	Upregulated/downregulated	miRNA sponge	Target gene/pathway	Reference
hsa_circ_0041103	TCF25	miRNA sponge	Upregulated	miR-103a, miR-107	CDK6	[108]
hsa_circ_0002768	MYLK	miRNA sponge	Upregulated	miR-29a	VEGFA/VEGFR2	[112]
circ-ITCH	ITCH	miRNA sponge	Downregulated	miR-17, miR-224	p21, PTEN	[113]
circ-BCRC4	BCRC4	miRNA sponge	Downregulated	miR-101	EZH2	[114]
circ-HIPK3	HIPK3	miRNA sponge	Downregulated	miR-558	HPSE	[110]

Table 10 circRNAs in pancreatic cancer

circBase ID (alias)	Host gene	Putative function	Upregulated/ downregulated	miRNA sponge	Target gene/ pathway	Reference
hsa_circ_0005397	RHOT1	miRNA sponge*	Upregulated	miR-26b, miR-125a, miR-181a, miR-330, miR-382	–	[118]
hsa_circ_0005785	ANAPC7	miRNA sponge*	Downregulated	miR-181a/b/d, miR-338, miR-526b	–	[118]
hsa_circ_0000977	NOL10	miRNA sponge*	Upregulated	miR-874	PLK1	[115]
circ-LDLRAD3	LDLRAD3	–	Upregulated	–	–	[116]
hsa_circ_0000284	HIPK3	miRNA sponge	Upregulated	miR-124	IL6/STAT	[117]

*Not validated experimentally

In addition, the levels of circRNAs in miliary tumors are lower than those of non-miliary tumors; however, it cannot be explained by the difference in proliferation rates.

Kidney cancer

In clear cell renal cell carcinoma (ccRCC) tissues, the circRNA (circ-HIAT1) derived from hippocampus-rich gene transcription protein 1 (HIAT1) is downregulated. Compared with metastatic ccRCC, circ-HIAT1 is expressed at a higher level in non-metastatic ccRCC. In addition, the OS rate of ccRCC patients with high expression of circ-RIAT1 is superior to that of patients with low circ-RIAT1. circ-HIAT1 can directly bind to miR-29a-3p, miR-29c-3p, and miR-195-5p and upregulate the expression of CDC42. Different from the classical function of miRNA sponges, circ-HIAT1 acts as a "miRNA reservoir," which increases miRNA stability, thereby reversing androgen receptor (AR)-mediated ccRCC migration and invasion. Inhibition of the miR-29a-3p/ 29c-3p/195-5p signaling pathway by circ-HIAT1 inhibits the migration and invasion of ccRCC cells [125]. The AR/ circHIAT1/CDC42 signaling pathway may become a new therapeutic target for metastatic ccRCC.

Thyroid cancer

Compared with normal thyroid tissues, researchers have found 88 significantly upregulated circRNAs and 10 downregulated circRNAs in papillary thyroid cancer (PTC) tissues. Based on the miRNA response elements (MREs) of these dysregulated circRNAs, a network of circRNA-miRNA interactions has been constructed by Cytoscape. The downregulated circRNA, hsa_circRNA_ 100395, has potential for interaction with two cancer-associated miRNAs, namely miR-141-3p and miR-200a-3p, suggesting that hsa_circRNA_100395- miR-141-3p/miR-200a-3p may be involved in the pathogenesis of PTC [126]. However, this hypothesis needs further verification.

BCC

Sand et al. identified 23 upregulated circRNAs and 48 downregulated circRNAs in BCC tissues [127]. Hsa_ circ_0022383 and hsa_circ_0022392 are the most significantly downregulated circRNAs and derived from FADS2 gene. Similarly, the two most significantly upregulated circRNAs are also encoded by the same host gene, namely, LINC00340.

CSCC

Sand et al. [128] identified 143 upregulated circRNAs and 179 downregulated circRNAs in CSCC. The two most significantly downregulated circRNAs (also most significantly downregulated in BCC) are from FADS2 gene, and the two most significantly upregulated circRNAs are encoded by LARP1B gene.

OSCC

Numerous circRNAs are differentially expressed in OSCC tissues and adjacent tissues. At present, 280 circRNAs have been identified with more than a twofold difference in OSCC, including 139 upregulated and 141 downregulated circRNAs. Among these circRNAs, hsa_ circ_0013339 (circRNA_100290) is derived from the SLC30A7 gene, and it is upregulated by approximately

Table 11 circRNAs in osteosarcoma

circBase ID (alias)	Host gene	Putative function	Upregulated/downregulated	miRNA sponge	Target gene/pathway	Reference
hsa_circ_0016347	KCNH1	miRNA sponge	Upregulated	–	–	[119]
circ-UBAP2	UBAP2	miRNA sponge	Upregulated	miR-143	–	[120]
hsa_circ_0001564	CANX	miRNA sponge	Upregulated	miR-29c	–	[121]
hsa_circ_0009910	MFN2	miRNA sponge	Upregulated	miR-449a	JAK1/STAT3	[122]
hsa_circRNA_103801	–	miRNA sponge*	Upregulated	miR-370	–	[123]
hsa_circRNA_104980	–	miRNA sponge*	Downregulated	–	–	[123]

*Not validated experimentally

Table 12 circRNAs in other tumors

circBase ID (alias)	Host gene	Putative function	Type of cancer	Upregulated/ downregulated	miRNA sponge	Target gene/ pathway	Reference
hsa_circ_0075828	LINC00340	miRNA sponge	BCC	Upregulated	–	–	[127]
hsa_circ_0075825	LINC00340	miRNA sponge	BCC	Upregulated	–	–	[127]
hsa_circ_0022383	FADS2	miRNA sponge	BCC	Downregulated	–	–	[127]
			CSCC	Downregulated	–	–	[128]
hsa_circ_0022392	FADS2	miRNA sponge	BCC	Downregulated	–	–	[127]
			CSCC	Downregulated	–	–	[128]
hsa_circ_0070933	LARP1B	miRNA sponge	CSCC	Upregulated	–	–	[128]
hsa_circ_0070934	LARP1B	miRNA sponge	CSCC	Upregulated	–	–	[128]
circ-DOCK1	DOCK1	miRNA sponge	OSCC	Upregulated	miR-196a	BIRC3	[130]
hsa_circ_0013339	SLC30A7	miRNA sponge	OSCC	Upregulated	miR-29b	CDK6	[129]
hsa_circ_0001649	SHPRH	miRNA sponge	Cholangiocarcinoma	Downregulated	–	MMP9	[134]
Cdr1as	CDR1	–	Cholangiocarcinoma	Upregulated	–	–	[133]
hsa_circ_0000284	HIPK3	miRNA sponge	Cervical cancer	Upregulated	miR-506	Snail-2	[135]
circ-SMARCA5	SMARCA5	–	Prostate cancer	Upregulated	–	–	[136]

sevenfold in OSCC compared to normal tissues. circRNA_100290 is a sponge of the miR-29 family. Functional analysis has revealed that knockdown of circRNA_100290 reduces CDK6 expression, induces G1/S arrest, and significantly inhibits the proliferation of SCC9 cell lines. In a nude mouse model, interference with circRNA_100290 also reduces tumor growth [129]. Moreover, circ-DOCK1 regulates BIRC3 expression through competitively binding to miR-196a as a ceRNA, and it is involved in the apoptosis of OSCC cells [130].

LSCC
In 698 dysregulated circRNAs in LSCC (302 upregulated cases and 396 downregulated cases), hsa_circ_100855 and hsa_circ_104912 are the two most significantly up- and downregulated circRNAs, respectively. High expression of hsa_circ_100855 and low expression of hsa_circ_104912 are associated with T3–4 stage, cervical lymph node metastasis, and later clinical stage of LSCC [131]. Researchers believe that the above circRNAs are involved in the initiation and development of LSCC and that they may be helpful for the diagnosis and prognosis in clinical practice.

Hypopharyngeal squamous cell carcinoma (HSCC)
Cao et al. showed that 2392 circRNAs are differentially expressed between HSCC and normal tissues [132]. Of these circRNAs, 1304 are upregulated, including hsa_circ_0024108, hsa_circ_0058106, and hsa_circ_0058107, while 1088 are downregulated, including hsa_circ_0001189, hsa_circ_0002260, and hsa_circ_0036722. However, the functions of these circRNAs in HSCC remain unexplored.

Cholangiocarcinoma
The expression of ciRS-7 (Cdr1as) in cholangiocarcinoma tissues is higher than that in adjacent normal tissues. Overexpression of ciRS-7 is closely related to later TNM staging, lymph node infiltration, and postoperative recurrence. The OS of cholangiocarcinoma patients with high ciRS-7 expression is inferior to that of patients with low ciRS-7 expression. Based on multivariate analysis, ciRS-7 is an independent prognostic biomarker with excellent sensitivity and specificity for cholangiocarcinoma [133]. Hsa_circ_0001649 is abnormally down-expressed in cholangiocarcinoma cells and tissues, and it is related to tumor size and differentiation grade of cholangiocarcinoma. Overexpression of hsa_circ_0001649 inhibits cell proliferation, migration, and invasion but induces apoptosis of KMBC and Huh-28 cells. Silencing hsa_circ_0001649 leads to the opposite effect. Therefore, hsa_circ_0001649 may be a potential diagnostic and therapeutic target for cholangiocarcinoma [134].

Cervical cancer
circRNA-000284 is significantly upregulated in cervical cancer cells. It promotes the proliferation and invasion of cervical cancer cells and that knockdown of circRNA-000284 causes G0/G1 cell cycle arrest, resulting in inhibition of cell proliferation and invasion. miR-506 is a miRNA related to circRNA-000284, and circRNA-000284 positively regulates the expression of Snail-2 which is a target gene of miR-506. However, co-expression of a miR-506 mimic or Snail-2 silencing vector eliminates the oncogenic effect of circRNA-000284. Thus, circRNA-000284 is expected to be a new therapeutic target for cervical cancer [135].

Prostate cancer

The role of circRNAs in prostate cancer is rarely explored. circ-SMARCA5 is significantly upregulated in prostate cancer tissues, and it promotes cell cycle process and inhibits apoptosis [136], acting as an oncogene.

Discussion

Recently, the clinical significance of circRNAs in a variety of tumors has been explored. circRNAs are generally superior to the corresponding linear RNAs in terms of stability. In addition, they represent the characteristics at different stages of tumor development [83, 84, 86, 91]. In addition, circRNAs can compensate for the defect of low organ specificity of traditional biomarkers. circ-CER may serve as a diagnostic marker for NSCLC, and its overexpression is significantly associated with local lymph node invasion, advanced tumor, and poor survival [20]. The combination of hsa_circ_006054, hsa_circ_100219, and hsa_circ_406697 is helpful for the diagnosis of breast cancer [30]. Hsa_circ_0067934, a potential prognostic marker for ESCC, is overexpressed in ESCC tissues and correlates with poor differentiation and more advanced TNM staging. The upregulation of circ-PVT1 and downregulation of circ-LARP4 in gastric cancer are independent prognostic factors [45, 53], and circ-PVT1 overexpression predicts better OS and DFS. The downregulation of circMTO1, circ-ITCH, and cSMARCA5 [87, 88, 90] or upregulation of circRNA_100338 in HCC [92] is associated with poor prognosis. Overexpression of ciRS-7 in HCC tissue is a risk factor for MVI [94], and the expression of hsa_circ_0005075 in HCC is positively correlated with tumor size, suggesting that it may be a potential biomarker of HCC. Overexpression of ciRS-7 in cholangiocarcinoma is significantly correlated with later TNM staging, lymph node infiltration, and postoperative recurrence, and it may be an independent negative prognostic biomarker with good sensitivity and specificity [133]. Hsa_circ_0001649 has been reported to have potential diagnostic and prognostic value in gastric cancer, CRC, HCC, and cholangiocarcinoma [57, 69, 85, 134], and it may be a sensitive indicator for distant metastasis in gastric cancer and HCC. High expression level of circ-BRAF is an independent marker for good prognosis in glioma patients [106]. Overexpression of circ-LDLRAD3 in pancreatic cancer is significantly correlated with venous and lymphatic infiltration as well as distant metastasis, and it is also a potential diagnostic marker for pancreatic cancer [116].

Another advantage of circRNAs is that they can be easily and reproducibly detected in human blood, saliva, and gastric juices, thus increasing its potential as a biomarker [48, 137–139]. In general, many circRNAs are expressed much higher in blood than the corresponding linear RNAs. Therefore, plasma circRNAs may provide additional information that cannot be revealed by routine RNA detection. For example, hsa_circ_002059, hsa_circ_0001017, and hsa_circ_0061276 can be stably detected in the plasma of gastric cancer patients [54]. These circRNAs are expected to become convenient diagnostic biomarkers for gastric cancer. Hsa_circ_0000190 is expressed at a low level both in gastric cancer plasma and tissues, and it is related to tumor size, lymph node and distant metastasis and TNM staging. The sensitivity and specificity of hsa_circ_0000190 as a diagnostic marker for gastric cancer are even better than that of CEA and CA19-9 [55]. The plasma level of hsa_circ_0000745 in gastric cancer patients is related to lymph node metastasis, and it has a good diagnostic value in combination with CEA [63]. The contents of circRNAs in exosomes are enriched more than twofold compared to their intracellular levels [140]. Bahn et al. found 422 circRNAs involved in intercellular signaling and inflammatory responses by bioinformatics analysis in human cell-free saliva [138]. Shao et al. demonstrated that hsa_circ_0014717 is stably detected in gastric juice, not affected by freeze-thaw for eight cycles or storage at 4 °C for 8 h [48]. The expression patterns and characteristics of circRNAs give them the potential to serve as a good biomarker in a variety of tumors.

The use of circRNAs as a therapeutic target or therapeutic vector will be a future trend. In therapeutic strategies targeting oncogenic circRNAs, exogenous siRNAs that are fully complementary to the back-splice junction can be used. Alternatively, it is possible to interfere with back-splicing by antisense oligonucleotides that are complementary to the back-splice signals in the precursor mRNA. It is necessary to avoid interfering with the expression of homologous linear mRNA. Another strategy is to induce tumor suppressor circRNA expression through gene therapy. In addition, some prefabricated circRNAs independent of nuclear splicing and output may also be used for the treatment of tumors. circRNAs have extremely high stability and the ability to adsorb miRNAs and proteins, suggesting that they can serve as delivery vehicles for certain treatments. circRNAs containing binding sites with oncogenic miRNAs and/or proteins can control the proliferation of tumor cells or induce apoptosis. Some strategies may help to achieve more precise treatment, for example, restricting the expression of circRNAs to certain types of cells by cell-specific promoters or designing different combinations of circRNAs and miRNAs and/or protein binding sites according to sponge maps to target specific carcinogenic factors. Because some circRNAs serve as a template for protein expression [8, 9, 141], cassettes containing tumor suppressor proteins can convert circRNAs into an effective treatment method for tumors.

At present, the exploration of the correlation between circRNAs and various diseases, including tumors, has become a new research field. Various methods have been developed for detecting circRNAs expression and biological functions. RNA-seq and microarrays are used to determine target circRNAs. The expression of circRNAs is mainly verified by real-time quantitative polymerase chain reaction (RT-qPCR), micro-drop digital PCR, Northern blotting, and FISH. For functional studies, overexpression and knockdown of genes are commonly used to regulate the expression of circRNAs. Bioinformatics predictions, luciferase reporter assays, RNA immunoprecipitation, and RNA pull-down experiments combined with mass spectrometry are utilized to reveal the interactions of circRNA-miRNA and circRNA-protein. M6A, IRES, and ORF in circRNAs can be predicted by bioinformatics analysis to investigate the protein-encoding ability of circRNAs. Ribosomal imprinting, ribosome IP, m6A IP, Western blotting, and mass spectrometry are commonly used in validation studies [142]. The development of high-throughput RNA-seq technology and bioinformatics methods enables accurate identification and quantification of circRNAs. Some online databases, such as circBase, CircInteractome, CircNet, and Circ2Traits, provide the basic information and potential regulatory networks of circRNAs. Continuous improvement of statistics and calculation methods will aid in a clearer and more comprehensive understanding of the expression patterns of circRNAs.

Conclusions

The present review introduced the biogenesis, characteristics, functions, and clinical value of circRNAs. circRNAs are closely related to a variety of physiological conditions and involved in certain diseases with a high degree of tissue and cell specificity. The biogenesis of circRNAs is a strictly controlled biological process, rather than a random splicing error. Although scientists have initially proposed a synthetic model for circRNAs, more research is needed to fully explore the mechanisms of circRNA generation, including the secondary structure of circRNAs, the initiation of novel circRNAs, the relationship among homologous RNA isomers, and the crosstalk between circRNAs and other molecules.

circRNAs have an extremely wide range of biological functions. As a miRNA sponge, circRNA makes the ceRNA network more complete and complicated. However, ceRNA does not represent all the functions of circRNAs. In the future, it is necessary to explore other mechanisms of circRNAs in tumors, such as regulating gene or protein activity.

The role of circRNAs in tumorigenesis and development has become the focus of oncology. circRNAs are considered as new diagnostic and prognostic biomarkers and potential therapeutic targets in the future. In the previous studies, the detection of circRNAs was mainly in tissues, but it is possible to detect the expressions of circRNAs in more accessible and less invasive samples (such as blood, urine, and saliva) or samples closely related to diseases (such as gastric juice, synovial effusion, and cerebrospinal fluid). It is necessary to develop circRNA as a clinical diagnostic biomarker based on the optimization of consistency and standardization of sample processing and detection. The combined detection of different circRNAs and traditional markers may have higher diagnostic efficiency. In addition, the potential of circRNAs in cancer therapy cannot be ignored. circRNA-targeted treatment may become a new mode of tumor therapy in the future.

Although increasingly more circRNAs have been discovered and investigated, the functions of thousands of circRNAs remain unclear. Research on circRNAs is still in its beginning stage, and only a small part of circRNA mechanism in tumorigenesis and progression has been clarified. With the efforts of scientists and application of new methods, more circRNAs will be discovered and applied in the diagnosis and treatment of related diseases, including tumors.

Abbreviation

AR: Androgen receptor; BCC: Basal cell carcinoma; BCSCs: Breast cancer stem cells; ccRCC: Clear cell renal cell carcinoma; ceRNA: Competing endogenous RNA; circRNA: Circular RNA; CIRI: circRNA identifier; ciRNAs: Circular intronic RNAs; CRC: Colorectal carcinoma; CSCC: Cutaneous squamous cell carcinoma; DCIS: Ductal carcinomas in situ; DFS: Disease-free survival; ecircRNA: Exonic circRNA; ElciRNA: Exon-intron circRNA; ER: Estrogen receptor; ESCC: Esophageal squamous cell carcinoma; FISH: Fluorescence in situ hybridization; GBM: Glioblastoma; HCC: Hepatocellular carcinoma; HIAT1: Hippocampus-rich gene transcription protein 1; HSCC: Hypopharyngeal squamous cell carcinoma; ICFs: Intronic circRNA fragments; IDC: Invasive ductal carcinoma; IRES: Internal ribosome entry site; LSCC: Laryngeal squamous cell cancer; miRNA: MicroRNA; MPP: Matrix metalloproteinase; MREs: miRNA response elements; MVI: Microvascular infiltration; ncRNAs: Non-coding RNAs; NSCLC: Non-small cell lung cancer; ORF: Open reading frame; OS: Overall survival; OSCC: Oral squamous cell carcinoma; PDAC: Pancreatic ductal adenocarcinoma; pre-mRNA: Precursor mRNA; PTC: Papillary thyroid cancer; RBPs: RNA-binding proteins; RNA-seq: RNA sequencing; RT-qPCR: Real-time quantitative polymerase chain reaction; SA: Splice acceptor; SD: Splice donor; TN: Triple negative; VEGF: Vascular endothelial growth factor

Funding

This work was financially supported by the National Key Technology R & D Program (No. 2015BAI12B12), National Natural Science Foundation of China (No. 31700792), and Changzhou Science and Technology Project (Applied Based Research, No. CJ20159021, CJ20179047).

Authors' contributions

YTG, JTJ, and CPW conceived and designed the study and helped to draft the manuscript. All authors read and approved the final manuscript.

Consent for publication

Not applicable.

Competing interests

The authors declare that they have no competing interests.

References

1. Djebali S, Davis CA, Merkel A, Dobin A, Lassmann T, Mortazavi A, et al. Landscape of transcription in human cells. Nature. 2012;489:101–8.
2. Hsu MT, Coca-Prados M. Electron microscopic evidence for the circular form of RNA in the cytoplasm of eukaryotic cells. Nature. 1979;280:339–40.
3. Wang F, Nazarali AJ, Ji S. Circular RNAs as potential biomarkers for cancer diagnosis and therapy. Am J Cancer Res. 2016;6:1167–76.
4. Zheng Q, Bao C, Guo W, Li S, Chen J, Chen B, et al. Circular RNA profiling reveals an abundant circHIPK3 that regulates cell growth by sponging multiple miRNAs. Nat Commun. 2016;7:11215.
5. Memczak S, Jens M, Elefsinioti A, Torti F, Krueger J, Rybak A, et al. Circular RNAs are a large class of animal RNAs with regulatory potency. Nature. 2013;495:333–8.
6. Hansen TB, Jensen TI, Clausen BH, Bramsen JB, Finsen B, Damgaard CK, et al. Natural RNA circles function as efficient microRNA sponges. Nature. 2013; 495:384–8.
7. Du WW, Yang W, Liu E, Yang Z, Dhaliwal P, Yang BB. Foxo3 circular RNA retards cell cycle progression via forming ternary complexes with p21 and CDK2. Nucleic Acids Res. 2016;44:2846–58.
8. Legnini I, Di Timoteo G, Rossi F, Morlando M, Briganti F, Sthandier O, et al. Circ-ZNF609 is a circular RNA that can be translated and functions in myogenesis. Mol Cell. 2017;66:22–37. e29
9. Pamudurti NR, Bartok O, Jens M, Ashwal-Fluss R, Stottmeister C, Ruhe L, et al. Translation of CircRNAs. Mol Cell. 2017;66:9–21. e27
10. Zhang Y, Zhang XO, Chen T, Xiang JF, Yin QF, Xing YH, et al. Circular intronic long noncoding RNAs. Mol Cell. 2013;51:792–806.
11. Li Z, Huang C, Bao C, Chen L, Lin M, Wang X, et al. Exon-intron circular RNAs regulate transcription in the nucleus. Nat Struct Mol Biol. 2015;22: 256–64.
12. Ashwal-Fluss R, Meyer M, Pamudurti NR, Ivanov A, Bartok O, Hanan M, et al. circRNA biogenesis competes with pre-mRNA splicing. Mol Cell. 2014;56:55–66.
13. Abdelmohsen K, Panda AC, Munk R, Grammatikakis I, Dudekula DB, De S, et al. Identification of HuR target circular RNAs uncovers suppression of PABPN1 translation by CircPABPN1. RNA Biol. 2017;14:361–9.
14. Du WW, Yang W, Chen Y, Wu ZK, Foster FS, Yang Z, et al. Foxo3 circular RNA promotes cardiac senescence by modulating multiple factors associated with stress and senescence responses. Eur Heart J. 2017;38:1402–12.
15. Kotake Y, Nakagawa T, Kitagawa K, Suzuki S, Liu N, Kitagawa M, et al. Long non-coding RNA ANRIL is required for the PRC2 recruitment to and silencing of p15(INK4B) tumor suppressor gene. Oncogene. 2011;30:1956–62.
16. Burd CE, Jeck WR, Liu Y, Sanoff HK, Wang Z, Sharpless NE. Expression of linear and novel circular forms of an INK4/ARF-associated non-coding RNA correlates with atherosclerosis risk. PLoS Genet. 2010;6:e1001233.
17. Holdt LM, Stahringer A, Sass K, Pichler G, Kulak NA, Wilfert W, et al. Circular non-coding RNA ANRIL modulates ribosomal RNA maturation and atherosclerosis in humans. Nat Commun. 2016;7:12429.
18. Zhao J, Li L, Wang Q, Han H, Zhan Q, Xu M. CircRNA expression profile in early-stage lung adenocarcinoma patients. Cell Physiol Biochem. 2017;44: 2138–46.
19. Wan L, Zhang L, Fan K, Cheng ZX, Sun QC, Wang JJ. Circular RNA-ITCH suppresses lung cancer proliferation via inhibiting the Wnt/beta-catenin pathway. Biomed Res Int. 2016;2016:1579490.
20. Yao JT, Zhao SH, Liu QP, Lv MQ, Zhou DX, Liao ZJ, et al. Over-expression of CircRNA_100876 in non-small cell lung cancer and its prognostic value. Pathol Res Pract. 2017;213:453–6.
21. Liu Q, Zhang X, Hu X, Dai L, Fu X, Zhang J, et al. Circular RNA related to the chondrocyte ECM regulates MMP13 expression by functioning as a MiR-136 'sponge' in human cartilage degradation. Sci Rep. 2016;6:22572.
22. Zhu X, Wang X, Wei S, Chen Y, Chen Y, Fan X, et al. hsa_circ_0013958: a circular RNA and potential novel biomarker for lung adenocarcinoma. FEBS J. 2017;284:2170–82.
23. Wang X, Zhu X, Zhang H, Wei S, Chen Y, Chen Y, et al. Increased circular RNA hsa_circ_0012673 acts as a sponge of miR-22 to promote lung adenocarcinoma proliferation. Biochem Biophys Res Commun. 2018;496:1069–75.
24. Jiang MM, Mai ZT, Wan SZ, Chi YM, Zhang X, Sun BH, et al. Microarray profiles reveal that circular RNA hsa_circ_0007385 functions as an oncogene in non-small cell lung cancer tumorigenesis. J Cancer Res Clin Oncol. 2018;144:667–74.
25. Zhang S, Zeng X, Ding T, Guo L, Li Y, Ou S, et al. Microarray profile of circular RNAs identifies hsa_circ_0014130 as a new circular RNA biomarker in non-small cell lung cancer. Sci Rep. 2018;8:2878.
26. Luo YH, Zhu XZ, Huang KW, Zhang Q, Fan YX, Yan PW, et al. Emerging roles of circular RNA hsa_circ_0000064 in the proliferation and metastasis of lung cancer. Biomed Pharmacother. 2017;96:892–8.
27. Pinder SE. Ductal carcinoma in situ (DCIS): pathological features, differential diagnosis, prognostic factors and specimen evaluation. Mod Pathol. 2010; 23(Suppl 2):S8–13.
28. Galasso M, Costantino G, Pasquali L, Minotti L, Baldassari F, Corra F, et al. Profiling of the predicted circular RNAs in ductal in situ and invasive breast cancer: a pilot study. Int J Genomics. 2016;2016:4503840.
29. Nair AA, Niu N, Tang X, Thompson KJ, Wang L, Kocher JP, et al. Circular RNAs and their associations with breast cancer subtypes. Oncotarget. 2016; 7:80967–79.
30. Lu L, Sun J, Shi P, Kong W, Xu K, He B, et al. Identification of circular RNAs as a promising new class of diagnostic biomarkers for human breast cancer. Oncotarget. 2017;8:44096–107.
31. Yin WB, Yan MG, Fang X, Guo JJ, Xiong W, Zhang RP. Circulating circular RNA hsa_circ_0001785 acts as a diagnostic biomarker for breast cancer detection. Clin Chim Acta. 2017. https://doi.org/10.1016/j.cca.2017.10.011
32. Du WW, Fang L, Yang W, Wu N, Awan FM, Yang Z, et al. Induction of tumor apoptosis through a circular RNA enhancing Foxo3 activity. Cell Death Differ. 2017;24:357–70.
33. Lu WY. Roles of the circular RNA circ-Foxo3 in breast cancer progression. Cell Cycle. 2017;16:589–90.
34. Yang W, Du WW, Li X, Yee AJ, Yang BB. Foxo3 activity promoted by non-coding effects of circular RNA and Foxo3 pseudogene in the inhibition of tumor growth and angiogenesis. Oncogene. 2016;35:3919–31.
35. Yan N, Xu H, Zhang J, Xu L, Zhang Y, Zhang L, et al. Circular RNA profile indicates circular RNA VRK1 is negatively related with breast cancer stem cells. Oncotarget. 2017;8:95704–18.
36. Wang H, Xiao Y, Wu L, Ma D. Comprehensive circular RNA profiling reveals the regulatory role of the circRNA-000911/miR-449a pathway in breast carcinogenesis. Int J Oncol. 2018;52:743–54.
37. Liang HF, Zhang XZ, Liu BG, Jia GT, Li WL. Circular RNA circ-ABCB10 promotes breast cancer proliferation and progression through sponging miR-1271. Am J Cancer Res. 2017;7:1566–76.
38. Tang YY, Zhao P, Zou TN, Duan JJ, Zhi R, Yang SY, et al. Circular RNA hsa_circ_0001982 promotes breast cancer cell carcinogenesis through decreasing miR-143. DNA Cell Biol. 2017;36:901–8.
39. He R, Liu P, Xie X, Zhou Y, Liao Q, Xiong W, et al. circGFRA1 and GFRA1 act as ceRNAs in triple negative breast cancer by regulating miR-34a. J Exp Clin Cancer Res. 2017;36:145.
40. Gao D, Zhang X, Liu B, Meng D, Fang K, Guo Z, et al. Screening circular RNA related to chemotherapeutic resistance in breast cancer. Epigenomics. 2017; 9:1175–88.
41. Liang G, Liu Z, Tan L, Su AN, Jiang WG, Gong C. HIF1alpha-associated circDENND4C promotes proliferation of breast cancer cells in hypoxic environment. Anticancer Res. 2017;37:4337–43.
42. Li F, Zhang L, Li W, Deng J, Zheng J, An M, et al. Circular RNA ITCH has inhibitory effect on ESCC by suppressing the Wnt/beta-catenin pathway. Oncotarget. 2015;6:6001–13.
43. Xia W, Qiu M, Chen R, Wang S, Leng X, Wang J, et al. Circular RNA has_circ_0067934 is upregulated in esophageal squamous cell carcinoma and promoted proliferation. Sci Rep. 2016;6:35576.
44. Su H, Lin F, Deng X, Shen L, Fang Y, Fei Z, et al. Profiling and bioinformatics analyses reveal differential circular RNA expression in radioresistant esophageal cancer cells. J Transl Med. 2016;14:225.
45. Chen J, Li Y, Zheng Q, Bao C, He J, Chen B, et al. Circular RNA profile identifies circPVT1 as a proliferative factor and prognostic marker in gastric cancer. Cancer Lett. 2017;388:208–19.

46. Huang YS, Jie N, Zou KJ, Weng Y. Expression profile of circular RNAs in human gastric cancer tissues. Mol Med Rep. 2017;16:2469–76.

47. Dang Y, Ouyang X, Zhang F, Wang K, Lin Y, Sun B, et al. Circular RNAs expression profiles in human gastric cancer. Sci Rep. 2017;7:9060.

48. Shao Y, Li J, Lu R, Li T, Yang Y, Xiao B, et al. Global circular RNA expression profile of human gastric cancer and its clinical significance. Cancer Med. 2017;6:1173–80.

49. Sui W, Shi Z, Xue W, Ou M, Zhu Y, Chen J, et al. Circular RNA and gene expression profiles in gastric cancer based on microarray chip technology. Oncol Rep. 2017;37:1804–14.

50. Lai Z, Yang Y, Yan Y, Li T, Li Y, Wang Z, et al. Analysis of co-expression networks for circular RNAs and mRNAs reveals that circular RNAs hsa_circ_0047905, hsa_circ_0138960 and has-circRNA7690-15 are candidate oncogenes in gastric cancer. Cell Cycle. 2017;16:2301–11.

51. Li P, Chen H, Chen S, Mo X, Li T, Xiao B, et al. Circular RNA 0000096 affects cell growth and migration in gastric cancer. Br J Cancer. 2017;116:626–33.

52. Zhang Y, Liu H, Li W, Yu J, Li J, Shen Z, et al. CircRNA_100269 is downregulated in gastric cancer and suppresses tumor cell growth by targeting miR-630. Aging (Albany NY). 2017;9:1585–94.

53. Zhang J, Liu H, Hou L, Wang G, Zhang R, Huang Y, et al. Circular RNA_LARP4 inhibits cell proliferation and invasion of gastric cancer by sponging miR-424-5p and regulating LATS1 expression. Mol Cancer. 2017;16:151.

54. Li P, Chen S, Chen H, Mo X, Li T, Shao Y, et al. Using circular RNA as a novel type of biomarker in the screening of gastric cancer. Clin Chim Acta. 2015; 444:132–6.

55. Chen S, Li T, Zhao Q, Xiao B, Guo J. Using circular RNA hsa_circ_0000190 as a new biomarker in the diagnosis of gastric cancer. Clin Chim Acta. 2017; 466:167–71.

56. Shao Y, Chen L, Lu R, Zhang X, Xiao B, Ye G, et al. Decreased expression of hsa_circ_0001895 in human gastric cancer and its clinical significances. Tumour Biol. 2017;39:1010428317699125.

57. Li WH, Song YC, Zhang H, Zhou ZJ, Xie X, Zeng QN, et al. Decreased expression of Hsa_circ_00001649 in gastric cancer and its clinical significance. Dis Markers. 2017;2017:4587698.

58. Xie Y, Shao Y, Sun W, Ye G, Zhang X, Xiao B, et al. Downregulated expression of hsa_circ_0074362 in gastric cancer and its potential diagnostic values. Biomark Med. 2018;12:11–20.

59. Sun H, Tang W, Rong D, Jin H, Fu K, Zhang W, et al. Hsa_circ_0000520, a potential new circular RNA biomarker, is involved in gastric carcinoma. Cancer Biomark. 2018;21:299–306.

60. Zhao Q, Chen S, Li T, Xiao B, Zhang X. Clinical values of circular RNA 0000181 in the screening of gastric cancer. J Clin Lab Anal. 2018;32(4): e22333. https://doi.org/10.1002/jcla.22333

61. Tian M, Chen R, Li T, Xiao B. Reduced expression of circRNA hsa_circ_0003159 in gastric cancer and its clinical significance. J Clin Lab Anal. 2018;32(3). https://doi.org/10.1002/jcla.22281

62. Li T, Shao Y, Fu L, Xie Y, Zhu L, Sun W, et al. Plasma circular RNA profiling of patients with gastric cancer and their droplet digital RT-PCR detection. J Mol Med (Berl). 2018;96:85–96.

63. Huang M, He YR, Liang LC, Huang Q, Zhu ZQ. Circular RNA hsa_circ_0000745 may serve as a diagnostic marker for gastric cancer. World J Gastroenterol. 2017;23:6330–8.

64. Zhang Y, Li J, Yu J, Liu H, Shen Z, Ye G, et al. Circular RNAs signature predicts the early recurrence of stage III gastric cancer after radical surgery. Oncotarget. 2017;8:22936–43.

65. Bachmayr-Heyda A, Reiner AT, Auer K, Sukhbaatar N, Aust S, Bachleitner-Hofmann T, et al. Correlation of circular RNA abundance with proliferation--exemplified with colorectal and ovarian cancer, idiopathic lung fibrosis, and normal human tissues. Sci Rep. 2015;5:8057.

66. Zhang P, Zuo Z, Shang W, Wu A, Bi R, Wu J, et al. Identification of differentially expressed circular RNAs in human colorectal cancer. Tumour Biol. 2017;39:1010428317694546.

67. Huang G, Zhu H, Shi Y, Wu W, Cai H, Chen X. cir-ITCH plays an inhibitory role in colorectal cancer by regulating the Wnt/beta-catenin pathway. PLoS One. 2015;10:e0131225.

68. Wang X, Zhang Y, Huang L, Zhang J, Pan F, Li B, et al. Decreased expression of hsa_circ_001988 in colorectal cancer and its clinical significances. Int J Clin Exp Pathol. 2015;8:16020–5.

69. Ji W, Qiu C, Wang M, Mao N, Wu S, Dai Y. Hsa_circ_0001649: a circular RNA and potential novel biomarker for colorectal cancer. Biochem Biophys Res Commun. 2018;497:122–6.

70. Zhuo F, Lin H, Chen Z, Huang Z, Hu J. The expression profile and clinical significance of circRNA0003906 in colorectal cancer. Onco Targets Ther. 2017;10:5187–93.

71. Weng W, Wei Q, Toden S, Yoshida K, Nagasaka T, Fujiwara T, et al. Circular RNA ciRS-7-a promising prognostic biomarker and a potential therapeutic target in colorectal cancer. Clin Cancer Res. 2017;23:3918–28.

72. Xie H, Ren X, Xin S, Lan X, Lu G, Lin Y, et al. Emerging roles of circRNA_001569 targeting miR-145 in the proliferation and invasion of colorectal cancer. Oncotarget. 2016;7:26680–91.

73. Ghosal S, Das S, Sen R, Basak P, Chakrabarti J. Circ2Traits: a comprehensive database for circular RNA potentially associated with disease and traits. Front Genet. 2013;4:283.

74. Guo JN, Li J, Zhu CL, Feng WT, Shao JX, Wan L, et al. Comprehensive profile of differentially expressed circular RNAs reveals that hsa_circ_0000069 is upregulated and promotes cell proliferation, migration, and invasion in colorectal cancer. Onco Targets Ther. 2016;9:7451–8.

75. Zhu M, Xu Y, Chen Y, Yan F. Circular BANP, an upregulated circular RNA that modulates cell proliferation in colorectal cancer. Biomed Pharmacother. 2017;88:138–44.

76. Zeng K, Chen X, Xu M, Liu X, Hu X, Xu T, et al. CircHIPK3 promotes colorectal cancer growth and metastasis by sponging miR-7. Cell Death Dis. 2018;9:417.

77. Zhang R, Xu J, Zhao J, Wang X. Silencing of hsa_circ_0007534 suppresses proliferation and induces apoptosis in colorectal cancer cells. Eur Rev Med Pharmacol Sci. 2018;22:118–26.

78. Xu XW, Zheng BA, Hu ZM, Qian ZY, Huang CJ, Liu XQ, et al. Circular RNA hsa_circ_000984 promotes colon cancer growth and metastasis by sponging miR-106b. Oncotarget. 2017;8:91674–83.

79. Zhang XL, Xu LL, Wang F. Hsa_circ_0020397 regulates colorectal cancer cell viability, apoptosis and invasion by promoting the expression of the miR-138 targets TERT and PD-L1. Cell Biol Int. 2017;41:1056–64.

80. Hsiao KY, Lin YC, Gupta SK, Chang N, Yen L, Sun HS, et al. Noncoding effects of circular RNA CCDC66 promote colon cancer growth and metastasis. Cancer Res. 2017;77:2339–50.

81. Dou Y, Cha DJ, Franklin JL, Higginbotham JN, Jeppesen DK, Weaver AM, et al. Circular RNAs are down-regulated in KRAS mutant colon cancer cells and can be transferred to exosomes. Sci Rep. 2016;6:37982.

82. Shang X, Li G, Liu H, Li T, Liu J, Zhao Q, et al. Comprehensive circular RNA profiling reveals that hsa_circ_0005075, a new circular RNA biomarker, is involved in hepatocellular crcinoma development. Medicine (Baltimore). 2016;95:e3811.

83. Fu L, Yao T, Chen Q, Mo X, Hu Y, Guo J. Screening differential circular RNA expression profiles reveals hsa_circ_0004018 is associated with hepatocellular carcinoma. Oncotarget. 2017;8:58405–16.

84. Fu L, Wu S, Yao T, Chen Q, Xie Y, Ying S, et al. Decreased expression of hsa_circ_0003570 in hepatocellular carcinoma and its clinical significance. J Clin Lab Anal. 2018;32(2). https://doi.org/10.1002/jcla.22239

85. Qin M, Liu G, Huo X, Tao X, Sun X, Ge Z, et al. Hsa_circ_0001649: a circular RNA and potential novel biomarker for hepatocellular carcinoma. Cancer Biomark. 2016;16:161–9.

86. Yao Z, Luo J, Hu K, Lin J, Huang H, Wang Q, et al. ZKSCAN1 gene and its related circular RNA (circZKSCAN1) both inhibit hepatocellular carcinoma cell growth, migration, and invasion but through different signaling pathways. Mol Oncol. 2017;11:422–37.

87. Han D, Li J, Wang H, Su X, Hou J, Gu Y, et al. Circular RNA circMTO1 acts as the sponge of microRNA-9 to suppress hepatocellular carcinoma progression. Hepatology. 2017;66:1151–64.

88. Guo W, Zhang J, Zhang D, Cao S, Li G, Zhang S, et al. Polymorphisms and expression pattern of circular RNA circ-ITCH contributes to the carcinogenesis of hepatocellular carcinoma. Oncotarget. 2017;8:48169–77.

89. Zhang K, Che S, Su Z, Zheng S, Zhang H, Yang S, et al. CD90 promotes cell migration, viability and sphereforming ability of hepatocellular carcinoma cells. Int J Mol Med. 2018;41:946–54.

90. Yu J, Xu QG, Wang ZG, Yang Y, Zhang L, Ma JZ, et al. Circular RNA cSMARCA5 inhibits growth and metastasis in hepatocellular carcinoma. J Hepatol. 2018;68(6):1214–27.

91. Fu L, Chen Q, Yao T, Li T, Ying S, Hu Y, et al. Hsa_circ_0005986 inhibits carcinogenesis by acting as a miR-129-5p sponge and is used as a novel biomarker for hepatocellular carcinoma. Oncotarget. 2017;8:43878–88.

92. Huang XY, Huang ZL, Xu YH, Zheng Q, Chen Z, Song W, et al. Comprehensive circular RNA profiling reveals the regulatory role of the circRNA-100338/miR-141-3p pathway in hepatitis B-related hepatocellular carcinoma. Sci Rep. 2017;7:5428.

93. Yu L, Gong X, Sun L, Zhou Q, Lu B, Zhu L. The circular RNA Cdr1as act as an oncogene in hepatocellular carcinoma through targeting miR-7 expression. PLoS One. 2016;11:e0158347.

94. Xu L, Zhang M, Zheng X, Yi P, Lan C, Xu M. The circular RNA ciRS-7 (Cdr1as) acts as a risk factor of hepatic microvascular invasion in hepatocellular carcinoma. J Cancer Res Clin Oncol. 2017;143:17–27.

95. Yang X, Xiong Q, Wu Y, Li S, Ge F. Quantitative proteomics reveals the regulatory networks of circular RNA CDR1as in hepatocellular carcinoma cells. J Proteome Res. 2017;16:3891–902.

96. Zhu Q, Lu G, Luo Z, Gui F, Wu J, Zhang D, et al. CircRNA circ_0067934 promotes tumor growth and metastasis in hepatocellular carcinoma through regulation of miR-1324/FZD5/Wnt/beta-catenin axis. Biochem Biophys Res Commun. 2018;497:626–32.

97. Song X, Zhang N, Han P, Moon BS, Lai RK, Wang K, et al. Circular RNA profile in gliomas revealed by identification tool UROBORUS. Nucleic Acids Res. 2016;44:e87.

98. Barbagallo D, Condorelli A, Ragusa M, Salito L, Sammito M, Banelli B, et al. Dysregulated miR-671-5p / CDR1-AS / CDR1 / VSNL1 axis is involved in glioblastoma multiforme. Oncotarget. 2016;7:4746–59.

99. Li G, Yang H, Han K, Zhu D, Lun P, Zhao Y. A novel circular RNA, hsa_circ_0046701, promotes carcinogenesis by increasing the expression of miR-142-3p target ITGB8 in glioma. Biochem Biophys Res Commun. 2018;498:254–61.

100. He Q, Zhao L, Liu Y, Liu X, Zheng J, Yu H, et al. circ-SHKBP1 regulates the angiogenesis of U87 glioma-exposed endothelial cells through miR-544a/FOXP1 and miR-379/FOXP2 pathways. Mol Ther Nucleic Acids. 2018;10:331–48.

101. Yang P, Qiu Z, Jiang Y, Dong L, Yang W, Gu C, et al. Silencing of cZNF292 circular RNA suppresses human glioma tube formation via the Wnt/beta-catenin signaling pathway. Oncotarget. 2016;7:63449–55.

102. Zheng J, Liu X, Xue Y, Gong W, Ma J, Xi Z, et al. TTBK2 circular RNA promotes glioma malignancy by regulating miR-217/HNF1beta/Derlin-1 pathway. J Hematol Oncol. 2017;10:52.

103. Yang Y, Gao X, Zhang M, Yan S, Sun C, Xiao F, et al. Novel role of FBXW7 circular RNA in repressing glioma tumorigenesis. J Natl Cancer Inst. 2018; 110(3). https://doi.org/10.1093/jnci/djx166

104. Barbagallo D, Caponnetto A, Cirnigliaro M, Brex D, Barbagallo C, D'Angeli F, et al. CircSMARCA5 inhibits migration of glioblastoma multiforme cells by regulating a molecular axis involving splicing factors SRSF1/SRSF3/PTB. Int J Mol Sci. 2018;19(2). https://doi.org/10.3390/ijms19020480

105. Zhang M, Huang N, Yang X, Luo J, Yan S, Xiao F, et al. A novel protein encoded by the circular form of the SHPRH gene suppresses glioma tumorigenesis. Oncogene. 2018;37:1805–14.

106. Zhu J, Ye J, Zhang L, Xia L, Hu H, Jiang H, et al. Differential expression of circular RNAs in glioblastoma multiforme and its correlation with prognosis. Transl Oncol. 2017;10:271–9.

107. Siegel RL, Miller KD, Jemal A. Cancer statistics, 2016. CA Cancer J Clin. 2016; 66:7–30.

108. Zhong Z, Lv M, Chen J. Screening differential circular RNA expression profiles reveals the regulatory role of circTCF25-miR-103a-3p/miR-107-CDK6 pathway in bladder carcinoma. Sci Rep. 2016;6:30919.

109. Cai D, Liu Z, Kong G. Molecular and bioinformatics analyses identify 7 circular RNAs involved in regulation of oncogenic transformation and cell proliferation in human bladder cancer. Med Sci Monit. 2018;24:1654–61.

110. Li Y, Zheng F, Xiao X, Xie F, Tao D, Huang C, et al. CircHIPK3 sponges miR-558 to suppress heparanase expression in bladder cancer cells. EMBO Rep. 2017;18:1646–59.

111. Huang M, Zhong Z, Lv M, Shu J, Tian Q, Chen J. Comprehensive analysis of differentially expressed profiles of lncRNAs and circRNAs with associated co-expression and ceRNA networks in bladder carcinoma. Oncotarget. 2016;7: 47186–200.

112. Zhong Z, Huang M, Lv M, He Y, Duan C, Zhang L, et al. Circular RNA MYLK as a competing endogenous RNA promotes bladder cancer progression through modulating VEGFA/VEGFR2 signaling pathway. Cancer Lett. 2017;403:305–17.

113. Yang C, Yuan W, Yang X, Li P, Wang J, Han J, et al. Circular RNA circ-ITCH inhibits bladder cancer progression by sponging miR-17/miR-224 and regulating p21, PTEN expression. Mol Cancer. 2018;17:19.

114. Li B, Xie F, Zheng FX, Jiang GS, Zeng FQ, Xiao XY. Overexpression of CircRNA BCRC4 regulates cell apoptosis and MicroRNA-101/EZH2 signaling in bladder cancer. J Huazhong Univ Sci Technolog Med Sci. 2017;37:886–90.

115. Huang WJ, Wang Y, Liu S, Yang J, Guo SX, Wang L, et al. Silencing circular RNA hsa_circ_0000977 suppresses pancreatic ductal adenocarcinoma progression by stimulating miR-874-3p and inhibiting PLK1 expression. Cancer Lett. 2018;422:70–80.

116. Yang F, Liu DY, Guo JT, Ge N, Zhu P, Liu X, et al. Circular RNA circ-LDLRAD3 as a biomarker in diagnosis of pancreatic cancer. World J Gastroenterol. 2017;23:45–8354.

117. Chen G, Shi Y, Zhang Y, Sun J. CircRNA_100782 regulates pancreatic carcinoma proliferation through the IL6-STAT3 pathway. Onco Targets Ther. 2017;10:5783–94.

118. Li H, Hao X, Wang H, Liu Z, He Y, Pu M, et al. Circular RNA expression profile of pancreatic ductal adenocarcinoma revealed by microarray. Cell Physiol Biochem. 2016;40:1334–44.

119. Jin H, Jin X, Zhang H, Wang W. Circular RNA hsa-circ-0016347 promotes proliferation, invasion and metastasis of osteosarcoma cells. Oncotarget. 2017;8:25571–81.

120. Zhang H, Wang G, Ding C, Liu P, Wang R, Ding W, et al. Increased circular RNA UBAP2 acts as a sponge of miR-143 to promote osteosarcoma progression. Oncotarget. 2017;8:61687–97.

121. Song YZ, Li JF. Circular RNA hsa_circ_0001564 regulates osteosarcoma proliferation and apoptosis by acting miRNA sponge. Biochem Biophys Res Commun. 2018;495:2369–75.

122. Deng N, Li L, Gao J, Zhou J, Wang Y, Wang C, et al. Hsa_circ_0009910 promotes carcinogenesis by promoting the expression of miR-449a target IL6R in osteosarcoma. Biochem Biophys Res Commun. 2018;495:189–96.

123. Liu W, Zhang J, Zou C, Xie X, Wang Y, Wang B, et al. Microarray expression profile and functional analysis of circular RNAs in osteosarcoma. Cell Physiol Biochem. 2017;43:969–85.

124. Ahmed I, Karedath T, Andrews SS, Al-Azwani IK, Mohamoud YA, Querleu D, et al. Altered expression pattern of circular RNAs in primary and metastatic sites of epithelial ovarian carcinoma. Oncotarget. 2016;7:36366–81.

125. Wang K, Sun Y, Tao W, Fei X, Chang C. Androgen receptor (AR) promotes clear cell renal cell carcinoma (ccRCC) migration and invasion via altering the circHIAT1/miR-195-5p/29a-3p/29c-3p/CDC42 signals. Cancer Lett. 2017; 394:1–12.

126. Peng N, Shi L, Zhang Q, Hu Y, Wang N, Ye H. Microarray profiling of circular RNAs in human papillary thyroid carcinoma. PLoS One. 2017;12:e0170287.

127. Sand M, Bechara FG, Sand D, Gambichler T, Hahn SA, Bromba M, et al. Circular RNA expression in basal cell carcinoma. Epigenomics. 2016;8:619–32.

128. Sand M, Bechara FG, Gambichler T, Sand D, Bromba M, Hahn SA, et al. Circular RNA expression in cutaneous squamous cell carcinoma. J Dermatol Sci. 2016;83:210–8.

129. Chen L, Zhang S, Wu J, Cui J, Zhong L, Zeng L, et al. circRNA_100290 plays a role in oral cancer by functioning as a sponge of the miR-29 family. Oncogene. 2017;36:4551–61.

130. Wang L, Wei Y, Yan Y, Wang H, Yang J, Zheng Z, et al. CircDOCK1 suppresses cell apoptosis via inhibition of miR196a5p by targeting BIRC3 in OSCC. Oncol Rep. 2018;39:951–66.

131. Xuan L, Qu L, Zhou H, Wang P, Yu H, Wu T, et al. Circular RNA: a novel biomarker for progressive laryngeal cancer. Am J Transl Res. 2016;8:932–9.

132. Cao S, Wei D, Li X, Zhou J, Li W, Qian Y, et al. Novel circular RNA expression profiles reflect progression of patients with hypopharyngeal squamous cell carcinoma. Oncotarget. 2017;8:45367–79.

133. Jiang XM, Li ZL, Li JL, Xu Y, Leng KM, Cui YF, et al. A novel prognostic biomarker for cholangiocarcinoma: circRNA Cdr1as. Eur Rev Med Pharmacol Sci. 2018;22:365–71.

134. Xu Y, Yao Y, Zhong X, Leng K, Qin W, Qu L, et al. Downregulated circular RNA hsa_circ_0001649 regulates proliferation, migration and invasion in cholangiocarcinoma cells. Biochem Biophys Res Commun. 2018;496:455–61.

135. Ma HB, Yao YN, Yu JJ, Chen XX, Li HF. Extensive profiling of circular RNAs and the potential regulatory role of circRNA-000284 in cell proliferation and invasion of cervical cancer via sponging miR-506. Am J Transl Res. 2018;10:592–604.

136. Kong Z, Wan X, Zhang Y, Zhang P, Zhang Y, Zhang X, et al. Androgen-responsive circular RNA circSMARCA5 is up-regulated and promotes cell proliferation in prostate cancer. Biochem Biophys Res Commun. 2017;493: 1217–23.

137. Memczak S, Papavasileiou P, Peters O, Rajewsky N. Identification and characterization of circular RNAs as a new class of putative biomarkers in human blood. PLoS One. 2015;10:e0141214.

138. Bahn JH, Zhang Q, Li F, Chan TM, Lin X, Kim Y, et al. The landscape of microRNA, Piwi-interacting RNA, and circular RNA in human saliva. Clin Chem. 2015;61:221–30.

139. Lasda E, Parker R. Circular RNAs co-precipitate with extracellular vesicles: a possible mechanism for circRNA clearance. PLoS One. 2016;11:e0148407.

140. Li Y, Zheng Q, Bao C, Li S, Guo W, Zhao J, et al. Circular RNA is enriched
     and stable in exosomes: a promising biomarker for cancer diagnosis. Cell
     Res. 2015;25:981–4.
141. Yang Y, Fan X, Mao M, Song X, Wu P, Zhang Y, et al. Extensive translation of
     circular RNAs driven by N (6)-methyladenosine. Cell Res. 2017;27:626–41.
142. Zhang Y, Liang W, Zhang P, Chen J, Qian H, Zhang X, et al. Circular RNAs:
     emerging cancer biomarkers and targets. J Exp Clin Cancer Res. 2017;36:152.

4

Abscopal effect of radiotherapy combined with immune checkpoint inhibitors

Yang Liu[1,2], Yinping Dong[1,2], Li Kong[2], Fang Shi[2], Hui Zhu[2,1*] and Jinming Yu[2,1*]

Abstract

Radiotherapy (RT) is used routinely as a standard treatment for more than 50% of patients with malignant tumors. The abscopal effect induced by local RT, which is considered as a systemic anti-tumor immune response, reflects the regression of non-irradiated metastatic lesions at a distance from the primary site of irradiation. Since the application of immunotherapy, especially with immune checkpoint inhibitors, can enhance the systemic anti-tumor response of RT, the combination of RT and immunotherapy has drawn extensive attention by oncologists and cancer researchers. Nevertheless, the exact underlying mechanism of the abscopal effect remains unclear. In general, we speculate that the immune mechanism of RT is responsible for, or at least associated with, this effect. In this review, we discuss the anti-tumor effect of RT and immune checkpoint blockade and discuss some published studies on the abscopal effect for this type of combination therapy. In addition, we also evaluate the most appropriate time window for the combination of RT and immune checkpoint blockade, as well as the optimal dose and fractionation of RT in the context of the combined treatment. Finally, the most significant purpose of this review is to identify the potential predictors of the abscopal effect to help identify the most appropriate patients who would most likely benefit from the combination treatment modality.

Keywords: Cancer, Radiotherapy, Immunotherapy, Abscopal effect

Background

Radiotherapy (RT) is a treatment for malignant tumors that has been used for the past century and has been applied to approximately 50% of all cancer patients [1–3], including patients with newly diagnosed cancers and those with persistent or recurrent tumors. Historically, radiation-induced deoxyribonucleic acid (DNA) damage, which leads to direct tumor cell death by the process of tumor cell apoptosis, senescence, and autophagy [4–6], is considered to be the major mechanism by which most solid tumors respond to clinical ionizing radiation [7]. Since these cytotoxic effects can also affect leukocytes, RT has been considered to be immunosuppressive. For example, the phenomenon of lymphopenia following RT has been observed in patients with solid tumors, including breast cancer, lung cancer, and head and neck tumors [8–10]. In addition, total body irradiation (TBI) has been widely used as a conditioning regimen for patients who require the treatment for bone marrow transplantation [11]. However, radiation-induced activation of the immune system has been increasingly recognized in recent years, an indication that RT could also elicit immune-mediated anti-tumor responses. In fact, the role of T cells in local tumor control induced by RT was demonstrated in a murine fibrosarcoma model over 30 years ago. The required radiation dose to control 50% of the tumors was much lower in immunocompetent mice compared to that of T cell-deficient mice (30 gray [Gy] vs. 64.5 Gy), and immunocompetent mice also had a lower incidence of metastases than immunosuppressed mice [12]. Similarly, in mouse melanoma tumor models, Lee et al. demonstrated that only immunocompetent hosts responded to 15–20 Gy radiation, while nude mice lacking T cells and B cells and wild-type mice depleted of CD8+ T cells did not respond to this high-dose radiation [13]. In patients, Holecek and Harwood reported that one Kaposi's sarcoma patient who previously received a kidney transplant and was treated with azathioprine to suppress kidney rejection responded less to irradiation than those who did not receive an exogenously administered immunosuppressive agent [14].

* Correspondence: drzhuh@126.com; sdyujinming@163.com
[2]Department of Radiation Oncology, Shandong Cancer Hospital affiliated to Shandong University, Shandong Academy of Medical Sciences, 440 Jiyan Road, Jinan 250117, Shandong, China
[1]School of Medicine and Life Sciences, University of Jinan-Shandong Academy of Medical Sciences, Jinan, Shandong, China

Furthermore, other studies have found that this immune-mediated anti-tumor effect of RT could also trigger the regression of metastatic tumors that were distant from the irradiated field, which is the so-called abscopal effect. This effect, initially defined by Mole in 1953 [15], was detected in renal cell carcinoma, melanoma, lymphomas, hepatocellular carcinoma, and other tumor types [16–23]. For instance, Stamell et al. reported a metastatic melanoma patient who received palliative RT to the primary tumor also experienced regression of non-irradiated metastases [17]. An abscopal effect has also been reported in mouse tumor models in which Demaria et al. observed that the abscopal effect was tumor-specific and only occurred in wild-type mice that were treated with a combination of RT and Flt3-L, a growth factor that stimulates the production of dendritic cells (DCs). But no growth delay of secondary non-irradiated tumors has been observed in immunodeficient athymic mice or in wild-type mice treated with single dose of RT alone, further confirming that the abscopal effect was mediated by immune mechanisms [24].

However, although the abscopal effect of RT alone has been reported by a growing number of trials and cases, the overall occurrence rate was relatively low. This may be explained by the insufficiency of RT alone to overcome the immunoresistance of malignant tumors. Given that immunotherapy can reduce host's immune tolerance toward tumors, it is possible that the combination of RT and immunotherapy can amplify the anti-tumor immune response, which is more likely to cause the occurrence of an abscopal effect [25–27]. In fact, this synergistic anti-tumor effect has been investigated in many clinical studies (Table 1). Nevertheless, the mechanism of the abscopal effect is not yet completely understood. Therefore, in this review, we describe the anti-tumor effect of RT and immune checkpoint blockade and discuss several publications on the abscopal effect of combination therapy, primarily to define the potential predictors of this effect so that the appropriate patients could receive more appropriate treatment. In addition, the second aim of this review is to evaluate the optimal timing for coupling RT with immune checkpoint blockade and to determine the most effective dose and fractionation of RT in the context of combination treatments.

RT reprograms the tumor microenvironment

Under the selective pressure of the immune system, cancer cells have evolved a series of immune resistance mechanisms to escape the elimination of the anti-tumor immune responses, which is known as immunoediting [28, 29]. Some tumors lack the appropriate inflammatory cytokines and chemokines to attract immune cells, such as DCs, macrophages, and cytotoxic T cells, to the tumor

site, and the expression of immunosuppressive ligands and death ligands inhibits the function and the activation of T cells. In addition, the downregulation of adhesion molecules, such as vascular cell adhesion molecule 1 (VCAM1) and intercellular adhesion molecule 1 (ICAM1), leads to an enhancement of a tumor vasculature barrier that inhibits T cell arrest and transmigration. Along with other immunosuppressive factors, such as the existence of inhibitory immune cells and the downregulation of the major histocompatibility complex (MHC), these complex interaction mechanisms contribute to cancer cell escape [30, 31]. However, although these immune escape mechanisms lead to the growth and invasion of tumors, the immune system can still recognize and clear tumor cells, and interventions such as RT that can promote the release of tumor neoantigens may potentially lead to effective immune responses and cancer control. Importantly, under certain conditions, RT can reprogram the anti-immunologic tumor microenvironment, making it more conducive for antigen-presenting cells (APCs) and T cells to recruit and function, thereby inducing tumor cells to be recognized and eradicated more easily by the immune system.

Radiation-induced release of cytokines and chemokines

Localized radiation induces a burst release of cytokines and chemokines, giving rise to an inflammatory tumor microenvironment. These factors are secreted by irradiated tumor cells and other cells such as fibroblasts, myeloid cells, and macrophages. Various types of cytokines and chemokines play different roles in modulating the immune response, either pro- or anti-immunogenic, and maintain a net balance in the tumor milieu.

Radiation-induced interferons (IFNs), which represent the main effector molecules of the anti-tumor immune response, play a significant role in the therapeutic effect of RT. The induction of type I IFN by RT is essential for the activation and function of DCs and T cells, which, in turn, is responsible for the release of IFN-γ and tumor control [32, 33]. IFN-γ (type II IFN) acts on tumor cells to induce the upregulation of VCAM-1 and MHC-I expression, thereby enhancing the presentation of tumor antigens [34]. Indeed, type I IFN non-responsive mice showed an abolished anti-tumor effect of RT, and an exogenous increase in type I IFN could mimic the therapeutic effect of RT on tumor regression [32]. The production of type I IFN after irradiation is mediated by the stimulator of interferon genes (STING) and its upstream cyclic guanosine monophosphate-adenosine monophosphate synthase (cGAS) signaling pathways by sensing cancer cell-derived cytosolic DNA [35]. This process can be detected in both cancer cells and in infiltrating DCs [36]. However, high-dose radiation, specifically a single dose above a threshold ranging from 12 to 18 Gy, would

Table 1 Some related clinical studies of RT combined with immunotherapy

Authors	Years	Tumors	Numbers of cases	Immunotherapy	RT	Sequence of RT and immunotherapy	Occurrence of abscopal effect
Roger et al. [157]	2018	Melanoma	25	Anti-PD-1 (pembrolizumab, 2 mg/kg/3 weeks or nivolumab, 3 mg/kg/2 weeks)	26 Gy/3–5 fractions	Concurrent and post-radiation	Observed
Formenti et al. [135]	2018	Metastatic breast cancer	23	Anti-TGFβ (fresolimumab, 1 mg/kg/3 weeks or 10 mg/kg/3 weeks)	22.5 Gy/3 fractions	Concurrent	Observed
Rodríguez-Ruiz et al. [136]	2018	Advanced cancer	15	DC vaccination and TLR-3 agonist	Stereotactic ablative RT	Concurrent	Observed
Aboudaram et al. [130]	2017	Melanoma	17	Anti-PD-1 (pembrolizumab, 2 mg/kg/3 weeks or nivolumab, 3 mg/kg/3 weeks)	30 Gy/10 fractions	Concurrent	Observed
Theurich et al. [158]	2016	Melanoma	45	Anti-CTLA-4 (ipilimumab, 3 mg/kg/3 weeks)	SBRT	Concurrent and post-radiation	Observed
Koller et al. [119]	2016	Melanoma	70	Anti-CTLA-4 (ipilimumab, 3 mg/kg/3 weeks)	Conventional external beam radiation and stereotactic radiosurgery	Concurrent	Observed
Twyman-Saint et al. [145]	2015	Melanoma	22	Anti-CTLA-4 (ipilimumab)	Lung/bone 8 Gy × 2 or 8 Gy × 3 Liver/subcutaneous 6 Gy × 2 or 6 Gy × 3	RT before ipilimumab	Observed
Golden et al. [107]	2015	Metastatic solid tumors	41	GM-CSF (125 µg/m²/2 weeks)	35 Gy/10 fractions	Concurrent	Observed
Grimaldi et al. [118]	2014	Melanoma	21	Anti-CTLA-4 (ipilimumab, 3 mg/kg/3 weeks)	RT of brain metastasis or extracranial sites	RT after ipilimumab	Observed
Hwang et al. [159]	2018	Metastatic lung cancer	164	Anti-PD-1/PD-L1	Thoracic RT	RT before or after immunotherapy	Non-observed
Shaverdian et al. [129]	2017	NSCLC	97	Anti-PD-1 (pembrolizumab, 2 mg/kg/3 weeks, 10 mg/kg/3 weeks, or 10 mg/kg/3 weeks)	Extracranial radiotherapy and thoracic radiotherapy	Ipilimumab after RT	Non-observed
Kropp et al. [160]	2016	Melanoma	16	Anti-CTLA-4 (ipilimumab, 3 mg/kg/3 weeks)	SBRT	RT after ipilimumab	Non-observed
Levy et al. [133]	2016	Metastatic tumors	10	Anti-PD-L1 (durvalumab, 10 mg/kg/3 weeks)	28 Gy/5 fractions (median)	Concurrent	Non-observed
Kwon et al. [121]	2014	Castration-resistant prostate cancer	799	Anti-CTLA-4 (ipilimumab, 10 mg/kg/3 weeks)	8 Gy/target bone lesion	Ipilimumab after RT	Non-observed
Slovin et al. [120]	2013	Castration-resistant prostate cancer	50	Anti-CTLA-4 (ipilimumab, 10 mg/kg/3 weeks)	8 Gy/target bone lesion	Concurrent	Non-observed

RT radiotherapy, *NSCLC* non-small cell lung cancer, *GM-CSF* granulocyte-macrophage colony-stimulating factor, *SBRT* stereotactic body radiotherapy

induce upregulation of the three prime repair exonuclease 1 (Trex 1) in tumor cells. Trex 1 is a DNA nuclease which can degrade cytoplasmic DNA and in turn preclude the induction of type I IFN mediated by the activation of the cGAS-STING pathway, demonstrating the radiation dose dependency of the activation of type I IFN signaling [37, 38].

Transforming growth factor beta (TGFβ), acting as a major immunosuppressive factor, is also released and activated during RT [39]. This radiation-induced pleiotropic cytokine is important in regulating tissue homeostasis in the tumor microenvironment that inhibits the immune response by reducing the antigen-presenting ability of DCs and the activation of effector T cells [40]. In addition, TGFβ also causes radioresistance of tumor cells and reduces their radiosensitivity [41]. Taken together, the RT-mediated release of TGFβ promotes tumorigenesis and metastasis and leads to poor clinical outcomes for patients [42].

The release of other radiation-induced cytokines in the tumor microenvironment also influences the delicate balance between immune clearance and immune tolerance. For instance, the induction of interleukin-6 (IL-6), IL-10, and colony stimulating factor 1 (CSF-1) contributes to the proliferation and invasion of tumor cells and thereby displays a pro-tumorigenic role [43–46]. In contrast, the secretion of pro-inflammatory IL-1β enhances the anti-tumor immune response [47, 48]. Furthermore, the differential expression of RT-induced chemokines determines the type of leukocyte infiltration in the tumor microenvironment. For example, the production of CXC-motif chemokine ligand 12 (CXCL12) results in chemotaxis of pro-tumorigenic CD11b+ myeloid-derived cells [49], whereas the upregulation of CXCL9, CXCL10, and CXCL16 can attract anti-tumor effector T cells [50–52]. These conflicting mechanisms reflect the complexity of the tumor microenvironment.

Radiation-induced infiltration of leukocytes

The radiation-induced release of inflammatory cytokines and chemokines increases tumor infiltration by various leukocytes including not only leukocytes that enhance anti-tumor immune responses, such as DCs, effector T cells, and natural killer (NK) cells [53–55], but also immunosuppressive cells such as regulatory T cells (Treg cells) and CD11b+ cells, including myeloid-derived suppressor cells (MDSCs) and tumor-associated macrophages (TAMs) [56–59].

RT can induce the maturation of DCs and facilitate their migration to draining lymph nodes. These migratory tumor-associated DCs are important in the presentation of tumor antigens, which endogenously trigger the priming of antigen-specific effector T cells and their subsequent infiltration into tumors [53, 54]. In addition, radiation-induced

normalization of the vasculature allows for more efficient infiltration of effector T cells [60]. In fact, the presence of tumor-infiltrating T cells has been shown to correlate with better clinical outcomes in patients with a variety of cancers such as colorectal cancer, ovarian cancer, and breast cancer [61–63]. In addition, NK cell-mediated cytotoxicity also plays a significant role in eliminating tumor cells, which can be enhanced by RT since radiation increases the expression of tumor ligands for NK cell-activating receptors, such as NKG2D and NKp30 [64–66].

Treg cells are a special type of CD4+ T cells, and they play a key role in maintaining tumor immune tolerance. In the tumor microenvironment, accumulated Treg cells can secrete relative immunosuppressive cytokines such as TGFβ and IL-10, which impair the antigen-presenting function of DCs and the activation of effector T cells. In addition, Treg cells can also promote tumor angiogenesis and enhance MDSCs to exert their immunosuppressive function, eventually leading to tumor progression [67]. MDSCs are heterogeneous myeloid cells consisting of two major subsets: granulocytic MDSC (G-MDSC) and monocytic MDSC (M-MDSC) [68, 69]. Both populations contribute to tumor progression not only by their negative regulatory effects on the immune system but also by promoting tumor cell invasion and metastasis [70]. Many studies have reported the presence of increased numbers of Treg cells and MDSCs after RT in the tumor microenvironment, which is associated with poor prognosis in cancer patients [56, 57, 71].

Macrophages are another type of leukocyte that can infiltrate the tumor microenvironment. They can be described by two phenotypes, M1 and M2 macrophages, that have different functions [72]. The classical activation of M1 macrophages can induce the release of pro-inflammatory cytokines such as IL-12 and tumor necrosis factor (TNF) and play a role in killing tumor cells. In contrast, M2 macrophages act as anti-immunogenic cells that express anti-inflammatory cytokines such as IL-10 and TGFβ, which subsequently inhibit the function of effector T cells and favor tumor progression [73]. Indeed, most TAMs are tumor-promoting M2 macrophages [74]. Interestingly, in a pancreatic tumor model, Klug et al. have reported that low-dose irradiation could reprogram the differentiation of TAMs to an M1 phenotype and enhance anti-tumor immunity [75]. Further studies are required to elucidate the effect of RT on TAMs.

Radiation-induced increased susceptibility of tumor cells

RT can also increase the susceptibility of tumor cells to immune-mediated tumor rejection. Upregulation of MHC-I molecules after RT has been observed in many studies. For example, Reits et al. observed that ionizing radiation, particularly at higher doses (10–26 Gy), could enhance the expression of MHC-I in a dose-dependent manner in both in vitro and in vivo studies, which increased the presentation of tumor antigens and rendered tumor cells more susceptible to T cell attack [76]. In addition, RT can induce the expression of Fas and ICAM-1 on tumor cells, rendering them more sensitive to T cell-mediated lysis, which can be blocked by the administration of anti-FasL [77]. Nevertheless, RT can also upregulate the expression of negative immune checkpoint ligands such as programmed death-ligand 1 (PD-L1) and impair the anti-tumor immune responses of effector T cells [78, 79]. Therefore, the influence of RT on the tumor microenvironment is very complex because of its dual effects on the host immune system. These opposing mechanisms for radiation are summarized in Table 2.

Anti-tumor immune effects of RT: from local to abscopal

RT generates in situ vaccination

RT can promote a special functional type of cell apoptosis named immunogenic cell death (ICD) [80–82] and can stimulate antigen-specific, adaptive immunity by some undetermined mechanisms [83]. ICD leads to subsequent anti-tumor immune responses including the release of tumor antigens by irradiated tumor cells, the cross-presentation of tumor-derived antigens to T cells by APCs, and the migration of effector T cells from the lymph nodes to distant tumor sites. These processes illustrate that irradiated tumors can act as an in situ vaccination [82, 84, 85].

Due to the stress response that is induced by irradiation, the dying tumor cells experience a series of

subtle changes involving the pre-apoptotic translocation of endoplasmic reticulum (ER) proteins, such as calreticulin (CRT) [82, 86], from the ER to the cell surface, and the release of damage-associated molecular pattern molecules (DAMPs) [87], such as high-mobility group box 1 (HMGB1) [88] and adenosine triphosphate (ATP) [89, 90] from the cytoplasm of stressed tumor cells to the outside environment. CRT, acting as an "eat-me" signal, promotes the uptake of irradiated tumor cells by APCs such as DCs and phagocytic cells [86, 90–92]. The release of DAMPs, including HMGB1 and ATP, is another characteristic change that occurs during cell death after exposure to radiation [93, 94]. Acting as a "find-me" signal to recruit APCs [95], ATP can attract monocytes and DCs to tumors by a purinergic receptor P2X7-dependent pathway and promote the secretion of pro-inflammatory cytokines such as IL-1β and IL-18 [96, 97]. HMGB1 is a histone chromatin-binding protein [98], and when it binds to the surface pattern recognition receptors (PRRs), such as Toll-like receptor (TLR) 2 and TLR 4, it exerts its potential pro-inflammatory effect [94]. This interaction drives downstream inflammation responses and promotes the processing and presentation of tumor antigens by host APCs [94, 98]. Additionally, HMGB1 can also facilitate the maturation of DCs, thereby enabling them to present antigens efficiently to T cells, a process that is mediated by type I IFNs [57]. As mentioned before, the production of type I IFNs depends on the activation of the cGAS-STING pathway by sensing cancer cell-derived DNA and can be impaired by the DNA nuclease Trex 1 [37, 38]. All of these processes contribute to the effective presentation of tumor antigens by DCs and exert potent immunomodulatory effects.

DCs interact with tumor antigens and then migrate to the lymph nodes where they present these antigens to T cells, a process that is mediated by the MHC pathway via recognition by the T cell receptor (TCR). Furthermore, the basic leucine zipper ATF-like transcription factor 3 (BATF3)-dependent DC subset has been recently shown to be essential for the cross-priming of CD8+ T cells, which are key effectors in anti-tumor immunity. These DCs can take up tumor antigens effectively and introduce these antigens by way of the MHC class I cross-presenting pathway. Indeed, Batf3$^{-/-}$ mice exhibit an impaired ability to cross-prime cytotoxic T lymphocytes against tumor antigens [99, 100].

However, antigen-MHC complex interactions alone are insufficient to lead to the activation of T cells; other co-stimulatory signals such as CD80, CD40 L, and CD28 are also required [84]. After activation by multiple signals, T cells, especially the CD8+ T cells that play a major role in the anti-tumor immune response, are activated and begin to propagate. As a result, activated effector T cells exit the lymph nodes and home to tumors to exert their effect of

Table 2 The dual effects of RT on tumor microenvironment

Effect of RT	Pro-immunogenic	Anti-immunogenic
Cytokine secretion	IFN I	TGF-β
	IFN II	CSF-1
	IL-1β	IL-6
	IL-18	IL-10
Chemokine secretion	CXCL9	CXCL12
	CXCL10	
	CXCL16	
Leukocyte infiltration	DCs	MDSCs
	Effector T cells	Treg cells
	M1 macrophages	M2 macrophages
Signal molecule expression	MHC-I	PD-L1
	STING	Trex 1
	Fas	

RT radiotherapy, *IFN* interferon, *IL* interleukin, *TGF* transforming growth factor, *CSF* colony-stimulating factor, *CXCL* CXC-motif chemokine ligand, *DCs* dendritic cells, *MDSCs* myeloid-derived suppressor cells, *Treg* regulatory T lymphocytes, *MHC* major histocompatibility complex, *STING* stimulator of interferon genes, *Trex* three prime repair exonuclease, *PD-L1* programmed cell death-ligand 1

killing tumor cells [101]. This mechanism can be used to explain the regression of distant metastatic tumor lesions combined with the locally irradiated tumors (Fig. 1). In fact, following the first report of the abscopal effect [15], the regression of distant tumor lesions after RT had been documented by many case reports of several malignant tumors such as melanoma, breast cancer, and lung cancer [18, 102, 103]. However, the overall incidence of the abscopal effect is low, and only 46 clinical cases of the abscopal effect due to RT alone have been reported from 1969 to 2014 [104]. This rare phenomenon can be explained by the insufficiency of RT alone to overcome the established immune tolerance mechanisms of tumor cells. Currently, many studies have shown that combining RT with immunotherapy can effectively overcome tumor immunosuppression and boost abscopal response rates compared with the use of RT alone [105–107].

Immunotherapy enhances the systemic anti-tumor response of RT

CTLA-4 and CTLA-4 blockade

As previously mentioned, the activation of T cells requires an interaction between the TCR and a peptide-MHC complex with APCs, as well as a dynamic balance between the co-stimulatory and inhibitory signals that regulate the effectiveness of the immune response. Among them, the binding of CD28 on T cells with the B7 family ligands CD80 and CD86 that are located on APCs is the dominating co-stimulatory signal. Because another trans-membrane receptor, cytotoxic T lymphocyte-associated antigen 4 (CTLA-4), can also combine with CD80/86, it has been considered as one of the major negative immunomodulatory receptors that attenuate T cell activation [108–110] (Fig. 1). Therefore, the blockade of CTLA-4 is considered to be a promising immunotherapeutic method for enhancing the anti-tumor immune response, and a series of preclinical and clinical trials have demonstrated the anti-tumor effect of the CTLA-4 blockade in solid tumors, largely in patients with malignant melanoma. For example, two clinical trials have demonstrated that treatment of patients with advanced melanoma using anti-CTLA-4 (ipilimumab) could lead to durable responses and improve the overall survival of patients [111, 112]. Furthermore, patients with ovarian cancer, prostate cancer, and renal cell carcinoma could also benefit from anti-CTLA-4 immunotherapy [113–115].

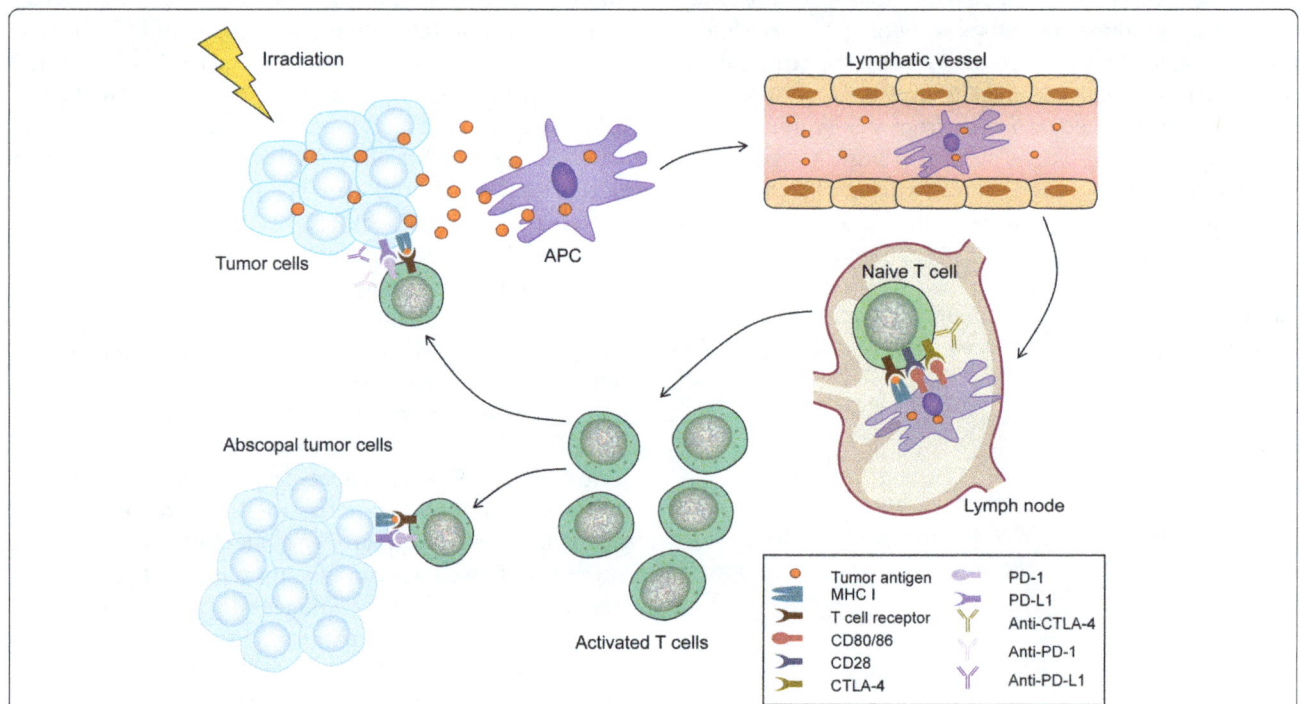

Fig. 1 Mechanism of the abscopal effect. Radiotherapy (RT) can lead to immunogenic cell death and the release of tumor antigens by irradiated tumor cells. These neoantigens are taken up by antigen-presenting cells (APCs), such as dendritic cells (DCs) and phagocytic cells. The APCs interact with tumor antigens and then migrate to the lymph nodes where they present antigens to T cells, a process that is mediated by the MHC pathway and other co-stimulatory signals, such as CD80 and CD28. After activation by multiple signals, T cells, especially the CD8+ T cells, are activated and begin to propagate. As a result, activated effector T cells exit the lymph nodes and home to tumors, including primary tumors and non-irradiated tumor metastases, to exert their effect of killing tumor cells. However, cytotoxic T lymphocyte-associated antigen 4 (CTLA-4) competitively combines with CD80/86 and inhibits the activation of T cells. Following T cell activation, programmed cell death 1 (PD-1) receptors that are expressed on the T cell surface bind primarily to programmed death-ligand 1 (PD-L1) and inhibit immune responses. The administration of immune checkpoint blockades of CTLA-1, PD-1, and PD-L1 can enhance the anti-tumor immunity of RT

However, the anti-tumor effect of CTLA-4 blockade alone is limited, and monotherapy may lead to serious autoimmune-related side effects such as dermatitis, colitis, hepatitis, and hypophysitis [116]. Given that blocking CTLA-4 could enhance the activation of T cells and increase the ratio of CD8+ T cells to Treg cells [117], which can strengthen the in situ vaccination effect of RT [110], the combined application of ipilimumab with RT has been increasingly valued by researchers and clinicians. In fact, this combination treatment strategy has achieved encouraging results in studies in both mice and humans and has been approved for the treatment of metastatic melanoma by the US Food and Drug Administration [111]. In a retrospective study, Grimaldi et al. documented a promising outcome for advanced melanoma patients treated with ipilimumab followed by RT. Among 21 patients, 11 patients (52%) experienced the abscopal effect, including 9 that had a partial response (PR) and 2 that had stable disease (SD). The median overall survival (OS) for patients with the abscopal effect was 22.4 months vs. 8.3 months for patients who did not experience this effect [118]. Consistently, in another retrospective analysis, Koller et al. demonstrated that advanced melanoma patients who received ipilimumab in combination with concurrent RT had a significantly increased median OS and complete response rates compared to those who did not [119]. Additionally, in a phase I/II study, Slovin et al. compared ipilimumab monotherapy with ipilimumab combined with RT (single fraction of 8 Gy) for patients with metastatic castration-resistant prostate cancer (mCRPC). The outcome was positive, in that among the 10 patients who received combination therapy, 1 had a PR and 6 had SD, and this combined approach of CTLA-4 blockade and RT could lead to durable disease control of mCRPC [120].

However, the outcomes were not always positive. In a clinical phase III trial, Kwon et al. also investigated the benefit of combination therapy with ipilimumab and RT in patients with mCRPC. Surprisingly, there were no differences in the median OS for the ipilimumab group compared to the placebo group, although reductions in prostate-specific antigen (PSA) concentration and improved progression-free survival (PFS) with ipilimumab treatment have been observed [121]. Therefore, additional studies are required to address this undetermined synergistic anti-tumor activity of combining RT with CTLA-4 blockade.

PD-1/PD-L1 and PD-1/PD-L1 blockade

Another co-inhibitory molecule, the inhibitory immune receptor programmed cell death 1 (PD-1), is expressed on the plasma membranes of T cells, DCs, and NK cells. PD-1 interferes with T cell-mediated signaling primarily through interactions with its two cognate ligands, PD-L1 and PD-L2, which are expressed by tumor cells. In fact, the expression of PD-L1 is upregulated in tumor cells, and PD-1 ligation by PD-L1 mainly promotes T cell apoptosis and leads to the elimination of activated T cells, thereby protecting tumor cells from T cell recognition and elimination [122–125]. Importantly, the upregulation of PD-L1 can be observed in experimental mouse tumor models after exposure to hypofractionated RT, which plays a key role in the RT resistance mechanism of tumor cells [79]. Consequently, we can hypothesize that the combination of the PD-1/PD-L1 blockade and RT may overcome tumor immunosuppression and improve the systemic effect of RT (Fig. 1). In fact, anti-PD-1/PD-L1 monoclonal antibodies (mAbs) have shown promising results in the treatment of non-small cell lung cancer (NSCLC), melanoma, and kidney cancer [126]. Additionally, two immune checkpoint inhibitors of PD-1, pembrolizumab and nivolumab, were approved by the US Food and Drug Administration for clinical application in patients with metastatic melanoma who experienced disease progression after prior treatment [127, 128].

In a secondary analysis of the KEYNOTE-001 phase trial, Shaverdian et al. assessed 97 advanced NSCLC patients who were treated with pembrolizumab. Patients who previously received RT achieved a significantly longer PFS (hazard ratio [HR] 0.56, $p = 0.019$; median PFS 4.4 vs. 2.1 months) and OS (HR 0.58, $p = 0.026$; median OS 10.7 vs. 5.3 months) than patients who did not previously receive RT [129]. Similarly, in a retrospective collection of consecutive patients with metastatic melanoma and who received PD-1 immune checkpoint inhibitors, Aboudaram et al. compared the survival data, overall response rates, and acute and delayed toxicities between patients receiving concurrent irradiation (IR) or no irradiation (NIR). Among 59 patients who received PD-1 blockade, 17 received palliative RT with a mean dose of 30 Gy that were delivered in 10 fractions. The objective response rate, including complete and partial response rates, was significantly higher in the IR group versus the NIR group (64.7 vs. 33.3%, $p = 0.02$) after a 10-month median follow-up and one complete responder experienced an abscopal effect. The 6-month disease-free survival (DFS) and OS rates were marginally increased in the IR group versus the NIR group (64.7% vs. 49.7%, $p = 0.32$; 76.4% vs. 58.8%, $p = 0.42$, respectively). Furthermore, no additional side effects were observed in the IR group, and the combination treatment was well tolerated [130]. In addition, abscopal effects have also been reported in patients with other malignant tumors, such as lung adenocarcinoma and Hodgkin's lymphoma [131, 132]. However, in a single-center subset analysis from a phase I/II trial, Levy et al. reported that among 10 patients with metastatic tumors who received palliative local RT for 15 isolated lesions, the objective response (OR) rate was 60%

after concurrent palliative RT and anti-PD-L1 durvalumab. Surprisingly, no outfield or abscopal effects were observed [133]. Therefore, although there are many encouraging reports concerning the combination of RT and anti-PD-1/PD-L1 mAbs, the rate of occurrence of abscopal effects is still undetermined. It is of significance to identify those patients who are most likely to respond, and additional or ongoing trials will hopefully elucidate their characteristics.

Other agents

Granulocyte-macrophage colony-stimulating factor (GM-CSF) is a potent stimulator of DC differentiation, proliferation, and maturation and facilitates the presentation of tumor antigens after cell death caused by RT [134]. In a prospective study conducted by Golden et al., the enrolled subjects were patients who had stable or advanced metastatic solid tumors after receiving single-agent chemotherapy or hormone therapy and had three distant measurable lesions. These patients were treated with RT (35 Gy in 10 fractions) to one metastatic site along with concurrent GM-CSF (125 μg/m^2). In the space of 9 years, abscopal effects were observed in 11 of 41 accrued patients (specifically in 2 patients with thymic cancer, 4 with NSCLC, and 5 with breast cancer). In addition, the risk of death for patients without an abscopal effect was more than twice that of patients with it. This prospective clinical trial first demonstrated that an abscopal effect could provide patients with a better survival benefit and suggested a promising combination of RT with GM-CSF to establish an in-site anti-tumor vaccine [107].

Other immunotherapy modalities are still under investigation. Recently, Formenti et al. examined the role of anti-TGFβ therapeutics during RT to induce an abscopal effect in metastatic breast cancer patients. Fresolimumab, a TGFβ-blocking antibody, was administered in two doses, along with focal radiation of 22.5 Gy in three fractions. Although there was a general lack of abscopal effects, patients who received a higher fresolimumab dose had a significantly lower risk of death and a longer OS (median OS 16.00 vs. 7.57 months, $p = 0.039$) than those receiving a lower dose [135]. In addition, in another phase I clinical trial, Rodríguez-Ruiz et al. evaluated an intensive treatment modality in advanced cancer patients, which combined RT with two immune interventions, namely, intradermal DC vaccinations and intratumoral injections of Hiltonol, a TLR-3 agonist that can activate elements of both innate and adaptive immunity. The results demonstrated that this combined treatment was well tolerated, and one prostate cancer patient experienced an abscopal response [136]. Many other immunotherapeutic agents such as agonistic CD40 mAb and anti-galectin-1 may also boost abscopal effects by targeting different aspects of the immune-mediated response [137, 138]. In summary, combining these cancer immunotherapy modalities with standard-of-care chemoradiotherapy is a new frontier for future cancer treatment that may provide better efficacy. A brief summary of the representative ongoing clinical trials concerning the combination treatment of RT and immunotherapy is shown in Table 3.

Future directions to improve abscopal effects of RT

Optimal dose and fractionation of RT in abscopal effects

There are three dominant schemes of RT: conventional fractionation schemes (1.8~2.2 Gy/fraction, one fraction/day, 5 days/week for 3~7 weeks), hypofractionation including stereotactic radiosurgery (3~20 Gy/fraction, one fraction/day), and hyperfractionation (0.5~2.2 Gy/fraction, two fractions/day, 2~5 fractions/week for 2~4 weeks). The dose and fractionation of RT can influence its modulatory effects on the immune system, but it is worth noting that immunological effects of different regimens are unpredictable. Given that repetitive daily delivery of irradiation can kill migrating immune lymphocytes, Siva et al. believe that conventional fractionation schemes of RT are negative for radiation-induced anti-tumor immune responses. Their group also determined that single high-dose (12 Gy) RT did not deplete established immune effector cells such as CD8+ T cells and NK cells and that it might be much more efficient to kill tumor cells when combined with immunotherapy [139]. Indeed, compared with conventional modalities, RT with ablative high-dose per fractionation has been considered as a better treatment protocol to enhance the anti-tumor immune response [140]. Furthermore, in murine breast and colon cancer models, Dewan et al. showed that 5 × 6 Gy and 3 × 8 Gy protocols of RT were more effective in inducing immune-mediated abscopal effects than a single ablative dose of 20 Gy when combined with anti-CTLA-4 hamster mAbs 9H10 [141]. Similarly, in a murine melanoma model, Schaue et al. found that fractionated treatment with medium-size radiation doses of 7.5 Gy/fraction produced the best tumor control and anti-tumor immune responses [142]. Based on these experiences, many clinical trials aiming to evaluate the systematic anti-tumor effect of combinatorial immunotherapy and RT are designed with hypofractionated RT. It is encouraging that some of these studies have achieved satisfactory results and have observed the occurrence of abscopal effects. However, although larger doses per fraction may boost abscopal responses, other clinical studies did not achieve good outcomes, implying that abscopal effects are influenced by multiple factors (Table 1). Based on the dose and the fractionation of RT, an optimal threshold or range of doses is likely to exist. In a recent study, Vanpouille-Box et al. found that a radiation dose

Table 3 Representative ongoing clinical trials using CTLA-4/PD-1/PD-L1 inhibitors and RT for malignant tumors

ClinicalTrials.gov identifier	Phase	Conditions	Drug classification	Interventions	Sponsors
NCT01996202	Phase 1	Melanoma	CTLA-4 inhibitors	Ipilimumab with radiation therapy	Duke University
NCT02642809	Phase 1	EC	PD-1 inhibitors	Pembrolizumab with brachytherapy (16 Gy in 2 fractions)	Washington University School of Medicine
NCT02837263	Phase 1	Colorectal cancer	PD-1 inhibitors	Pembrolizumab with SBRT (40–60 Gy in 5 fractions)	University of Wisconsin, Madison
NCT02587455	Phase 1	Thoracic tumors	PD-1 inhibitors	Arm I: pembrolizumab with low-dose radiation therapy Arm II: pembrolizumab with high-dose radiation therapy	Royal Marsden NHS Foundation Trust
NCT03151447	Phase 1	TNBC	PD-L1 inhibitors	JS001 with SBRT	Fudan University
NCT02868632	Phase 1	Pancreatic cancer	PD-L1 and CTLA-4 inhibitors	Durvalumab or/and tremelimumab with SBRT (30 Gy in 5 fractions)	New York University School of Medicine
NCT03275597	Phase 1	NSCLC	PD-L1 and CTLA-4 inhibitors	Durvalumab and tremelimumab with SBRT (30–50 Gy in 5 fractions)	University of Wisconsin, Madison
NCT02239900	Phase 1/2	Liver cancer, lung cancer	CTLA-4 inhibitors	Ipilimumab with SBRT	M.D. Anderson Cancer Center
NCT03050554	Phase 1/2	NSCLC	PD-L1 inhibitors	Avelumab with SBRT (48 Gy in 4 fractions or 50 Gy in 5 fractions)	Andrew Sharabi
NCT02696993	Phase 1/2	Brain metastases (NSCLC)	PD-1 and CTLA-4 inhibitors	Arm I: nivolumab with stereotactic radiosurgery Arm II: nivolumab with whole brain radiation therapy Arm III: nivolumab and ipilimumab with stereotactic radiosurgeryArm IV: nivolumab and ipilimumab with whole brain radiation therapy	M.D. Anderson Cancer Center
NCT01970527	Phase 2	Melanoma	CTLA-4 inhibitors	Ipilimumab with SBRT	University of Washington
NCT02609503	Phase 2	Head and neck cancer	PD-1 inhibitors	Pembrolizumab with radiation therapy	UNC Lineberger Comprehensive Cancer Center
NCT02730130	Phase 2	Metastatic breast cancer	PD-1 inhibitors	Pembrolizumab with radiation therapy	Memorial Sloan Kettering Cancer Center
NCT02992912	Phase 2	Metastatic tumors	PD-L1 inhibitors	Atezolizumab with SBRT (45 Gy in 3 fractions)	Gustave Roussy, Cancer Campus, Grand Paris
NCT03122509	Phase 2	Metastatic colorectal cancer	PD-L1 and CTLA-4 inhibitors	Tremelimumab and durvalumab with radiation therapy	Memorial Sloan Kettering Cancer Center
NCT02888743	Phase 2	Colorectal cancer and NSCLC	PD-L1 and CTLA-4 inhibitors	Arm I: tremelimumab and durvalumab Arm II: tremelimumab and durvalumab with high-dose radiation therapy Arm III: tremelimumab and durvalumab with low-dose radiation therapy	National Cancer Institute (NCI)
NCT02701400	Phase 2	Recurrent SCLC	PD-L1 and CTLA-4 inhibitors	Arm I: tremelimumab and durvalumab Arm II: tremelimumab and durvalumab with SBRT	Emory University

Table 3 Representative ongoing clinical trials using CTLA-4/PD-1/PD-L1 inhibitors and RT for malignant tumors *(Continued)*

ClinicalTrials.gov identifier	Phase	Conditions	Drug classification	Interventions	Sponsors
NCT02617589	Phase 3	Brain Cancer	PD-1 inhibitors	Arm I: nivolumab with radiation therapy Arm II: temozolomide with radiation therapy	Bristol-Myers Squibb
NCT02768558	Phase 3	NSCLC	PD-1 inhibitors	Cisplatin and etoposide plus radiation followed by nivolumab	RTOG Foundation, Inc.

SCLC small cell lung cancer, *NSCLC* non-small cell lung cancer, *TNBC* triple-negative breast cancer, *EC* esophageal cancer, *SBRT* stereotactic body radiation therapy

above a threshold of 10–12 Gy per fraction could attenuate the immunogenicity of cancer cells because of the induced upregulation of the DNA nuclease Trex 1, which can degrade cytoplasmic DNA and inhibit immune activation [37]. Thus, researchers should take these different data into a careful consideration in order to develop an optimal dose and fractionation scheme for RT in the context of radioimmunotherapy combinations to induce anti-tumor abscopal effects efficiently.

Combination time window for RT and immunotherapy
The optimal schedule for the administration of RT relative to the immune checkpoint inhibitors is currently unclear. Should immune inhibitors of checkpoints be given concomitantly or sequentially with RT, and in which order? This time window may significantly influence the therapeutic anti-tumor response of this combination treatment.

Indeed, different combinatorial schedules have been evaluated in some preclinical studies. For instance, in mouse colon carcinoma models, in which a fractionated RT cycle of 2 Gy × 5 fractions was administered, Dovedi et al. evaluated three different schedules including the administration of anti-PD-L1 mAbs on day 1 of the RT cycle (schedule A), day 5 of the cycle (schedule B), or 7 days after the completion of RT (schedule C). Interestingly, both schedule A and schedule B achieved increased OS compared with RT alone, and there was no significant difference in the OS between these two subgroups. In contrast, sequential treatments with delayed administration of anti-PD-L1 mAbs at 7 days after RT completion (schedule C) were completely ineffective for improving the OS when compared with RT alone [143]. Similarly, in a murine breast model, Dewan et al. showed that the administration of anti-CTLA-4 mAbs at 2 days before or on the day of RT achieved a better therapeutic efficacy when compared with the delayed administration of mAbs at 2 days after RT [141]. Furthermore, some clinical case reports also imply the optimal time window of combining RT with immunotherapy. Golden et al. reported an abscopal effect in a treatment-refractory lung cancer patient treated with four three-weekly cycles of ipilimumab (3 mg/kg) and concurrent RT [144]. In

addition, in a melanoma patient, Stamell et al. also observed an abscopal effect after combining ipilimumab with stereotactic RT concurrently [17]. Similarly, in the published clinical studies of radioimmunotherapy combinations, abscopal effects were mostly reported in patients who received RT while receiving concomitant immunotherapy (Table 1). Given the experience of preclinical and clinical trials in which abscopal effects were observed, although there is no consensus yet, the administration of immunotherapy initiated before or at the time of delivering RT may be preferred. However, in a phase I clinical trial of 22 advanced melanoma patients, Twyman-Saint et al. found that hypofractionated radiation followed by a treatment with the anti-CTLA4 antibody ipilimumab could also lead to partial responses in the non-irradiated lesions [145]. In addition, the potential toxicity of combination therapy, especially combinatorial radioimmunotherapy with concurrent regimens, limits their clinical application and should be investigated in further studies.

Biomarkers for predicting the abscopal effect
Although a combination of immunotherapy and RT has achieved promising results in multiple solid tumors, not all of the patients experienced an abscopal effect. Therefore, it is necessary to identify efficient and effective biomarkers that can predict abscopal responses in patients who received combinatorial therapeutic regimens of immunotherapy and RT. In addition, validated biomarkers would be helpful in selecting suitable patients, identifying optimal therapeutic strategies, and predicting treatment responses.

As a tumor suppressor gene, p53 plays an important role in regulating the proliferation, apoptosis, and DNA repair of tumor cells, and its encoded protein P53 is a transcription factor that influences the onset of the cell cycle. As a guardian of the genome, p53 can inhibit the growth of tumors by obstructing the replication of damaged DNA, which acts as a major culprit inducing the abnormal proliferation of tumor cells [146]. However, the probability of a p53 mutation is greater than 50% among patients with malignant tumors, and a mutant p53 would lose its ability to inhibit the proliferation of tumor cells. In recent years, many studies have revealed that the status of p53 could regulate the abscopal anti-tumor effect of RT. In a mouse model system, Strigari et al. demonstrated growth inhibition of non-irradiated wild-type p53 tumors after irradiation of 20 Gy or 10 Gy. However, no significant tumor growth delay was observed in non-irradiated p53-null tumors regardless of the dose delivered [147]. Consistently, Camphausen et al. observed a similar result, in that the abscopal anti-tumor effect was observed neither in p53-null mice nor in mice in which p53 was inhibited by pifithrin-α, a drug that can block the p53 pathway [148]. Therefore, we can hypothesize that p53-dependent signals might be responsible for the systemic anti-tumor effect of RT, and an evaluation of the status of p53 in vivo might be used to predict the possibility of the occurrence of abscopal effects for cancer patients treated with RT regimens and thus provide better treatment administration.

In the Grimaldi et al. report on advanced melanoma, an abscopal effect was observed in 11 patients who were treated with ipilimumab followed by RT. Importantly, all patients who achieved an immune-related abscopal effect displayed a local response to RT. Thus, it is reasonable to speculate that a local response to RT could be of use to prognosticate abscopal effects. Furthermore, patients with an abscopal effect had a significantly higher median absolute lymphocyte count (ALC) before RT than those without an abscopal response, implying that lymphocyte counts preceding RT might be another patient parameter that can predict the occurrence of the abscopal effect. Nevertheless, given the limited number of patients in this retrospective study, further investigations are required to evaluate the predictive role of the local response to RT and the ALC on systemic abscopal effects [118].

Calreticulin expression may act as another potential marker to predict the response to combination treatments. As mentioned above, the radiation-induced translocation of calreticulin would promote the uptake of irradiated tumor cells by APCs and enhance the killing effect of T cells [86]. Furthermore, knockdown of calreticulin would impair the T cell recognition of tumor cells [149]. Therefore, the expression of calreticulin after RT implies susceptibility of tumor cells to T cell killing and can be used as a biomarker for the response to immunotherapy and RT. In addition, a recent preclinical study indicated that Trex 1 can be used as a potential biomarker to guide the administration of an optimal dose and fractionation of RT, which would be helpful in providing a better combination treatment strategy that might overcome the immunosuppression of tumor cells and facilitate the occurrence of abscopal effects [37, 38].

In addition, other biomarkers for immunotherapy have also been widely investigated. For instance, the tumor mutation burden (TMB) is closely related to the anti-cancer effect of immune checkpoint inhibitors, and patients with a high mutation burden experienced a long-term clinical benefit [150–152]. The PD-L1 expression can serve as a potential biomarker for the prediction of response to immunotherapies that target PD-1/PD-L1 [153–156]. However, a predictive role for them in the systemic abscopal effects of combinatorial immunotherapy and RT has yet to be defined. Furthermore, no specific sensitive biomarkers have been determined that can exclusively predict the abscopal responses in patients who experienced combined treatment regimens, and this is still an active area that needs to be further investigated.

Conclusion

The abscopal effects of RT have been extensively reported in preclinical and clinical studies, and irradiated tumor cell death can stimulate anti-tumor adaptive immunity by promoting the release of tumor antigens and the cross-presentation of tumor-derived antigens to T cells. However, it is difficult for RT alone to overcome the immunoresistance of malignant tumors. With the development of cancer immunotherapy, especially immune checkpoint inhibitors, the abscopal effect of RT has become more meaningful, since the in situ vaccination that is generated by RT can be substantially potentiated by immunotherapy. Exploiting the synergistic anti-tumor effect of these two treatments is encouraging because of its effective potential to improve the OS and PFS of patients with malignant tumors. However, many challenges remain for this combination treatment, including the determination of optimal dose/fractionation schemes for RT, the administration of optimal time points for these two treatment modalities, and the identification of relative biomarkers for the prediction of treatment efficacy. These challenges need to be addressed in future preclinical and clinical trials. In addition, translating these preclinical data into relevant and clinically efficient treatments and developing evidence-based consensus guidelines for RT and immunotherapy will also be required.

Abbreviations

ALC: Absolute lymphocyte count; APCs: Antigen-presenting cells; ATP: Adenosine triphosphate; BATF3: Basic leucine zipper ATF-like transcription factor 3; cGAS: Cyclic guanosine monophosphate-adenosine monophosphate synthase; CRT: Calreticulin; CSF-1: Colony stimulating factor 1; CTLA-4: Cytotoxic T lymphocyte-associated antigen 4; CXCL12: CXC-motif chemokine ligand 12; DAMPs: Damage-associated molecular pattern molecules; DCs: Dendritic cells; DFS: Disease-free survival; DNA: Deoxyribonucleic acid; ER: Endoplasmic reticulum; GM-CSF: Granulocyte-macrophage colony-stimulating factor; G-MDSC: Granulocytic MDSC; Gy: Gray; HMGB1: High-mobility group box 1; ICAM1: Intercellular adhesion molecule 1; ICD: Immunogenic cell death; IFNs: Interferons; IL-6: Interleukin-6; IR: Irradiation; mAbs: Monoclonal antibodies; mCRPC: Metastatic castration-resistant prostate cancer; MDSCs: Myeloid-derived suppressor cells; MHC: Major histocompatibility complex; M-MDSC: Monocytic MDSC; NIR: No irradiation; NK cells: Natural killer cells; NSCLC: Non-small cell lung cancer; OR: Objective response; OS: Overall survival; PD-1: Programmed cell death 1; PD-L1: Programmed death-ligand 1; PD-L2: Programmed death-ligand 2; PFS: Progression-free survival; PR: Partial response; PRRs: Pattern recognition receptors; PSA: Prostate-specific antigen; RT: Radiotherapy; SD: Stable disease; STING: Stimulator of interferon genes; TAMs: Tumor-associated macrophages; TBI: Total body irradiation; TCR: T cell receptor; TGFβ: Transforming growth factor beta; TLR: Toll-like receptor; TMB: Tumor mutation burden; TNF: Tumor necrosis factor; Treg cells: Regulatory T cells; Trex 1: Three prime repair exonuclease 1; VCAM1: Vascular cell adhesion molecule 1

Acknowledgements

The authors would such as to express their great thanks to the Innovation Project of the Shandong Academy of Medical Science.

Funding

This work was supported by the Key Research and Development Program of Shandong Province (grant numbers 2016GSF201148 and 2016CYJS01A03).

Authors' contributions

HZ and JMY designed the study. YL drafted the manuscript. YL, YPD, LK, and FS coordinated, edited, and finalized the drafting of the manuscript. All authors read and approved the final manuscript.

Consent for publication

Not applicable.

Competing interests

The authors declare that they have no competing interests.

References

1. Möller TR, Einhorn N, Lindholm C, Ringborg U, Svensson H. Radiotherapy and cancer care in Sweden. Acta Oncol. 2009;42:366–75.
2. Delaney G, Jacob S, Featherstone C, Barton M. The role of radiotherapy in cancer treatment: estimating optimal utilization from a review of evidence-based clinical guidelines. Cancer. 2005;104:1129–37.
3. Jaffray DA. Image-guided radiotherapy: from current concept to future perspectives. Nat Rev Clin Oncol. 2012;9:688–99.
4. Rupnow BA, Murtha AD, Alarcon RM, Giaccia AJ, Knox SJ. Direct evidence that apoptosis enhances tumor responses to fractionated radiotherapy. Cancer Res. 1998;58:1779–84.
5. Dewey WC, Ling CC, Meyn RE. Radiation-induced apoptosis: relevance to radiotherapy. Int J Radiat Oncol Biol Phys. 1995;33:781–96.
6. Eriksson D, Stigbrand T. Radiation-induced cell death mechanisms. Tumour Biol. 2010;31:363–72.
7. Ross G. Induction of cell death by radiotherapy. Endocrine Related Cancer. 1999;6:41–4.
8. Blomgren H, Glas U, Melén B, Wasserman J. Blood lymphocytes after radiation therapy of mammary carcinoma. Acta Radiol Ther Phys Biol. 1974; 13:185–200.
9. Campian JL, Ye X, Brock M, Grossman SA. Treatment-related lymphopenia in patients with stage III non-small-cell lung cancer. Cancer Investig. 2013;31: 183–8.
10. Harisiadis L, Kopelson G, Chang CH. Lymphopenia caused by cranial irradiation in children receiving craniospinal radiotherapy. Cancer. 1977;40: 1102–8.
11. Hill-Kayser CE, Plastaras JP, Tochner Z, Glatstein E. TBI during BM and SCT: review of the past, discussion of the present and consideration of future directions. Bone Marrow Transplant. 2011;46:475–84.
12. Stone HB, Peters LJ, Milas L. Effect of host immune capability on

radiocurability and subsequent transplantability of a murine fibrosarcoma. J Natl Cancer Inst. 1979;63:1229–35.
13. Lee Y, Auh SL, Wang Y, Burnette B, Wang Y, Meng Y, et al. Therapeutic effects of ablative radiation on local tumor require CD8+ T cells: changing strategies for cancer treatment. Blood. 2009;114:589–95.
14. Holecek MJ, Harwood AR. Radiotherapy of Kaposi's sarcoma. Cancer. 1978; 41:1733–8.
15. Mole RH. Whole body irradiation—radiobiology or medicine? Br J Radiol. 1953;26:234–41.
16. Poleszczuk JT, Luddy KA, Prokopiou S, Robertson-Tessi M, Moros EG, Fishman M, et al. Abscopal benefits of localized radiotherapy depend on activated T-cell trafficking and distribution between metastatic lesions. Cancer Res. 2016;76:1009–18.
17. Stamell EF, Wolchok JD, Gnjatic S, Lee NY, Brownell I. The abscopal effect associated with a systemic anti-melanoma immune response. Int J Radiat Oncol Biol Phys. 2013;85:293–5.
18. Postow MA, Callahan MK, Barker CA, Yamada Y, Yuan J, Kitano S, et al. Immunologic correlates of the abscopal effect in a patient with melanoma. N Engl J Med. 2012;366:925–31.
19. Antoniades J, Brady LW, Lightfoot DA. Lymphangiographic demonstration of the abscopal effect in patients with malignant lymphomas. Int J Radiat Oncol Biol Phys. 1977;2:141–7.
20. Robins HI, Buchon JA, Varanasi VR, Weinstein AB. The abscopal effect: demonstration in lymphomatous involvement of kidneys. Med Pediatr Oncol. 1981;9:473–6.
21. Kingsley DP. An interesting case of possible abscopal effect in malignant melanoma. Br J Radiol. 1975;48:863–6.
22. Reynders K, Illidge T, Siva S, Chang JY, De Ruysscher D. The abscopal effect of local radiotherapy: using immunotherapy to make a rare event clinically relevant. Cancer Treat Rev. 2015;41:503–10.
23. O'Regan B, Hirshberg C. Spontaneous remission: an annotated bibliography. Petaluma: Institute of Noetic Sciences Sausalito; 1993.
24. Demaria S, Ng B, Devitt ML, Babb JS, Kawashima N, Liebes L, et al. Ionizing radiation inhibition of distant untreated tumors (abscopal effect) is immune mediated. Int J Radiat Oncol Biol Phys. 2004;58:862–70.
25. Hodge JW, Sharp HJ, Gameiro SR. Abscopal regression of antigen disparate tumors by antigen cascade after systemic tumor vaccination in combination with local tumor radiation. Cancer Biother Radiopharm. 2012;27:12–22.
26. Demaria S, Kawashima N, Yang AM, Devitt ML, Babb JS, Allison JP, et al. Immune-mediated inhibition of metastases after treatment with local radiation and CTLA-4 blockade in a mouse model of breast cancer. Clin Cancer Res. 2005;11:728–34.
27. Vatner RE, Cooper BT, Vanpouille-Box C, Demaria S, Formenti SC. Combinations of immunotherapy and radiation in cancer therapy. Front Oncol. 2014;4:325.
28. Dunn GP, Bruce AT, Ikeda H, Old LJ, Schreiber RD. Cancer immunoediting: from immunosurveillance to tumor escape. Nat Immunol. 2002;3:991–8.
29. Schreiber RD, Old LJ, Smyth MJ. Cancer immunoediting: integrating immunity's roles in cancer suppression and promotion. Science. 2011;331: 1565–70.
30. Vesely MD, Kershaw MH, Schreiber RD, Smyth MJ. Natural innate and adaptive immunity to cancer. Annu Rev Immunol. 2011;29:235–71.
31. Dunn GP, Old LJ, Schreiber RD. The three Es of cancer immunoediting. Annu Rev Immunol. 2004;22:329–60.
32. Burnette BC, Liang H, Lee Y, Chlewicki L, Khodarev NN, Weichselbaum RR, et al. The efficacy of radiotherapy relies upon induction of type I interferon-dependent innate and adaptive immunity. Cancer Res. 2011;71:2488–96.
33. Fuertes MB, Kacha AK, Kline J, Woo SR, Kranz DM, Murphy KM, et al. Host type I IFN signals are required for antitumor CD8+ T cell responses through CD8{alpha}+ dendritic cells. J Exp Med. 2011;208: 2005–16.
34. Lugade AA, Sorensen EW, Gerber SA, Moran JP, Frelinger JG, Lord EM. Radiation-induced IFN- production within the tumor microenvironment influences antitumor immunity. J Immunol. 2008;180:3132–9.
35. Deng L, Liang H, Xu M, Yang X, Burnette B, Arina A, et al. STING-dependent cytosolic DNA sensing promotes radiation-induced type I interferon-dependent antitumor immunity in immunogenic tumors. Immunity. 2014;41:843–52.
36. Woo SR, Fuertes MB, Corrales L, Spranger S, Furdyna MJ, Leung MY, et al. STING-dependent cytosolic DNA sensing mediates innate immune recognition of immunogenic tumors. Immunity. 2014;41:830–42.

37. Vanpouille-Box C, Alard A, Aryankalayil MJ, Sarfraz Y, Diamond JM, Schneider RJ, et al. DNA exonuclease Trex1 regulates radiotherapy-induced tumour immunogenicity. Nat Commun. 2017;8:15618.

38. Vanpouille-Box C, Formenti SC, Demaria S. TREX1 dictates the immune fate of irradiated cancer cells. Oncoimmunology. 2017;6:e1339857.

39. Vanpouille-Box C, Diamond JM, Pilones KA, Zavadil J, Babb JS, Formenti SC, et al. TGFbeta is a master regulator of radiation therapy-induced antitumor immunity. Cancer Res. 2015;75:2232–42.

40. Wrzesinski SH, Wan YY, Flavell RA. Transforming growth factor-beta and the immune response: implications for anticancer therapy. Clin Cancer Res. 2007;13:5262–70.

41. Bouquet F, Pal A, Pilones KA, Demaria S, Hann B, Akhurst RJ, et al. TGFbeta1 inhibition increases the radiosensitivity of breast cancer cells in vitro and promotes tumor control by radiation in vivo. Clin Cancer Res. 2011;17:6754–65.

42. Saito H, Tsujitani S, Oka S, Kondo A, Ikeguchi M, Maeta M, et al. An elevated serum level of transforming growth factor-beta 1 (TGF-beta 1) significantly correlated with lymph node metastasis and poor prognosis in patients with gastric carcinoma. Anticancer Res. 2000;20:4489–93.

43. Matsuoka Y, Nakayama H, Yoshida R, Hirosue A, Nagata M, Tanaka T, et al. IL-6 controls resistance to radiation by suppressing oxidative stress via the Nrf2-antioxidant pathway in oral squamous cell carcinoma. Br J Cancer. 2016;115:1234–44.

44. Wojciechowska-Lacka A, Matecka-Nowak M, Adamiak E, Lacki JK, Cerkaska-Gluszak B. Serum levels of interleukin-10 and interleukin-6 in patients with lung cancer. Neoplasma. 1996;43:155–8.

45. Visco C, Vassilakopoulos TP, Kliche KO, Nadali G, Viviani S, Bonfante V, et al. Elevated serum levels of IL-10 are associated with inferior progression-free survival in patients with Hodgkin's disease treated with radiotherapy. Leuk Lymphoma. 2004;45:2085–92.

46. Xu J, Escamilla J, Mok S, David J, Priceman S, West B, et al. CSF1R signaling blockade stanches tumor-infiltrating myeloid cells and improves the efficacy of radiotherapy in prostate cancer. Cancer Res. 2013;73:2782–94.

47. Ghiringhelli F, Apetoh L, Tesniere A, Aymeric L, Ma Y, Ortiz C, et al. Activation of the NLRP3 inflammasome in dendritic cells induces IL-1beta-dependent adaptive immunity against tumors. Nat Med. 2009;15:1170–8.

48. Calveley VL, Khan MA, Yeung IW, Vandyk J, Hill RP. Partial volume rat lung irradiation: temporal fluctuations of in-field and out-of-field DNA damage and inflammatory cytokines following irradiation. Int J Radiat Biol. 2005;81:887–99.

49. Kozin SV, Kamoun WS, Huang Y, Dawson MR, Jain RK, Duda DG. Recruitment of myeloid but not endothelial precursor cells facilitates tumor regrowth after local irradiation. Cancer Res. 2010;70:5679–85.

50. Matsumura S, Wang B, Kawashima N, Braunstein S, Badura M, Cameron TO, et al. Radiation-induced CXCL16 release by breast cancer cells attracts effector T cells. J Immunol. 2008;181:3099–107.

51. Lim JY, Gerber SA, Murphy SP, Lord EM. Type I interferons induced by radiation therapy mediate recruitment and effector function of CD8(+) T cells. Cancer Immunol Immunother. 2014;63:259–71.

52. Meng Y, Mauceri HJ, Khodarev NN, Darga TE, Pitroda SP, Beckett MA, et al. Ad.Egr-TNF and local ionizing radiation suppress metastases by interferon-beta-dependent activation of antigen-specific CD8+ T cells. Mol Ther. 2010;18:912–20.

53. Lugade AA, Moran JP, Gerber SA, Rose RC, Frelinger JG, Lord EM. Local radiation therapy of B16 melanoma tumors increases the generation of tumor antigen-specific effector cells that traffic to the tumor. J Immunol. 2005;174:7516–23.

54. Gupta A, Probst HC, Vuong V, Landshammer A, Muth S, Yagita H, et al. Radiotherapy promotes tumor-specific effector CD8+ T cells via dendritic cell activation. J Immunol. 2012;189:558–66.

55. Ni J, Miller M, Stojanovic A, Garbi N, Cerwenka A. Sustained effector function of IL-12/15/18-preactivated NK cells against established tumors. J Exp Med. 2012;209:2351–65.

56. Kachikwu EL, Iwamoto KS, Liao YP, DeMarco JJ, Agazaryan N, Economou JS, et al. Radiation enhances regulatory T cell representation. Int J Radiat Oncol Biol Phys. 2011;81:1128–35.

57. Wu CY, Yang LH, Yang HY, Knoff J, Peng S, Lin YH, et al. Enhanced cancer radiotherapy through immunosuppressive stromal cell destruction in tumors. Clin Cancer Res. 2014;20:644–57.

58. Du R, Lu KV, Petritsch C, Liu P, Ganss R, Passegue E, et al. HIF1alpha induces the recruitment of bone marrow-derived vascular modulatory cells to regulate tumor angiogenesis and invasion. Cancer Cell. 2008;13:206–20.

59. Laoui D, Van Overmeire E, De Baetselier P, Van Ginderachter JA, Raes G. Functional relationship between tumor-associated macrophages and macrophage colony-stimulating factor as contributors to cancer progression. Front Immunol. 2014;5:489.

60. Barker HE, Paget JT, Khan AA, Harrington KJ. The tumour microenvironment after radiotherapy: mechanisms of resistance and recurrence. Nat Rev Cancer. 2015;15:409–25.

61. Galon J, Costes A, Sanchez-Cabo F, Kirilovsky A, Mlecnik B, Lagorce-Pages C, et al. Type, density, and location of immune cells within human colorectal tumors predict clinical outcome. Science. 2006;313:1960–4.

62. Hwang WT, Adams SF, Tahirovic E, Hagemann IS, Coukos G. Prognostic significance of tumor-infiltrating T cells in ovarian cancer: a meta-analysis. Gynecol Oncol. 2012;124:192–8.

63. Mahmoud SM, Paish EC, Powe DG, Macmillan RD, Grainge MJ, Lee AH, et al. Tumor-infiltrating CD8+ lymphocytes predict clinical outcome in breast cancer. J Clin Oncol Off J Am Soc Clin Oncol. 2011;29:1949–55.

64. Morvan MG, Lanier LL. NK cells and cancer: you can teach innate cells new tricks. Nat Rev Cancer. 2016;16:7–19.

65. Kim JY, Son YO, Park SW, Bae JH, Chung JS, Kim HH, et al. Increase of NKG2D ligands and sensitivity to NK cell-mediated cytotoxicity of tumor cells by heat shock and ionizing radiation. Exp Mol Med. 2006;38:474–84.

66. Matta J, Baratin M, Chiche L, Forel JM, Cognet C, Thomas G, et al. Induction of B7-H6, a ligand for the natural killer cell-activating receptor NKp30, in inflammatory conditions. Blood. 2013;122:394–404.

67. Facciabene A, Motz GT, Coukos G. T-regulatory cells: key players in tumor immune escape and angiogenesis. Cancer Res. 2012;72:2162–71.

68. Youn JI, Gabrilovich DI. The biology of myeloid-derived suppressor cells: the blessing and the curse of morphological and functional heterogeneity. Eur J Immunol. 2010;40:2969–75.

69. Movahedi K, Guilliams M, Van den Bossche J, Van den Bergh R, Gysemans C, Beschin A, et al. Identification of discrete tumor-induced myeloid-derived suppressor cell subpopulations with distinct T cell-suppressive activity. Blood. 2008;111:4233–44.

70. Condamine T, Ramachandran I, Youn JI, Gabrilovich DI. Regulation of tumor metastasis by myeloid-derived suppressor cells. Annu Rev Med. 2015;66:97–110.

71. Kumar V, Patel S, Tcyganov E, Gabrilovich DI. The nature of myeloid-derived suppressor cells in the tumor microenvironment. Trends Immunol. 2016;37:208–20.

72. Mantovani A, Bottazzi B, Colotta F, Sozzani S, Ruco L. The origin and function of tumor-associated macrophages. Cell Mol Immunol. 1992;265:265–70.

73. Mantovani A, Sozzani S, Locati M, Allavena P, Sica A. Macrophage polarization: tumor-associated macrophages as a paradigm for polarized M2 mononuclear phagocytes. Trends Immunol. 2002;23:549–55.

74. Huang Y, Snuderl M, Jain RK. Polarization of tumor-associated macrophages: a novel strategy for vascular normalization and antitumor immunity. Cancer Cell. 2011;19:1–2.

75. Klug F, Prakash H, Huber PE, Seibel T, Bender N, Halama N, et al. Low-dose irradiation programs macrophage differentiation to an iNOS(+)/M1 phenotype that orchestrates effective T cell immunotherapy. Cancer Cell. 2013;24:589–602.

76. Reits EA, Hodge JW, Herberts CA, Groothuis TA, Chakraborty M, Wansley EK, et al. Radiation modulates the peptide repertoire, enhances MHC class I expression, and induces successful antitumor immunotherapy. J Exp Med. 2006;203:1259–71.

77. Chakraborty M, Abrams SI, Camphausen K, Liu K, Scott T, Coleman CN, et al. Irradiation of tumor cells up-regulates Fas and enhances CTL lytic activity and CTL adoptive immunotherapy. J Immunol. 2003;170:6338–47.

78. Verbrugge I, Hagekyriakou J, Sharp LL, Galli M, West A, McLaughlin NM, et al. Radiotherapy increases the permissiveness of established mammary tumors to rejection by immunomodulatory antibodies. Cancer Res. 2012;72:3163–74.

79. Deng L, Liang H, Burnette B, Beckett M, Darga T, Weichselbaum RR, et al. Irradiation and anti-PD-L1 treatment synergistically promote antitumor immunity in mice. J Clin Invest. 2014;124:687–95.

80. Galluzzi L, Kepp O, Kroemer G. Immunogenic cell death in radiation therapy. Oncoimmunology. 2013;2:e26536.

81. Kepp O, Galluzzi L, Martins I, Schlemmer F, Adjemian S, Michaud M, et al. Molecular determinants of immunogenic cell death elicited by anticancer chemotherapy. Cancer Metastasis Rev. 2011;30:61–9.

82. Kroemer G, Galluzzi L, Kepp O, Zitvogel L. Immunogenic cell death in cancer therapy. Annu Rev Immunol. 2013;31:51–72.

83. Zelenay S, Reis e Sousa C. Adaptive immunity after cell death. Trends Immunol. 2013;34:329–35.

84. Herrera FG, Bourhis J, Coukos G. Radiotherapy combination opportunities leveraging immunity for the next oncology practice. CA Cancer J Clin. 2017;67:65–85.

85. Vanpouille-Box C, Pilones KA, Wennerberg E, Formenti SC, Demaria S. In situ vaccination by radiotherapy to improve responses to anti-CTLA-4 treatment. Vaccine. 2015;33:7415–22.

86. Obeid M, Tesniere A, Ghiringhelli F, Fimia GM, Apetoh L, Perfettini JL, et al. Calreticulin exposure dictates the immunogenicity of cancer cell death. Nat Med. 2007;13:54–61.

87. Boone BA, Lotze MT. Targeting damage-associated molecular pattern molecules (DAMPs) and DAMP receptors in melanoma. Methods Mol Biol. 2014;1102:537–52.

88. Tang D, Kang R, Zeh HJ 3rd, Lotze MT. High-mobility group box 1, oxidative stress, and disease. Antioxid Redox Signal. 2011;14:1315–35.

89. Elliott MR, Chekeni FB, Trampont PC, Lazarowski ER, Kadl A, Walk SF, et al. Nucleotides released by apoptotic cells act as a find-me signal to promote phagocytic clearance. Nature. 2009;461:282–6.

90. Garg AD, Krysko DV, Verfaillie T, Kaczmarek A, Ferreira GB, Marysael T, et al. A novel pathway combining calreticulin exposure and ATP secretion in immunogenic cancer cell death. EMBO J. 2012;31:1062–79.

91. Gardai SJ, McPhillips KA, Frasch SC, Janssen WJ, Starefeldt A, Murphy-Ullrich JE, et al. Cell-surface calreticulin initiates clearance of viable or apoptotic cells through trans-activation of LRP on the phagocyte. Cell. 2005;123:321–34.

92. Panaretakis T, Kepp O, Brockmeier U, Tesniere A, Bjorklund AC, Chapman DC, et al. Mechanisms of pre-apoptotic calreticulin exposure in immunogenic cell death. EMBO J. 2009;28:578–90.

93. Matzinger P. Tolerance, danger, and the extended family. Annu Rev Immunol. 1994;12:991–1045.

94. Marshak-Rothstein A. Toll-like receptors in systemic autoimmune disease. Nat Rev Immunol. 2006;6:823–35.

95. Chekeni FB, Elliott MR, Sandilos JK, Walk SF, Kinchen JM, Lazarowski ER, et al. Pannexin 1 channels mediate 'find-me' signal release and membrane permeability during apoptosis. Nature. 2010;467:863–7.

96. Perregaux DG, McNiff P, Laliberte R, Conklyn M, Gabel CA. ATP acts as an agonist to promote stimulus-induced secretion of IL-1 and IL-18 in human blood. J Immunol. 2000;165:4615–23.

97. Gorbunov NV, Garrison BR, Kiang JG. Response of crypt paneth cells in the small intestine following total-body gamma-irradiation. Int J Immunopathol Pharmacol. 2010;23:1111–23.

98. Apetoh L, Ghiringhelli F, Tesniere A, Criollo A, Ortiz C, Lidereau R, et al. The interaction between HMGB1 and TLR4 dictates the outcome of anticancer chemotherapy and radiotherapy. Immunol Rev. 2007;220:47–59.

99. Sanchez-Paulete AR, Cueto FJ, Martinez-Lopez M, Labiano S, Morales-Kastresana A, Rodriguez-Ruiz ME, et al. Cancer immunotherapy with immunomodulatory anti-CD137 and anti-PD-1 monoclonal antibodies requires BATF3-dependent dendritic cells. Cancer Discov. 2016;6:71–9.

100. Hildner K, Edelson BT, Purtha WE, Diamond M, Matsushita H, Kohyama M, et al. Batf3 deficiency reveals a critical role for CD8alpha+ dendritic cells in cytotoxic T cell immunity. Science. 2008;322:1097–100.

101. Tabi Z, Spary LK, Coleman S, Clayton A, Mason MD, Staffurth J. Resistance of CD45RA- T cells to apoptosis and functional impairment, and activation of tumor-antigen specific T cells during radiation therapy of prostate cancer. J Immunol. 2010;185:1330–9.

102. Hu ZI, McArthur HL, Ho AY. The abscopal effect of radiation therapy: what is it and how can we use it in breast cancer? Curr Breast Cancer Rep. 2017;9:45–51.

103. Siva S, Callahan J, MacManus MP, Martin O, Hicks RJ, Ball DL. Abscopal [corrected] effects after conventional and stereotactic lung irradiation of non-small-cell lung cancer. J Thorac Oncol. 2013;8:e71–2.

104. Abuodeh Y, Venkat P, Kim S. Systematic review of case reports on the abscopal effect. Curr Probl Cancer. 2016;40:25–37.

105. Rodriguez-Ruiz ME, Rodriguez I, Barbes B, Mayorga L, Sanchez-Paulete AR, Ponz-Sarvise M, et al. Brachytherapy attains abscopal effects when combined with immunostimulatory monoclonal antibodies. Brachytherapy. 2017;16:1246–51.

106. Ngwa W, Irabor OC, Schoenfeld JD, Hesser J, Demaria S, Formenti SC. Using immunotherapy to boost the abscopal effect. Nat Rev Cancer. 2018;18:313–22.

107. Golden EB, Chhabra A, Chachoua A, Adams S, Donach M, Fenton-Kerimian M, et al. Local radiotherapy and granulocyte-macrophage colony-stimulating factor to generate abscopal responses in patients with metastatic solid tumours: a proof-of-principle trial. Lancet Oncol. 2015;16:795–803.

108. Grosso JF, Jure-Kunkel MN. CTLA-4 blockade in tumor models: an overview of preclinical and translational research. Cancer Immun Arch. 2013;13:5.

109. Salama AK, Hodi FS. Cytotoxic T-lymphocyte-associated antigen-4. Clin Cancer Res. 2011;17:4622–8.

110. Pedicord VA, Montalvo W, Leiner IM, Allison JP. Single dose of anti-CTLA-4 enhances CD8+ T-cell memory formation, function, and maintenance. Proc Natl Acad Sci U S A. 2011;108:266–71.

111. Hodi FS, O'Day SJ, McDermott DF, Weber RW, Sosman JA, Haanen JB, et al. Improved survival with ipilimumab in patients with metastatic melanoma. N Engl J Med. 2010;363:711–23.

112. Robert C, Thomas L, Bondarenko I, O'Day S, Weber J, Garbe C, et al. Ipilimumab plus dacarbazine for previously untreated metastatic melanoma. N Engl J Med. 2011;364:2517–26.

113. Hodi FS, Mihm MC, Soiffer RJ, Haluska FG, Butler M, Seiden MV, et al. Biologic activity of cytotoxic T lymphocyte-associated antigen 4 antibody blockade in previously vaccinated metastatic melanoma and ovarian carcinoma patients. Proc Natl Acad Sci U S A. 2003;100:4712–7.

114. Small EJ, Tchekmedyian NS, Rini BI, Fong L, Lowy I, Allison JP. A pilot trial of CTLA-4 blockade with human anti-CTLA-4 in patients with hormone-refractory prostate cancer. Clin Cancer Res. 2007;13:1810–5.

115. Blansfield JA, Beck KE, Tran K, Yang JC, Hughes MS, Kammula US, et al. Cytotoxic T-lymphocyte-associated antigen-4 blockage can induce autoimmune hypophysitis in patients with metastatic melanoma and renal cancer. J Immunother. 2005;28:593–8.

116. Scalapino KJ, Daikh DI. CTLA-4: a key regulatory point in the control of autoimmune disease. Immunol Rev. 2008;223:143–55.

117. Wing K, Onishi Y, Prieto-Martin P, Yamaguchi T, Miyara M, Fehervari Z, et al. CTLA-4 control over Foxp3+ regulatory T cell function. Science. 2008;322:271–5.

118. Grimaldi AM, Simeone E, Giannarelli D, Muto P, Falivene S, Borzillo V, et al. Abscopal effects of radiotherapy on advanced melanoma patients who progressed after ipilimumab immunotherapy. Oncoimmunology. 2014;3:e28780.

119. Koller KM, Mackley HB, Liu J, Wagner H, Talamo G, Schell TD, et al. Improved survival and complete response rates in patients with advanced melanoma treated with concurrent ipilimumab and radiotherapy versus ipilimumab alone. Cancer Biol Ther. 2017;18:36–42.

120. Slovin SF, Higano CS, Hamid O, Tejwani S, Harzstark A, Alumkal JJ, et al. Ipilimumab alone or in combination with radiotherapy in metastatic castration-resistant prostate cancer: results from an open-label, multicenter phase I/II study. Ann Oncol. 2013;24:1813–21.

121. Kwon ED, Drake CG, Scher HI, Fizazi K, Bossi A, van den Eertwegh AJM, et al. Ipilimumab versus placebo after radiotherapy in patients with metastatic castration-resistant prostate cancer that had progressed after docetaxel chemotherapy (CA184-043): a multicentre, randomised, double-blind, phase 3 trial. Lancet Oncol. 2014;15:700–12.

122. Dong H, Zhu G, Tamada K, Chen L. B7-H1, a third member of the B7 family, co-stimulates T-cell proliferation and interleukin-10 secretion. Nat Med. 1999;5:1365–9.

123. Latchman Y, Wood CR, Chernova T, Chaudhary D, Borde M, Chernova I, et al. PD-L2 is a second ligand for PD-1 and inhibits T cell activation. Nat Immunol. 2001;2:261–8.

124. Greenwald RJ, Freeman GJ, Sharpe AH. The B7 family revisited. Annu Rev Immunol. 2005;23:515–48.

125. Callahan MK, Wolchok JD. At the bedside: CTLA-4- and PD-1-blocking antibodies in cancer immunotherapy. J Leukoc Biol. 2013;94:41–53.

126. Teng F, Kong L, Meng X, Yang J, Yu J. Radiotherapy combined with immune checkpoint blockade immunotherapy: achievements and challenges. Cancer Lett. 2015;365:23–9.

127. Robert C, Schachter J, Long GV, Arance A, Grob JJ, Mortier L, et al. Pembrolizumab versus ipilimumab in advanced melanoma. N Engl J Med. 2015;372:2521–32.

128. Weber JS, D'Angelo SP, Minor D, Hodi FS, Gutzmer R, Neyns B, et al. Nivolumab versus chemotherapy in patients with advanced melanoma who progressed after anti-CTLA-4 treatment (CheckMate 037): a randomised, controlled, open-label, phase 3 trial. Lancet Oncol. 2015;16:375–84.

129. Shaverdian N, Lisberg AE, Bornazyan K, Veruttipong D, Goldman JW, Formenti SC, et al. Previous radiotherapy and the clinical activity and toxicity of pembrolizumab in the treatment of non-small-cell lung cancer: a secondary analysis of the KEYNOTE-001 phase 1 trial. Lancet Oncol. 2017;18:895–903.

130. Aboudaram A, Modesto A, Chaltiel L, Gomez-Roca C, Boulinguez S, Sibaud V, et al. Concurrent radiotherapy for patients with metastatic melanoma and receiving anti-programmed-death 1 therapy: a safe and effective combination. Melanoma Res. 2017;27:485–91.

131. Komatsu T, Nakamura K, Kawase A. Abscopal effect of nivolumab in a patient with primary lung cancer. J Thorac Oncol. 2017;12:e143–e4.

132. Michot JM, Mazeron R, Dercle L, Ammari S, Canova C, Marabelle A, et al. Abscopal effect in a Hodgkin lymphoma patient treated by an anti-programmed death 1 antibody. Eur J Cancer. 2016;66:91–4.

133. Levy A, Massard C, Soria JC, Deutsch E. Concurrent irradiation with the anti-programmed cell death ligand-1 immune checkpoint blocker durvalumab: single centre subset analysis from a phase 1/2 trial. Eur J Cancer. 2016;68:156–62.

134. Inaba K. Generation of large numbers of dendritic cells from mouse bone marrow cultures supplemented with granulocyte/macrophage colony-stimulating factor. J Exp Med. 1992;176:1693–702.

135. Formenti SC, Lee P, Adams S, Goldberg JD, Li X, Xie MW, et al. Focal irradiation and systemic TGFbeta blockade in metastatic breast cancer. Clin Cancer Res. 2018;24:2493–504.

136. Rodriguez-Ruiz ME, Perez-Gracia JL, Rodriguez I, Alfaro C, Onate C, Perez G, et al. Combined immunotherapy encompassing intratumoral poly-ICLC, dendritic-cell vaccination and radiotherapy in advanced cancer patients. Ann Oncol. 2018;29:1312–9.

137. Vonderheide RH, Glennie MJ. Agonistic CD40 antibodies and cancer therapy. Clin Cancer Res. 2013;19:1035–43.

138. Dalotto-Moreno T, Croci DO, Cerliani JP, Martinez-Allo VC, Dergan-Dylon S, Mendez-Huergo SP, et al. Targeting galectin-1 overcomes breast cancer-associated immunosuppression and prevents metastatic disease. Cancer Res. 2013;73:1107–17.

139. Siva S, MacManus MP, Martin RF, Martin OA. Abscopal effects of radiation therapy: a clinical review for the radiobiologist. Cancer Lett. 2015;356:82–90.

140. Finkelstein SE, Timmerman R, McBride WH, Schaue D, Hoffe SE, Mantz CA, et al. The confluence of stereotactic ablative radiotherapy and tumor immunology. Clin Dev Immunol. 2011;2011:439752.

141. Dewan MZ, Galloway AE, Kawashima N, Dewyngaert JK, Babb JS, Formenti SC, et al. Fractionated but not single-dose radiotherapy induces an immune-mediated abscopal effect when combined with anti-CTLA-4 antibody. Clin Cancer Res. 2009;15:5379–88.

142. Schaue D, Ratikan JA, Iwamoto KS, McBride WH. Maximizing tumor immunity with fractionated radiation. Int J Radiat Oncol Biol Phys. 2012;83:1306–10.

143. Dovedi SJ, Adlard AL, Lipowska-Bhalla G, McKenna C, Jones S, Cheadle EJ, et al. Acquired resistance to fractionated radiotherapy can be overcome by concurrent PD-L1 blockade. Cancer Res. 2014;74:5458–68.

144. Golden EB, Demaria S, Schiff PB, Chachoua A, Formenti SC. An abscopal response to radiation and ipilimumab in a patient with metastatic non-small cell lung cancer. Cancer Immunol Res. 2013;1:365–72.

145. Twyman-Saint Victor C, Rech AJ, Maity A, Rengan R, Pauken KE, Stelekati E, et al. Radiation and dual checkpoint blockade activate non-redundant immune mechanisms in cancer. Nature. 2015;520:373–7.

146. Lane DP. Cancer. p53, guardian of the genome. Nature. 1992;358:15–6.

147. Strigari L, Mancuso M, Ubertini V, Soriani A, Giardullo P, Benassi M, et al. Abscopal effect of radiation therapy: interplay between radiation dose and p53 status. Int J Radiat Biol. 2014;90:248–55.

148. Camphausen K, Moses MA, Ménard C, Sproull M, Beecken W-D, Folkman J, et al. Radiation abscopal antitumor effect is mediated through p53. Cancer Res. 2003;63:1990–3.

149. Gameiro SR, Jammeh ML, Wattenberg MM, Tsang KY, Ferrone S, Hodge JW. Radiation-induced immunogenic modulation of tumor enhances antigen processing and calreticulin exposure, resulting in enhanced T-cell killing. Oncotarget. 2014;5:403–16.

150. Snyder A, Makarov V, Merghoub T, Yuan J, Zaretsky JM, Desrichard A, et al. Genetic basis for clinical response to CTLA-4 blockade in melanoma. N Engl J Med. 2014;371:2189–99.

151. Rizvi NA, Hellmann MD, Snyder A, Kvistborg P, Makarov V, Havel JJ, et al. Mutational landscape determines sensitivity to PD-1 blockade in non-small cell lung cancer. Science. 2015;348:124–8.

152. Johnson DB, Frampton GM, Rioth MJ, Yusko E, Ennis R, Fabrizio D, et al. Hybrid capture-based next-generation sequencing (HC NGS) in melanoma to identify markers of response to anti-PD-1/PD-L1. J Clin Oncol. 2016;34:105.

153. Garon EB, Rizvi NA, Hui R, Leighl N, Balmanoukian AS, Eder JP, et al. Pembrolizumab for the treatment of non-small-cell lung cancer. N Engl J Med. 2015;372:2018–28.

154. Herbst RS, Baas P, Kim D-W, Felip E, Pérez-Gracia JL, Han J-Y, et al. Pembrolizumab versus docetaxel for previously treated, PD-L1-positive, advanced non-small-cell lung cancer (KEYNOTE-010): a randomised controlled trial. Lancet. 2016;387:1540–50.

155. Reck M, Rodriguez-Abreu D, Robinson AG, Hui R, Csoszi T, Fulop A, et al. Pembrolizumab versus chemotherapy for PD-L1-positive non-small-cell lung cancer. N Engl J Med. 2016;375:1823–33.

156. Topalian SL, Hodi FS, Brahmer JR, Gettinger SN, Smith DC, McDermott DF, et al. Safety, activity, and immune correlates of anti-PD-1 antibody in cancer. N Engl J Med. 2012;366:2443–54.

157. Roger A, Finet A, Boru B, Beauchet A, Mazeron J-J, Otzmeguine Y, et al. Efficacy of combined hypo-fractionated radiotherapy and anti-PD-1 monotherapy in difficult-to-treat advanced melanoma patients. Oncoimmunology. 2018;7:e1442166.

158. Theurich S, Rothschild SI, Hoffmann M, Fabri M, Sommer A, Garcia-Marquez M, et al. Local tumor treatment in combination with systemic ipilimumab immunotherapy prolongs overall survival in patients with advanced malignant melanoma. Cancer Immunol Res. 2016;4:744–54.

159. Hwang WL, Niemierko A, Hwang KL, Hubbeling H, Schapira E, Gainor JF, et al. Clinical outcomes in patients with metastatic lung cancer treated with PD-1/PD-L1 inhibitors and thoracic radiotherapy. JAMA Oncol. 2018;4:253–5.

160. Kropp LM, De Los Santos JF, McKee SB, Conry RM. Radiotherapy to control limited melanoma progression following ipilimumab. J Immunother. 2016; 39:373–8.

5

Haploidentical transplantation is associated with better overall survival when compared to single cord blood transplantation: an EBMT-Eurocord study of acute leukemia patients conditioned with thiotepa, busulfan, and fludarabine

Federica Giannotti[1†], Myriam Labopin[1,2†], Roni Shouval[3,4*†] (iD), Jaime Sanz[5,6], William Arcese[7], Emanuele Angelucci[8], Jorge Sierra[9], Josep-Maria Ribera Santasusana[10], Stella Santarone[11], Bruno Benedetto[12], Alessandro Rambaldi[13], Riccardo Saccardi[14], Didier Blaise[15], Michele Angelo Carella[16], Vanderson Rocha[17,18,19], Frederic Baron[20], Mohamad Mohty[1,2], Annalisa Ruggeri[1,21] and Arnon Nagler[2,3]

Abstract

Background: Thiotepa-busulfan-fludarabine (TBF) is a widely used conditioning regimen in single umbilical cord blood transplantation (SUCBT). More recently, it was introduced in the setting of non-T cell depleted haploidentical stem cell transplantation (NTD-Haplo). Whether TBF based conditioning provides additional benefit in transplantation from a particular alternative donor type remains to be established.

Methods: This was a retrospective study based on an international European registry. We compared outcomes of de-novo acute myeloid leukemia patients in complete remission receiving NTD-Haplo ($n = 186$) vs. SUCBT ($n = 147$) following myeloablative conditioning (MAC) with TBF. Median follow-up was 23 months. Treatment groups resembled in baseline characteristics.

Results: SUCBT was associated with delayed engraftment and higher graft failure. In multivariate analysis no statistically significant differences were observed between the two groups in terms of acute or chronic graft-versus-host disease (GvHD) (HR = 1.03, $p = 0.92$ or HR = 1.86, $p = 0.21$) and relapse incidence (HR = 0.8, $p = 0.65$). Non-relapse mortality (NRM) was significantly higher in SUCBT as compared to NTD-Haplo (HR = 2.63, $p = 0.001$); moreover, SUCBT did worse in terms of overall survival (HR = 2.18, $p = 0.002$), leukemia-free survival (HR = 1.94, $p = 0.007$), and GvHD relapse-free survival (HR = 2.38, $p = 0.0002$).

(Continued on next page)

* Correspondence: shouval@gmail.com
[†]Federica Giannotti, Myriam Labopin and Roni Shouval contributed equally to this work.
[3]Division of Hematology and Bone Marrow Transplantation Division, Chaim Sheba Medical Center, Tel-Hashomer, Sackler School of Medicine, Tel-Aviv University, 52621 Ramat-Gan, Israel
[4]Dr. Pinchas Bornstein Talpiot Medical Leadership Program, Chaim Sheba Medical Center, Tel-Hashomer, Israel
Full list of author information is available at the end of the article

(Continued from previous page)

Conclusions: Our results suggest that TBF-MAC might allow for a potent graft-versus-leukemia, regardless of the alternative donor type. Furthermore, in patients receiving TBF-MAC, survival with NTD-Haplo may be better compared to SUCBT due to decreased NRM.

Keywords: Acute myeloid leukemia, Stem cell transplantation, Conditioning regimens, Thiotepa-busulfan-fludarabine, Haploidentical stem cell transplantation, Umbilical cord blood transplantation,

Background

Allogeneic hematopoietic stem cell transplantation (HSCT) is a potential curative treatment for patients with acute myeloid leukemia (AML) [1]. The introduction of transplantation from alternative donors, i.e., unrelated umbilical cord blood transplantation (UCBT) and haploidentical transplantation (Haplo), has increased the availability of this treatment. UCBT and Haplo are considered a valid option for patients with acute leukemia lacking a human leukocyte antigen (HLA) matched sibling or unrelated donor, or when transplantation cannot be delayed [2–6]. Stem cells from both types of donors are readily available. In the UCBT setting the process of stem cell collection is risk-free to the donor, and the graft is relatively permissive to HLA incompatibility [7–11]. Contemporary transplantation practice involving the use of double cord blood units in case that there are not enough stem cells in a single cord, flexible conditioning regimens, effective graft-versus-host disease (GvHD) prophylaxis platforms with non-T cell depleted (NTD) Haplo, and improved management of post-transplant complications, have brought improvement in outcomes of alternative donor transplantations [3, 7, 12]. Several studies have reported that results with UCBT and Haplo are comparable with those of transplants from HLA identical or matched unrelated donors [13–22].

Conditioning regimens are administered as part of the transplant procedure to prevent graft rejection by immunoablation and in order to reduce the tumor burden. As the graft versus tumor effect was recognized to contribute to the effectiveness of HSCT, reduced-intensity and non-myeloablative conditioning regimens have been developed, making HSCT applicable to older or unfit patients [23]. Still, myeloablative conditioning (MAC) regimens remain the preferred option in adult patients (age ≤ 55 years) with high-risk acute leukemia [24]. Despite the availability of various effective conditioning protocols, standard regimens have yet to be established for the different types of HSCT in the various malignancies, leading to high heterogeneity in clinical practice [25]. Therefore, characterizing the effects of a specific regimen in a particular disease category is of major clinical importance.

The use of thiotepa–IV busulfan–fludarabine (TBF) at a myeloablative dose in single unit UCBT (SUCBT) was pioneered by the Valencia group, which reported high rates of engraftment and long-term disease-free survival in patients transplant at early disease stage of hematological malignancies [26]. TBF is widely applied in UCBT and its efficacy is well established [27]. Conditioning protocols in the Haplo setting are more heterogeneous and often determined according to institutional policies [2, 28–32]. More recently, TBF has been increasingly employed in Haplo transplantation with favorable outcomes [31, 32]. Comparing the outcome between patients receiving an allogeneic HSCT from alternative donors is an unmet need. Therefore, we retrospectively analyzed and compared the results of allogeneic HSCT with myeloablative TBF-based conditioning, in a homogeneous population of AML adult patients in complete remission (CR) receiving either NTD-Haplo ($n = 186$) or SUCBT ($n = 147$). The analysis was based on data reported to the European Society for Blood and Marrow Transplantation (EBMT) Acute Leukemia Working Party (ALWP), Cellular Therapy and Immunobiology Working Party, and the Eurocord registry.

Methods

Study design and definition

We retrospectively analyzed patients aged ≥18 years diagnosed with de novo AML, who received a first HSCT either from an NTD haploidentical-related donor (recipient-donor number of mismatches ≥ 2) ($n = 186$) or an unmanipulated single cord blood unit ($n = 147$). Data were reported by the ALWP of the EBMT and EUROCORD, between January 2007 and December 2015. Minimal HLA typing requirements for UCBT followed the current practice of antigen level typing for HLA-A and -B and allele-level typing of HLA-DRB1. For patients receiving Haplo, peripheral blood or bone marrow was used as a stem cell source, without ex vivo T cell depletion. Transplants were performed in 75 EBMT transplant centers: 17 performed only SUCBT, 44 only Haplo, and 14 centers performed both procedures. All patients were given a myeloablative reduced toxicity conditioning regimen consisting of thiotepa, IV busulfan, and fludarabine. TBF-MAC was defined as a regimen containing a total dose of IV busulfan ≥ 9.6 mg/kg [33]. Cytogenetic risk groups were defined according to the Medical Research Council (MRC) classification system [34].

All patients provided informed consent for transplants according to the Declaration of Helsinki. The Review Boards of the ALWP of EBMT, and Eurocord approved this study.

Endpoints

The primary endpoint was leukemia-free survival (LFS). LFS was defined as survival without leukemia or relapse following transplantation. GvHD-free relapse-free survival (GRFS) events were defined as grade 3–4 acute GvHD, extensive chronic GvHD, disease relapse, or death from any cause [35]. Overall survival (OS) was calculated from the date of transplant until death from any cause or last observation alive. Relapse incidence (RI) was defined as the occurrence of disease after transplantation, determined by morphological evidence of the disease in bone marrow, blood, or extramedullary organs. Non-relapse mortality (NRM) was defined as death without prior relapse.

Neutrophil recovery was defined as achieving absolute neutrophil count of 0.5×10^9/l for three consecutive days. Acute and chronic GvHD was defined using the standard criteria [36, 37].

Statistical analysis

Median values and ranges were used for continuous variables and percentages for categorical variables. For each continuous variable, the study population was initially split into quartiles and into two groups by the median. Patient-, disease-, and transplant-related variables of the groups were compared using chi-square or Fischer's exact test for categorical variables, and the Mann–Whitney test for continuous variables. The probabilities of OS, LFS, and GRFS were calculated using the Kaplan–Meier method and the log-rank test for univariate comparisons [38]. The probabilities of neutrophil engraftment, grade II–IV acute and chronic GvHD, relapse, and NRM were calculated with the cumulative incidence method and Gray test for comparisons. Multivariate analyses adjusted for differences between the groups were performed using the Cox proportional hazards regression model for LFS and OS, and for engraftment, GvHD, NRM, and relapse [39].

The final model was adjusted for the following variables: transplant strategy (Haplo or SUCBT), disease status at HSCT (first or second CR), time from diagnosis to HSCT, age at transplant, year of HSCT, donor/recipient sex match, Karnofsky performance status (KPS), and center effect. p values were two-sided. Statistical analyses were performed with the SPSS 22 (SPSS Inc./IBM, Armonk, NY, USA) and R 3.0 (R Development Core Team, Vienna, Austria) software packages.

Results

Patients, disease, and transplant characteristics

Patient and disease characteristics are summarized in Table 1. Per protocol, all patients received a TBF-MAC-based regimen. The two populations were overall homogeneous in terms of patients and disease characteristics, except for median age at transplant which was older for NTD-Haplo (44 [range, 19–66] vs. 42 [range, 18–68], $p = 0.046$). Most patients were in first CR (NTD-Haplo, 70% vs. SUCBT, 77% $p = 0.14$); median interval from diagnosis to transplant was also similar (176 vs. 194 days; $p = 0.09$). Cytogenetic risk groups were alike between the Haplo and SUCBT groups ($p = 0.76$), with intermediate risk being most prevalent (36% vs. 41%, respectively). Haplo transplantations were performed in more recent years (median year of transplantation was 2014 vs. 2011; $p < 0.001$). As expected, anti-thymocyte globulin (ATG) was mostly used in SUCBT (91% vs. 29% in NTD-Haplo; $p < 0.001$). For SUCBT, the median dose of total nucleated cells at collection was 3.3×10^7/kg (range, 1.7–8.4), and 80% of the patients received $\geq 2.5 \times 10^7$/kg. Cord blood units were HLA matched with the recipient at a level of at least 4/6 in 68% of the cases. Among NTD-Haplo patients, 80% received bone marrow as stem cell source, and post-transplant cyclophosphamide (PTCY) was administrated in 71% of the cases (Additional file 1: Table S1). Further details about transplant procedures and GvHD prophylaxis are provided in (Additional file 1: Tables S2, S3). The median follow-up was 22 (range, 1–96) and 24 (range, 1–83) months for NTD-Haplo and SUCBT, respectively.

Engraftment

The cumulative incidence of neutrophil engraftment at day 60 after NTD-Haplo and SUCBT was 96% vs. 86% ($p < 0.001$), respectively. The median time for neutrophil recovery was 18 (range – 8-38) days for Haplo and 21 (range 11–57) days for SUCBT, ($p < 0.001$). Twenty patients did not engraft after SUCBT; of these, two are alive at 10 and 62 months, respectively, both after salvage with a second transplant from a haploidentical-related donor. The remaining 18 patients died in a median time of 1 month (range, 0–7), one patient after an autologous back-up. Among the seven patients who did not engraft after NTD-Haplo, none are alive, with a median time to death of 1.74 months (range, 0.3–17.22). Three of these patients received a second allogeneic transplantation, and only one engrafted, surviving more than 1 year.

Acute and chronic GvHD

The cumulative incidence of day 100 grade II–IV acute GvHD was 26% and 29% after NTD-Haplo and SUCBT ($p = 0.85$), respectively (Table 2). Cumulative incidence

Table 1 Population characteristics

	NTD-Haplo (n = 186)	SUCBT (n = 147)	p value
Follow-up, months median (range)	22.07 (0–96.3)	24.42 (0–83.1)	
HSCT year, median (range)	2014 (2008–2015)	2011 (2007–2015)	< 0.001
Age, years. median (range)	44.3 (18.5–66.1)	42.6 (18–67.9)	0.046
Recipient sex			
Male	85 (45.7%)	65 (44.2%)	0.787
Female	101 (54.3%)	82 (55.8%)	
Missing	0	6	
Karnofsky performance status			
< 90	21 (12.5%)	15 (15.31%)	0.519
≥ 90	147 (87.5%)	83 (84.69%)	
Missing	18	49	
Interval from diagnosis to HSCT, months, median (range)	6.6 (2.1–189.6)	6 (3–214.2)	0.097
Disease status at HSCT			
CR1	130 (69.9%)	113 (76.9%)	0.154
CR2	56 (30.1%)	34 (23.1%)	
MRC risk classification			
Good	16 (8.6%)	13 (8.8%)	0.762
Intermediate	67 (36.0%)	60 (40.8%)	
Poor	19 (10.2%)	16 (10.9%)	
Missing	84 (45.2%)	58 (39.5%)	
Female donor to male recipient			
No	143 (76.9%)	108 (76.6%)	0.952
Yes	43 (23.1%)	33 (23.4%)	
Recipient CMV serostatus			< 0.001
Negative	35 (19.1%)	29 (25.9%)	
Positive	148 (80.9%)	83 (74.1%)	
Missing	3	35	
In-vivo T cell depletion (ATG)			
No	131 (71.2%)	13 (9.0%)	< 0.001
Yes	53 (28.8%)	131 (91.0%)	
Missing	2	3	

NTD-Haplo Non-T cell depleted haploidentical transplantation, *SUCBT* single umbilical cord blood transplantation, *HSCT* hematopoietic stem cell transplantation, *CR* complete remission, *MRC* Medical Research Council, *CMV* cytomegalovirus, *ATG* antithymocyte globulin

of grade III–IV acute GvHD was 7% in both groups ($p = 0.99$). The cumulative incidence of chronic GvHD was 33% after NTD-Haplo and 37% after SUCBT ($p = 0.49$). In the multivariate analysis (Table 3), no significant difference was found between the two groups in terms of acute or chronic GvHD (hazard ratio (HR) = 1.03, $p = 0.92$; HR = 1.86, $p = 0.92$, respectively). A center effect was found for chronic GvHD ($p < 0.001$).

Relapse and NRM

The 2-year RI was 17% for NTD-Haplo vs. 12% for SUCBT ($p = 0.7$) (Fig. 1a, Table 2). In the multivariate analysis (Table 3), relapse was not statistically different

between the two groups of patients (HR = 0.8, $p = 0.65$). However, it was lower in patients who had a good KPS (≥ 90) at transplant (HR = 0.35, $p = 0.01$). NRM at 2 years was 21% and 48% for NTD-Haplo and SUCBT ($p < 0.001$), respectively (Fig. 1b, Table 2). The causes of death are listed in Additional file 1: Table S4. The multivariate model confirmed a significantly higher risk of NRM in the SUCBT group (HR = 2.63, $p = 0.002$). Also, NRM was higher in male recipients receiving a female donor (HR 1.84, $p = 0.015$), independently of the stem cell source. Infections and GvHD were the most common causes of transplant-related deaths in both groups (NTD-Haplo vs. SUCBT, infections 35% vs. 45%; GvHD

Table 2 Univariate analysis

	Acute GvHD II–IV [95% CI]	Acute GvHD III–IV [95% CI]	2-year chronic GvHD [95% CI]	2-year relapse [95% CI]	2-year NRM [95% CI]	2-year LFS [95% CI]	2-years OS [95% CI]	2-year GRFS [95% CI]
Donor type								
NTD-Haplo	25.6% [19.4–32.2]	6.8% [3.7–11.2]	33% [25.2–40.9]	16.6% [11.1–23.1]	20.6% [14.7–27.2]	62.8% [55.1–70.6]	69.2% [61.9–76.6]	55.5% [47.5–63.5]
SUCBT	28.5% [21.3–36]	7% [3.6–12]	37.1% [27–47.2]	11.6% [6.9–17.6]	48.4% [39.4–56.8]	40% [31.5–48.6]	41.7% [33–50.4]	30.3% [22.3–38.3]
p value	0.853	0.997	0.492	0.709	< 0.001	< 0.001	< 0.001	< 0.001
HSCT year								
≤ 2013	26.5% [20.6–32.9]	6.2% [3.4–10.2]	37.1% [29.4–44.8]	14.1% [9.6–19.4]	37.4% [30.5–44.3]	48.5% [41.4–55.7]	52.8% [45.7–59.9]	41.1% [34.1–48.1]
> 2013	27.4% [19.8–35.4]	8% [4.1–13.6]	27.6% [18.4–37.6]	14.6% [8.3–22.7]	26.3% [17.4–36]	59.1% [48.5–69.7]	61.4% [50.1–72.8]	49.5% [38.9–60.2]
p value	0.780	0.483	0.278	0.834	0.027	0.022	0.023	0.142
Age, years								
< 44	30.7% [23.7–37.9]	6.3% [3.2–10.8]	32.6% [24.1–41.3]	16.5% [10.9–23.1]	28% [20.9–35.5]	55.5% [47.2–63.7]	61% [53–69]	48.2% [39.9–56.6]
≥ 44	23% [16.8–29.8]	7.5% [4.1–12.2]	36.3% [27.4–45.2]	11.8% [7.2–17.8]	38.6% [30.5–46.6]	49.6% [41.2–57.9]	52.2% [43.7–60.7]	39.2% [30.9–47.4]
p value	0.133	0.683	0.355	0.576	0.043	0.137	0.089	0.090
Karnofsky performance status								
< 90	31.6% [16.9–47.3]	14.4% [5.1–28.2]	33.4% [14.7–53.4]	20.5% [8.8–35.6]	49.2% [29.9–65.9]	30.2% [13.5–47]	41.1% [23.4–58.8]	22.9% [7.1–38.7]
≥ 90	26.3% [20.7–32.3]	5% [2.6–8.4]	32.2% [25–39.6]	12.9% [8.6–18.1]	29.1% [22.9–35.7]	58% [50.9–65]	59.8% [52.8–66.8]	49.2% [42–56.5]
p value	0.634	0.042	0.880	0.085	0.017	< 0.001	0.007	0.002
Interval from diagnosis to HSCT, months								
≤ 6.3	25.2% [18.7–32.2]	6.3% [3.2–10.9]	33.9% [25.3–42.7]	15.9% [10.1–22.8]	33.3% [25.4–41.3]	50.8% [42.2–59.5]	56.4% [47.8–65]	40% [31.4–48.5]
> 6.3	28% [21.3–35.1]	7.5% [4.1–12.3]	34.8% [25.9–43.8]	12.9% [8.2–18.8]	33.4% [26–41]	53.7% [45.7–61.7]	56.7% [48.7–64.7]	47.7% [39.6–55.7]
p value	0.502	0.665	0.955	0.718	0.713	0.830	0.676	0.576
Disease status at HSCT								
CR1	26.8% [21.3–32.6]	7.3% [4.4–11.1]	36% [28.8–43.2]	13.9% [9.6–19.1]	33.2% [26.9–39.7]	52.9% [45.9–59.8]	57.7% [50.8–64.5]	42.8% [35.8–49.7]
CR2	26.8% [17.9–36.6]	5.8% [2.1–12.2]	29.8% [18.3–42.2]	15% [8.2–23.9]	33.3% [23.1–43.9]	51.6% [40.4–62.9]	54.1% [42.9–65.2]	46.2% [35.1–57.3]
p value	0.965	0.654	0.367	0.591	0.906	0.618	0.376	0.960
Female donor to male recipient								
No	25.7% [20.4–31.4]	5.4% [3–8.8]	32.1% [25.1–39.2]	14% [9.7–19.1]	30.2% [24.2–36.5]	55.8% [49–62.6]	60.2% [53.6–66.9]	46.8% [39.9–53.7]
Yes	31.5% [21.2–42.3]	12.3% [6–21]	42.4% [29–55.2]	13.3% [6.4–22.6]	41.9% [29.8–53.5]	44.8% [32.7–57]	48.5% [36.2–60.8]	36.2% [24.6–47.8]
p value	0.295	0.041	0.133	0.485	0.073	0.035	0.055	0.063

GvHD Graft-versus-host disease, *NRM* non-relapse mortality, *LFS* leukemia-free survival, *OS* overall survival, *GRFS* GvHD-free relapse-free survival, *CI* confidence interval, *NTD-Haplo* non-T cell depleted Haploidentical transplantation, *SUCBT* single umbilical cord blood transplantation, *HSCT* hematopoietic stem cell transplantation, *CR* complete remission

20% vs. 19%). Disease recurrence accounted for 27% and 16% of deaths after NTD-Haplo and SUCBT, respectively.

OS, LFS, and GRFS

The probability of 2-year OS, LFS, and GRFS in the NTD-Haplo vs. SUCBT groups were 69% vs. 42% ($p <$ 0.001), 63% vs. 40% ($p <$ 0.001), and 56% vs. 30% ($p <$ 0.001), respectively (Table 2). The benefit of NTD-Haplo was maintained in a sub-analysis restricted to patients with intermediate cytogenetic risk (Additional file 1: Table S5). In the multivariate analysis (Table 3), the type of donor had a statistically significant impact on OS, LFS, and GRFS, which were significantly lower in SUCBT as compared to NTD-Haplo (OS, HR = 2.18, $p =$ 0.003; LFS, HR = 1.93, $p =$ 0.007; GRFS, HR = 2.38, $p =$ 0.0002). The use of female donors for male recipients was independently associated with lower OS, LFS overall survival (HR = 2.18, $p =$ 0.002) and GRFS (HR = 1.67,

$p =$ 0.02; HR = 1.67, $p =$ 0.014; and HR = 1.54, $p =$ 0.026), while a KPS ≥ 90 at transplant was associated with higher LFS and GRFS (HR = 0.5, $p =$ 0.004 and HR = 0.57, $p =$ 0.02) Fig. 2.

Discussion

TBF is a well-established conditioning regimen in SUCBT and has more recently brought into use in Haplo transplantations [26, 27, 31, 32]. In this retrospective analysis, we compare outcomes of NTD-Haplo and SUCBT in a population of AML patients conditioned with TBF at a myeloablative dose. Overall, the treatment groups resembled with regard to baseline characteristics. The risk for relapse and acute and chronic GvHD were similar regardless of donor type. Engraftment was faster with a Haplo donor. Importantly, the risk of NRM, death, or having a GRFS-related event was all higher in UCBT patients.

Table 3 Multivariable analysis

	Acute GvHD II-IV		Chronic GvHD		Relapse		NRM		LFS		OS		GRFS	
	HR (95% CI)	p	HR (95% CI)	p	HR (95% CI)	p	HR (95% CI)	p	HR (95% CI)	p	HR (95%CI)	p	HR (95% CI)	p
Donor type														
SUCBT vs. Haplo	1.03 (0.56–1.89)	0.923	1.86 (0.70–4.95)	0.21	0.81 (0.32–2.04)	0.65	2.63 (1.44–4.83)	0.002	1.95 (1.20–3.16)	0.007	2.19 (1.31–3.65)	0.003	2.39 (1.51–3.79)	<0.001
Year of HSCT	0.97 (0.85–1.11)	0.677	0.91 (0.77–1.08)	0.30	0.93 (0.76–1.14)	0.50	1.01 (0.88–1.15)	0.925	0.98 (0.88–1.10)	0.772	1.00 (0.89–1.12)	1.000	1.07 (0.97–1.189)	0.197
Age (per 10 years)	0.89 (0.72–1.08)	0.236	1.17 (0.93–1.47)	0.19	1.07 (0.80–1.42)	0.66	1.20 (0.99–1.47)	0.071	1.15 (0.98–1.35)	0.096	1.18 (0.99–1.40)	0.055	1.11 (0.96–1.29)	0.164
Karnofsky PS														
≥ 90 vs. < 90	0.67 (0.35–1.31)	0.243	1.05 (0.44–2.55)	0.91	0.35 (0.15–0.81)	0.01	0.60 (0.33–1.09)	0.094	0.50 (0.31–0.81)	0.005	0.60 (0.36–1.00)	0.053	0.58 (0.36–0.92)	0.020
Disease status at HSCT														
CR2 vs. CR1	1.16 (0.68–1.98)	0.582	0.89 (0.44–1.79)	0.74	0.79 (0.34–1.84)	0.59	1.19 (0.70–1.20)	0.524	1.07 (0.69–1.66)	0.760	1.19 (0.76–1.87)	0.457	0.92 (0.61–1.39)	0.703
Female donor to male recipient														
Yes vs. No	1.63 (0.97–2.73)	0.064	1.15 (0.60–2.18)	0.67	1.25 (0.57–2.73)	0.58	1.84 (1.12–3.02)	0.016	1.67 (1.11–2.53)	0.014	1.67 (1.08–2.58)	0.020	1.55 (1.05–2.28)	0.027
Center		0.935		<0.001		0.94		0.262		0.924		0.278		0.206

GvHD Graft-versus-host disease, NRM non-relapse mortality, LFS leukemia-free survival, OS overall survival, GRFS GvHD-free relapse-free survival, CI confidence interval, SUCBT single umbilical cord blood transplantation, NTD-Haplo non-T cell depleted Haploidentical transplantation, HSCT hematopoietic stem cell transplantation, CR complete remission

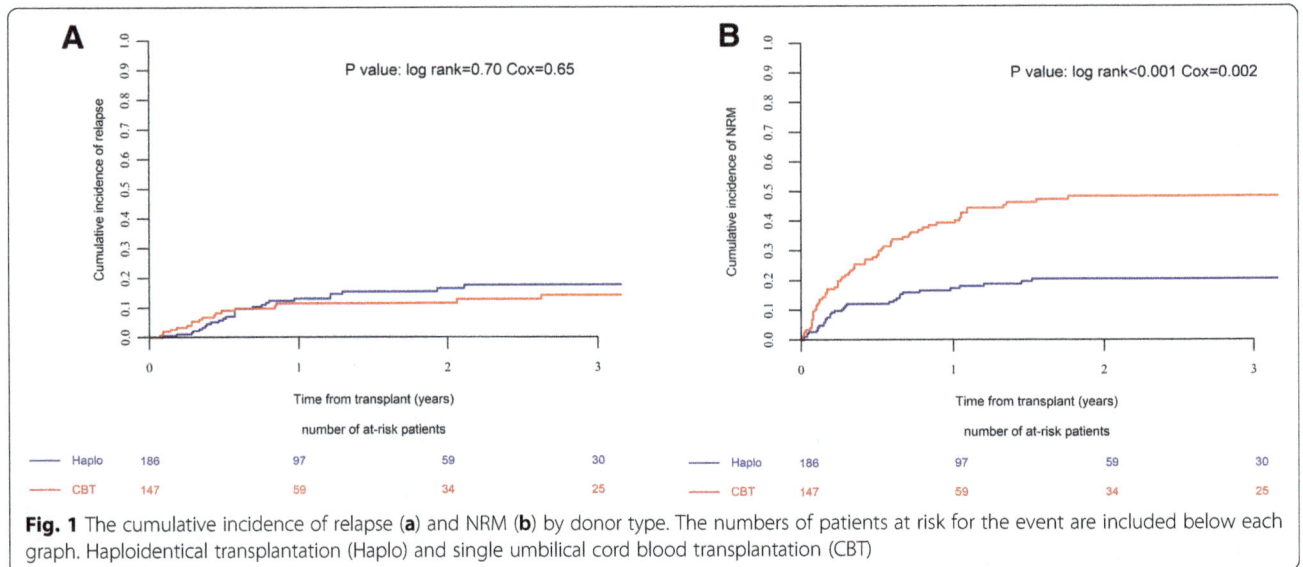

Fig. 1 The cumulative incidence of relapse (**a**) and NRM (**b**) by donor type. The numbers of patients at risk for the event are included below each graph. Haploidentical transplantation (Haplo) and single umbilical cord blood transplantation (CBT)

Differences in OS and LFS in favor of Haplo transplantation are the results of increased NRM with SUCBT. The difference in NRM was mainly driven by infectious complications since the incidence of acute and chronic GvHD was similar between groups. Several factors might have contributed to the excess NRM observed in the SUCBT. First, consistent with previous publication, engraftment with CB was inferior [40]. These issues could translate to an incidence of life-threatening infections. Indeed, infection accounted for 45% of deaths in the SUCBT vs. 35% in NTD-Haplo transplantation. Novel strategies for CB stem cell expansion and others facilitating engraftment kinetics equivalent to other graft sources may help to overcome this limitation [41]. Another important difference is the use of ATG, mainly in patients undergoing SUCBT. Retrospective analyses have found ATG to be associated with worse outcomes after myeloablative and reduced intensity conditioning in the setting of UCBT [42–44]; possibly due to a delayed immune recovery with ATG and

increased incidence of post-transplantation lymphoproliferative disorder and infections [43, 45–48].

Finally, Haplo transplantations were performed more recently compared to SUCBT (median year of transplantation 2014 vs. 2011, $p < 0.001$), possibly accounting for lower rates of NRM in the former (20.6% vs. 48.4%, $p < 0.001$) due to improvements in supportive care. Still, one would not expect such a major difference solely on the basis of year of transplantation. Furthermore, in a multivariable analysis, adjusting for transplantation year, the benefit of Haplo was maintained.

TBF is widely used in the setting of SUCBT. Sanz et al. reported in 2012 on a single center experience of 88 patients with hematologic malignancies, who were treated with a SUCBT after conditioning with TBF-MAC [26]. Over 90% of patients engrafted at a median of 19 days. Furthermore, the 5-year cumulative incidence of NRM and relapse were 44% and 18%, respectively. Ruggeri et al. have found a similar incidence of relapse and lower NRM (33%) in acute leukemia patients treated

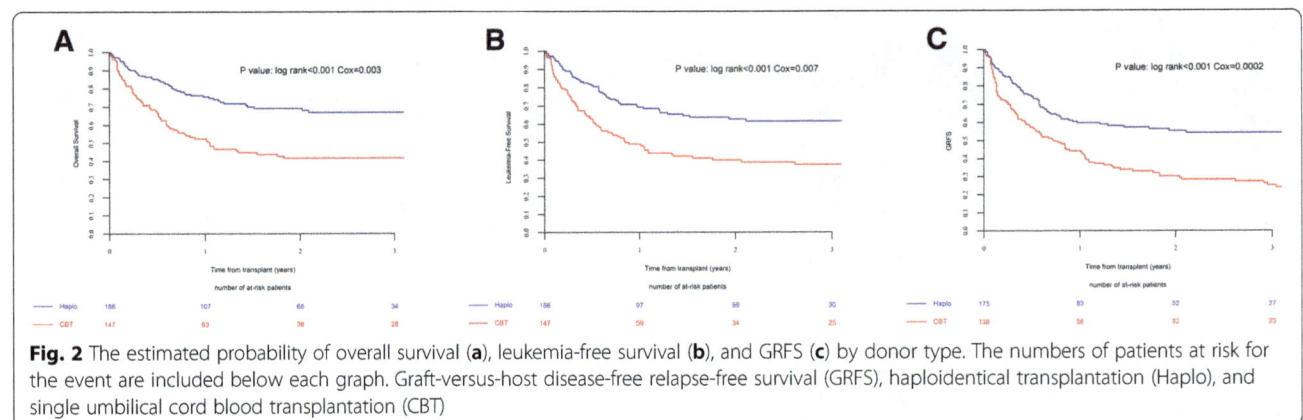

Fig. 2 The estimated probability of overall survival (**a**), leukemia-free survival (**b**), and GRFS (**c**) by donor type. The numbers of patients at risk for the event are included below each graph. Graft-versus-host disease-free relapse-free survival (GRFS), haploidentical transplantation (Haplo), and single umbilical cord blood transplantation (CBT)

with SUCBT and TBF-MAC [27]; outcomes were evaluated at 2 years following transplantation. The rather low relapse rates reported in these two analyses have paved the way for the increasing use of TBF-MAC for SUCBT. Indeed, our results further support the anti-leukemia effect of TBF not only in SUCBT but also with Haplo transplantations, both groups experiencing relatively low relapse rates. The effectiveness of the TBF regimen may be related to the combination of two alkylating agents, as shown in other regimens (e.g., busulfan and melphalan or carmustine [BCNU] and melphalan) [49]. More recently, our group compared TBF to a fludarabine-busulfan protocol in AML patients. Relapse rate was lower in the former, suggesting a stronger anti-leukemic effect with two alkylating agents [33]. In an additional study, the likelihood of relapse was lower with TBF compared to busulfan-cyclophosphamide, indicating that even within possible combinations of alkylating agents, thiotepa confers an additional anti-leukemia advantage [50].

Aside from donor type, additional prognostic factors were observed in our population. Low-performance status was a major predictor of relapse, decreased LFS and GRFS. Poor performance status may be a confounder of disease aggressiveness and exposure to multiple treatments. Therefore, it is difficult to determine its independent merit. Our analysis was not designed to study the importance of donor–recipient sex mismatch in the alternative donor setting. However, we found that transplantation from a female donor to male recipients was associated with an increase in NRM risk, without an apparent reduction of relapse. The results are in line with findings described by Wang and others [51–53].

The current study has several limitations. First, being a retrospective registry-based study, unknown or unmeasured factors could influence the results. However, such studies provide useful guidelines for clinical practice while waiting for randomized trials comparing specific conditionings in defined transplant settings Second, the GvHD prophylaxis strategy varied within each transplantation type. Nonetheless, both the ATG and PTCY are established options in the setting of NTD-Haplo [31, 32, 54]. Finally, a minority of patients in the SUCBT group received grafts with a total nucleated cell dose below 3×10^7/kg, thereby, possibly contributing to the higher incidence of NRM in this group [55]. Yet, since only 20% grafts with less than 2.5×10^7/kg, it is unlikely that changes in NRM can be entirely attributed to the cell dose.

The results of the current analysis validate the effectiveness of TBF-MAC as a potent conditioning platform allowing for graft-versus-leukemia, regardless of the type of alternative donor. While 2-year relapse risk was similar between NTD-Haplo and SUCBT in the current analysis, OS, GRFS, and NRM were superior with the former. Efforts to decrease toxicity and transplant-related mortality needs to be done to further improve outcomes. Nonetheless, a decisive conclusion that NTD-Haplo is preferable is still premature. Prospective trials comparing the two donor types are currently ongoing, and the results will help to clarify the place of the type of graft in the algorithm of donor selection. Second, UCBT safety is likely to improve with the introduction of novel technologies for stem cell expansion and better graft selection. Third, the selection of an alternative donor is mostly dependent on center preference. Currently, most institutions performing these types of transplantation are highly experienced.

Conclusion

This retrospetive analysis suggest that TBF conditioning at a myeloablative dose enables a potent graft-versus-leukemia, regardless of the alternative donor type. Furthermore, in patients receiving TBF, survival with NTD-Haplo may be better compared to SUCBT due to decreased NRM.

Additional file

Additional file 1: Table S1. HLA haploidentical transplantation strategy. **Table S2.** GvHD prophylaxis in patients receiving NTD-Haplo. **Table S3.** GvHD prophylaxis in patients receiving single umbilical cord blood transplantation. **Table S4.** Causes of Death. **Table S5.** The impact of MRC cytogenetic risk groups. (DOCX 19 kb)

Abbreviations

ALWP: Acute Leukemia Working Party; AML: Acute myeloid leukemia; ATG: Anti-thymocyte globulin; CBUs: Cord blood units; CR: Complete remission; EBMT: European Society for Blood and Marrow Transplantation; GRFS: GvHD-free relapse-free survival; GvHD: Graft-versus-host disease; Haplo: Haploidentical stem cell transplantation; HLA: Human leukocyte antigen; HR: Hazard ratio; HSCT: Hematopoietic stem cell transplantation; KPS: Karnofsky performance status; LFS: Leukemia-free survival; MAC: Myeloablative conditioning; NRM: Non-relapse mortality; NTD: Non-T cell depleted; OS: Overall survival; PTCY: Post-transplant cyclophosphamide; RI: Relapse incidence; SUCBT: Single unit umbilical cord blood transplantation; TBF: Thiotepa–IV busulfan–fludarabine; UCBT: Unrelated umbilical cord blood transplantation

Acknowledgements

The authors thank Emmanuelle Polge from the ALWP EBMT and Chantal Kenzey from Eurocord for data management, and all participating centres and patients.

Authors' contributions

FG and ML designed the study. FG, RoS, AR, and AN wrote the manuscript. ML performed the statistical analysis. JaS, WA, EA, JoS. JMRS, SS, BB, AR, RiS, and DB provided cases for the study. All authors read and approved the final manuscript.

Consent for publication

Not applicable.

Competing interests

The authors declare that they have no competing interests.

Author details

[1]Department of Hematology and Cell Therapy, Saint-Antoine Hospital, Paris, France. [2]Acute Leukemia Working Party EBMT Paris Office, Hospital Saint-Antoine, Paris, France. [3]Division of Hematology and Bone Marrow Transplantation Division, Chaim Sheba Medical Center, Tel-Hashomer, Sackler School of Medicine, Tel-Aviv University, 52621 Ramat-Gan, Israel. [4]Dr. Pinchas Bornstein Talpiot Medical Leadership Program, Chaim Sheba Medical Center, Tel-Hashomer, Israel. [5]Hospital Universitari y Politecnic La Fe, Valencia, Spain. [6]Instituto Carlos III, CIBERONC, Madrid, Spain. [7]Rome Transplant Network, "Tor Vergata" University of Rome, Stem Cell Transplant Unit, Policlinico Universitario Tor Vergata, Rome, Italy. [8]Hematology and transplant Unit, Ospedale Policlinico San Martino, Genoa, Italy. [9]Hematology Department, Hospital Santa Creu i Sant Pau, Barcelona, Spain. [10]ICO-Hospital Universitari Germans Trias i Pujol, Josep Carreras Research Institute, Badalona, Spain. [11]Ospedale Civile, Dipartimento di Ematologia, Medicina Trasfusionale e Biotecnologie, Pescara, Italy. [12]S.S.C.V.D Trapianto di Cellule Staminali A.O.U Citta della Salute e della Scienza di Torino, Torino, Italy. [13]Azienda Ospedaliera Papa Giovanni XXIII, Hematology and Bone Marrow Transplant Unit, Bergamo, Italy. [14]Azienda Ospedaliera Universitaria Careggi, Cell Therapy and Transfusion Medicine Unit, Florence, Italy. [15]Programme de Transplantation&Therapie Cellulaire, Centre de Recherche en Cancérologie de Marseille, Institut Paoli Calmettes, Marseille, France. [16]IRCCS, Casa Sollievo della Sofferenza, Department of Hemato-Oncology, Setm Cell Transplant Unit, San Giovanni Rotondo, Italy. [17]Eurocord, Hôpital Saint Louis, Université Paris-Diderot, Paris, France. [18]Department of Hematology, Churchill Hospital, NHS BT, Oxford University, Oxford, UK. [19]Serviço de Hematologia, Hemoterapia e Terapia Celular, Universidade de São Paulo, São Paulo, SP, Brazil. [20]GIGA-I3, University of Liege, Liege, Belgium. [21]Department of Pediatric Hematology and Oncology, IRCCS Bambino Gesù Children's Hospital, Piazza S Onofrio, 4, 00165 Rome, Italy.

References

1. Cornelissen JJ, Blaise D. Hematopoietic stem cell transplantation for patients with AML in first complete remission. Blood. 2016;127(1):62–70.
2. Aversa F, Terenzi A, Tabilio A, Falzetti F, Carotti A, Ballanti S, et al. Full haplotype-mismatched hematopoietic stem-cell transplantation: a phase II study in patients with acute leukemia at high risk of relapse. J Clin Oncol. 2005;23(15):3447–54.
3. Ballen KK, Spitzer TR. The great debate: haploidentical or cord blood transplant. Bone Marrow Transplant. 2011;46(3):323–9.
4. Ciceri F, Labopin M, Aversa F, Rowe JM, Bunjes D, Lewalle P, et al. A survey of fully haploidentical hematopoietic stem cell transplantation in adults with high-risk acute leukemia: a risk factor analysis of outcomes for patients in remission at transplantation. Blood. 2008;112(9):3574–81.
5. Gluckman E, Rocha V, Arcese W, Michel G, Sanz G, Chan KW, et al. Factors associated with outcomes of unrelated cord blood transplant: guidelines for donor choice. Exp Hematol. 2004;32(4):397–407.
6. Rocha V, Labopin M, Sanz G, Arcese W, Schwerdtfeger R, Bosi A, et al. Transplants of umbilical-cord blood or bone marrow from unrelated donors in adults with acute leukemia. N Engl J Med. 2004;351(22):2276–85.
7. Shouval R, Nagler A. From patient centered risk factors to comprehensive prognostic models: a suggested framework for outcome prediction in umbilical cord blood transplantation. Stem Cell Investig. 2017;4:39.
8. Ruggeri A. Alternative donors: cord blood for adults. Semin Hematol. 2016; 53(2):65–73.
9. Querol S, Rubinstein P, Marsh SG, Goldman J, Madrigal JA. Cord blood banking: "providing cord blood banking for a nation". Br J Haematol. 2009; 147(2):227–35.
10. MacMillan ML, Weisdorf DJ, Brunstein CG, Cao Q, DeFor TE, Verneris MR, et al. Acute graft-versus-host disease after unrelated donor umbilical cord blood transplantation: analysis of risk factors. Blood. 2009;113(11):2410–5.
11. Rocha V, Wagner JE Jr, Sobocinski KA, Klein JP, Zhang MJ, Horowitz MM, et al. Graft-versus-host disease in children who have received a cord-blood or bone marrow transplant from an HLA-identical sibling. Eurocord and International Bone Marrow Transplant Registry Working Committee on Alternative Donor and Stem Cell Sources. N Engl J Med. 2000;342(25):1846–54.
12. Bregante S, Dominietto A, Ghiso A, Raiola AM, Gualandi F, Varaldo R, et al. Improved outcome of alternative donor transplantations in patients with myelofibrosis: from unrelated to haploidentical family donors. Biol Blood Marrow Transplant. 2016;22(2):324–9.
13. Laughlin MJ, Eapen M, Rubinstein P, Wagner JE, Zhang MJ, Champlin RE, et al. Outcomes after transplantation of cord blood or bone marrow from unrelated donors in adults with leukemia. N Engl J Med. 2004;351(22):2265–75.
14. Lu DP, Dong L, Wu T, Huang XJ, Zhang MJ, Han W, et al. Conditioning including antithymocyte globulin followed by unmanipulated HLA-mismatched/haploidentical blood and marrow transplantation can achieve comparable outcomes with HLA-identical sibling transplantation. Blood. 2006;107(8):3065–73.
15. Eapen M, Rocha V, Sanz G, Scaradavou A, Zhang MJ, Arcese W, et al. Effect of graft source on unrelated donor haemopoietic stem-cell transplantation in adults with acute leukaemia: a retrospective analysis. Lancet Oncol. 2010; 11(7):653–60.
16. Brunstein CG, Eapen M, Ahn KW, Appelbaum FR, Ballen KK, Champlin RE, et al. Reduced-intensity conditioning transplantation in acute leukemia: the effect of source of unrelated donor stem cells on outcomes. Blood. 2012; 119(23):5591–8.
17. Bashey A, Zhang X, Sizemore CA, Manion K, Brown S, Holland HK, et al. T-cell-replete HLA-haploidentical hematopoietic transplantation for hematologic malignancies using post-transplantation cyclophosphamide results in outcomes equivalent to those of contemporaneous HLA-matched related and unrelated donor transplantation. J Clin Oncol. 2013;31(10):1310–6.
18. Raiola AM, Dominietto A, di Grazia C, Lamparelli T, Gualandi F, Ibatici A, et al. Unmanipulated haploidentical transplants compared with other alternative donors and matched sibling grafts. Biol Blood Marrow Transplant. 2014;20(10):1573–9.
19. Wang Y, Liu QF, Xu LP, Liu KY, Zhang XH, Ma X, et al. Haploidentical vs identical-sibling transplant for AML in remission: a multicenter, prospective study. Blood. 2015;125(25):3956–62.
20. Wang Y, Liu QF, Xu LP, Liu KY, Zhang XH, Ma X, et al. Haploidentical versus matched-sibling transplant in adults with Philadelphia-negative high-risk acute lymphoblastic leukemia: a biologically phase III randomized study. Clin Cancer Res. 2016;22(14):3467–76.
21. Wang Y, Wang HX, Lai YR, Sun ZM, Wu DP, Jiang M, et al. Haploidentical transplant for myelodysplastic syndrome: registry-based comparison with identical sibling transplant. Leukemia. 2016;30(10):2055–63.
22. Mo XD, Tang BL, Zhang XH, Zheng CC, Xu LP, Zhu XY, et al. Comparison of outcomes after umbilical cord blood and unmanipulated haploidentical hematopoietic stem cell transplantation in children with high-risk acute lymphoblastic leukemia. Int J Cancer. 2016;139(9):2106–15.
23. Ringden O, Labopin M, Ehninger G, Niederwieser D, Olsson R, Basara N, et al. Reduced intensity conditioning compared with myeloablative conditioning using unrelated donor transplants in patients with acute myeloid leukemia. J Clin Oncol. 2009;27(27):4570–7.
24. Scott BL, Pasquini MC, Logan BR, Wu J, Devine SM, Porter DL, et al. Myeloablative versus reduced-intensity hematopoietic cell transplantation for acute myeloid leukemia and myelodysplastic syndromes. J Clin Oncol. 2017;35(11):1154–61.
25. Gyurkocza B, Sandmaier BM. Conditioning regimens for hematopoietic cell transplantation: one size does not fit all. Blood. 2014;124(3):344–53.
26. Sanz J, Boluda JC, Martin C, Gonzalez M, Ferra C, Serrano D, et al. Single-unit umbilical cord blood transplantation from unrelated donors in patients with hematological malignancy using busulfan, thiotepa, fludarabine and ATG as myeloablative conditioning regimen. Bone Marrow Transplant. 2012;47(10):1287–93.
27. Ruggeri A, Sanz G, Bittencourt H, Sanz J, Rambaldi A, Volt F, et al. Comparison of outcomes after single or double cord blood transplantation in adults with acute leukemia using different types of myeloablative conditioning regimen, a retrospective study on behalf of

Eurocord and the Acute Leukemia Working Party of EBMT. Leukemia. 2014;28(4):779–86.

28. Huang XJ, Liu DH, Liu KY, Xu LP, Chen H, Han W, et al. Treatment of acute leukemia with unmanipulated HLA-mismatched/haploidentical blood and bone marrow transplantation. Biol Blood Marrow Transplant. 2009;15(2):257–65.

29. Lee KH, Lee JH, Lee JH, Kim DY, Kim SH, Shin HJ, et al. Hematopoietic cell transplantation from an HLA-mismatched familial donor is feasible without ex vivo-T cell depletion after reduced-intensity conditioning with busulfan, fludarabine, and antithymocyte globulin. Biol Blood Marrow Transplant. 2009;15(1):61–72.

30. Luznik L, Bolanos-Meade J, Zahurak M, Chen AR, Smith BD, Brodsky R, et al. High-dose cyclophosphamide as single-agent, short-course prophylaxis of graft-versus-host disease. Blood. 2010;115(16):3224–30.

31. Di Bartolomeo P, Santarone S, De Angelis G, Picardi A, Cudillo L, Cerretti R, et al. Haploidentical, unmanipulated, G-CSF-primed bone marrow transplantation for patients with high-risk hematologic malignancies. Blood. 2013;121(5):849–57.

32. Raiola AM, Dominietto A, Ghiso A, Di Grazia C, Lamparelli T, Gualandi F, et al. Unmanipulated haploidentical bone marrow transplantation and posttransplantation cyclophosphamide for hematologic malignancies after myeloablative conditioning. Biol Blood Marrow Transplant. 2013;19(1):117–22.

33. Saraceni F, Labopin M, Hamladji RM, Mufti G, Socie G, Shimoni A, et al. Thiotepa-busulfan-fludarabine compared to busulfan-fludarabine for sibling and unrelated donor transplant in acute myeloid leukemia in first remission. Oncotarget. 2018;9(3):3379–93.

34. Grimwade D, Walker H, Oliver F, Wheatley K, Harrison C, Harrison G, et al. The importance of diagnostic cytogenetics on outcome in AML: analysis of 1,612 patients entered into the MRC AML 10 trial. The Medical Research Council Adult and Children's Leukaemia Working Parties. Blood. 1998;92(7):2322–33.

35. Ruggeri A, Labopin M, Ciceri F, Mohty M, Nagler A. Definition of GvHD-free, relapse-free survival for registry-based studies: an ALWP-EBMT analysis on patients with AML in remission. Bone Marrow Transplant. 2016;51(4):610–1.

36. Glucksberg H, Storb R, Fefer A, Buckner CD, Neiman PE, Clift RA, et al. Clinical manifestations of graft-versus-host disease in human recipients of marrow from HL-A-matched sibling donors. Transplantation. 1974;18(4):295–304.

37. Terwey TH, Vega-Ruiz A, Hemmati PG, Martus P, Dietz E, le Coutre P, et al. NIH-defined graft-versus-host disease after reduced intensity or myeloablative conditioning in patients with acute myeloid leukemia. Leukemia. 2012;26(3):536–42.

38. Kaplan EL, Meier P. Nonparametric estimation from incomplete observations. J Am Stat Assoc. 1958;53(282):457–81.

39. Cox DR. Regression models and life-tables. In Breakthroughs in statistics. New York: Springer; 1992. p. 527–41.

40. Ruggeri A, Labopin M, Sanz G, Piemontese S, Arcese W, Bacigalupo A, et al. Comparison of outcomes after unrelated cord blood and unmanipulated haploidentical stem cell transplantation in adults with acute leukemia. Leukemia. 2015;29(9):1891–900.

41. Baron F, Ruggeri A, Nagler A. Methods of ex vivo expansion of human cord blood cells: challenges, successes and clinical implications. Expert Rev Hematol. 2016;9(3):297–314.

42. Shouval R, Ruggeri A, Labopin M, Mohty M, Sanz G, Michel G, et al. An integrative scoring system for survival prediction following umbilical cord blood transplantation in acute leukemia. Clin Cancer Res. 2017;23(21):6478–86.

43. Pascal L, Tucunduva L, Ruggeri A, Blaise D, Ceballos P, Chevallier P, et al. Impact of ATG-containing reduced-intensity conditioning after single- or double-unit allogeneic cord blood transplantation. Blood. 2015;126(8):1027–32.

44. Pascal L, Mohty M, Ruggeri A, Tucunduva L, Milpied N, Chevallier P, et al. Impact of rabbit ATG-containing myeloablative conditioning regimens on the outcome of patients undergoing unrelated single-unit cord blood transplantation for hematological malignancies. Bone Marrow Transplant. 2015;50(1):45–50.

45. Admiraal R, Lindemans CA, van Kesteren C, Bierings MB, Versluijs AB, Nierkens S, et al. Excellent T-cell reconstitution and survival depend on low ATG exposure after pediatric cord blood transplantation. Blood. 2016; 128(23):2734–41.

46. Sanz J, Arango M, Senent L, Jarque I, Montesinos P, Sempere A, et al. EBV-associated post-transplant lymphoproliferative disorder after umbilical cord blood transplantation in adults with hematological diseases. Bone Marrow Transplant. 2014;49(3):397–402.

47. Dumas PY, Ruggeri A, Robin M, Crotta A, Abraham J, Forcade E, et al. Incidence and risk factors of EBV reactivation after unrelated cord blood transplantation:

a Eurocord and Societe Francaise de Greffe de Moelle-Therapie Cellulaire collaborative study. Bone Marrow Transplant. 2013;48(2):253–6.

48. Brunstein CG, Weisdorf DJ, DeFor T, Barker JN, Tolar J, van Burik JA, et al. Marked increased risk of Epstein-Barr virus-related complications with the addition of antithymocyte globulin to a nonmyeloablative conditioning prior to unrelated umbilical cord blood transplantation. Blood. 2006;108(8):2874–80.

49. Bertz H, Potthoff K, Finke J. Allogeneic stem-cell transplantation from related and unrelated donors in older patients with myeloid leukemia. J Clin Oncol. 2003;21(8):1480–4.

50. Saraceni F, Beohou E, Labopin M, Arcese W, Bonifazi F, Stepensky P, et al. Thiotepa, busulfan and fludarabine compared to busulfan and cyclophosphamide as conditioning regimen for allogeneic stem cell transplant from matched siblings and unrelated donors for acute myeloid leukemia. Am J Hematol. 2018. https://doi.org/10.1002/ajh.25225. [Epub ahead of print].

51. Wang Y, Chang YJ, Xu LP, Liu KY, Liu DH, Zhang XH, et al. Who is the best donor for a related HLA haplotype-mismatched transplant? Blood. 2014; 124(6):843–50.

52. Luo Y, Xiao H, Lai X, Shi J, Tan Y, He J, et al. T-cell-replete haploidentical HSCT with low-dose anti-T-lymphocyte globulin compared with matched sibling HSCT and unrelated HSCT. Blood. 2014;124(17):2735–43.

53. McCurdy SR, Kanakry JA, Showel MM, Tsai HL, Bolanos-Meade J, Rosner GL, et al. Risk-stratified outcomes of nonmyeloablative HLA-haploidentical BMT with high-dose posttransplantation cyclophosphamide. Blood. 2015;125(19):3024–31.

54. Bacigalupo A, Dominietto A, Ghiso A, Di Grazia C, Lamparelli T, Gualandi F, et al. Unmanipulated haploidentical bone marrow transplantation and post-transplant cyclophosphamide for hematologic malignanices following a myeloablative conditioning: an update. Bone Marrow Transplant. 2015; 50(Suppl 2):S37–9.

55. Barker JN, Scaradavou A, Stevens CE. Combined effect of total nucleated cell dose and HLA match on transplantation outcome in 1061 cord blood recipients with hematologic malignancies. Blood. 2010;115(9):1843–9.

6

Exosomes released by hepatocarcinoma cells endow adipocytes with tumor-promoting properties

Shihua Wang[1†], Meiqian Xu[1†], Xiaoxia Li[2], Xiaodong Su[1], Xian Xiao[1], Armand Keating[3,4,5*] and Robert Chunhua Zhao[1*]

Abstract

Background: The initiation and progression of hepatocellular carcinoma (HCC) are largely dependent on its local microenvironment. Adipocytes are an important component of hepatic microenvironment in nonalcoholic fatty liver disease (NAFLD), which is a significant risk factor for HCC. Given the global prevalence of NAFLD, a better understanding of the interplay between HCC cells and adipocytes is urgently needed. Exosomes, released by malignant cells, represent a novel way of cell-cell interaction and have been shown to play an important role in cancer cell communication with their microenvironment. Here, we explore the role of HCC-derived exosomes in the cellular and molecular conversion of adipocytes into tumor-promoting cells.

Methods: Exosomes were isolated from HCC cell line HepG2 and added to adipocytes. Transcriptomic alterations of exosome-stimulated adipocytes were analyzed using gene expression profiling, and secretion of inflammation-associated cytokines was detected by RT-PCR and ELISA. In vivo mouse xenograft model was used to evaluate the growth-promoting and angiogenesis-enhancing effects of exosome-treated adipocytes. Protein content of tumor exosomes was analyzed by mass spectrometry. Activated phospho-kinases involved in exosome-treated adipocytes were detected by phospho-kinase antibody array and Western blot.

Results: Our results demonstrated that HCC cell HepG2-derived exosomes could be actively internalized by adipocytes and caused significant transcriptomic alterations and in particular induced an inflammatory phenotype in adipocytes. The tumor exosome-treated adipocytes, named exo-adipocytes, promoted tumor growth, enhanced angiogenesis, and recruited more macrophages in mouse xenograft model. In vitro, conditioned medium from exo-adipocytes promoted HepG2 cell migration and increased tube formation of human umbilical vein endothelial cells (HUVECs). Mechanistically, we found HepG2 exosomes activated several phopho-kinases and NF-κB signaling pathway in exo-adipocytes. Additionally, a total of 1428 proteins were identified in HepG2 exosomes by mass spectrometry.

Conclusions: Our results provide new insights into the concept that tumor cell-derived exosomes can educate surrounding adipocytes to create a favorable microenvironment for tumor progression.

Keywords: Exosomes, Adipocyte, HCC, MSCs, NF-κB

* Correspondence: armand.keating@uhn.ca; zhaochunhua@ibms.pumc.edu.cn
†Shihua Wang and Meiqian Xu contributed equally to this work.
³Cell Therapy Translational Research Laboratory, Princess Margaret Cancer Centre, Toronto, Ontario M5G 2M9, Canada
¹Center of Excellence in Tissue Engineering, Institute of Basic Medical Sciences, Peking Union Medical College Hospital, Chinese Academy of Medical Sciences, School of Basic Medicine Peking Union Medical College, Beijing 100005, China
Full list of author information is available at the end of the article

Background

Hepatocellular carcinoma (HCC) now represents the fifth most common cancer worldwide and the third leading cause of cancer-related mortality [1, 2]. Although both diagnostic and therapeutic strategies for HCC have improved over the past decades, the 5-year survival rate only is around 10%, and HCC continues to be a global health issue, especially in Asian countries [3, 4]. Emerging evidence suggested that nonalcoholic fatty liver disease (NAFLD), a common disorder in obese people, is a significant risk factor for HCC [5, 6]. Given the global prevalence of obesity, there is the looming threat of a rapidly rising occurrence of NAFLD-related HCC. Therefore, it is urgent and paramount to understand the mechanisms by which NAFLD contributes to HCC development.

Tumor behavior is determined by not only the malignant potential of tumor cell itself but also the signals from its microenvironment. Thus, it is clear that the crosstalk between tumor cells and their surrounding microenvironment is crucial for HCC development. In NAFLD, the hepatic microenvironment comprises multiple cell lineages including endothelial cells, hepatic satellite cells, immune cells, and adipocytes [7, 8]. Previous studies have focused intensively on the interactions between HCC cells and a wide variety of immune cells such as Kupffer cells, NK cells, T cells, and several antigen-presenting cells. For example, necrotic debris of HCC cells can induce potent IL-1β release by macrophages which subsequently promote HCC metastasis in mouse models [9]. The work done by Wolf et al. showed that hepatic NKT cells promoted NAFLD by secreting LIGHT and activated NF-κB signaling in hepatocytes to enhance malignant transformation [10]. However, the interplay between the HCC cells and adjacent adipocytes remains poorly understood so far.

Currently, how cancer cells communicate with their local and distant microenvironment is undergoing a re-evaluation with the discovery of a novel way of cell-cell interaction exosomes [11, 12]. In addition to diffusible factors, such as growth factors, cytokines, and extracellular bioactive molecules, exosomes are small membrane vesicles that are released by many different cell types, including cancer cells. Increasing evidence suggests that tumor-derived exosomes support tumor development and progression by generating a favorable milieu through immune suppression, angiogenesis enhancement, extracellular matrix remodeling, and stromal cell conversion [13–15]. Exosome-mediated transfer of proteins, DNA, noncoding RNAs, and mRNAs could induce phenotypic changes in target cells [16]. In melanoma, the tumor-derived exosomes educated bone marrow progenitors toward a pro-metastatic phenotype through the receptor tyrosine kinase MET [17]. In pancreatic cancer, the secreted exosomes induced lipolysis in subcutaneous adipose tissue [18]. In HCC, exosomes derived from metastatic HCC cell lines significantly enhanced the migratory and invasive abilities of nonmotile hepatocytes [19]. However, to our knowledge, no study has reported on the effects of tumor-derived exosomes on adipocytes, which represent an abundant cell type within tumor microenvironment in overweight patients.

In this study, we explored the role of HCC-derived exosomes in the cellular and molecular conversion of adipocytes into tumor-promoting cells. Our results demonstrated that HCC cell line HepG2-derived exosomes could be actively internalized by adipocytes differentiated from mesenchymal stem cells (MSCs) and caused significant transcriptomic alterations, and in particular, induced an inflammatory phenotype in adipocytes. The tumor exosome-treated adipocytes, named exo-adipocytes, promoted tumor growth, enhanced angiogenesis, and recruited more macrophages in mouse xenograft model. In vitro, conditioned medium from exo-adipocytes promoted HepG2 cell migration and increased tube formation of human umbilical vein endothelial cells (HUVECs). Mechanistically, we found HepG2 exosomes activated several kinases and NF-κB signaling pathway in exo-adipocytes. Our findings showed for the first time that HCC-derived exosomes could convert adipocytes into tumor-promoting cells, which may provide new insights into understanding the interactions between tumor cells and surrounding microenvironment.

Methods

Cell culture

Human adipose tissues and umbilical cords were obtained according to the procedures approved by the Ethics Committee at the Chinese Academy of Medical Sciences and Peking Union Medical College. MSCs were isolated and culture-expanded from healthy volunteers as previously reported [20]. Passage 3 MSCs were used for following experiments. To obtain adipocytes, MSCs were induced under adipogenic differentiation medium, which is high glucose of Dulbecco's modified Eagle's medium (H-DMEM) supplemented with 10% FBS, 1 μM dexamethasone, 0.5 mM 3-isobutyl-1-methylxanthine, and 5 μg/mL 0.1 mM L-ascorbic acid. Adipocytes were characterized by Oil Red O staining according to the manufacture's (Beyotime Biotechnology) instructions. HUVECs were isolated and cultured as routinely described [21]. HCC cell line HepG2 was purchased from cell bank at the Chinese Academy of Medical Sciences and cultured in DF12 containing 10% FBS, penicillin (100 U/mL), and streptomycin (100lg/mL) at 37 °C with 5% CO_2.

Exosomes isolation

Exosome extraction was performed as previously described [22]. Briefly, HepG2 cells were cultured in serum-free DF12 medium for 24 h. Then, the culture medium was collected and centrifuged at 800g for 5 min and additional 2000g for 10 min to remove lifted cells. The supernatant was subjected to filtration on a 0.1-mm-pore polyethersulfone membrane filter (Corning) to remove cell debris and large vesicles, followed by concentration by a 100,000-Mw cutoff membrane (CentriPlus-70, Millipore). The volume of supernatant was reduced from approximately 250–500 mL to less than 5 mL. The supernatant was then ultracentrifuged at 100,000g for 1 h at 4 °C using 70Ti Rotor (Beckman Coulter). The resulting pellets were resuspended in 6 mL PBS and ultracentrifuged at 100,000g for 1 h at 4 °C using 100Ti Rotor (Beckman Coulter). In the experiments involving HepG2 exosomes, we use PBS as a negative control.

Transmission electron microscopy

Purified exosomes were fixed with 1% glutaraldehyde in PBS (pH 7.4). After rinsing, a 20-uL drop of the suspension was loaded onto a formvar/carbon-coated grid, negatively stained with 3% (w/v) aqueous phosphotungstic acid for 1 min, and observed by transmission electron microscope.

Quantitative real-time polymerase chain reaction

Total RNA was extracted using TRIzol (Invitrogen) according to the manufacturer's instruction, and cDNA was prepared. Real-time PCR amplification was performed in triplicates according to the procedures reported previously [23]. Relative expression of mRNA was evaluated by the 2-$\Delta\Delta$Ct method and normalized to the expression of GAPDH.

Western blotting

Proteins were extracted with radioimmunoprecipitation (RIPA) lysis buffer with PMSF, quantified by BCA Protein Assay Kit (Beyotime). Western blot was performed in triplicates according to the procedures reported previously [24]. GAPDH was used as an internal control. We used the following antibodies: p-AKT (1:2000; rabbit IgG, CST, 4060T), p-ERK1/2 (1:5000; rabbit IgG, Abcam, ab76299), p-STAT5α (1:1000; rabbit IgG, Abcam, ab30648), p-GSK (1:5000; rabbit IgG, Abcam, ab75814), AKT (1:1000; mouse IgG, proteintech, 60203-2-Ig), ERK1/2 (1:1000; rabbit IgG, proteintech, 16443-1-AP), STAT5α (1:1000; rabbit IgG, Abcam, ab32043), GSK3β (1:1000, rabbit IgG, proteintech, 22104-1-AP), CD63 (1:500; rabbit IgG, proteintech, 25682-1-AP), TSG101 (1:500; rabbit IgG, Abcam, ab83), HSP70 (1:100; rabbit IgG, SBI, EXOAB-KIT-1), calnexin (1:2000; rabbit IgG, CST, 2433s), GAPDH (1:10000; rabbit IgG, proteintech, 10494-1-AP) (1:10000; mouse IgG, proteintech, 60004-1-Ig), HRP-conjugated anti-rabbit-IgG (NeoBioscience), HRP-conjugated anti-goat-IgG (NeoBioscience), and HRP-conjugated anti-mouse-IgG (NeoBioscience).

Cytokine analysis

Culture medium was collected 24 h after the treatment with or without exosomes. The concentrations of all cell cytokines in supernatants were measured using ELISA kits (BD Technologies).

Immunofluorescence staining

The cultured cells were fixed at 4 °C in ice-cold methanol for 10 min, washed three times in phosphate-buffered saline (PBS), and then permeabilized in 0.1% Triton X-100/PBS for 10 min at room temperature. Nonspecific binding was blocked with 0.5% Tween-20/PBS containing 1% bovine serum albumin (BSA) for 30 min. The primary antibodies were incubated at 4 °C overnight. The secondary antibodies were incubated for 1 h at room temperature. The incubated cells were washed in PBS, and Hoechst 33342 (Sigma-Aldrich) was used to visualize nuclei. p65 antibody (10745-1-AP) was purchased from Proteintech.

Mouse xenograft experiments

Nude mice were purchased from the Laboratory Animal Center of the Chinese Academy of Medical Sciences (Beijing, China). Animal use and experimental procedures were approved by the Animal Care and Use Committee of the Chinese Academy of Medical Sciences. Mice were randomly divided into three groups, one group received a subcutaneous injection of 2×10^5 exo-adipocytes and 2×10^6 HepG2 cells, one group received 2×10^5 adipocytes and 2×10^6 HepG2 cells, and the last one received 2×10^6 HepG2 cells. The tumor weight was measured after 4 weeks. The tumor tissues were fixed with 10% PFA. Each group was treated with HE, IL-6, Ki67, CD31, and F4/80 staining.

Tube formation assay in Matrigel

In vitro capillary network formation was determined by performing a tube formation assay in Matrigel (BD Biosciences). 1×10^4 HUVECs were plated on a growth factor-reduced Matrigel (BD)-coated 96-well plate in triplicates with 100 uL serum-free medium (control), exo-adipocyte-conditioned medium, or adipocyte-conditioned medium. After 8 h of incubation, tube formation was examined by microscopy (Olympus, Tokyo, Japan), and the branch density and tube length were quantified by randomly selecting three fields per well.

Statistical analysis

Data are presented as mean ± SD. Comparisons between groups were analyzed via Student's t test. Differences were considered statistically significant at *$P < 0.05$, **$P < 0.01$, and ***$P < 0.001$.

Results

HepG2 exosomes are actively internalized by adipocytes

To investigate whether exosomes are secreted by hepatocarcinoma cell HepG2 and play a role in their communication with adipocytes, we used differential centrifugation to purify exosomes from the supernatant of HepG2 cells. Isolated particles were observed under transmission electron microscopy and found to present characteristics of exosomes, with typical appearance and diameter ranging from 30 to 200 nm (Fig. 1a). The nanoparticle size distribution for the HepG2 exosomes was further obtained by NTA, and the peaks of particle size were ~ 100 nm, within the expected size of exosomes (Fig. 1b). Enrichment for exosome marker CD63, TSG101, and the absence of the cell-specific marker calnexin was demonstrated by Western blot (Fig. 1c). Adipocytes were differentiated from human mesenchymal stem cells (MSCs) under adipogenic induction conditions. Figure 1d characterizes the MSC-derived adipocytes by morphology, Oil Red O staining, BODIPY staining, and expression of specific adipogenic marker genes during adipogenic differentiation of MSCs. To examine if adipocytes might be targets of HepG2-derived exosomes, a lipid-associating fluorescent dye, PKH67, was used to label exosome preparations and then incubated with adipocytes. Exosome incorporation was observed 0.5 h after treatment, and exosomes accumulated in adipocytes over time (Fig. 1e). Collectively, we show that HepG2 cells secrete exosomes, which are actively incorporated in vitro by adipocytes.

HepG2 exosomes induce an inflammatory phenotype in adipocytes

To determine the effects of HepG2 exosomes on adipocytes, we exposed adipocytes to 25 μg/mL HepG2 exosomes for 24 h and evaluated the transcriptomic alterations using gene expression profiling. Seven hundred twenty-five upregulated and 648 downregulated genes were identified (Fig. 2a), and the top 10 up- and downregulated genes in HepG2 exosome-treated adipocytes (exo-adipocytes) compared to control are shown in Fig. 2b. Interestingly, unsupervised clustering identified expression changes in gene signatures related to inflammation in exosome-treated adipocytes (Fig. 2c). Considering that cancer is often associated with an inflammatory milieu, we began to explore whether HepG2 exosomes could change inflammatory response

in adipocytes. In our previous report, we found that lung tumor exosomes trigger the release of cytokines including IL-6, IL-8, and MCP-1 in MSC [24]. Therefore, we extended this analysis in adipocytes and confirmed the enhanced release of IL-6, IL-8, and MCP-1 by qRT-PCR (Fig. 2d left) and ELISA (Fig. 2d right). To determine whether increased expression of cytokines in exosome-treated adipocytes was concentration-dependent, we treated adipocytes with different concentrations of HepG2 exosomes for 24 h and found a partial dose-dependent effect of exosomes on the secretion of IL-6, IL-8, and MCP-1 (Fig. 2e).

exo-adipocytes promote tumor growth in vivo

Considering the important role of inflammatory cytokines in tumor development, we next analyzed whether exo-adipocytes affected HepG2 cells and provided a benefit for tumor growth by using a nude mouse xenograft tumor model. HepG2 cells were subcutaneously co-implanted with exo-adipocytes, adipocytes, or PBS at a ratio of 10:1. Coinjection with exo-adipocytes resulted in an increased tumor weight compared with tumor cells injected with adipocytes or PBS (Fig. 3a). To determine the effect of exo-adipocytes on angiogenesis and proliferation of tumor cells in vivo, we performed IHC staining to detect CD31 and Ki67. Coinjected exo-adipocytes could enhance the vascular density as demonstrated by the increased expression of CD31 (Fig. 3b,c). Figure 3d, e revealed that the numbers of Ki67-positive cells were increased significantly in the presence of exo-adipocytes. When the tumors were excised for assessment of immune cell infiltration, we observed that the number of F4/80 macrophages was higher in tumors receiving exo-adipocytes than those receiving control adipocytes (Fig. 3f, g). Previous studies suggest IL-6 to be a major regulator of tumor-stroma interaction in cancer microenvironment [25]. Here, we examined IL-6 expression levels in tumor sections and found increased IL-6 protein levels (Fig. 3h, i), consistent with the upregulation of IL-6 genes shown in Fig. 2e. In addition, we observed the appearance of adipocytes among cancer cells in the tumor sections, suggesting that adipocytes were not consumed by neighboring cancer cells during the 4-week tumorigenesis process (Fig. 3j). Taken together, exo-adipocytes were endowed with a capability by tumor exosomes to promote tumor growth, enhance angiogenesis, and recruit macrophages in vivo.

exo-adipocyte-conditioned medium is chemotaxic and promotes HepG2 migration

The increased number of F4/80 macrophages in tumors receiving exo-adipocytes prompted us to investigate the effect of exo-adipocyte-conditioned medium on THP-1 cells in vitro as THP-1 cells are one of the

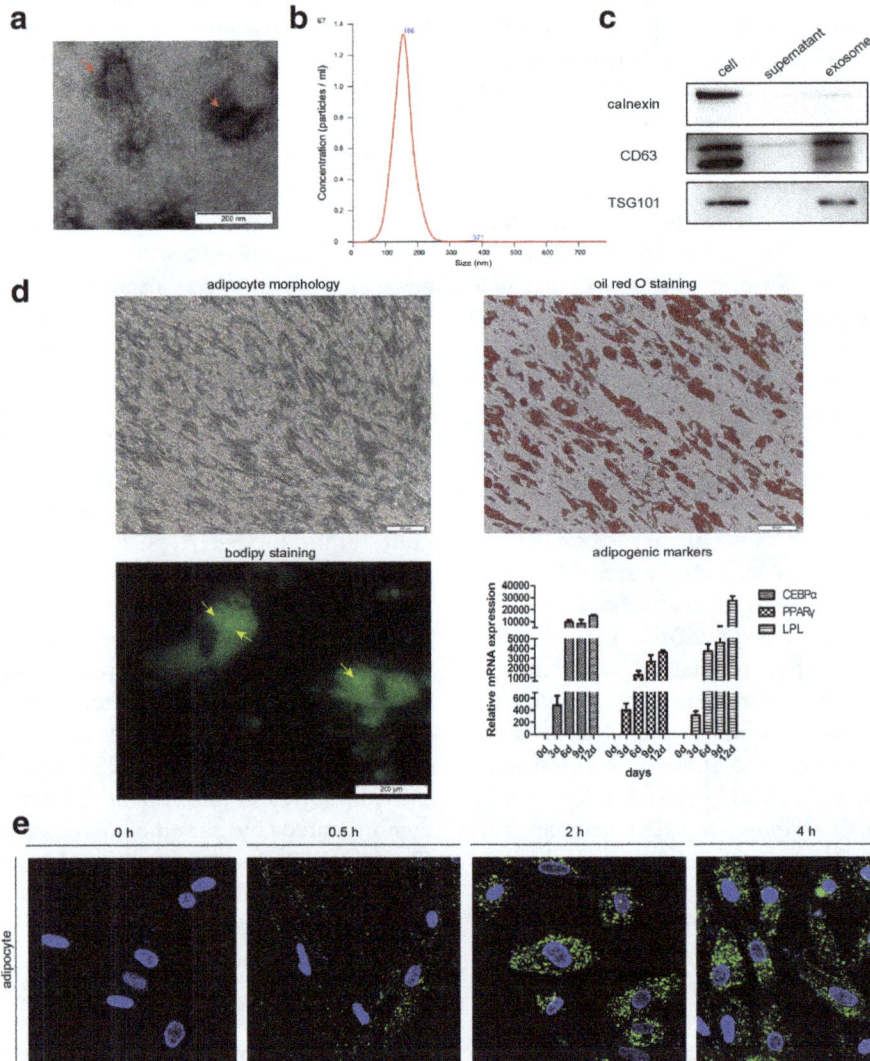

Fig. 1 HepG2 cell-secreted exosomes are actively incorporated by adipocytes in culture. **a** A representative electron microscopy image of purified HepG2 exosomes showed morphology. Scale bar, 200 nm. **b** The nanoparticle size distribution for HepG2 exosomes was obtained by NTA. The particle size is between 0 and 300, with a peak around 100 nm. **c** Western blot analysis of exosome marker CD63, TSG101, and cell-specific marker calnexin. Positive control was HepG2 cell lysate, and negative control was culture medium. **d** Characterization of adipocytes differentiated from MSCs by morphology, Oil Red O staining, BODIPY staining, and expression of specific adipogenic marker genes CEBPα, PPARγ, and LPL. **e** Adipocytes were incubated with 70 ng/mL PKH67-labeled HepG2 exosomes for the indicated times, and uptake of exosomes was determined by fluorescence confocal microscopy

most widely used cell lines to investigate the function and regulation of macrophages [26, 27]. We found that exo-adipocyte-conditioned medium was more chemotactic than adipocyte-conditioned medium for THP-1 cells (Fig. 4a). Additionally, a similar effect was observed for HepG2 tumor cells (Fig. 4b). We then examined whether exo-adipocyte-conditioned medium could affect tumor cell migration. As expected, compared with the adipocyte-conditioned medium, exo-adipocyte-conditioned medium increased the migration capacity of HepG2 (Fig. 4c).

exo-adipocyte-conditioned medium enhanced tube formation of HUVECs

To confirm our in vivo findings that exo-adipocytes promote angiogenesis in tumors, we examined the effect of exo-adipocyte-conditioned medium on HUVECs. Forty-eight hours after exposure to exo-adipocyte-conditioned medium, HUVECs exhibited upregulated expression of pro-angiogenic genes Ang1 and Flk1 as well as downregulated the expression of anti-angiogenic genes Vash1 and TSP1 (Fig. 5a). We

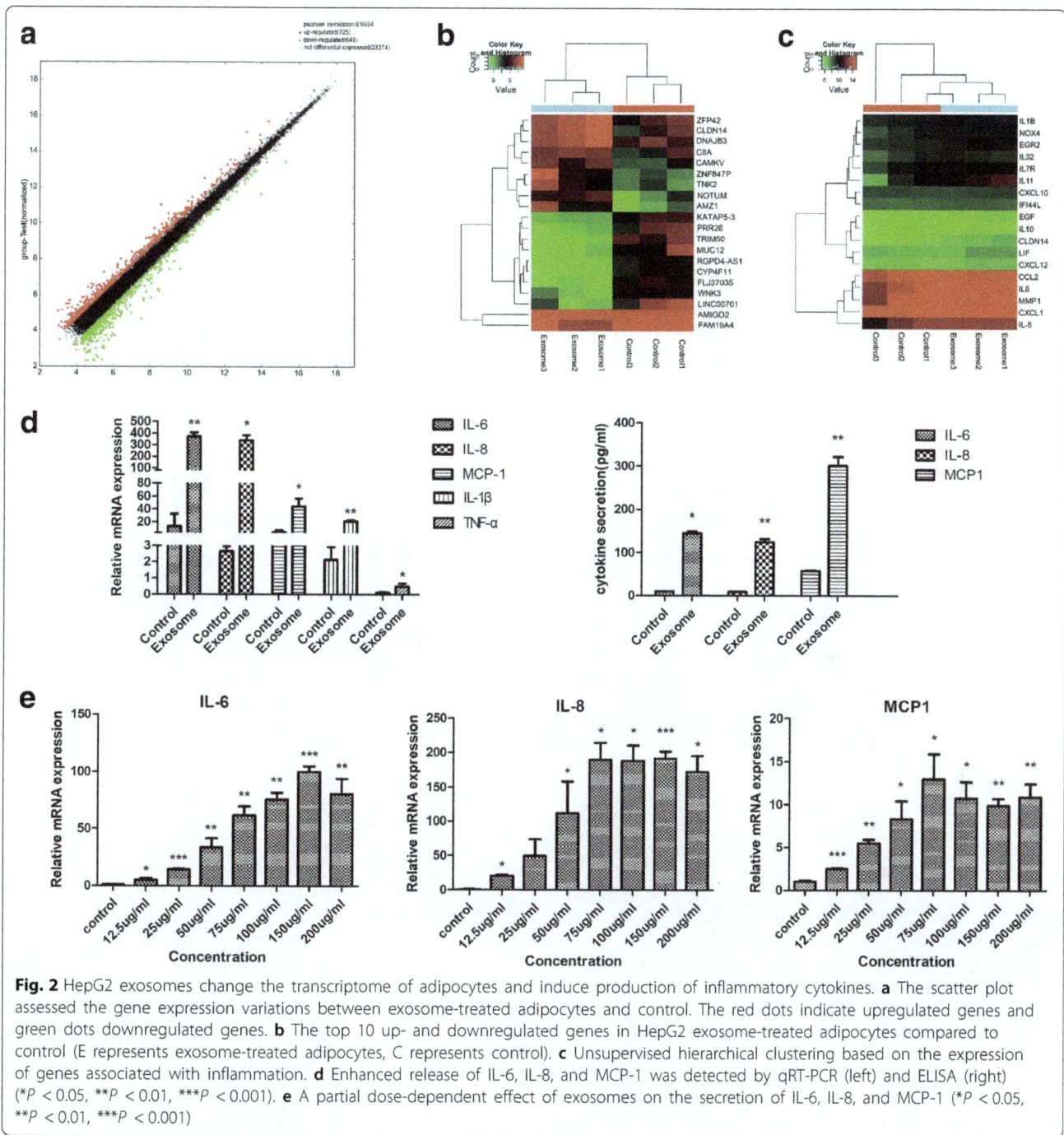

Fig. 2 HepG2 exosomes change the transcriptome of adipocytes and induce production of inflammatory cytokines. **a** The scatter plot assessed the gene expression variations between exosome-treated adipocytes and control. The red dots indicate upregulated genes and green dots downregulated genes. **b** The top 10 up- and downregulated genes in HepG2 exosome-treated adipocytes compared to control (E represents exosome-treated adipocytes, C represents control). **c** Unsupervised hierarchical clustering based on the expression of genes associated with inflammation. **d** Enhanced release of IL-6, IL-8, and MCP-1 was detected by qRT-PCR (left) and ELISA (right) (*$P < 0.05$, **$P < 0.01$, ***$P < 0.001$). **e** A partial dose-dependent effect of exosomes on the secretion of IL-6, IL-8, and MCP-1 (*$P < 0.05$, **$P < 0.01$, ***$P < 0.001$)

further evaluated the effects of exo-adipocyte-conditioned medium on HUVECs tube formation. As expected, tube formation of HUVECs was significantly increased in the presence of exo-adipocyte-conditioned medium as demonstrated by the increase in tube lengths and areas (Fig. 5b). Collectively, our results suggest that exo-adipocyte-conditioned medium promoted angiogenesis of endothelial cells both in vitro and in vivo.

HepG2 exosomes activate various kinases and NF-κB signaling pathway in adipocytes

To identify which signaling pathways were activated by HepG2 exosomes, we performed phospho-kinase antibody array in adipocytes treated with or without HepG2 exosomes for 1 h. As shown in Fig. 6a, of the 43 kinases examined, 15 was detected to have an increase of phosphorylation in exo-adipocytes. The top 5 increased

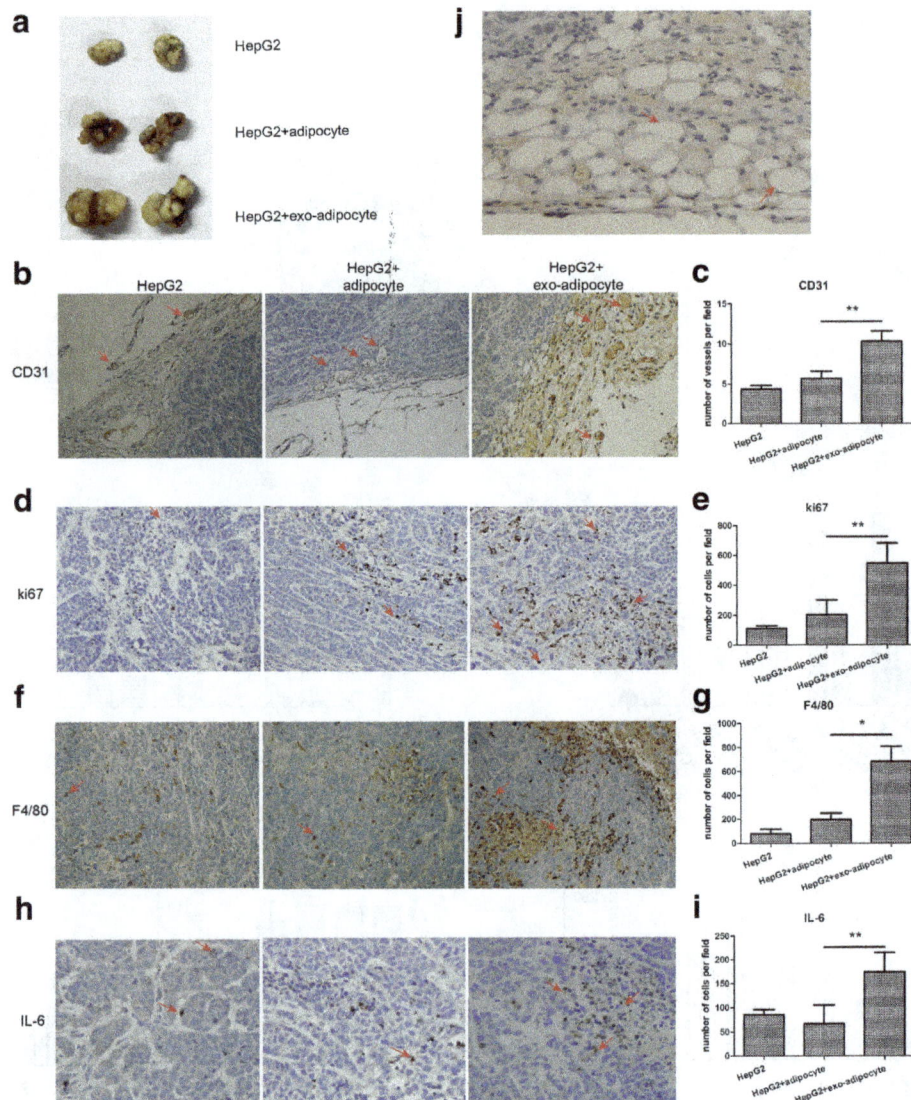

Fig. 3 exo-adipocytes promote tumor growth, enhance angiogenesis, and recruited macrophages in vivo. **a** Representative photographs of HepG2 tumors generated from nude mice injected with tumor cells alone or co-injected with exo-adipocytes or control adipocytes at a ratio of 10:1. **b** IHC staining of blood vessel density in tumor sections from xenografts by staining with anti-CD31 antibody. **c** CD31-positive cells were quantified, and the data represents the mean number of CD31 + cells per 200× field (three fields per group). **d** Detection of proliferating cells in tumors with IHC staining using the anti-Ki67 antibody. Representatives of Ki67 staining from each group are shown (magnification × 200). **e** Ki67 staining-positive cells were quantified, and the data represent the mean number per 200× field (three fields per group). **f** The macrophage infiltration was examined by detecting the number of F4/80-positive cells using immunohistochemical staining in the tumor tissues harvested. Representatives of F4/80 staining from each group are shown (magnification × 200). **g** F4/80 + macrophages were quantified, and the data represent the mean number of F4/80+ macrophages per 200× field (three fields per group). **h** Detection of IL-6 expression in tumors. **i** IL-6 expression was quantified, and the data represent the mean number of IL-6+ cells per 200× field (three fields per group). **j** A representative H&E staining of tumor sections demonstrated presence of adipocytes in mice injected with exo-adipocytes or adipocytes

kinases were AKT, STAT5α, GSK3 alpha/beta, p38 alpha, and ERK1/2. Using Western blot, we confirmed the strong and rapid activation of AKT, STAT5α, ERK1/2, and GSK3β (Fig. 6b). Since several kinases activated in adipocytes such as AKT, ERK1/2, and GSK3β are closely associated with NF-κB signaling pathway, we investigated

the possible activation of NF-κB after HepG2 exosome treatment. Figure 6c showed the translocation of active p65 from the cytoplasm to the nucleus.

Moreover, when NFκB inhibitor PDTC was added, the enhanced expression of IL-6, IL-8, and MCP-1 induced by HepG2 exosomes in adipocytes was reduced (Fig. 6d).

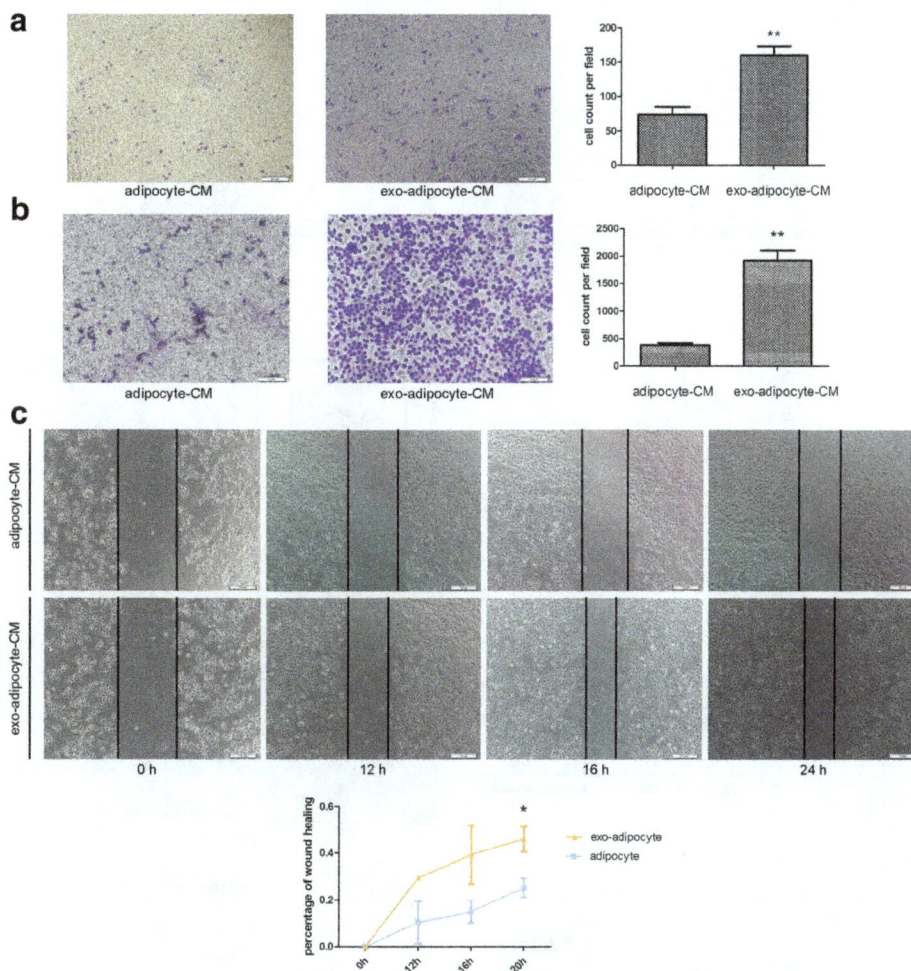

Fig. 4 exo-adipocyte-conditioned medium is chemotactic and promotes HepG2 migration. **a** Transwell migration assays showed that THP-1 cells were more chemotactic toward exo-adipocyte-conditioned medium than adipocyte-conditioned medium. Left is a representative microscopic image of crystal violet staining; right shows the statistical results. **b** Transwell migration assays showed that HepG2 cells were more chemotactic toward exo-adipocyte-conditioned medium than adipocyte-conditioned medium. Left is a representative microscopic image of crystal violet staining; right shows the statistical results. **c** Migratory abilities of HepG2 co-cultured with exo-adipocyte-conditioned medium or adipocyte-conditioned medium were determined by wound healing assay

Taken together, these results demonstrated that HepG2 exosomes are able to activate various kinases and NF-κB signaling pathway in adipocytes.

Proteomic analysis of HepG2 exosomes

Finally, we used mass spectrometry to characterize proteins contained within HepG2 exosomes. One thousand four hundred twenty-eight proteins were detected in exosomes, which were classified by GO annotation according to biological process, cellular component, and molecular function. The results showed a high prevalence of proteins involved in immune responses ("biological process," Fig. 7a), proteins with binding activity ("molecular function," Fig. 7b), and a high proportion of proteins associated with vesicle and granule ("cellular compartment," Fig. 7c). We selected 32 proteins with known functions according to Exocarta (http://www.exocarta.org/). As demonstrated in Fig. 7d, these selected proteins included common exosomal markers, structure or surface proteins, exosomal formation or secretion-related proteins, and oncogenic proteins. Future studies are required to identify which proteins are involved in the modification of adipocytes into tumor-promoting cells.

Discussion

Tumor initiation and progression rely on the dynamic interactions between malignant tumor cells and multiple normal cell types within its microenvironment such as fibroblasts, various immune cells, endothelial

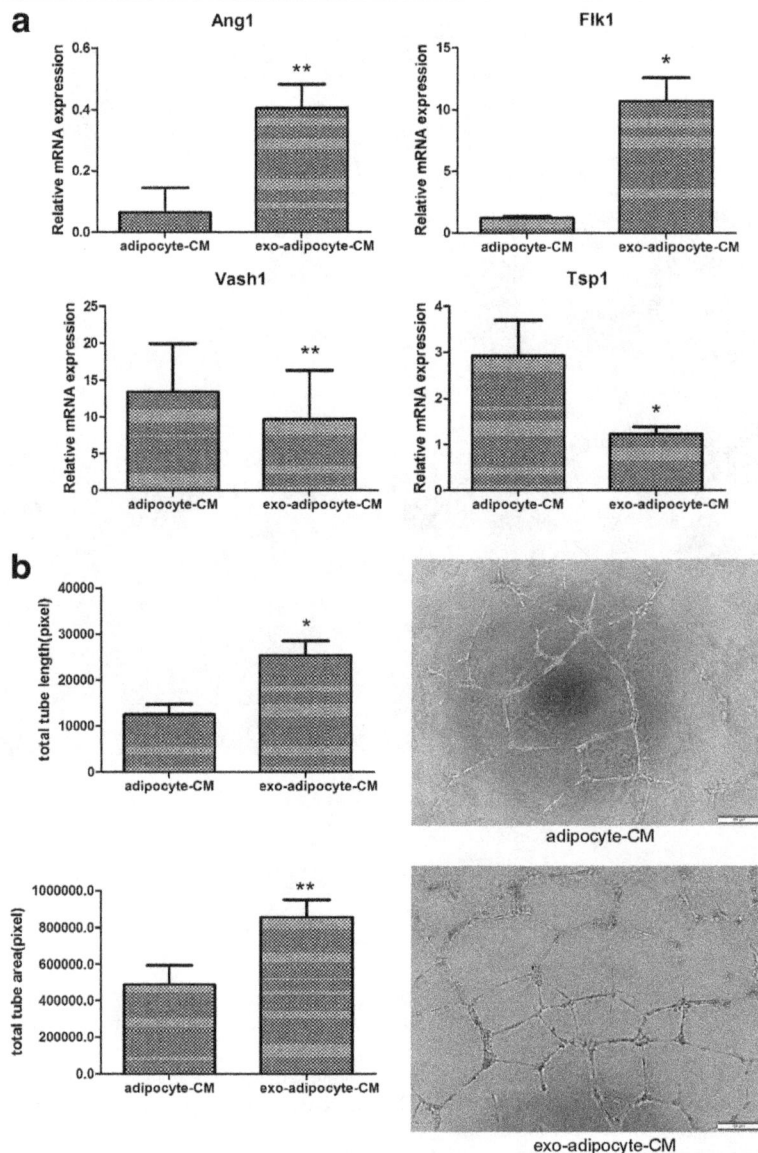

Fig. 5 exo-adipocyte-conditioned medium enhances tube formation of HUVECs. **a** HUVECs were incubated with exo-adipocyte-conditioned medium or adipocyte-conditioned medium for 48 h. The mRNA levels of Ang1, Flk1, Vash1, and TSP1 were evaluated by qRT-PCR. Results are mean ± SD ($n = 3$ for each group). **b** Compared with adipocyte-conditioned medium, exo-adipocyte-conditioned medium increased HUVEC tube formation in vitro. Scale bar, 100 μm. Right—representative photograph of tube formation. Left—calculations in three randomly selected fields. Results are mean ± SD (Student's t test)

cells, and adipocytes. Of these cell types, adipocytes are probably the least well studied, although they represent a significant part of the tissue surrounding a tumor [28]. Emerging evidence suggests that adipocytes should not be considered simply as an energy-storage depot. Instead, adipose tissue can play a central role in both endocrine and metabolic processes by producing a battery of factors including growth factors and adipokines [29]. Thus, understanding how obesity and adipose tissue-related factors

are connected to tumor development is paramount. In 2010, Dirat's group coined the term "cancer-associated adipocytes (CAA)" to demonstrate the bidirectional crosstalk between breast cancer cells and tumor-surrounding adipocytes and that CAA are a key player in tumor progression [30]. Subsequently, several studies also showed the existence of the putative CAA in the vicinity of cancer cells [31, 32]. Here, we chose adipocytes as a cellular model which are differentiated by culturing human MSCs under

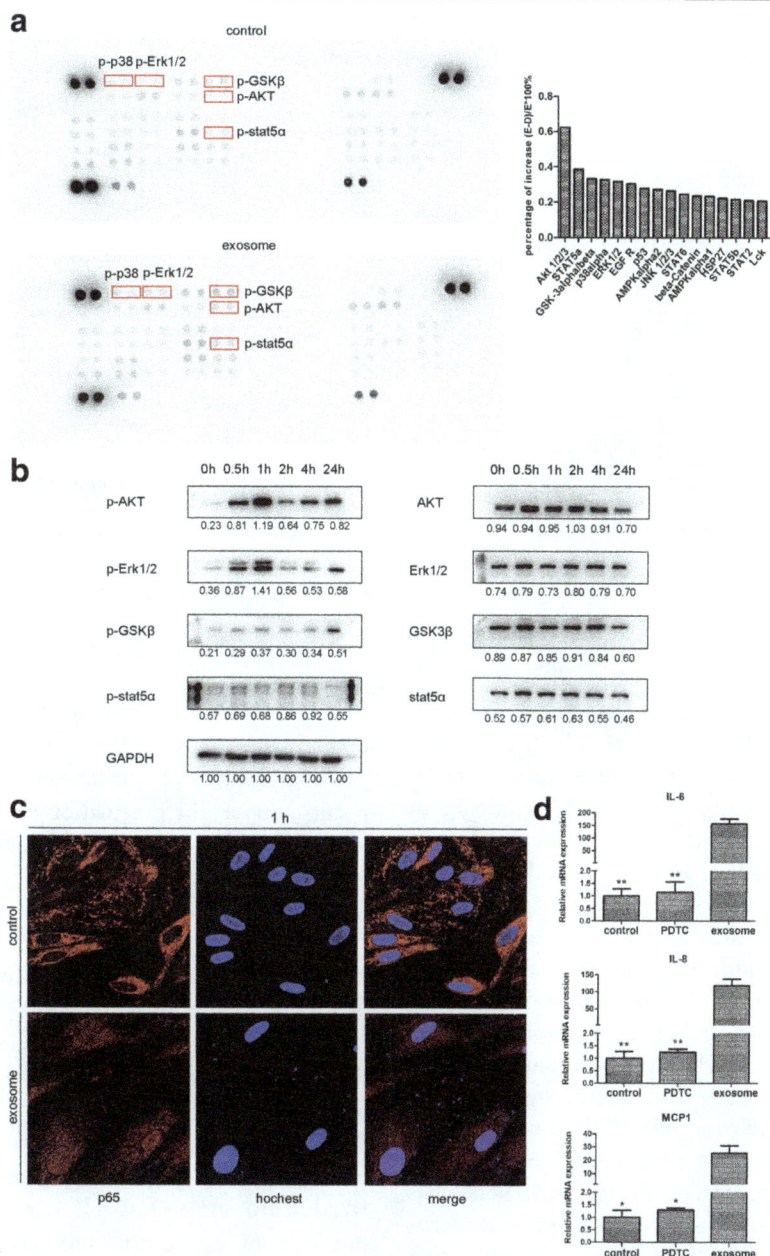

Fig. 6 HepG2 exosomes activate several kinases and NF-κB in adipocytes. **a** Phospho-kinase antibody array was performed on protein lysates from adipocytes treated with or without HepG2 exosomes. Data (right) are reported as percentage of increase. The percentage was calculated as (exosome − control)/exosome × 100%, and percentage over 20% is considered statistically significant. The top 5 kinases with an increased phosphorylation were highlighted by red boxes in the left panel. **b** Phosphorylation of AKT, ERK1/2, STAT5α, and GSK3β was confirmed by Western blot. GAPDH was used as loading control. **c** Representative immunofluorescence staining images of nuclear translocation of p65 in HepG2 exosome-treated adipocytes. Red (anti-p65 antibody), blue (Hochest). **d** Relative mRNA expression of IL-6, IL-8, and MCP-1 in adipocytes treated with exosome in the presence or absence of NF-κB inhibitor (*$P < 0.05$, **$P < 0.01$)

adipogenic conditions and are fully characterized by morphology, staining, and marker gene expression. We demonstrated that HCC cell line HepG2-derived exosomes could be actively incorporated by adipocytes and convert adipocytes into tumor-promoting cells (exo-adipocytes). In the mouse xenograft model, we found that exo-adipocytes promoted tumor growth and enhanced angiogenesis. Fujisaki et al. reported that in the presence of breast cancer cell lines MCF7 and MDA-MB-231, adipocytes reverted to an immature and

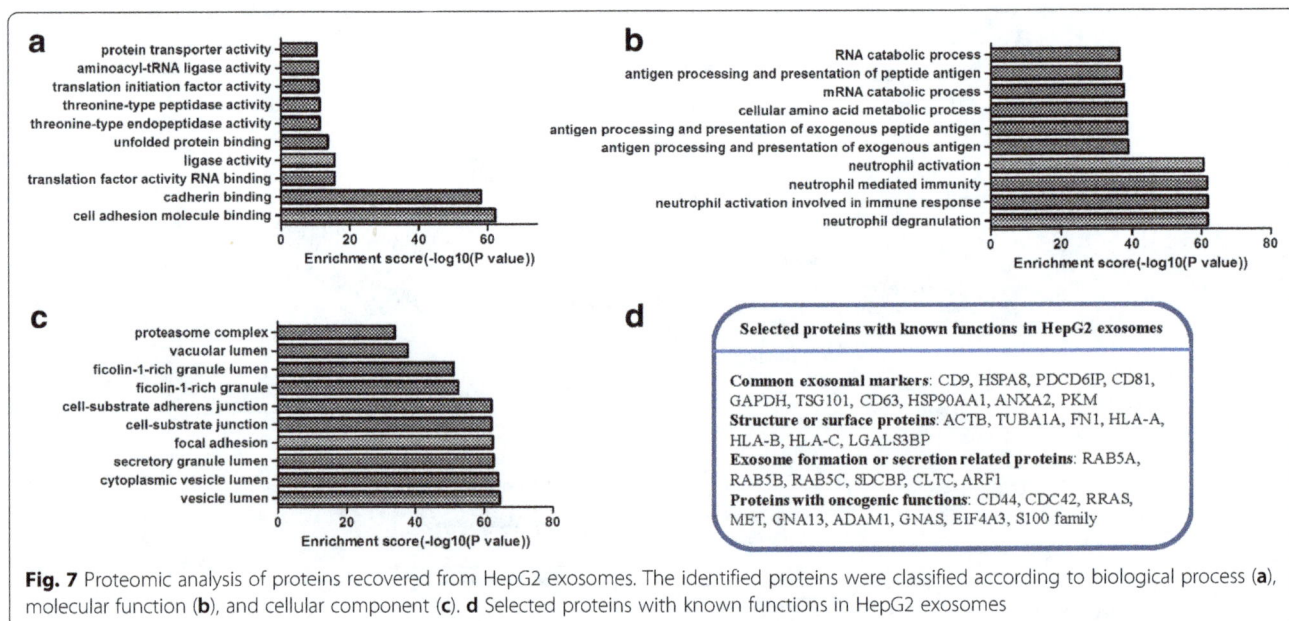

Fig. 7 Proteomic analysis of proteins recovered from HepG2 exosomes. The identified proteins were classified according to biological process (**a**), molecular function (**b**), and cellular component (**c**). **d** Selected proteins with known functions in HepG2 exosomes

proliferative phenotype of CAA that could promote cancer cell migration [33]. Lee et al. found that when indirectly co-cultured with breast cancer cells, adipocytes would be transited into CAA, resulting in proliferation-enhancing effect in ER-positive breast cancer cells such as MCF7 and ZR-75-1 but not in ER-negative cells [34]. Thus, we postulate that the exo-adipocytes in our study are a kind of CAA as they exhibit tumor-promoting capacity and higher expression of pro-inflammatory factors such as IL-6, IL-8, and MCP-1 whose higher expression in CAA has been reported [33, 34]. IL-6 plays diverse regulatory roles in cancer pathogenesis including remodeling the tumor microenvironment, activation of EMT process, and promoting drug resistance [35, 36]. IL-8 is known to be a stimulatory factor for tumor angiogenesis [37], and MCP-1 promotes the recruitment of macrophages into tumors [38]. These cytokines may be at least partially responsible for the tumor-promoting and angiogenesis-enhancing effects of exo-adipocytes.

The regulatory mechanisms of the CAA transition are not clearly understood. In this study, we explored the role of HCC-derived exosomes on the cellular and molecular changes of exo-adipocytes, which further confirmed that tumor cells could use exosomes as a novel way of cell-cell communication. Our study is consistent with previous findings that tumor exosomes from various cancer types can "educate" neighboring cells such as MSCs [39], endothelial cells [40], monocytes [41], and dendritic cells [42]. For example, exosomes from ovarian and breast cancer cells can convert adipose-derived MSCs (AMSC) into myofibroblast-like

cells [43, 44] while prostate cancer cell-derived exosomes trigger bone marrow MSCs (BMSC) to differentiate into pro-angiogenic and pro-invasive myofibroblasts [45]. Our results support the postulation that the elements of adipose tissue can also be modified by cancer cells and participate in a highly complex vicious cycle to form a tumor-favorable microenvironment.

How exosomes cause significant cellular and molecular changes in target cells remains an area of intensive research. Using microarray, Fang et al. found that HCC exosomes could deliver miR-1247-3p into fibroblasts and converted them into cancer-associated fibroblast to foster lung metastasis [46]. Using proteomic analysis, He et al. revealed that exosomes derived from metastatic HCC cell lines carried a large number of protumorigenic proteins, such as MET protooncogene, S100 family members, and the caveolins [19]. Here, we also detected common exosomal markers, structure or surface proteins, exosomal formation or secretion-related proteins, and oncogenic proteins in HepG2 exosomes. Upon taking up HCC exosomes, 725 upregulated and 648 downregulated genes were identified, and several cell signaling pathways were activated. In our previous study [24], we found that lung tumor exosomes could activate NFκB signaling pathway through HSP70/TLR2. Here, we also detected the activation of the NFκB signaling pathway. However, several questions remain for future investigation, including which receptors on the surface of adipocytes participated in HCC exosome in-

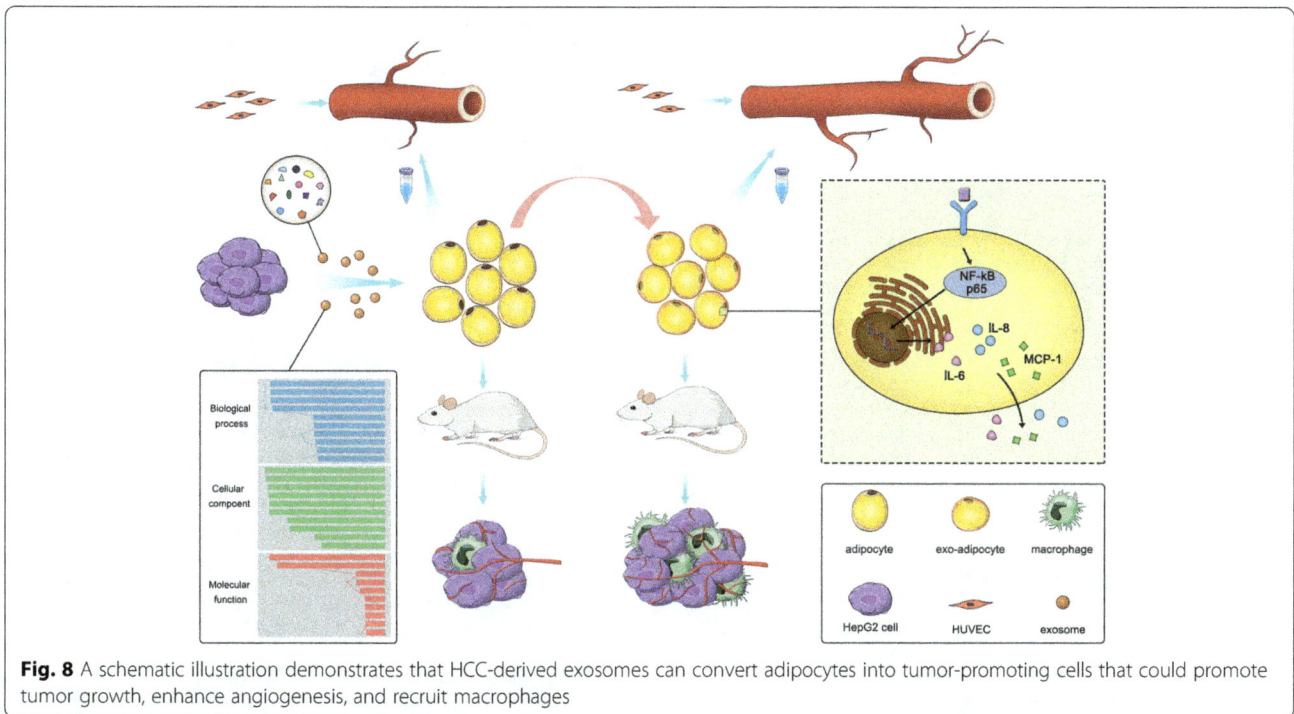

Fig. 8 A schematic illustration demonstrates that HCC-derived exosomes can convert adipocytes into tumor-promoting cells that could promote tumor growth, enhance angiogenesis, and recruit macrophages

ternalization and how the internalized exosome cargos activated the downstream signaling pathways.

Conclusions

Collectively, our data indicated that (i) HCC tumor-derived exosomes were actively incorporated into adipocytes and dramatically changed adipocytes transcripome and cytokine secretion; (ii) exo-adipocytes strongly supported tumor growth, enhanced angiogenesis, and recruited more macrophages; and (iii) several kinases and NF-κB signaling pathway were activated in exo-adipocytes (Fig. 8). Our results provide new insights into the concept that tumor cell can educate surrounding adipocytes to create a favorable microenvironment for tumor progression and that this effect might be amplified in overweight patients.

Abbreviations
EDTA: Ethylenediaminetetraacetic acid; ELISA: Enzyme-linked immunosorbent assay; exo-adipocytes: Exosome-treated adipocytes; FBS: Fetal bovine serum; H-DMEM: High glucose of Dulbecco's modified Eagle's medium; HE: Hematoxylin-eosin; MCP-1: Monocyte chemotactic protein 1; MSCs: Mesenchymal stem cells; NF-κB: Nuclear factor kappa-light-chain-enhancer of activated B cells; IL: Interleukin; qRT-PCR: Quantitative real-time PCR

Funding
This study was supported by CAMS Innovation Fund for Medical Sciences (2017-I2M-3-007), The National Key Research and Development Program of China (2016YFA0101000, 2016YFA0101003), Beijing Key Laboratory of New Drug Development and Clinical Trial of Stem Cell Therapy (BZ0381), and National Natural Science Foundation of China (81473450).

Authors' contributions
SHW designed and analyzed the experiments and wrote the manuscript. MQX performed and analyzed the experiments and prepared the figures. XXL, XDS, and XX performed the experiments. AK and RCHZ designed the experiment. All authors have read and approved the final manuscript.

Competing interests
The authors declare that they have no competing interests.

Author details
[1]Center of Excellence in Tissue Engineering, Institute of Basic Medical Sciences, Peking Union Medical College Hospital, Chinese Academy of Medical Sciences, School of Basic Medicine Peking Union Medical College, Beijing 100005, China. [2]Department of Genetics and Cell Biology, Basic Medical College, Qingdao University, 308 Ningxia Road, Qingdao 266071, China. [3]Cell Therapy Translational Research Laboratory, Princess Margaret Cancer Centre, Toronto, Ontario M5G 2M9, Canada. [4]Institute of Biomaterials and Biomedical Engineering, University of Toronto, Toronto, Ontario M5G 2M9, Canada. [5]Institute of Medical Science, University of Toronto, Toronto, Ontario M5G 2M9, Canada.

References
1. Giannelli G, Villa E, Lahn M. Transforming growth factor-beta as a therapeutic target in hepatocellular carcinoma. Cancer Res. 2014;74(7):1890–4.
2. Ferlay J, Soerjomataram I, Dikshit R, Eser S, Mathers C, Rebelo M, Parkin DM, Forman D, Bray F. Cancer incidence and mortality worldwide: sources, methods and major patterns in GLOBOCAN 2012. Int J Cancer. 2015; 136(5):E359–86.
3. Bray F, Ren JS, Masuyer E, Ferlay J. Global estimates of cancer prevalence for 27 sites in the adult population in 2008. Int J Cancer. 2013;132(5):1133–45.

4. Villanueva A, Llovet JM. Liver cancer in 2013: mutational landscape of HCC—the end of the beginning. Nat Rev Clin Oncol. 2014;11(2):73–4.

5. Shen ZQ, Chen YF, Chen JR, Jou YS, Wu PC, Kao CH, Wang CH, Huang YL, Chen CF, Huang TS, et al. CISD2 haploinsufficiency disrupts calcium homeostasis, causes nonalcoholic fatty liver disease, and promotes hepatocellular carcinoma. Cell Rep. 2017;21(8):2198–211.

6. Kim GA, Lee HC, Choe J, Kim MJ, Lee MJ, Chang HS, Bae IY, Kim HK, An J, Shim JH, et al. Association between non-alcoholic fatty liver disease and cancer incidence rate. J Hepatol. 2017; https://doi.org/10.1016/j.jhep.2017.09.012.

7. Van den Eynden GG, Majeed AW, Illemann M, Vermeulen PB, Bird NC, Hoyer-Hansen G, Eefsen RL, Reynolds AR, Brodt P. The multifaceted role of the microenvironment in liver metastasis: biology and clinical implications. Cancer Res. 2013;73(7):2031–43.

8. Starley BQ, Calcagno CJ, Harrison SA. Nonalcoholic fatty liver disease and hepatocellular carcinoma: a weighty connection. Hepatology. 2010; 51(5):1820–32.

9. Zhang J, Zhang Q, Lou Y, Fu Q, Chen Q, Wei T, Yang J, Tang J, Wang J, Chen Y, et al. HIF-1alpha/IL-1beta signaling enhances hepatoma epithelial-mesenchymal transition via macrophages in a hypoxic-inflammatory microenvironment. Hepatol. 2018;67(5):1872-89.

10. Wolf MJ, Adili A, Piotrowitz K, Abdullah Z, Boege Y, Stemmer K, Ringelhan M, Simonavicius N, Egger M, Wohlleber D, et al. Metabolic activation of intrahepatic CD8+ T cells and NKT cells causes nonalcoholic steatohepatitis and liver cancer via cross-talk with hepatocytes. Cancer Cell. 2014;26(4):549–64.

11. Li A, Zhang T, Zheng M, Liu Y, Chen Z. Exosomal proteins as potential markers of tumor diagnosis. J Hematol Oncol. 2017;10(1):175.

12. Ruivo CF, Adem B, Silva M, Melo SA. The biology of Cancer exosomes: insights and new perspectives. Cancer Res. 2017;77(23):6480–8.

13. Chen W, Jiang J, Xia W, Huang J. Tumor-related exosomes contribute to tumor-promoting microenvironment: an immunological perspective. J Immunol Res. 2017;2017:1073947.

14. Sharma A. Role of stem cell derived exosomes in tumor biology. Int J Cancer. 2018;142(6):1086-92.

15. Hood JL, San RS, Wickline SA. Exosomes released by melanoma cells prepare sentinel lymph nodes for tumor metastasis. Cancer Res. 2011;71(11): 3792–801.

16. Ma P, Pan Y, Li W, Sun C, Liu J, Xu T, Shu Y. Extracellular vesicles-mediated noncoding RNAs transfer in cancer. J Hematol Oncol. 2017;10(1):57.

17. Peinado H, Aleckovic M, Lavotshkin S, Matei I, Costa-Silva B, Moreno-Bueno G, Hergueta-Redondo M, Williams C, Garcia-Santos G, Ghajar C, et al. Melanoma exosomes educate bone marrow progenitor cells toward a pro-metastatic phenotype through MET. Nat Med. 2012;18(6):883–91.

18. Sagar G, Sah RP, Javeed N, Dutta SK, Smyrk TC, Lau JS, Giorgadze N, Tchkonia T, Kirkland JL, Chari ST, et al. Pathogenesis of pancreatic cancer exosome-induced lipolysis in adipose tissue. Gut. 2016;65(7):1165–74.

19. He M, Qin H, Poon TC, Sze SC, Ding X, Co NN, Ngai SM, Chan TF, Wong N. Hepatocellular carcinoma-derived exosomes promote motility of immortalized hepatocyte through transfer of oncogenic proteins and RNAs. Carcinogenesis. 2015;36(9):1008–18.

20. Cao Y, Sun Z, Liao L, Meng Y, Han Q, Zhao RC. Human adipose tissue-derived stem cells differentiate into endothelial cells in vitro and improve postnatal neovascularization in vivo. Biochem Biophys Res Commun. 2005; 332(2):370–9.

21. Baudin B, Bruneel A, Bosselut N, Vaubourdolle M. A protocol for isolation and culture of human umbilical vein endothelial cells. Nat Protoc. 2007;2(3):481–5.

22. Lin R, Wang S, Zhao RC. Exosomes from human adipose-derived mesenchymal stem cells promote migration through Wnt signaling pathway in a breast cancer cell model. Mol Cell Biochem. 2013;383(1–2):13–20.

23. Yang Z, Bian C, Zhou H, Huang S, Wang S, Liao L, Zhao RC. MicroRNA hsa-miR-138 inhibits adipogenic differentiation of human adipose tissue-derived mesenchymal stem cells through adenovirus EID-1. Stem Cells Dev. 2011; 20(2):259–67.

24. Li X, Wang S, Zhu R, Li H, Han Q, Zhao RC. Lung tumor exosomes induce a pro-inflammatory phenotype in mesenchymal stem cells via NFkappaB-TLR signaling pathway. J Hematol Oncol. 2016;9:42.

25. Dirat B, Bochet L, Dabek M, Daviaud D, Dauvillier S, Majed B, Wang YY, Meulle A, Salles B, Le Gonidec S, et al. Cancer-associated adipocytes exhibit an activated phenotype and contribute to breast cancer invasion. Cancer Res. 2011;71(7):2455–65.

26. Chanput W, Mes JJ, Wichers HJ. THP-1 cell line: an in vitro cell model for immune modulation approach. Int Immunopharmacol. 2014;23(1):37–45.

27. Qin Z. The use of THP-1 cells as a model for mimicking the function and regulation of monocytes and macrophages in the vasculature. Atherosclerosis. 2012;221(1):2–11.

28. Robado de Lope L, Alcibar OL, Amor Lopez A, Hergueta-Redondo M, Peinado H. Tumour-adipose tissue crosstalk: fuelling tumour metastasis by extracellular vesicles. Philos Trans R Soc Lond Ser B Biol Sci. 2018;373(1737) https://doi.org/10.1098/rstb.2016.0485.

29. Chkourko Gusky H, Diedrich J, MacDougald OA, Podgorski I. Omentum and bone marrow: how adipocyte-rich organs create tumour microenvironments conducive for metastatic progression. Obes Rev. 2016; 17(11):1015–29.

30. Dirat B, Bochet L, Escourrou G, Valet P, Muller C. Unraveling the obesity and breast cancer links: a role for cancer-associated adipocytes? Endocr Dev. 2010;19:45–52.

31. Nieman KM, Kenny HA, Penicka CV, Ladanyi A, Buell-Gutbrod R, Zillhardt MR, Romero IL, Carey MS, Mills GB, Hotamisligil GS, et al. Adipocytes promote ovarian cancer metastasis and provide energy for rapid tumor growth. Nat Med. 2011;17(11):1498–503.

32. Wang C, Gao C, Meng K, Qiao H, Wang Y. Human adipocytes stimulate invasion of breast cancer MCF-7 cells by secreting IGFBP-2. PLoS One. 2015; 10(3):e0119348.

33. Fujisaki K, Fujimoto H, Sangai T, Nagashima T, Sakakibara M, Shiina N, Kuroda M, Aoyagi Y, Miyazaki M. Cancer-mediated adipose reversion promotes cancer cell migration via IL-6 and MCP-1. Breast Cancer Res Treat. 2015;150(2):255–63.

34. Lee J, Hong BS, Ryu HS, Lee HB, Lee M, Park IA, Kim J, Han W, Noh DY, Moon HG. Transition into inflammatory cancer-associated adipocytes in breast cancer microenvironment requires microRNA regulatory mechanism. PLoS One. 2017;12(3):e0174126.

35. Yang L, Han S, Sun Y. An IL6-STAT3 loop mediates resistance to PI3K inhibitors by inducing epithelial-mesenchymal transition and cancer stem cell expansion in human breast cancer cells. Biochem Biophys Res Commun. 2014;453(3):582–7.

36. Ara T, Nakata R, Sheard MA, Shimada H, Buettner R, Groshen SG, Ji L, Yu H, Jove R, Seeger RC, et al. Critical role of STAT3 in IL-6-mediated drug resistance in human neuroblastoma. Cancer Res. 2013;73(13):3852–64.

37. Paggetti J, Haderk F, Seiffert M, Janji B, Distler U, Ammerlaan W, Kim YJ, Adam J, Lichter P, Solary E, et al. Exosomes released by chronic lymphocytic leukemia cells induce the transition of stromal cells into cancer-associated fibroblasts. Blood. 2015;126(9):1106–17.

38. Sierra-Filardi E, Nieto C, Dominguez-Soto A, Barroso R, Sanchez-Mateos P, Puig-Kroger A, Lopez-Bravo M, Joven J, Ardavin C, Rodriguez-Fernandez JL, et al. CCL2 shapes macrophage polarization by GM-CSF and M-CSF: identification of CCL2/CCR2-dependent gene expression profile. J Immunol. 2014;192(8):3858–67.

39. Nakata R, Shimada H, Fernandez GE, Fanter R, Fabbri M, Malvar J, Zimmermann P, DeClerck YA. Contribution of neuroblastoma-derived exosomes to the production of pro-tumorigenic signals by bone marrow mesenchymal stromal cells. J Extracell Vesicles. 2017;6(1):1332941.

40. Schillaci O, Fontana S, Monteleone F, Taverna S, Di Bella MA, Di Vizio D, Alessandro R. Exosomes from metastatic cancer cells transfer amoeboid phenotype to non-metastatic cells and increase endothelial permeability: their emerging role in tumor heterogeneity. Sci Rep. 2017;7(1):4711.

41. Haderk F, Schulz R, Iskar M, Cid LL, Worst T, Willmund KV, Schulz A, Warnken U, Seiler J, Benner A, et al. Tumor-derived exosomes modulate PD-L1 expression in monocytes. Sci Immunol. 2017;2(13) https://doi.org/10.1126/sciimmunol.aah5509.

42. Yu S, Liu C, Su K, Wang J, Liu Y, Zhang L, Li C, Cong Y, Kimberly R, Grizzle WE, et al. Tumor exosomes inhibit differentiation of bone marrow dendritic cells. J Immunol. 2007;178(11):6867–75.

43. Cho JA, Park H, Lim EH, Kim KH, Choi JS, Lee JH, Shin JW, Lee KW. Exosomes from ovarian cancer cells induce adipose tissue-derived mesenchymal stem cells to acquire the physical and functional characteristics of tumor-supporting myofibroblasts. Gynecol Oncol. 2011;123(2):379–86.

44. Cho JA, Park H, Lim EH, Lee KW. Exosomes from breast cancer cells can convert adipose tissue-derived mesenchymal stem cells into myofibroblast-like cells. Int J Oncol. 2012; 40(1):130-8.

45. Chandler EM, Seo BR, Califano JP, Andresen Eguiluz RC, Lee JS, Yoon CJ, Tims DT, Wang JX, Cheng L, Mohanan S, et al. Implanted adipose

progenitor cells as physicochemical regulators of breast cancer. Proc Natl Acad Sci U S A. 2012;109(25):9786–91.

46. Fang T, Lv H, Lv G, Li T, Wang C, Han Q, Yu L, Su B, Guo L, Huang S, et al. Tumor-derived exosomal miR-1247-3p induces cancer-associated fibroblast activation to foster lung metastasis of liver cancer. Nat Commun. 2018;9(1):191.

7

Organoid technology and applications in cancer research

Hanxiao Xu[1], Xiaodong Lyu[2], Ming Yi[1], Weiheng Zhao[1], Yongping Song[3] and Kongming Wu[1]*(iD)

Abstract

During the past decade, the three-dimensional organoid technology has sprung up and become more and more popular among researchers. Organoids are the miniatures of in vivo tissues and organs, and faithfully recapitulate the architectures and distinctive functions of a specific organ.

These amazing three-dimensional constructs represent a promising, near-physiological model for human cancers, and tremendously support diverse potential applications in cancer research. Up to now, highly efficient establishment of organoids can be achieved from both normal and malignant tissues of patients. Using this bioengineered platform, the links of infection-cancer progression and mutation-carcinogenesis are feasible to be modeled. Another potential application is that organoid technology facilitates drug testing and guides personalized therapy. Although organoids still fail to model immune system accurately, co-cultures of organoids and lymphocytes have been reported in several studies, bringing hope for further application of this technology in immunotherapy. In addition, the potential value in regeneration medicine might be another paramount branch of organoid technology, which might refine current transplantation therapy through the replacement of irreversibly progressively diseased organs with isogenic healthy organoids.

In conclusion, organoids represent an excellent preclinical model for human tumors, promoting the translation from basic cancer research to clinical practice. In this review, we outline organoid technology and summarize its applications in cancer research.

Keywords: Organoid, Cancer, Drug development, Drug efficacy, Drug toxicity, Personalized medicine, Immunotherapy, Regeneration medicine

Background

During the past decades, enormous efforts have been exerted to cancer research [1, 2] and substantial progresses have been achieved in diagnosis [3, 4] and treatment [5–12]. However, cancer still represents a major worldwide health concern and many obstacles remain to be solved for further improving life quality and prolonging survival of cancer patients. The development of effective treatment regimens is among the major hurdles. Due to poor recapitulation of human tumors by conventional cancer models, numerous drugs working in these cancer models are finally eliminated in clinical trials because of either ineffectiveness or unbearable side effects.

Traditional two-dimensional (2D) cell line cultures and patient-derived tumor xenografts (PDTXs) have long been employed as tumor models and have made tremendous contribution to cancer research. However, many drawbacks hamper these two models for clinical use. 2D cell line cultures show their inability in simulating some vital subjects, such as the immune system, microenvironment, stromal compartments, and organ-specific functions. Other limitations include the lack of genetic heterogeneity of original tumors after many passages for cancer cell lines [13] as well as experiencing mouse-specific tumor evolution [14] and being consuming in money, time, and resources for PDTXs [15].

Organoid technology springs up and becomes an independent research tool. Organoids are three-dimensional (3D) constructs and can be developed from embryonic stem cells (ESCs), induced pluripotent stem cells (iPSCs), somatic SCs, and cancer cells in specific 3D culture

* Correspondence: kmwu@tjh.tjmu.edu.cn
[1]Department of Oncology, Tongji Hospital of Tongji Medical College, Huazhong University of Science and Technology, 1095 Jiefang Avenue, Wuhan 430030, Hubei, China
Full list of author information is available at the end of the article

system (Fig. 1). Stem cells are a class of under-differentiated cells with self-renewing capacity and the potential to regenerate various tissues and organs. According to the developmental stage in which stem cells are located, they are divided into embryonic stem cells and adult stem cells. Embryonic stem cells are a type of cells isolated from early embryos with the ability of unlimited proliferation, self-renewal, and multi-directional differentiation. Progenitor cells belong to adult stem cells and are undifferentiated pluripotent or multipotent stem cells. Progenitor cells are present in various adult tissues of organisms and are responsible for the repair and regeneration process after tissue damage.

These amazing 3D tissues in small scale are fabricated in the laboratory and resemble the parent organ in vivo in terms of structure and function. Three basic features are as follows: firstly, it contains multiple cell types of the in vivo counterpart; secondly, the cells organize similarly to the primary tissue; thirdly, it functions specifically to the parent organ [16]. This powerful technology bridges the conventional 2D in vitro models and in vivo models, and exerts great potential for clinical applications (Fig. 2), especially in cancer research [17]. Tumor modeling might be a pivotal branch of organoid technology [18, 19], including modeling infection-cancer development [20, 21], mutation-tumorigenesis processes [22, 23] and genetic carcinoma [24, 25]. Apart from cancer modeling, organoid technology also exerts enormous potential in evaluation of efficacy and toxicity of drugs [26],

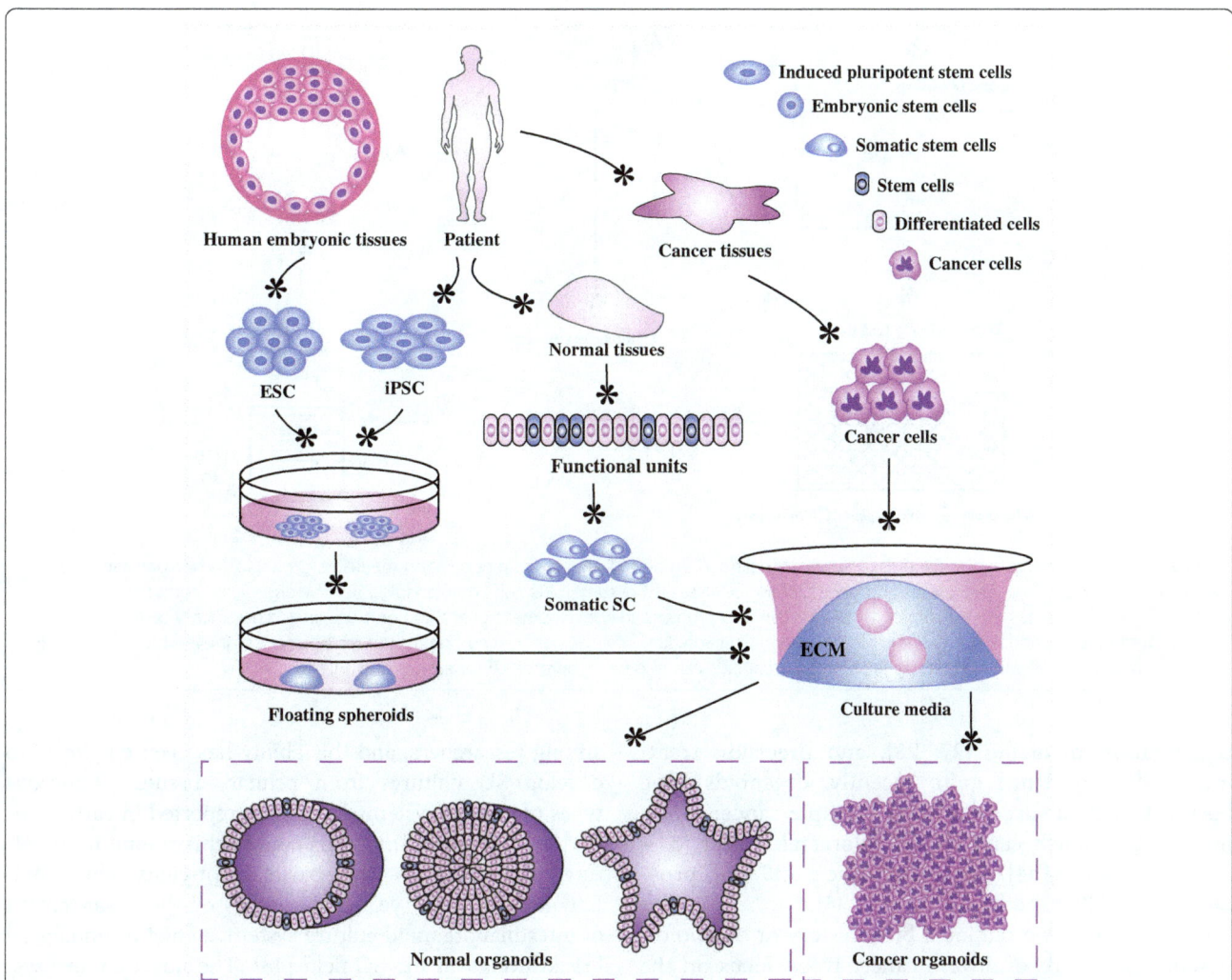

Fig. 1 Organoid establishment from stem cells and cancer cells. Embryonic stem cells from human embryonic tissues and induced pluripotent stem cells from adult tissues firstly experience directed differentiation, generate floating spheroids, and subsequently are planted on extracellular matrix in specific culture medium to initiate organoid culture. Primary tissues from patients can be dissociated into functional units, which contain somatic stem cells. These somatic stem cells are enriched and cultured in three-dimensional medium to form organoids. Tumor cells isolated from cancer tissues can also form tumoroids in well-defined three-dimensional culture

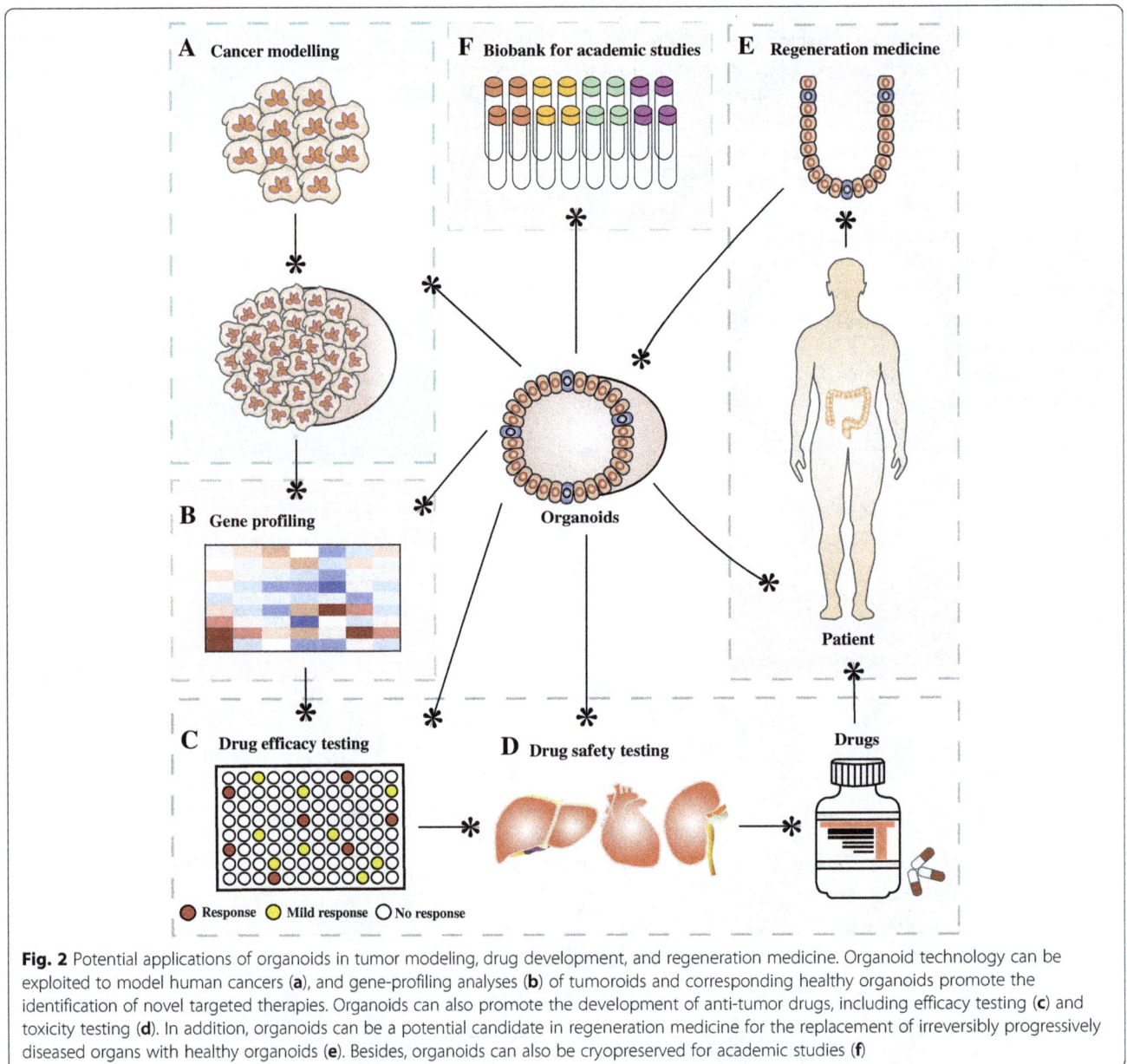

Fig. 2 Potential applications of organoids in tumor modeling, drug development, and regeneration medicine. Organoid technology can be exploited to model human cancers (**a**), and gene-profiling analyses (**b**) of tumoroids and corresponding healthy organoids promote the identification of novel targeted therapies. Organoids can also promote the development of anti-tumor drugs, including efficacy testing (**c**) and toxicity testing (**d**). In addition, organoids can be a potential candidate in regeneration medicine for the replacement of irreversibly progressively diseased organs with healthy organoids (**e**). Besides, organoids can also be cryopreserved for academic studies (**f**)

regeneration medicine [27, 28], and precision treatment [29, 30]. Until quite recently, organoids have been established successfully for multiple cancer types, including stomach cancer [26], colorectal cancer [31–33], liver cancer [34], pancreatic cancer [35, 36], prostate cancer [37], and breast cancer [38].

In this review, we outline a brief history of organoids, describe organoids of diverse cancer types, focus on the potential applications of this promising technology in oncology, and finally discuss the current limitations.

The history of organoids

The notion that mammalian cells are inherently endowed with self-organizing capacity has long been widely known

among researchers, and this ability has been employed to develop 3D cultures from primary tissues. Numerous types of culture systems have been reported in early studies [39–42], but no methods could achieve long-term culture and maintain the basic crypt-villus physiology. Encouragingly, the year 2009 witnessed the advancement of intestinal organoid culture system, a chief technological breakthrough in the SC field [43]. The novel culture system contained laminin-rich Matrigel replacing extracellular matrix (ECM) and growth factors including epidermal growth factor (EGF), Noggin, Wnt, and R-spondin. 3D mouse crypt structures in which continuously renewing epithelial layer exhausted apoptotic cells into a central lumen lined by crypt-like and villus-like sections were established in this 3D culture system, and these features remained when cultured for 8 months [43]. Subsequently, this culture system was adapted for the establishment of human intestinal organoids and other organ 3D architectures, such as the liver, stomach, and colon [44–46]. The organoid technology has become widely accepted in recent years, since these 3D cultures faithfully recapitulate the genotype, phenotype, and cellular behaviors of parent tissues [47].

Breast organoid cultures also experience a gradual evolution from the earliest attempts of in vitro cultivation of organ explants to the current relatively refined versions [48–50]. Mammary gland explants of from virgin mice could be cultivated in a serum-free medium, which consists of four major components: aldosterone, prolactin, insulin, and cortisol [48]. Through testing the mammary-derived growth inhibitor (MDGI) in mammary explants in vitro from mice at different development stages, it was demonstrated that MDGI expression was correlated with functional differentiation of normal mammary gland [48]. Next, mouse mammary gland cultivated in organ culture containing MRG protein showed a differentiated morphology with the upregulation of beta-casein [49]. Recently, it has been indicated that 3D cultures of breast cancer could more accurately model the structural and functional changes during the conversion from breast ductal carcinoma in situ to invasive carcinoma [50]. Up to now, breast cancer organoids have been efficiently established for studying breast cancer biology, and efforts are still in need for further improving culture conditions in order to overcome the current limitations.

Early in the 1980s, organotypic cultures have been employed to cultivate embryonic kidney, which allowed accurate manipulation of diversity developmental events in vivo in comparison with monolayer cell cultures [51]. However, the in vitro conditions led to metabolic changes, and it was difficult to realize long-term cultures because of the nutrition insufficiency-induced tissue damage [51]. When fetal murine metanephric tissues were isolated and incubated in serum-free medium, organotypic proximal tubular and glomerular epithelial differentiation were observed but without perfusion, urine production, and vascularization [52]. Quite recently, it was reported that host-derived vascularization formed in iPSC-derived kidney organoids in fully defined conditions without any exogenous vascular endothelial growth factor [53]. Progressive morphogenesis, including functional glomerular perfusion in function as well as connection to pre-existing vascular system, glomerular basement membrane, and fenestrated endothelial cells in structure, was observed in these organoids after transplanted under the kidney capsule [53].

Isolated brain cells, cultured in serum-free medium with classical hormones, EGF, fibroblast growth factor (FGF), attachment factors/basal membrane components, transport proteins, transferrin, albumin, vitamins, experienced morphological, bioelectrical, and biochemical differentiation [54–56]. During the past a few years, a variety of neural organoids have been established from ESCs or iPSCs in refined 3D culture systems which faithfully manipulated brain structures and some specific functions, including the whole brain [57] and sub-brain regions, such as hypothalamus [58], adenohypophysis [59], midbrain [60], cerebellum [61], and hippocampus [62].

Establishment of cancer organoids

The poverty of in vitro tumor models that mimic the heterogenicity of human cancers has impeded the full understanding on tumor pathogenesis, therapeutic responses, and adverse reactions. The 3D organoid system draws researchers' attention and has tremendous potential for modeling human cancers [63–65]. Major establishment procedures for each cancer organoid type were showed in Fig. 3. 3D culture system for organoid establishment consists of Matrigel or basement membrane extract as ECM substitutes and specific culture medium. Components in organoid culture medium majorly include advanced Dulbecco's modified Eagle's medium (ADMEM)/F12, penicillin/streptomycin, primocin, GlutaMAX, HEPES, B27, N2, EGF, FGF10, FGF7, hepatocyte growth factor (HGF), Wnt3A, Noggin, R-spondin-1, gastrin, prostaglandin E_2, nicotinamide, neuregulin 1, N-acetylcysteine, Y27632 (a Rho kinase inhibitor), A-83-01 (a transforming growth factor-beta inhibitor), and SB202190 (a p38 inhibitor) (Table 1). There are minor differences in medium components among different tumoroid types [26, 34, 38, 66–68], shown in Table 2. Compared with conventional 2D cultures of cell lines, the most outstanding feature is the addition of ECM substitutes in 3D cultures.

Stomach cancer

Organoid technology has been applied to model gastric cancer [26, 69]. There are some subtle differences among studies in detailed manipulation. The proliferation rates of gastric cancer organoids were significantly higher than normal controls in vitro, and tumor growth of organoid engrafts in vivo was consistent with the expansion rates of corresponding organoids in vitro [69]. The organoids faithfully recapitulated important characteristics of the corresponding parent tumors as exemplified by architectures, the expression of typical gastric cancer markers including carcinoembryonal antigen, cadherin 17, cytokeratin 7 (KRT7), and periodic acid Schiff reaction [69]. These organoids harbored diverse mutations, which were prevalent in gastric cancer and could be detected in corresponding

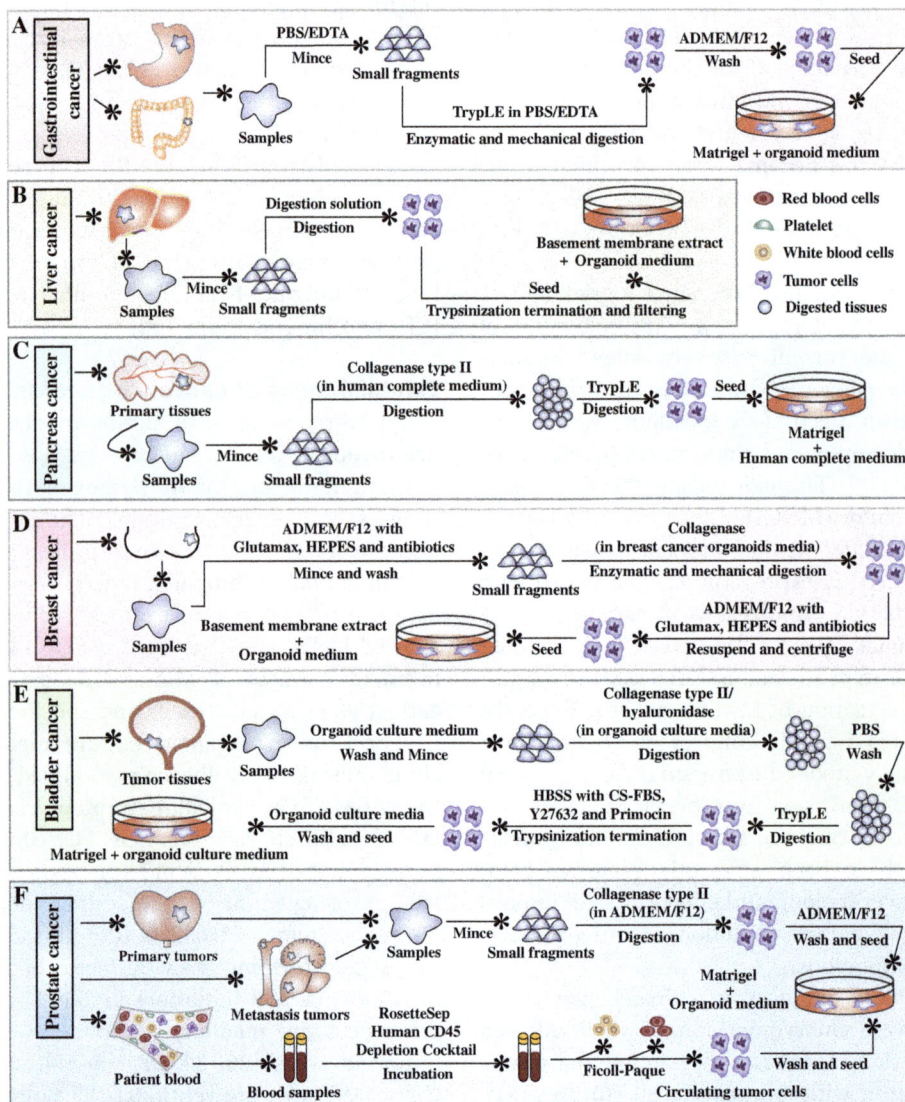

Fig. 3 Flow charts for tumoroid establishment processes. Major steps during tumoroid establishment of gastrointestinal cancer (**a**), liver cancer (**b**), pancreatic cancer (**c**), breast cancer (**d**), bladder cancer (**e**), and prostate cancer (**f**) are shown

primary tumors, such as mutations in *mutL homolog 1*, *mutS homologs 6*, *phosphatidylinositol 3-kinase catalytic subunit*, *ERBB2*, and *TP53* [69].

Intestinal cancer

Intestinal cancer organoids have been successfully developed in several studies [26, 31–33]. Sato T and colleagues demonstrated that colorectal cancer organoids responded diversely to Wnt3A/R-spondin-1, oxygen concentration, and SB202190 in organoid proliferation in consideration of the phenomenon that some tumoroids needed Wnt activators, some required hypoxia, and some showed growth suppression in reaction to SB212090 exposure [31]. Colorectal cancer organoids

have been successfully propagated from different anatomical sites (right-sided, left-sided, and rectal tumors) and rare histological subtypes (mucinous adenocarcinoma and neuroendocrine carcinoma) [31]. Colorectal cancer organoids showed remarkable resemblance with the primary tumors in the aspects of histological subtypes, differentiation hierarchies, mutational landscape, and transcriptomic profiling [26, 31]. It was noted that colorectal cancer organoids in combination with an orthotopic transplantation system could more accurately model tumor formation and liver metastasis in the native colon environment [70]. Proteomic analyses on colorectal cancer organoids showed each organoid from distinct patients harbored different proteomic profiles,

Table 1 Growth factors and small molecule inhibitors applied in organoid cultures

	Function
Growth factors	
EGF	◆ A well-known growth factor for epithelial tissues; ◆ EGF, binding to EGF receptors, induces hyperplasic changes; ◆ EGF promotes tumor growth through stimulating the proliferation of cancer cells.
FGF10	◆ FGF10/FGF receptor 2IIIb axis is important for the organ development, including the stomach, liver, breast, and prostate; ◆ FGF10 promotes migration and invasion of pancreatic cancer cells and drives tumorigenesis of breast cancer;
FGF7	◆ FGF7/FGF receptor 2 signaling promotes growth, invasion, and migration of tumors.
HGF	◆ HGF/Met signaling promoted oncogenesis, tumor angiogenesis, tumor invasion of multiple tumor types;
Wnt	◆ A master regulator in regulation of cell development, proliferation, differentiation, adhesion, and polarity; ◆ The aberrant activation of Wnt signaling promotes carcinogenesis and progression of cancers.
Noggin	◆ An inhibitor of bone morphogenetic proteins that modulates cellular differentiation, proliferation, and apoptosis; ◆ Noggin promotes bone metastasis of some cancers and is associated with tumorigenesis of primary bone malignancies.
R-spondin-1	◆ The ligand of Lgr5 and a niche factor that is required for the self-renewal of stem cells and activates Wnt signaling; ◆ R-spondin-1facilitates the growth and metastasis of cancer cells.
Gastrin	◆ Gastrin stimulates tumor growth through promoting the proliferation and suppressing the apoptosis of cancer cells;
Prostaglandin E_2	◆ Prostaglandin E_2 promotes angiogenesis in gastric cancer through the up-regulation of vascular endothelial growth factor.
Nicotinamide	◆ Vitamin PP is a nutrient that is required for long-term culture of organoids.
Neuregulin 1	◆ It is a ligand of human EGF receptor tyrosine kinases-3 and -4; ◆ It is involved in mammary development and tumorigenesis.
Molecule inhibitors	
Y27632	◆ A Rho kinase inhibitor that effectively reduces the anoikis of dissociated stem cells; ◆ Y27632 improves culture media and promotes proliferation of tumor epithelial cells for long-term in vitro;
A-83-01	◆ A transforming growth factor-beta inhibitor; ◆ Transforming growth factor-beta inhibitor suppresses the proliferation of organoids;
SB202190	◆ It is a p38 inhibitor and suppresses the proliferation and migration of cancer cells; ◆ High concentration of SB202190 contributes to relatively lower efficiency of the establishment of breast tumoroids.

which signifies that specific organoid proteome profile from patients can guide precision management [71].

Liver cancer

Human liver cancer organoids have been established in several studies [72]. Primary liver cancer organoids of three major types including hepatocellular carcinoma (HCC), cholangiocarcinoma (CC), and combined hepatocellular-CC (CHC) have been successfully developed in specific isolated medium and passaged in expansion medium [34]. Specific isolated medium used during the establishment of liver cancer organoids includes two types: classical human liver organoid isolation medium and tumoroid-specific isolation medium [34]. Some organoids needed tumoroid-specific isolation medium, while some other organoids required classical isolation medium [34]. It was observed that one CC organoid only grew in classical human liver organoid isolation medium due to the need of R-spondin-1 for growth [34]. Y27632 is only required during the first 2–3 weeks of culture. At histological level, these primary liver cancer organoids recapitulated their parent tumors to a great degree even after long-term expansion [34]. The organoids of HCC and CHC were solid architectures filled with HCCs, in which a histological characteristic of HCC

(pseudoglandular rosettes) was observed [34]. Just as found in patients' tissues, it was also noted that CC tumoroids contained a great many glandular regions with cancer cells, which invaded the lumen and grew in a cribriform manner [34]. For expression profile, alfa-fetoprotein and glypican-3, markers of HCC, were upregulated in HCC tumoroids but the levels of CC markers remained low [34]. Conversely, CC markers (epithelial cell adhesion molecules, KRT19, and S100 Calcium Binding Protein A11 were enhanced in CC organoids but HCC markers were remarkably downregulated [34]. For transcriptional level, these organoids faithfully recapitulated transcriptomic alterations, which were identified in corresponding original tissues [34].

Pancreatic cancer

Pancreatic tumor organoids have been successfully established in a flurry of studies [36, 66, 73]. For long-term maintenance and enrichment of *KRAS*-mutant pancreatic ductal adenocarcinoma (PDAC) organoids, serum and EGF were eliminated from the culture medium [36]. For the organoids that were sensitive to the removal of EGF, an inhibitor of murine double minute 2 Nutlin3 or Noggin elimination could be employed to select possible existing organoids with *TP53* or *SMAD4*-mutants, respectively

Table 2 Culture systems of multiple tumoroids

Tumoroid type	Culture components			Ref
	Extracellular matrix	Growth factors	Molecule inhibitors	
Stomach cancer Intestinal cancer	Matrigel (growth factor reduced)	ADMEM/F12, penicillin/streptomycin, L-glutamine, B27, N2, bovine serum albumin, EGF, Noggin, R-spondin-1, gastrin, FGF10, FGF-basic, Wnt3A, prostaglandin E_2, and nicotinamide	A-83-01 Y27632 SB202190	[26]
Liver cancer	Basement membrane extract	Classical human liver organoid isolation medium: ADMEM/F12, penicillin/streptomycin, GlutaMAX, HEPES, B27 (without vitamin A), N2, N-acetylcysteine, nicotinamide, gastrin 1, EGF, FGF10, HGF, forskolin, R-spondin-1, Wnt3A, and Noggin Tumoroid-specific isolation medium: Classical human liver organoid isolation medium with the elimination of R-spondin-1, Wnt3A, and Noggin as well as addition of dexamethasone Human healthy liver-derived organoids expansion medium Classical human liver organoid isolation medium with the elimination of Y27632, Wnt3A, and Noggin	A-83-01 Y27632	[34]
Pancreatic cancer	Matrigel	ADMEM/F12, penicillin/streptomycin, GlutaMAX, HEPES, B27, N-acetylcysteine, EGF, R-spondin-1, gastrin 1, Wnt3A, Noggin, and FGF	A-83-01	[66]
Breast cancer	Basement membrane extract (reduced growth factor)	ADMEM/F12, penicillin/streptomycin, GlutaMAX, HEPES, B27, N-acetylcysteine, R-spondin-1, FGF7, FGF10, nicotinamide, Noggin, primocin, and neuregulin 1	A-83-01 Y27632	[38]
Bladder cancer	Matrigel	Hepatocyte media with EGF, FBS, GlutaMAX, and primocin	Y27632	[67]
Prostate cancer	Matrigel (growth factor reduced)	ADMEM, penicillin/streptomycin, primocin, GlutaMAX, B27, EGF, N-acetylcysteine, FGF10, FGF-basic, nicotinamide, testosterone, prostaglandin E_2, Noggin, and R-spondin	A-83-01 SB202190	[68]

[36]. Driver-gene alterations including *KRAS*, *cyclin-dependent kinase inhibitor 2A*, *TP53*, and *SMAD4*, which are common in human pancreatic carcinoma, were detected in corresponding organoids. When transplanted into mice, the organoids formed tumors in vivo like the derived PDAC [36]. Optical metabolic imaging of PDAC organoids is quite sensitive to metabolic changes induced by anti-cancer drugs. The combination of this nondestructive method and cancer organoid platform help better monitoring of dynamic drug response for patients in vitro [74].

Breast cancer

Breast cancer organoid models have been successfully achieved to study breast carcinoma biology [38, 75, 76]. Hans Clevers, et al. highlighted that (1) neuregulin 1 was an essential element for efficient generation and long-term expansion for breast cancer organoids; (2) Wnt3A was not essential for culture conditions; (3) EGF was a double-edged sword for low concentration impeding proliferation and high concentration leading to organoid sinking and gradual loss of 3D organization; (4) SB202190 at high concentration was detrimental to effective establishment of breast cancer organoids [38]. The breast cancer organoid lines were consistent with the parent tumors in morphology, histopathology, hormone receptor status, human epidermal growth factor receptor 2 (Her2) status, mutational landscape, and DNA CNAs [38]. Organoids

represent a valuable tool for evaluating local tumor invasion of breast cancer, which is the basis for distant metastasis and involves the interactions between tumor, ECM, and stromal cells [75].

Bladder cancer

The culture system of bladder cancer organoids has been reported in many studies [67, 77]. A biobank of patient-derived bladder cancer organoids has been established by Suk Hyung Lee and colleagues, who reported a well-defined culture protocol for propagation of bladder cancer organoids [67]. Histological analysis demonstrated the remarkable similarity between these organoids and the corresponding derived tumors [67]. In terms of the mutational profiles for 468 tumor-related genes, high concordance was observed between bladder cancer organoids and their parental tumors [67]. However, there were some genomic changes in organoids, which accompanied with cancer evolution in culture [67]. According to the deep sequencing analysis, some mutations were lost or gained during the continuous process in organoid cultures [67]. Using bladder tumoroids as a platform, drug response was partly associated with mutational profiles, signifying the feasibility that bladder tumor organoids derived from patients can be employed to predict treatment response and guide personalized therapies for each individual patient [67].

Prostate cancer

Prostate cancer organoids from patients have been reported in multiple studies [37, 68, 78]. Dong Gao's group provided a detailed protocol for the metastatic prostate cancer organoid establishment from metastatic tumor cells and circulating tumor cells [37]. A diversity of characteristic copy number alterations (CNAs) in prostate cancer were detected in the prostate tumoroid lines, including deletions of SHQ1, transmembrane protease, serine 2/erythroblast transformation-specific-related gene and phosphatase and tensin homolog (PTEN) as well as the amplification of androgen receptor (AR) [37]. Furthermore, mutation profile detected in organoid lines overlaid the prevalent mutations in prostate cancer, such as mutations in TP53, forkhead box A1, phosphoinositide-3-kinase regulatory subunit 1 (PIK3R1), alpha thalassemia/mental retardation syndrome X-linked, checkpoint kinase 2, KDM4C, KDM4D, and MLL2 [37]. When transplanted into severe combined immunodeficient mice, organoid lines displayed histological patterns found in parent tumors [37]. The 3D co-cultures of bone stroma cells and prostate cancer cells not only induced cytogenetic and gene expression changes in stromal cells but also fueled growth and metastasis of prostate tumoroids, which indicated the co-evolution of cancer and stroma as well as the significance of tumor-stroma interaction [79].

Other cancer types

Organoids of other cancer types have also been faithfully established, such as CC [26], thyroid cancer [80], ovarian cancer (OC) [81], and brain cancer [82]. CC organoids derived from human metastatic CC biopsies retained rearrangements of fibroblast growth factor receptor 2 that parent tumors harbored [26]. Mouse models of poorly differentiated thyroid tumors has been established through the transplantation of the thyroid organoids with enhanced expression of oncogene neuroblastoma RAS derived from mouse with P53 knockout [80]. In addition, OC cell lines from patients were planted on Matrigel in cancer SC medium containing Gentamicin, Fungizone, and Y27632, and formed organoids with the expression of tumor marker carbohydrate antigen 125 [81]. The infiltration capacity of glioblastoma multiforme cell into healthy brain parenchyma partly accounts for that high-grade of this tumor type cannot benefit much from surgical management [82]. Human glioblastoma multiforme spheroids could spontaneously infiltrate early-stage brain organoids and form hybrid organoids, demonstrating an invasive tumor phenotype and helping explore anti-invasion strategies for this refractory disease [82].

However, organoid models of some cancer types have not been reported as exemplified by lung cancer. Lung normal organoids can be developed from basal cells derived from trachea or large airways or even nasal epithelium, commonly containing TRP63$^+$and KRT5$^+$ basal cells, secretory goblet cells, and functional multiciliated cells [83, 84]. Through clustered regularly interspersed short palindromic repeats (CRISPR)/CRISPR-associated protein 9 (Cas9) gene editing technology, organoid can be employed as a platform to identify genes that modulate vital airway functions, such as selective permeability, barrier formation, fluid transport, innate immunity, and ciliogenesis [85, 86]. According to these findings, we can suppose that oncogene-activated mutations introduced by CRISPR/Cas9 might drive tumorigenesis in primary normal lung organoids. Further efforts are in need for application of organoid technology in lung cancer.

Organoid in cancer modeling

Some infectious pathogens are identified to be significant risk factors of cancer, such as Helicobacter pylori in gastric cancer, Salmonella enterica in gallbladder carcinoma, hepatitis virus in HCC, and Epstein-Barr virus (EBV) in gastric cancer, nasopharyngeal carcinoma, and lymphoma. However, there is still a lack of extensive understanding of the direct relationships and causal mechanisms between the infectious pathogens and corresponding cancers. Organoids can serve as a potential excellent model for studying these processes through co-culture systems with different pathogens. Neefjes J and colleagues employed co-cultures of murine-derived genetically predisposed gallbladder organoids and Salmonella enterica to explore the epidemiological association between gallbladder carcinoma and Salmonella Typhi infection, and supported that Salmonella enterica triggered and maintained malignant transformation accompanied by TP53 mutations and c-Myc amplification through Salmonella enterica effectors-induced activation of mitogen-activated protein kinase and AKT pathways [20]. Besides, viral infectious organoid models can also be established as exemplified by intestinal organoids with rotavirus infection [21], indicating that the virus-tumor relationship can also be simulated by co-culture systems, such as hepatitis virus versus liver cancer and EBV versus nasopharyngeal carcinoma. Modeling of the transition from infection to tumor formation and progression of organoids might help to reveal pathogenic mechanisms and find potential anti-tumor targets during this process.

Cancers occur on the genetic basis of sequential accumulation of mutations, signifying that it is pivotal to throw light upon the mutational processes during homeostasis and tumorigenesis. Knowledge of original mutation profile has been demonstrated to be of importance [22], for which healthy organoids provide a platform. Whole genome sequencing on human colon organoids with knockout of DNA repair genes through CRISPA-Cas9 technology revealed that the deficiency in mismatch repair genes contributed to mutation accumulation through replication errors, and deficiency in the cancer-predisposition gene DNA glycosylase led to mutation profile previously noted in cancer patients [23]. In addition, understanding of heterogeneous mutational signatures underlying tumor progression is also of great significance, which can also be prompted by organoid technology. Remarkably increased mutation rates and acquisition of new mutational profile were observed during development of colorectal tumoroids, and the diverse contributions of mutational processes in different regions of the same tumor were demonstrated by Roerink SF and colleagues [87]. It is interesting and feasible to employ organoid platform to evaluate the impact of drugs and irradiation on mutation profiles of cancer and normal cells as well as explore the mutational differences between sensitive and resistant organoids towards treatments.

Genetic cancer modeling is another paramount potential application of tumoroids [24, 25, 88, 89]. The conversion from healthy human intestinal organoids to colorectal progressive tumoroids has been achieved through the introduction of a set of common driver mutations in colorectal cancer via CRISPR-Cas9 gene editing technology, indicating tumor growth as a consequence of cancer driver mutations was independent of SC niche factors and identifying loss of *adenomatosis polyposis coli* (*APC*) and *TP53* as pivotal contributors for chromosome instability and aneuploidy [24, 90]. Using organoid models, it was demonstrated that *ring finger protein 43* mutations positively regulated Wnt-β-catenin signaling in human serrated colon adenoma [91], and loss of mutations in *caudal type homeobox2* and *BRAF*^{V600E} synergistically drove progression of serrated colorectal cancer [89]. Organoids facilitate better understanding of tumor initiation and progression of cancers at the genetic level.

Organoids in drug development

During the past decades, numerous anti-cancer drugs developed from screening on conventional 2D culture of large standard cell lines failed in clinical studies [92, 93]. For most cytotoxic agents, broad activity was observed across tumor cell lines, but clinical efficiency noted in patients was in more limited settings [93]. Voskoglou-Nomikos T evaluated whether in vitro cell lines were reliable in predicting clinical utility. The results showed that in vitro cell line model was predictive for non-small cell lung cancer under the disease-oriented approach, but not for colon cancer [94]. Since cancer organoids are near-physiological architectures, retain specific functions of the parent tumors and can faithfully recapitulate drug responses, the organoid technology fills the gap between drug screening based on classical 2D cell lines and clinical trials. Numerous studies have demonstrated that organoid can serve as

an excellent model for evaluating specific responses of cancer patients [26, 69, 81, 95, 96]. Besides, it also can be an extraordinary alternative to explore the detailed causal epigenetic and genetic alterations underlying drug resistance [97]. Several organoid biobanks of cancers so far have been established for the purposes of identifying and testing novel drugs [37, 38, 98], and healthy organoids can be utilized to test toxicology.

Drug efficacy testing

Recently, metastatic gastrointestinal cancer (colorectal cancer and gastroesophageal cancer) organoids derived from patients have been established and employed to identify whether organoids can forecast treatment response among patients. In this study, a wide spectrum of anti-tumor drugs, including used in clinical practice and currently in phases of clinical trials, were enrolled for testing drug sensitivity [26]. The results reflected that organoids cancer faithfully recapitulated treatment responses of gastrointestinal cancers with high sensitivity (100%), specificity (93%), positive predictive value (88%), and negative predictive value (100%) in predicting response to chemotherapy in patients [26]. For instance, there was a remarkable association between retinoblastoma 1 amplification and the sensitivity of tumor organoids to cyclin dependent kinase 4/6 inhibitor palbociclib, which was in line with previously published data [26, 99]. Another example was that patient-derived organoids with *BRAF*^{V600E} mutation exhibited dramatically reduced viability but no differences in apoptosis after the exposure of the *BRAF* inhibitor vemurafenib in comparison with the organoids with no mutations in *BRAF* gene, which was consistent with the ineffectiveness of monotherapy with *BRAF* inhibitors in metastatic colorectal cancer [26]. By conducting drug screening on human gastric cancer organoids, Therese Seidlitz and colleagues identified organoids recapitulated the divergent responses to conventional chemotherapeutics, including 5-fluorouracil (5-FU), irinotecan, epirubicin, oxaliplantin, and docetaxel [69]. Furthermore, these organoid lines can be employed to test not only the efficacy of a known mutation-targeted therapy for an individual patient but also the effectiveness of treatment on unknown mutations, as exemplified by trastuzumab treatment for *ERBB2* amplifications/*ERBB2* mutations and imatinib treatment for an unknown mutation in exon 3 of the *KIT* receptor [69].

A panel of human colorectal cancer organoids has been assembled for assessing mutation-targeted inhibitors and drug combination therapy, including irreversible epidermal growth factor receptor/Her2 inhibitor afatinib, MEK inhibitor selumetinib, and ERK inhibitor SCH772984 [100]. The results reflected that both the combinations of afatinib plus selumetinib and SCH772984 plus selumetinib significantly inhibited growth of *RAS*-mutant tumor organoids with obvious cell cycle block but no impact on cell death. After these drugs were withdrawn, tumor cells could restore proliferation activity, which might hamper the effectiveness of the combination therapy among patients with RAS-mutant colorectal cancer [100]. However, the combination of a preclinical B-cell lymphoma 2 (BCL-2)/BCL-xL inhibitor navitoclax, afatinib, and selumetinib potently promoted cell death in comparison with monotherapy of these drugs, indicating a possible alternative treatment strategy [100].

Huch M, et al. has propagated primary liver tumoroids, which faithfully recapitulated histology, expression patterns and genetic alterations of corresponding original tumors [34]. A total of 29 anti-cancer drugs were enrolled in the proof-of-concept testing of drug sensitivity using organoid model, and the results indicated that these tumoroids facilitated identification of drug sensitivity in individual patient. Intriguingly, it was identified that ERK signaling could be a potential therapeutic target for primary liver cancer patients [34].

A living biobank of primary breast cancer organoids and metastatic breast cancer organoids can also be employed as an excellent platform for drug screening, supported by that responses to afatinib or tamoxifen of organoids showed remarkably similarity to patients [38]. As another example, standard OC cells from patients were cultured to differentiate into organoids [81]. The responses to multiple OC drugs and the association with genomic alterations in organoids were assessed through *DeathPro* assay for improving drug screening [81]. A diversity of drug responses were observed in OC organoids and drug effects in organoids resembled the findings in clinical trials [81]. For instance, a majority of OC patients failed to response to paclitaxel, and the addition of paclitaxel to carboplatin did not refine efficacy in comparison to carboplatin monotherapy [81]. Compared with 2D cultures, the responses to drugs of organoids were more similar to the parent tumors. Dasatinib, to which recurrent OC is resistant at clinical phase II, was also ineffective in 3D culture but effective in 2D culture [81].

Because of the extraordinary recapitulation of responses to drugs for original tumors in vivo, prostate cancer organoid lines have also been exploited to help the screening of anti-cancer drugs [37]. For instance, *AR*-amplified prostate cancer organoids were exquisitely sensitive to the AR inhibitor enzalutamide, while *AR*-negative prostate cancer organoids responded to this drug in an opposite manner [37]. Besides, prostate cancer organoid lines harboring both *PTEN* loss and *PIK3R1* mutation were sensitive to everolinus and BKM120 [37].

Pharmacokinetic

Organoids technology can also be employed in pharmacokinetic testing, which is a pivotal thing during drug development. Human iPSCs-derived intestinal organoids have been generated through appropriate methods with a variety of intestinal cells [101], and these organoids were endowed with pharmacokinetic function [101]. In the condition of some small-molecular compounds, organoids expressed drug transporters, efflux transport activity, and the activation of drug-metabolizing enzyme cytochrome P450 [101]. The results indicated that these organoids could be employed for pharmacokinetic assessment in drug development [101].

Drug toxicity testing

Another major advantage of organoid technology in drug development is that normal organoids can be generated and exploited for screening of drugs which exclusively target tumor cells without harming healthy cells. Intolerant side effects majorly lead to drug failure in clinical trials, including hepatotoxicity, cardiotoxicity, and nephrotoxicity. Hepatic organoid represents an extraordinary model for hepatotoxicity testing of experimental compounds [102–104]. Drug-related hepatotoxicity is mostly mediated through cytochrome P450 enzymes, which is inspiringly observed in hepatic organoids at near-physiological levels [104, 105]. Cardiac adverse effects such as arrhythmias and cardiotoxic effects can also be tested in 3D cultures [96, 106]. Besides, kidney organoids has also been employed for toxicological research [107].

Immunotherapy

Immunotherapy, which is among the chief novel and promising strategies, employs the patient's own immune system to kill tumor cells. A prerequisite for immunotherapy is that malignant cells exhibit sufficient immunogenicity to trigger adequate immune response [108, 109]. Mutational status of cancer cells, which contribute to neo-antigens production, is responsible for immune responses [109, 110]. However, the intensity of immune response induced by neo-antigens of carcinoma is insufficient, which can be addressed through activating and expanding immune cells in vitro for in vivo application in patients.

Multiple studies have brought new hope for the application of organoid technology in immunotherapy, as exemplified by functional maintenance of intraepithelial lymphocytes being co-cultured with mouse intestinal organoids at the presence of interleukin-2 (IL-2), IL7, and IL-15 in the culture medium [111]. Another example is that the short-term maintenance of CD45-positive lymphocytes can be achieved through co-culture with patient-derived organoids of air-liquid interface tumors [112]. Encouragingly, co-cultures of $V\delta2^+$ T lymphocytes and organoids of primary human breast epithelial have been developed successfully, and these T lymphocytes could potently eradicate triple-negative breast cancer cells [113]. These findings signify the possibility that T lymphocytes from healthy blood donors can be expanded and activated with organoids and subsequently utilized to treat patients, and the possibility that the cytotoxic effects of healthy donor-derived T cells on patient-derived tumoroids can be tested in vitro.

Personalized medicine

Personalized medicine, also called precision medicine, aims to identify effective treatment strategies for each patient through better characterization of diseases at molecular and pharmacogenomics levels. As an excellent minute incarnation of an in vivo organ, organoids are superior to conventional models, because this easily established model can better recapitulate in vivo characteristics in phenotype, genotype, and specific functions as well as physiological and pathological changes even after many generations. Organoids are endowed with enormous potential to identify the feasible optimized treatment strategy for the individual patient [29, 30, 114, 115].

Rubin MA and colleagues applied the organoid platform to identify the optimized combination therapy options for some cancer types as exemplified by uterine carcinosarcoma and endometrial adenocarcinoma harboring similar driver mutations in *PIK3 catalytic subunit alpha* and *PTEN* [29]. The uterine carcinosarcoma organoid receiving combination treatment of vorinostat and buparlisib showed strongest inhibition in comparison with other combination strategies, while the combination of buparlisib andolaparib was among the most effective strategies for the endometrial adenocarcinoma organoid [29].

Another example was that the *KRAS* and *TP53*-mutant organoid of stage IV colorectal cancer only showed notable response to trametinib, and the combination of trametinib and celecoxib was among the chief strongly effective combinational options [29]. Besides, it was also demonstrated that the novel combination of afatinib and histone deacetylase inhibitors contributed to dramatically enhanced growth suppression of colorectal tumoroids with *APC* mutations, even greater than the standard FOLFOX (oxaliplatin, FU and leucovorin) regimen did [29]. In addition, drug screening was also conducted on human colorectal organoids from patients, containing many cancer SCs and being resistant to 5-FU and irinotecan [116]. Organoids treated with hedgehog signal inhibitors (AY9944 and GANT61) exhibited reduced cell viability with downregulation of c-Myc, CD44, and Nanog [116], and organoids treated with the combination of AY9944 or GANT61 with 5-FU or irinotecan showed impaired cell viability in comparison to each drug alone [116]. These results reflected that inhibitors of hedgehog signaling could serve as an effective combinational candidate for the treatment of 5-FU or irinotecan-resistant colorectal tumors [116]. Based on the phenomenon that anaplastic lymphoma kinase (ALK) mutation (F1174C) promoted growth and upregulated the expression of neuroendocrine marker neuron-specific enolase in the organoids of prostate small cell carcinoma, alectinic showed more significant effects than crizotinibin terms of inhibiting ALKF1174C-expressing cell expansion [117].

Photodynamic therapy, known as a light-activated cancer therapy, supplements conventional chemotherapies and brings clinical promise for pancreatic cancer treatment [118]. As observed in organoids of metastatic pancreatic carcinoma, intelligent combination of oxaliplatin and neoadjuvant photodynamic therapy exhibited remarkably enhanced anti-tumor efficacy in comparison with any therapy alone, without augment of toxicity [118].

Although it is still in an immature stage of organoid technology in personalized medicine, further efforts can refine this model and broaden horizon in personalized medicine in replacement for conventional "one-size-fits-all" treatments.

Current limitations

Although organoids have a wide range of potential applications, the current version still represents a somewhat rough model, and researchers still grapple with obstacles of this technology. Firstly, organoids are imperfect reproductions. The "tissues in a dish" comprise only epithelial layer without native microenvironment including surrounding mesenchyme, immune cells, nervous system, or muscular layer [81]. Possible solutions to this limitation are to further refine organotypic culture system or to co-culture with additional cellular elements such as immune cells, stromal cells, or neural cells, as exemplified by iPSC-derived intestinal organoids containing a functional nervous system [119] and co-culture of PDAC organoids with mouse pancreatic stellate cells which differentiated into cancer-related fibroblasts [120]. In spite of these encouraging findings, an immune microenvironment around a tumor is difficult to be modeled. Immune niche of tumors is a complicated system composed of diverse immune cells including cytotoxic lymphocytes, tumor infiltrating dendritic cells, regulatory T cells, tumor-associated macrophage, and myeloid-derived suppressor cells, and tumor immune microenvironment is in dynamic changes, and there may be differences between different tumor types as well as individual patients. Secondly, fully maturation is an obstacle required to be tackled, which might affect the therapeutic potential. Thirdly, some organoid lines still cannot be expanded for long term, which could be disposed through improvement of culture medium. Fourthly, cancer organoids tend to grow more slowly than corresponding organoids from normal epithelial, thus probably contributing to the outgrowth of tumor organoids by contaminating normal epithelial cells. This problem might be addressed through improving the tissue extraction process to minimize the contaminating normal cells. Fifthly, current organoids are majorly derived from epithelium, and further investigation of cultures of non-epithelial organoids is needed, taking the recent advances in establishment of organoids induced from primary glioblastoma as an example. Lastly, the growth factors or small molecular inhibitors in culture medium may have significant effects on gene expression and signaling pathways in organoids, and may affect drug sensitivity. Further efforts are in need for addressing this problem.

Conclusion

In spite of these limitations, the exciting and promising organoid technology holds enormous potential to more accurately model human tumors. Up to now, highly efficient establishment of organoids has been achieved from both normal and malignant tissues. Using these amazing 3D cultures, both drug screening and personalized medicine can be prompted dramatically to better predict drug responses and guide optimized therapy strategies for an individual patient. Future efforts will doubtless bring this novel technique closer to clinical practice.

Abbreviations

2D: Two-dimensional; 3D: Three-dimensional; 5-FU: 5-fluorouracil; ADMEM: Advanced Dulbecco's modified Eagle's medium; ALK: Anaplastic lymphoma kinase; APC: Adenomatosis polyposis coli; AR: Androgen receptor; BCL-2: B-cell lymphoma 2; Cas9: CRISPR-associated protein 9; CC: Cholangiocarcinoma; CD45: Cluster of differentiation 45; CHC: Combined hepatocellular-cholangiocarcinoma; CNAs: Copy number alterations; CRISPR: Clustered regularly interspersed short palindromic repeats; EBV: Epstein-Barr virus; ECM: Extracellular matrix; EGF: Epidermal growth factor; ESCs: Embryonic stem cells; FBS: Fetal bovine serum; FGF10: Fibroblast growth factor 10; HBSS: Hank's balanced salt solution; HCC: Hepatocellular carcinoma; Her2: Human epidermal growth factor receptor 2; HGF: Hepatocyte growth factor; IL-2: Interleukin-2; iPSCs: Induced pluripotent stem cells; KRT7: Cytokeratin 7; MDGI: Mammary-derived growth inhibitor; OC: Ovarian cancer; PBS: Phosphate-buffered saline; PDAC: Pancreatic ductal adenocarcinoma; PDTXs: Patient-derived tumor xenografts; PIK3R1: Phosphoinositide-3-kinase regulatory subunit 1; PTEN: Phosphatase and tensin homolog; SCs: Stem cells

Funding

This work was supported by the National Natural Science Foundation of China (nos. 81572608, 81172422 and 81874120) and supported by Wuhan Science and Technology Bureau (no. 2017060201010170).

Authors' contributions

HX performed the selection of literature, drafted the manuscript, and prepared the figures. XL, MY, and WZ collected the related references. YS and KW carried out the design of this review and revised the manuscript. All authors contributed to this manuscript. All authors read and approved the final manuscript.

Consent for publication

Not applicable.

Competing interests

The authors declare that they have no competing interests.

Author details

[1]Department of Oncology, Tongji Hospital of Tongji Medical College, Huazhong University of Science and Technology, 1095 Jiefang Avenue, Wuhan 430030, Hubei, China. [2]Central Laboratory, the Affiliated Cancer Hospital of Zhengzhou University, Henan Cancer Hospital, Zhengzhou 450000, Henan, China. [3]Department of Hematology, the Affiliated Cancer Hospital of Zhengzhou University, Henan Cancer Hospital, Zhengzhou 450000, Henan, China.

References

1. Lai YH, Lin SY, Wu YS, Chen HW, Chen JJW. AC-93253 iodide, a novel Src inhibitor, suppresses NSCLC progression by modulating multiple Src-related signaling pathways. J Hematol Oncol. 2017;10:172.
2. Lai Y, Wei X, Lin S, Qin L, Cheng L, Li P. Current status and perspectives of patient-derived xenograft models in cancer research. J Hematol Oncol. 2017;10:106.
3. Meng S, Zhou H, Feng Z, Xu Z, Tang Y, Li P, et al. CircRNA: functions and properties of a novel potential biomarker for cancer. Mol Cancer. 2017;16:94.
4. Li A, Zhang T, Zheng M, Liu Y, Chen Z. Exosomal proteins as potential markers of tumor diagnosis. J Hematol Oncol. 2017;10:175.
5. Viardot A, Bargou R. Bispecific antibodies in haematological malignances. Cancer Treat Rev. 2018;65:87–95.
6. Yu S, Liu Q, Han X, Qin S, Zhao W, Li A, et al. Development and clinical application of anti-HER2 monoclonal and bispecific antibodies for cancer treatment. Exp Hematol Oncol. 2017;6:31.
7. Yu S, Li A, Liu Q, Yuan X, Xu H, Jiao D, et al. Recent advances of bispecific antibodies in solid tumors. J Hematol Oncol. 2017;10:155.
8. Yi M, Jiao D, Xu H, Liu Q, Zhao W, Han X, et al. Biomarkers for predicting efficacy of PD-1/PD-L1 inhibitors. Mol Cancer. 2018;17:129.
9. Wei G, Ding L, Wang J, Hu Y, Huang H. Advances of CD19-directed chimeric antigen receptor-modified T cells in refractory/relapsed acute lymphoblastic leukemia. Exp Hematol Oncol. 2017;6:10.
10. Xu H, Yu S, Liu Q, Yuan X, Mani S, Pestell RG, et al. Recent advances of highly selective CDK4/6 inhibitors in breast cancer. J Hematol Oncol. 2017;10:97.
11. Pang Y, Hou X, Yang C, Liu Y, Jiang G. Advances on chimeric antigen receptor-modified T-cell therapy for oncotherapy. Mol Cancer. 2018;17:91.
12. Liu B, Song Y, Liu D. Recent development in clinical applications of PD-1 and PD-L1 antibodies for cancer immunotherapy. J Hematol Oncol. 2017;10:174.
13. Zhou J, Su J, Fu X, Zheng L, Yin Z. Microfluidic device for primary tumor spheroid isolation. Exp Hematol Oncol. 2017;6:22.
14. Ben-David U, Ha G, Tseng YY, Greenwald NF, Oh C, Shih J, et al. Patient-derived xenografts undergo mouse-specific tumor evolution. Nat Genet. 2017;49:1567–75.
15. Byrne AT, Alferez DG, Amant F, Annibali D, Arribas J, Biankin AV, et al. Interrogating open issues in cancer medicine with patient-derived xenografts. Nat Rev Cancer. 2017;17:632.
16. Lancaster MA, Knoblich JA. Organogenesis in a dish: modeling development and disease using organoid technologies. Science. 2014;345:1247125.
17. Drost J, Clevers H. Organoids in cancer research. Nat Rev Cancer. 2018;18: 407–18.
18. Yeung TM, Gandhi SC, Wilding JL, Muschel R, Bodmer WF. Cancer stem cells from colorectal cancer-derived cell lines. Proc Natl Acad Sci U S A. 2010;107: 3722–7.
19. Onuma K, Ochiai M, Orihashi K, Takahashi M, Imai T, Nakagama H, et al. Genetic reconstitution of tumorigenesis in primary intestinal cells. Proc Natl Acad Sci U S A. 2013;110:11127–32.
20. Scanu T, Spaapen RM, Bakker JM, Pratap CB, Wu LE, Hofland I, et al. Salmonella manipulation of host signaling pathways provokes cellular transformation associated with gallbladder carcinoma. Cell Host Microbe. 2015;17:763–74.

21. Yin Y, Bijvelds M, Dang W, Xu L, van der Eijk AA, Knipping K, et al. Modeling rotavirus infection and antiviral therapy using primary intestinal organoids. Antivir Res. 2015;123:120–31.

22. Davies H, Glodzik D, Morganella S, Yates LR, Staaf J, Zou X, et al. HRDetect is a predictor of BRCA1 and BRCA2 deficiency based on mutational signatures. Nat Med. 2017;23:517–25.

23. Drost J, van Boxtel R, Blokzijl F, Mizutani T, Sasaki N, Sasselli V, et al. Use of CRISPR-modified human stem cell organoids to study the origin of mutational signatures in cancer. Science. 2017;358:234–8.

24. Matano M, Date S, Shimokawa M, Takano A, Fujii M, Ohta Y, et al. Modeling colorectal cancer using CRISPR-Cas9-mediated engineering of human intestinal organoids. Nat Med. 2015;21:256–62.

25. Li X, Nadauld L, Ootani A, Corney DC, Pai RK, Gevaert O, et al. Oncogenic transformation of diverse gastrointestinal tissues in primary organoid culture. Nat Med. 2014;20:769–77.

26. Vlachogiannis G, Hedayat S, Vatsiou A, Jamin Y, Fernandez-Mateos J, Khan K, et al. Patient-derived organoids model treatment response of metastatic gastrointestinal cancers. Science. 2018;359:920–6.

27. Sampaziotis F, Justin AW, Tysoe OC, Sawiak S, Godfrey EM, Upponi SS, et al. Reconstruction of the mouse extrahepatic biliary tree using primary human extrahepatic cholangiocyte organoids. Nat Med. 2017;23:954–63.

28. Ramsden CM, Powner MB, Carr AJ, Smart MJ, da Cruz L, Coffey PJ. Stem cells in retinal regeneration: past, present and future. Development. 2013; 140:2576–85.

29. Pauli C, Hopkins BD, Prandi D, Shaw R, Fedrizzi T, Sboner A, et al. Personalized in vitro and in vivo Cancer models to guide precision medicine. Cancer Discov. 2017;7:462–77.

30. Papapetrou EP. Patient-derived induced pluripotent stem cells in cancer research and precision oncology. Nat Med. 2016;22:1392–401.

31. Fujii M, Shimokawa M, Date S, Takano A, Matano M, Nanki K, et al. A colorectal tumor organoid library demonstrates progressive loss of niche factor requirements during tumorigenesis. Cell Stem Cell. 2016;18:827–38.

32. Schutte M, Risch T, Abdavi-Azar N, Boehnke K, Schumacher D, Keil M, et al. Molecular dissection of colorectal cancer in pre-clinical models identifies biomarkers predicting sensitivity to EGFR inhibitors. Nat Commun. 2017;8:14262.

33. Weeber F, van de Wetering M, Hoogstraat M, Dijkstra KK, Krijgsman O, Kuilman T, et al. Preserved genetic diversity in organoids cultured from biopsies of human colorectal cancer metastases. Proc Natl Acad Sci U S A. 2015;112:13308–11.

34. Broutier L, Mastrogiovanni G, Verstegen MM, Francies HE, Gavarro LM, Bradshaw CR, et al. Human primary liver cancer-derived organoid cultures for disease modeling and drug screening. Nat Med. 2017;23:1424–35.

35. Huang L, Holtzinger A, Jagan I, BeGora M, Lohse I, Ngai N, et al. Ductal pancreatic cancer modeling and drug screening using human pluripotent stem cell- and patient-derived tumor organoids. Nat Med. 2015;21:1364–71.

36. Seino T, Kawasaki S, Shimokawa M, Tamagawa H, Toshimitsu K, Fujii M, et al. Human pancreatic tumor organoids reveal loss of stem cell niche factor dependence during disease progression. Cell Stem Cell. 2018;22:454–67.e6.

37. Gao D, Vela I, Sboner A, Iaquinta PJ, Karthaus WR, Gopalan A, et al. Organoid cultures derived from patients with advanced prostate cancer. Cell. 2014;159:176–87.

38. Sachs N, de Ligt J, Kopper O, Gogola E, Bounova G, Weeber F, et al. A living biobank of breast Cancer organoids captures disease heterogeneity. Cell. 2018;172:373–86.e10.

39. Evans GS, Flint N, Somers AS, Eyden B, Potten CS. The development of a method for the preparation of rat intestinal epithelial cell primary cultures. J Cell Sci. 1992;101:219–31.

40. Whitehead RH, Demmler K, Rockman SP, Watson NK. Clonogenic growth of epithelial cells from normal colonic mucosa from both mice and humans. Gastroenterology. 1999;117:858–65.

41. Fukamachi H. Proliferation and differentiation of fetal rat intestinal epithelial cells in primary serum-free culture. J Cell Sci. 1992;103:511–9.

42. Perreault N, Beaulieu JF. Use of the dissociating enzyme thermolysin to generate viable human normal intestinal epithelial cell cultures. Exp Cell Res. 1996;224:354–64.

43. Sato T, Vries RG, Snippert HJ, van de Wetering M, Barker N, Stange DE, et al. Single Lgr5 stem cells build crypt-villus structures in vitro without a mesenchymal niche. Nature. 2009;459:262–5.

44. Sato T, Stange DE, Ferrante M, Vries RG, Van Es JH, Van den Brink S, et al. Long-term expansion of epithelial organoids from human colon,

adenoma, adenocarcinoma, and Barrett's epithelium. Gastroenterology. 2011;141:1762–72.

45. Stange DE, Koo BK, Huch M, Sibbel G, Basak O, Lyubimova A, et al. Differentiated troy+ chief cells act as reserve stem cells to generate all lineages of the stomach epithelium. Cell. 2013;155:357–68.

46. Huch M, Dorrell C, Boj SF, van Es JH, Li VS, van de Wetering M, et al. In vitro expansion of single Lgr5+ liver stem cells induced by Wnt-driven regeneration. Nature. 2013;494:247–50.

47. Messner S, Agarkova I, Moritz W, Kelm JM. Multi-cell type human liver microtissues for hepatotoxicity testing. Arch Toxicol. 2013;87:209–13.

48. Binas B, Spitzer E, Zschiesche W, Erdmann B, Kurtz A, Muller T, et al. Hormonal induction of functional differentiation and mammary-derived growth inhibitor expression in cultured mouse mammary gland explants. In Vitro Cell Dev Biol. 1992;28a:625–34.

49. Wang M, Liu YE, Ni J, Aygun B, Goldberg ID, Shi YE. Induction of mammary differentiation by mammary-derived growth inhibitor-related gene that interacts with an omega-3 fatty acid on growth inhibition of breast cancer cells. Cancer Res. 2000;60:6482–7.

50. Brock EJ, Ji K, Shah S, Mattingly RR, Sloane BF. In vitro models for studying invasive transitions of ductal carcinoma in situ. J Mammary Gland Biol Neoplasia. 2018. https://doi.org/10.1007/s10911-018-9405-3.

51. Saxen L, Lehtonen E. Embryonic kidney in organ culture. Differentiation. 1987;36:2–11.

52. Avner ED, Piesco NP, Sweeney WE Jr, Ellis D. Renal epithelial development in organotypic culture. Pediatr Nephrol. 1988;2:92–9.

53. van den Berg CW, Ritsma L, Avramut MC, Wiersma LE, van den Berg BM, Leuning DG, et al. Renal subcapsular transplantation of PSC-derived kidney organoids induces neo-vasculogenesis and significant glomerular and tubular maturation in vivo. Stem Cell Reports. 2018;10:751–65.

54. Bottenstein JE, Sato GH. Growth of a rat neuroblastoma cell line in serum-free supplemented medium. Proc Natl Acad Sci U S A. 1979;76:514–7.

55. Honegger P, Lenoir D, Favrod P. Growth and differentiation of aggregating fetal brain cells in a serum-free defined medium. Nature. 1979;282:305–8.

56. Snyder EY, Kim SU. Hormonal requirements for neuronal survival in culture. Neurosci Lett. 1979;13:225–30.

57. Pasca SP. Building three-dimensional human brain organoids. Nat Neurosci. 2018. https://doi.org/10.1038/s41593-018-0107-3.

58. Qian X, Nguyen HN, Song MM, Hadiono C, Ogden SC, Hammack C, et al. Brain-region-specific organoids using mini-bioreactors for modeling ZIKV exposure. Cell. 2016;165:1238–54.

59. Suga H, Kadoshima T, Minaguchi M, Ohgushi M, Soen M, Nakano T, et al. Self-formation of functional adenohypophysis in three-dimensional culture. Nature. 2011;480:57–62.

60. Jo J, Xiao Y, Sun AX, Cukuroglu E, Tran HD, Goke J, et al. Midbrain-like organoids from human pluripotent stem cells contain functional dopaminergic and neuromelanin-producing neurons. Cell Stem Cell. 2016;19:248–57.

61. Muguruma K, Nishiyama A, Kawakami H, Hashimoto K, Sasai Y. Self-organization of polarized cerebellar tissue in 3D culture of human pluripotent stem cells. Cell Rep. 2015;10:537–50.

62. Sakaguchi H, Kadoshima T, Soen M, Narii N, Ishida Y, Ohgushi M, et al. Generation of functional hippocampal neurons from self-organizing human embryonic stem cell-derived dorsomedial telencephalic tissue. Nat Commun. 2015;6:8896.

63. Kuo CJ, Curtis C. Organoids reveal cancer dynamics. Nature. 2018;556:441–2.

64. Muthuswamy SK. Organoid models of cancer explode with possibilities. Cell Stem Cell. 2018;22:290–1.

65. Crespo M, Vilar E, Tsai SY, Chang K, Amin S, Srinivasan T, et al. Colonic organoids derived from human induced pluripotent stem cells for modeling colorectal cancer and drug testing. Nat Med. 2017;23:878–84.

66. Boj SF, Hwang CI, Baker LA, Chio II, Engle DD, Corbo V, et al. Organoid models of human and mouse ductal pancreatic cancer. Cell. 2015;160: 324–38.

67. Lee SH, Hu W, Matulay JT, Silva MV, Owczarek TB, Kim K, et al. Tumor evolution and drug response in patient-derived organoid models of bladder cancer. Cell. 2018;173:515–28.e17.

68. Puca L, Bareja R, Prandi D, Shaw R, Benelli M, Karthaus WR, et al. Patient derived organoids to model rare prostate cancer phenotypes. Nat Commun. 2018;9:2404.

69. Seidlitz T, Merker SR, Rothe A, Zakrzewski F, von Neubeck C, Grutzmann K, et al. Human gastric cancer modelling using organoids. Gut. 2018. https://doi.org/10.1136/gutjnl-2017-314549.

70. Roper J, Tammela T, Cetinbas NM, Akkad A, Roghanian A, Rickelt S, et al. In vivo genome editing and organoid transplantation models of colorectal cancer and metastasis. Nat Biotechnol. 2017;35:569–76.

71. Cristobal A, van den Toorn HWP, van de Wetering M, Clevers H, Heck AJR, Mohammed S. Personalized proteome profiles of healthy and tumor human colon organoids reveal both individual diversity and basic features of colorectal cancer. Cell Rep. 2017;18:263–74.

72. Nuciforo S, Fofana I, Matter MS, Blumer T, Calabrese D, Boldanova T, et al. Organoid models of human liver cancers derived from tumor needle biopsies. Cell Rep. 2018;24:1363–76.

73. Zhang HC, Kuo CJ. Personalizing pancreatic cancer organoids with hPSCs. Nat Med. 2015;21:1249–51.

74. Walsh AJ, Castellanos JA, Nagathihalli NS, Merchant NB, Skala MC. Optical imaging of drug-induced metabolism changes in murine and human pancreatic cancer organoids reveals heterogeneous drug response. Pancreas. 2016;45:863–9.

75. Ranftl RE, Calvo F. Analysis of breast Cancer cell invasion using an Organotypic culture system. Methods Mol Biol. 2017;1612:199–212.

76. Duarte AA, Gogola E, Sachs N, Barazas M, Annunziato S, de Ruiter JR, et al. BRCA-deficient mouse mammary tumor organoids to study cancer-drug resistance. Nat Methods. 2018;15:134–40.

77. Yoshida T, Sopko NA, Kates M, Liu X, Joice G, McConkey DJ, et al. Three-dimensional organoid culture reveals involvement of Wnt/beta-catenin pathway in proliferation of bladder cancer cells. Oncotarget. 2018;9:11060–70.

78. Shenoy TR, Boysen G, Wang MY, Xu QZ, Guo W, Koh FM, et al. CHD1 loss sensitizes prostate cancer to DNA damaging therapy by promoting error-prone double-strand break repair. Ann Oncol. 2017;28:1495–507.

79. Sung SY, Hsieh CL, Law A, Zhau HE, Pathak S, Multani AS, et al. Coevolution of prostate cancer and bone stroma in three-dimensional coculture: implications for cancer growth and metastasis. Cancer Res. 2008;68:9996–10003.

80. Saito Y, Onishi N, Takami H, Seishima R, Inoue H, Hirata Y, et al. Development of a functional thyroid model based on an organoid culture system. Biochem Biophys Res Commun. 2018;497:783–9.

81. Jabs J, Zickgraf FM, Park J, Wagner S, Jiang X, Jechow K, et al. Screening drug effects in patient-derived cancer cells links organoid responses to genome alterations. Mol Syst Biol. 2017;13:955.

82. da Silva B, Mathew RK, Polson ES, Williams J, Wurdak H. Spontaneous glioblastoma spheroid infiltration of early-stage cerebral organoids models brain tumor invasion. SLAS Discov. 2018;23:862–8.

83. Butler CR, Hynds RE, Gowers KH, Lee Ddo H, Brown JM, Crowley C, et al. Rapid expansion of human epithelial stem cells suitable for airway tissue engineering. Am J Respir Crit Care Med. 2016;194:156–68.

84. Hild M, Jaffe AB. Production of 3-D airway organoids from primary human airway basal cells and their use in high-throughput screening. Curr Protoc Stem Cell Biol. 2016;37:Ie.9.1–ie.9.15.

85. Chu HW, Rios C, Huang C, Wesolowska-Andersen A, Burchard EG, O'Connor BP, et al. CRISPR-Cas9-mediated gene knockout in primary human airway epithelial cells reveals a proinflammatory role for MUC18. Gene Ther. 2015; 22:822–9.

86. Gao X, Bali AS, Randell SH, Hogan BL. GRHL2 coordinates regeneration of a polarized mucociliary epithelium from basal stem cells. J Cell Biol. 2015;211: 669–82.

87. Roerink SF, Sasaki N, Lee-Six H, Young MD, Alexandrov LB, Behjati S, et al. Intra-tumour diversification in colorectal cancer at the single-cell level. Nature. 2018;556:457–62.

88. Fessler E, Drost J, van Hooff SR, Linnekamp JF, Wang X, Jansen M, et al. TGFbeta signaling directs serrated adenomas to the mesenchymal colorectal cancer subtype. EMBO Mol Med. 2016;8:745–60.

89. Sakamoto N, Feng Y, Stolfi C, Kurosu Y, Green M, Lin J, et al. BRAF(V600E) cooperates with CDX2 inactivation to promote serrated colorectal tumorigenesis. Elife. 2017;6. https://doi.org/10.7554/eLife.20331.

90. Drost J, van Jaarsveld RH, Ponsioen B, Zimberlin C, van Boxtel R, Buijs A, et al. Sequential cancer mutations in cultured human intestinal stem cells. Nature. 2015;521:43–7.

91. Yan HHN, Lai JCW, Ho SL, Leung WK, Law WL, Lee JFY, et al. RNF43 germline and somatic mutation in serrated neoplasia pathway and its association with BRAF mutation. Gut. 2017;66:1645–56.

92. Kamb A. What's wrong with our cancer models? Nat Rev Drug Discov. 2005; 4:161–5.

93. Caponigro G, Sellers WR. Advances in the preclinical testing of cancer therapeutic hypotheses. Nat Rev Drug Discov. 2011;10:179–87.

94. Voskoglou-Nomikos T, Pater JL, Seymour L. Clinical predictive value of the in vitro cell line, human xenograft, and mouse allograft preclinical cancer models. Clin Cancer Res. 2003;9:4227–39.

95. Abbasi J. Patient-derived organoids predict cancer treatment response. JAMA. 2018;319:1427.

96. Eder A, Vollert I, Hansen A, Eschenhagen T. Human engineered heart tissue as a model system for drug testing. Adv Drug Deliv Rev. 2016;96:214–24.

97. Duong HQ, Nemazanyy I, Rambow F, Tang SC, Delaunay S, Tharun L, et al. The endosomal protein CEMIP links Wnt signaling to MEK1-ERK1/2 activation in Selumetinib-resistant intestinal organoids. Cancer Res. 2018; 78:4533–48.

98. van de Wetering M, Francies HE, Francis JM, Bounova G, Iorio F, Pronk A, et al. Prospective derivation of a living organoid biobank of colorectal cancer patients. Cell. 2015;161:933–45.

99. Sherr CJ, Beach D, Shapiro GI. Targeting CDK4 and CDK6: from discovery to therapy. Cancer Discov. 2016;6:353–67.

100. Verissimo CS, Overmeer RM, Ponsioen B, Drost J, Mertens S, Verlaan-Klink I, et al. Targeting mutant RAS in patient-derived colorectal cancer organoids by combinatorial drug screening. elife. 2016;5. https://doi.org/10.7554/eLife.18489.

101. Onozato D, Yamashita M, Nakanishi A, Akagawa T, Kida Y, Ogawa I, et al. Generation of intestinal organoids suitable for pharmacokinetic studies from human induced pluripotent stem cells. Drug Metab Dispos. 2018. https://doi.org/10.1124/dmd.118.080374.

102. Kostadinova R, Boess F, Applegate D, Suter L, Weiser T, Singer T, et al. A long-term three dimensional liver co-culture system for improved prediction of clinically relevant drug-induced hepatotoxicity. Toxicol Appl Pharmacol. 2013;268:1–16.

103. Meng Q. Three-dimensional culture of hepatocytes for prediction of drug-induced hepatotoxicity. Expert Opin Drug Metab Toxicol. 2010;6:733–46.

104. Katsuda T, Kawamata M, Hagiwara K, Takahashi RU, Yamamoto Y, Camargo FD, et al. Conversion of terminally committed hepatocytes to culturable bipotent progenitor cells with regenerative capacity. Cell Stem Cell. 2017;20: 41–55.

105. Huch M, Gehart H, van Boxtel R, Hamer K, Blokzijl F, Verstegen MM, et al. Long-term culture of genome-stable bipotent stem cells from adult human liver. Cell. 2015;160:299–312.

106. Voges HK, Mills RJ, Elliott DA, Parton RG, Porrello ER, Hudson JE. Development of a human cardiac organoid injury model reveals innate regenerative potential. Development. 2017;144:1118–27.

107. Takasato M, Er PX, Chiu HS, Maier B, Baillie GJ, Ferguson C, et al. Kidney organoids from human iPS cells contain multiple lineages and model human nephrogenesis. Nature. 2015;526:564–8.

108. Sato T, Clevers H. SnapShot: growing organoids from stem cells. Cell. 2015; 161:1700-.e1.

109. Rizvi NA, Hellmann MD, Snyder A, Kvistborg P, Makarov V, Havel JJ, et al. Cancer immunology. Mutational landscape determines sensitivity to PD-1 blockade in non-small cell lung cancer. Science. 2015;348:124–8.

110. Asaoka Y, Ijichi H, Koike K. PD-1 blockade in tumors with mismatch-repair deficiency. N Engl J Med. 2015;373:1979.

111. Nozaki K, Mochizuki W, Matsumoto Y, Matsumoto T, Fukuda M, Mizutani T, et al. Co-culture with intestinal epithelial organoids allows efficient expansion and motility analysis of intraepithelial lymphocytes. J Gastroenterol. 2016;51:206–13.

112. Finnberg NK, Gokare P, Lev A, Grivennikov SI, AWt MF, Campbell KS, et al. Application of 3D tumoroid systems to define immune and cytotoxic therapeutic responses based on tumoroid and tissue slice culture molecular signatures. Oncotarget. 2017;8:66747–57.

113. Zumwalde NA, Haag JD, Sharma D, Mirrielees JA, Wilke LG, Gould MN, et al. Analysis of immune cells from human mammary ductal epithelial organoids reveals Vdelta2+ T cells that efficiently target breast carcinoma cells in the presence of bisphosphonate. Cancer Prev Res (Phila). 2016;9:305–16.

114. Tiriac H, Bucobo JC, Tzimas D, Grewel S, Lacomb JF, Rowehl LM, et al. Successful creation of pancreatic cancer organoids by means of EUS-guided fine-needle biopsy sampling for personalized cancer treatment. Gastrointest Endosc. 2018;87:1474–80.

115. Organoids May Point to Best Therapy. Cancer Discov. 2018;8:524.

116. Usui T, Sakurai M, Umata K, Elbadawy M, Ohama T, Yamawaki H, et al. Hedgehog signals mediate anti-cancer drug resistance in three-dimensional

primary colorectal cancer organoid culture. Int J Mol Sci. 2018;19(4). https://doi.org/10.3390/ijms19041098.

117. Carneiro BA, Pamarthy S, Shah AN, Sagar V, Unno K, Han H, et al. Anaplastic lymphoma kinase mutation (ALK F1174C) in small cell carcinoma of the prostate and molecular response to alectinib. Clin Cancer Res. 2018;24:2732–9.

118. Broekgaarden M, Rizvi I, Bulin AL, Petrovic L, Goldschmidt R, Massodi I, et al. Neoadjuvant photodynamic therapy augments immediate and prolonged oxaliplatin efficacy in metastatic pancreatic cancer organoids. Oncotarget. 2018;9:13009–22.

119. Workman MJ, Mahe MM, Trisno S, Poling HM, Watson CL, Sundaram N, et al. Engineered human pluripotent-stem-cell-derived intestinal tissues with a functional enteric nervous system. Nat Med. 2017;23:49–59.

120. Ohlund D, Handly-Santana A, Biffi G, Elyada E, Almeida AS, Ponz-Sarvise M, et al. Distinct populations of inflammatory fibroblasts and myofibroblasts in pancreatic cancer. J Exp Med. 2017;214:579–96.

8

Simple deep sequencing-based post-remission MRD surveillance predicts clinical relapse in B-ALL

Shuhua Cheng[1], Giorgio Inghirami[1], Shuo Cheng[2] and Wayne Tam[1*]

Abstract

Background: Next-generation sequencing (NGS) of the rearranged immunoglobulin heavy-chain gene has emerged as a highly sensitive method to detect minimal residual disease (MRD) in B acute lymphoblastic leukemia/lymphoma (B-ALL). However, a sensitive and easily implemented NGS methodology for routine clinical laboratories is lacking and clinical utility of NGS-MRD surveillance in a post-remission setting to predict clinical relapse has not been determined.

Methods: Here we described a simple and quantitative NGS platform and assessed its performance characteristics, quantified NGS-MRD levels in 122 B-ALL samples from 30 B-ALL patients, and explored the clinical merit of NGS-based MRD surveillance.

Results: The current NGS platform has an analytic sensitivity of 0.0001% with excellent specificity and reproducibility. Overall, it performs better than routine multi-color flow cytometry (MCF) in detecting MRD. Utilizing this assay in MRD surveillance in a post-remission setting showed that it detected conversion to positive MRD (CPMRD) in patients with NGS-based molecular remission much earlier than MCF, and that positive MRD conversion could be detected as early as 25.6 weeks prior to clinical relapse in closely surveilled patients. Post-remission CPMRD, but not NGS-based MRD positivity at end of induction, can accurately predict clinical relapse in our limited cohort of B-ALL patients.

Conclusions: This pilot proof-of-concept study illustrates the clinical utility of a simple, sensitive, and clinically feasible MRD detection platform in post-remission NGS-based MRD surveillance and early relapse detection in B-ALL patients.

Keywords: NGS, MRD surveillance, B lymphoblastic leukemia/lymphoma, Relapse, Post-remission setting

Background

Minimal residual disease has emerged to be an important biomarker for risk stratification and individual risk-directed treatment decision in B acute lymphoblastic leukemia/lymphoma (B-ALL). Studies with large cohort of pediatric B-ALL patients demonstrated that minimal residual disease (MRD) status is a powerful predictor for relapse and clinical outcome [1–4]. In adults with relapsed/refractory B-ALL, MRD negativity after salvage therapy is associated with significantly longer overall survival (OS) [5]. Protocols of high-risk patients designed based on MRD readouts led to a fivefold increase of 5-year event-free survival (EFS) rate

without recurrence. Two conventional approaches for detection of MRD in B-ALL have been multi-parameter flow cytometry (MFC) and qPCR, each of which has distinct limitations [6]. MFC is a relatively simple procedure with short turnaround time, and it is currently the most frequently applied modality to quantify MRD in clinical laboratories across the USA. However, technical constraints, for example, sample availability, low tumor burden, immunophenotypic shifts, and clonal selection, can decrease its sensitivity leading to false negative results, as suggested by the higher than expected rate of relapses in negative MFC-MRD [3, 7]. The second conventional method is the allele-specific oligonucleotide PCR (ASO-PCR). This methodology requires the design of customized patient-specific primers in the VDJ junctions of the *IGH* gene and individual optimization of testing conditions to monitor MRD; thus, the procedure is laborious and time-consuming, and

* Correspondence: wtam@med.cornell.edu
[1]Department of Pathology and Laboratory Medicine, Weill Cornell Medicine, New York, NY 10021, USA

not routinely available in the USA. Importantly, some adult patients with flow or qPCR-based MRD negativity at the end of induction or after consolidation treatment relapse clinically and a fraction of the patients with flow or qPCR-based MRD positivity remained in complete remission (CR) without hematologic recurrence [8, 9]. A more reliable, sensitive, and dynamic MRD detection methodology is needed.

Recently, several studies have explored next-generation sequencing (NGS)-based deep sequencing assays for the determination of MRD in B-ALL patients [10–17]. Similar to ASO-PCR, this method utilizes the unique sequences within the VDJ junctions in B-lymphocytes as unique/clonal markers to identify and track MRD [18–20]. However, unlike ASO-PCR, the NGS-based VDJ deep sequencing method interrogates leukemic-specific (*IGH*) VDJ gene rearrangement without a need of customized PCR primers and conditions. Pioneering studies demonstrated excellent sensitivity and reliability of the NGS-MRD detection method [10–17]. Prognostic significance and predictive power of NGS-MRD status during induction therapy or at the end of induction or in bone marrow transplantation setting have been confirmed in B-ALL, particularly for pediatric patients [11, 13, 14, 21]. Besides MRD monitoring after induction, MRD monitoring in a post-remission setting may become increasingly relevant. This is evidenced by recent findings which showed a correlation between favorable clinical outcome and low disease burden in relapsed B-ALL patients treated with pre-emptive therapy like CAR T immunotherapy [22], which imply that early relapse detection might be beneficial. The clinical relevance and utility of NGS-based MRD surveillance in a post-remission setting has not been previously determined. Though the NGS-based MRD test described in recent studies is commercially available, its accessibility is limited to sample send-out to a central laboratory. The methodology is proprietary, not easily replicable, and cannot be easily adopted in routine clinical molecular pathology laboratories. Thus the development of a highly sensitive, reproducible, quantitative assay that can be readily implemented and adopted for routine MRD surveillance seems warranted.

Here we describe a simple, ultrasensitive, and easily applicable NGS assay with excellent performance. We also explore the clinical utility and merit of this assay in post-remission MRD surveillance to generate biomarkers for early relapse detection.

Methods
Sample preparation
A total of 128 cryopreserved clinical samples from 32 B-ALL patients (32 initial diagnostic, relapse, and additional 96 post-treatment specimens) were initially retrieved from the biobank of the Department of Pathology and Laboratory Medicine at Weill Cornell Medicine and evaluated by this study. Clinical Information was obtained from electronic clinical records. This study was conducted in accordance with the Declaration of Helsinki regulations of the protocols approved by the Institutional Review Board of Weill Cornell Medicine, New York, USA. Written consent for use of the samples for research was obtained from patients or their guardians.

DNA extraction and concentration
Genomic DNA was extracted from bone marrow and PBMC cell pellets following manufacturer's instructions (QIAamp DNA Mini Kit, Qiagen, Germantown). If necessary, DNA samples were concentrated using a Genomic DNA Clean & Concentrator-10 column (D4010, Zymo Research, Irvine). DNA samples and sequencing libraries were quantitated by Tape Station (Agilent Technologies, Santa Clara) and Qubit (Thermo Fisher Scientific, Singapore).

MRD detection by conventional flow cytometry
MRD by MFC was assessed using the Euroflow 8-color panel on bone marrow specimens obtained at clinical remission and at approximately 1–6-month intervals. For each of the specimens tested, between 400,000 and 1 million events (excluding debris) were initially acquired. Doublet exclusion was performed by plotting the height against the area for forward scatter and single cells (singlets) were accordingly gated for further analysis.

MRD detection with LymphoTrack-Miseq platform
Deep sequencing by LymphoTrack® IGHV Leader Somatic Hypermutation Assay-MiSeq/IGH FR1/2/3 Panel-MiSeq (71,210,069/71210139, Invivoscribe) (LIGV-Miseq) was performed following the manufacturer's instructions with modifications to improve the MRD quantification. The overall methodology of the assay is summarized in Additional file 1. Briefly, a set of primers targeting the Leader (VHL) or FR1/3 and J_H gene regions of *IGH* were contained in a single multiplex master mix in which the designed primers included unique Illumina adaptor index. For diagnostic samples, 0.02–0.5 µg of genomic DNA was used in a 29–31 µl one-step PCR reaction (25 µl Master mix+4 µl genomic DNA, or 25 µl Master mix+4 µl genomic DNA + 1–2 µl MRD control spike-in). For any given follow-up samples, all available amounts of DNA with a range of 0.5 to 5 µg of genomic DNA were used in a 45–47 µl one-step PCR reaction (39 µl Master mix+6 µl genomic DNA, or 39 µl Master mix+6 µl genomic DNA + 2 µl MRD control spike-in). MRD control spike-in contained the equivalent amount of DNA from 50 to 500 B-lymphoid cells with monoclonal *IGH* rearrangement. After PCR reaction, amplified VDJ amplicons were mixed with 1 volume of Agencourt AMPure XP beads (Beckman Coulter) for 5 min at room

temperature. Mixed samples were placed on a DynaMag 96-well plate (5 min) and then washed with 200 µl of 80% ethanol twice, following by elution with 20 µl of 10 mM Tris buffer (pH 8.0). The eluted libraries then were mixed with 18 µl of AMPure XP beads again, and the binding and washing procedures were repeated. The second elution was conducted with 15 µl of 10 mM Tris buffer. Quality and quantity of purified VDJ sequencing libraries were assessed with Tape station system (Agilent Technologies) and Qubit (Thermo Fisher Scientific). Pooled libraries (10~15 pM) were loaded into Reagent Cartridge (MiSeq Reagent Kits v3, Illumina) and sequenced (600 cycles) using a Miseq unit (Illumina). Libraries generated from the diagnostic samples are sequenced separately in different runs from those generated from post-treatment samples to avoid bioinformatics contamination due to read mis-assignment.

Sequencing data analysis

Fastq files were initially analyzed with the LymphoTrack-Miseq software from Invivoscribe following the manufacturer's guideline. This analysis identifies VDJ sequences from diagnostic samples and creates an output that includes all unique VDJ sequences and their corresponding abundance. The dominant B-ALL tumor clone, as well as any minor subclones that generated 5% or more of total reads, was identified from these sequences. We developed a custom algorithm that used leukemia-specific VDJ junction sequences, defined as the complementarity-determining region 3 (CDR3) of the dominant B-cell tumor clone and subclones (if present) to identify MRD in post-treatment samples with ultra-high sensitivity. The algorithm does not tolerate any mismatch in the junction sequences for MRD detection. Although theoretically the entire VDJ sequence can also be used for MRD tracking, we found that the use of VDJ junction sequence had superior sensitivity. If more than one clone is identified in a diagnostic sample, the same algorithm run will be repeated for each of the independent leukemia-specific VDJ junctions in any follow-up samples. Matched reads of more than two were considered positive. Tumor load was calculated based on one of the two methods: (1) MRD% = (number of leukemia cell-specific VDJ reads/total numbers of VDJ read mapped in a sample) × (corresponding fraction of B cells defined as CD19 + % in the total mononuclear cell population as determined by flow cytometry) × 100; (2) MRD% = (number of leukemia cell-specific VDJ reads/number of VDJ reads generated from MRD control spike-in) × (number of cells corresponding to MRD control spike-in input (50–500))/ total number of cells tested in a given sample × 100. The current assay along with the LymphoTrack-Miseq software might not completely exclude potential multiplex PCR amplification bias (i.e., over- or under-representation of certain VDJ recombination) due to unknown and proprietary primer sequences and analysis strategy Invivoscribe applied.

Definition and assessment of negative and positive MRD conversion status

To investigate the clinical predictive value of post remission MRD surveillance in B-ALL patients, MRD trends during the post remission period was divided into two categories: conversion to positive MRD (CPMRD), and negative for MRD conversion (NMRDC). CPMRD was defined when the NGS-MRD became detectable any time post-treatment after initially achieving negative MRD by NGS, and NMRDC was defined when patient's NGS-MRD levels reached undetectable levels and remained as such in the post-treatment period up to Jan. 20, 2018. Categorization to NMRDC or CPMRD was only possible when two or more sequential clinical follow-up samples for each of the B-ALL patients were available.

Statistical methods

Linear regression and Pearson correlation were used to analyze the sensitivity of the NGS test and to compare tumor burden measurements obtained by multi-color flow cytometry (MCF) and NGS. Relapse-free survival comparison between patient groups (CPMRD vs NMRDC) was performed using Kaplan-Meier curves (log-rank test, significance defined as $p < 0.05$). Significant differences between categorical variables, clinical specificity, clinical sensitivity, positive predictive value (PPV), and negative predictive value (NPV) were calculated with contingency 2×2 table. Survival graphs and linear plots were generated using GraphPad/Prism 5 software.

Results

Performance characteristic of LIGV-Miseq MRD detection method

To assess the sensitivity of our NGS-MRD assay and to define an optimal amount of input DNA, serially diluted clinical samples containing a broad range of leukemic cells from 0.1 to 0.00005% were subjected to sequencing library preparation with different amounts of DNA input (0.5 µg, 2.5 µg, and 5µg) and MRD level quantification in duplicate or triplicate. As shown in Fig. 1a, the sensitivity of the assay was enhanced with increased DNA input. Specifically, inputs of 0.5 µg, 2.5 µg, and 5 µg resulted in analytical sensitivities of ~ 0.004%, ~ 0.001%, and ~ 0.0001%, respectively, corresponding to the capability of the assay to detect 50, 10, and 1 leukemic cells among 1 million normal leukocytes. Therefore, ~ 5 µg DNA is recommended as the input amount for routine clinical testing to maximize sensitivity if enough DNA material is available. With this DNA input, the assay

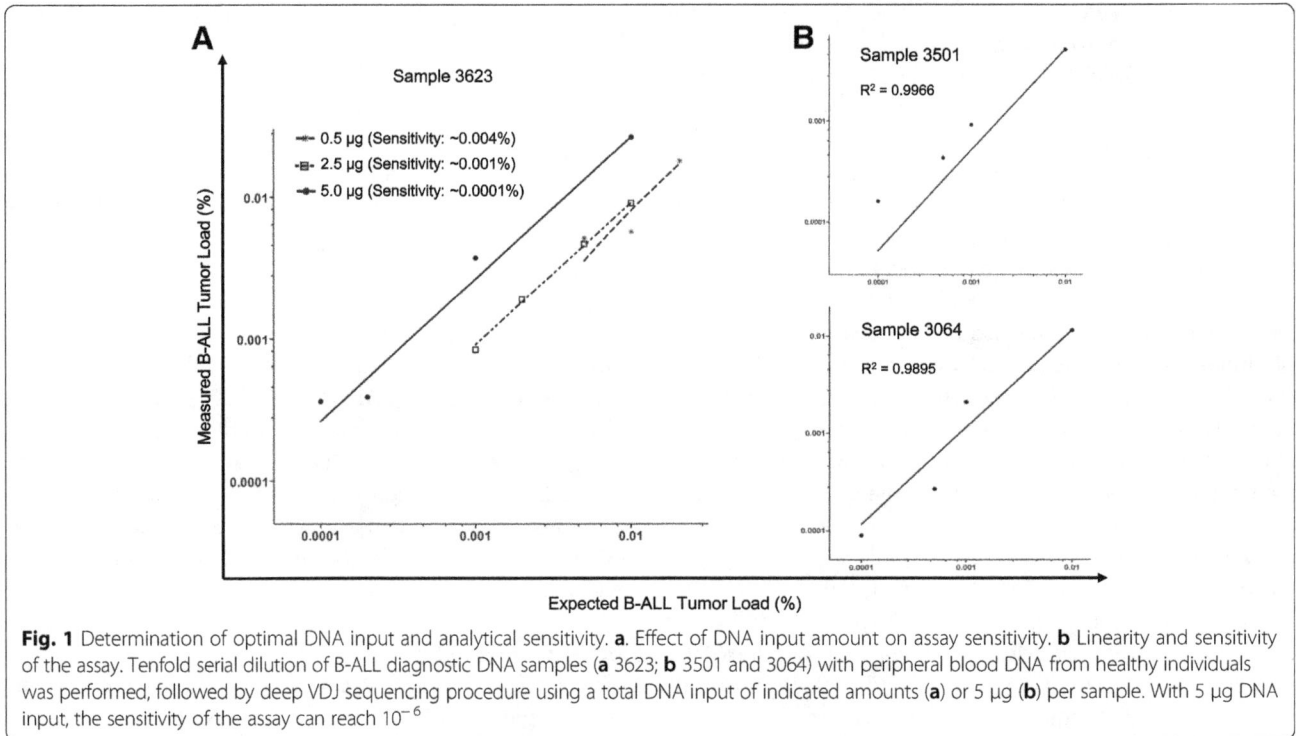

Fig. 1 Determination of optimal DNA input and analytical sensitivity. **a.** Effect of DNA input amount on assay sensitivity. **b** Linearity and sensitivity of the assay. Tenfold serial dilution of B-ALL diagnostic DNA samples (**a** 3623; **b** 3501 and 3064) with peripheral blood DNA from healthy individuals was performed, followed by deep VDJ sequencing procedure using a total DNA input of indicated amounts (**a**) or 5 μg (**b**) per sample. With 5 μg DNA input, the sensitivity of the assay can reach 10^{-6}

reproducibly detected in all three samples the leukemic clone-specific *IGH* rearrangements with a sensitivity of 2×10^{-6}, and in at least one of the replica at the 1×10^{-6} dilution (Fig. 1b and Additional file 2). Overall, the dilution test showed an excellent linearity and high correlation between expected and observed clonal frequencies ($r^2 > 0.98$), as well as superior sensitivity ($\sim 0.0001\%$) in the presence of adequate DNA input.

To investigate the intra-run reproducibility of the assay, the same B-ALL samples diluted to 2×10^{-6}, which is near the limit of detection of the assay, and MRD levels were measured in triplicate in a single run. Our results showed that the intra-run variation was relatively small (Fig. 2 and Additional file 3). Specifically, for samples 3623, 3501, and 3064, the mean ± SD of the MRD levels were $0.00116\% \pm 0.000689\%$, $0.00032 \pm 0.00020\%$, and $0.00048 \pm 0.000289\%$, respectively. All the MRD values measured were within 2SD from mean with a median coverage of 432,556×. To evaluate the inter-run reproducibility, a B-ALL sample (3623) with a MRD level of $\sim 0.001\%$ was repeatedly measured in five independent runs on five separate days. The mean value for the five separate runs is $0.00088\% \pm 0.000275\%$ (mean ± SD) with a median coverage of 129,000× (Fig. 2 and Additional file 4). These data support a high precision of the assay in both intra-run and inter-run settings.

The diagnostic accuracy of the assay was evaluated by performing comparative studies between the NGS and conventional eight-color MCF assays. For this purpose,

a total number of 128 B-ALL samples from 32 B-ALL patients, including diagnostic (Dx, $n = 22$), 10 relapse, and 96 post-treatment follow-up specimens, were selected. Among these 128 samples, 6 samples from 2 patients were excluded because clonal *IGH* sequences could not be identified for their diagnostic samples. The remaining 122 specimens (Dx, 20, follow-up, 92, relapse, 10) from 30 patients (93.8% of the patients tested, see Additional file 5 for patient characteristics) were analyzed by both eight-color MFC and NGS for tumor content (%). Two independent methods were available to calculate MRD levels (flow cytometry vs spike-in) depending on whether the flow cytometry data for B cell fraction in a given sample was available. A comparison study with 20 B-ALL samples from 7 patients showed that these two calculation methods produced comparable results with excellent correlation and linearity ($r = 0.99$, $p < 0.0001$) (Additional file 6).Overall, there was excellent concordance between the NGS and MFC assays for tumor burden levels (Fig. 3a and Additional file 7). Of the 122 evaluable samples from 30 patients with a median coverage of 395,542 reads per sample, 98 (80.3%), consisting of 45 (36.9%) positive and 53 (43.4%) negative samples, were qualitatively (positive vs negative) and quantitatively concordant. Correlation of the measured tumor burdens between the two methods in the entire cohort as well as in the concordant cases was very high ($p < 0.0001$, $r = 0.971$ and 0.973, respectively) (Fig. 3a, b). This rate of concordance is consistent with previously reported results [17, 23].

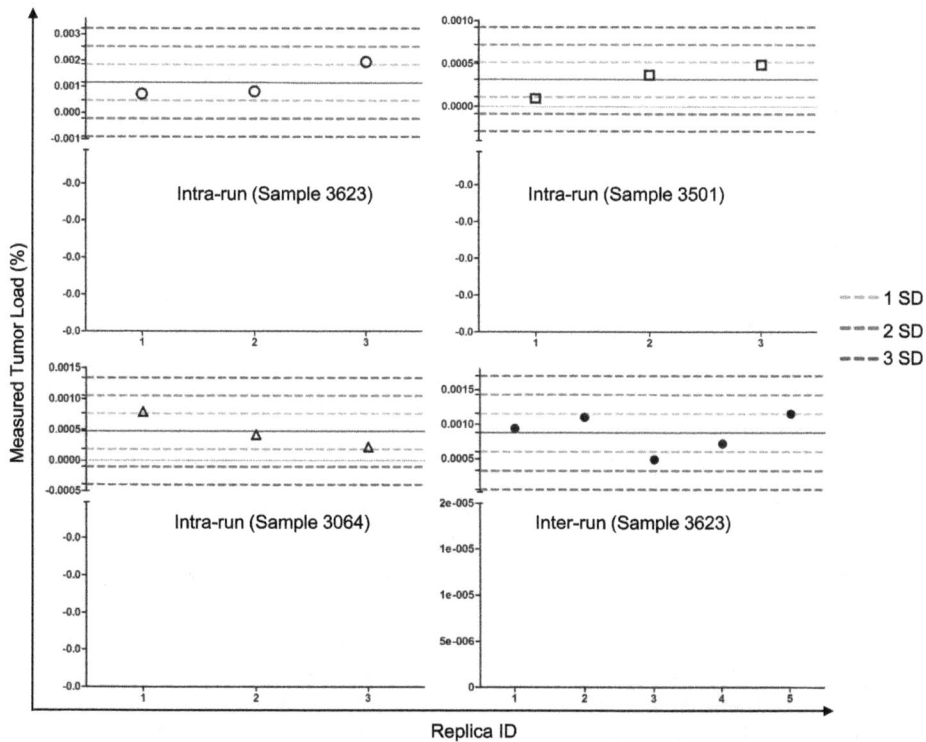

Fig. 2 Assessment of intra-run and inter-run reproducibility. Three samples (3623, 3064, and 3501) were run in triplicates to measure intra-run reproducibility. Sample 3623 was assayed in five separate runs to measure inter-run reproducibility. SD, standard deviation. All values obtained are within 2 SD of the mean

Discordant results were observed in the remaining 25 follow-up samples. Among those specimens, 22 (18.03%) were MRD negative by MFC but positive by the NGS test, at very low levels ranging from 0.000174 to 0.30% with a median of 0.02242% (Fig. 3c and Additional file 7, the samples marked as red). MFC+/NGS- discordance was observed in the other three samples (Additional file 7, the samples marked as blue). This difference possibly represents false positivity by MFC, supported by the

observation that these "MRD positive" cases have not been associated with any clinical relapses to date (Fig. 4).

The specificity of the assay was assessed by performing the MRD testing in patient-specific follow-up vs unrelated B-ALL samples. For this purpose, four patients who had both an identifiable leukemic-specific *IGH* clonotype as well as one diagnostic plus three follow-up samples available including relapsed specimens, were selected (Additional file 8). Besides four samples for each individual patient, additional

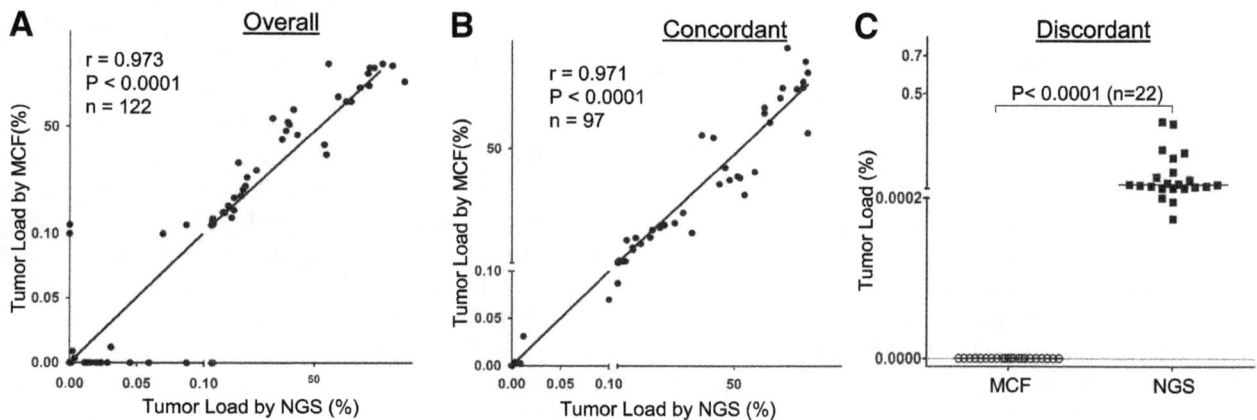

Fig. 3 Comparison of tumor load determined by the NGS and MCF assays. Correlation between NGS and MCF-based measurement of tumor load is illustrated for all samples (**a**), the concordant samples (**b**), and the MCF-negative/NGS-positive discordant samples (**c**). r, correlation coefficient, n, number of samples, p, *p* value

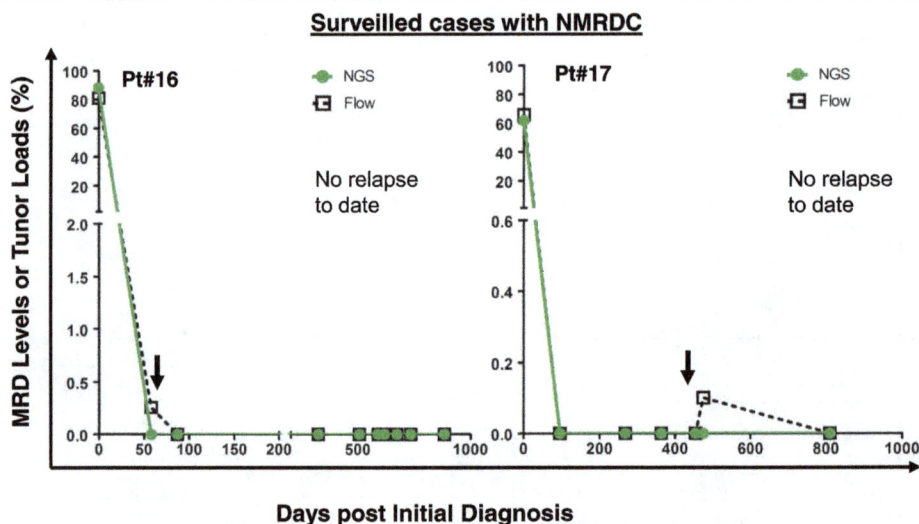

Fig. 4 Representative surveilled B-ALL cases negative for MRD conversion (NMRDC). Dynamic changes in tumor load were measured by both the LIGV assay and MCF. Arrows indicate discordant MRD values where there was detectable MRD by MCF but negative NGS-MRD

15 unrelated B-ALL and 5 normal PBMC control samples were assayed for the patient-specific tumor burdens. As shown in Additional file 8, while the leukemia-specific *IGH* clonotypes were detectable in diagnostic and/or other follow-up samples for each individual patient, no such clones were detected in all the unrelated B-ALL and normal PBMC samples (Additional file 8), demonstrating 100% specificity for the NGS assay as well as absence of experimental or bioinformatics contamination.

Post remission MRD surveillance by NGS but not MCF can detect early conversion to positive MRD (CPMRD) before clinical relapse

We hypothesized that this NGS test, with its superior sensitivity as compared to the MCF, can detect conversion to positive MRD (CPMRD) from undetectable MRD with MRD surveillance at a much earlier stage of relapse. To test this hypothesis and also to determine whether CPMRD may be useful to predict eventual relapse, 10 patients were selected for this comparison study according to the following four criteria: (1) positive identification of leukemia-specific clonotypes; (2) achievement of complete molecular remission defined as undetectable MRD by NGS before relapse; (3) availability of sufficient amount (minimum 500 ng) of DNA from post CR, pre-relapse specimens; and (4) symptomatic clinical relapse after achieving CR as described above. All patients were initially treated by conventional chemotherapy, with patients #4, #5, and #14 further undergoing stem cell transplantation. These patients were classified into two groups, surveilled (*n* = 5) and non-surveilled (*n* = 5), according to whether any post-treatment bone marrow specimens for ILGV assay are available within 6–7 months prior to clinical relapse

(Fig. 5). The leukemic contents at different time points are shown in Fig. 6.

All surveilled patients achieved MRD negativity based on MCF and NGS post-chemotherapy. In patient #4, at day 186 post-initial diagnosis (day 37 post-matched unrelated donor (MUD) stem cell transplantation), the patient achieved molecular MRD response (Figs. 5 and 6a). The tumor burden then started to increase slowly, with the MRD levels increasing two folds (0.0113% vs 0.0238%) during the 4-month interval (day 334 to day 446). Then the tumor appeared to grow more rapidly, with a 3336.5-fold increase in tumor content in a span of 80 days (Fig. 6a). In patient #5, CPMRD was detected by NGS at day 358. From days 358 to 408, patient #5's tumor burden increased 304 folds from 0.000195 to 0.0593%, with an average daily increase of 6.1 folds, followed by clinical relapse on day 413 (Fig. 6b). In patients #6–8, CPMRDs were also captured early by NGS. Patients #6, #7, and #8 achieved molecular remission on days 36, 171, and 160 post initial diagnosis and were converted to NGS-MRD positivity on days 212, 338, and 333 post initial diagnosis, respectively (Figs. 5 and 6c–e), each having 324-, 1063.8-, and 6.2-fold increase in leukemic burden before hematologic relapse. All patients with CPMRD eventually relapsed, and the median interval between CPMRD to clinical relapse in the surveilled cases is 4.7 months (1 to 6.4 months, Fig. 5). In all these patients, the emergence of relapsed tumor clones were detected earlier by NGS compared to MCF. In fact, MCF provided false negative results in all measurable time points before clinical relapse.

On the other hand, among the non-surveilled cases (patients # 10–14), all the patients had relapses despite the lack of demonstrable CPMRD. In this group of

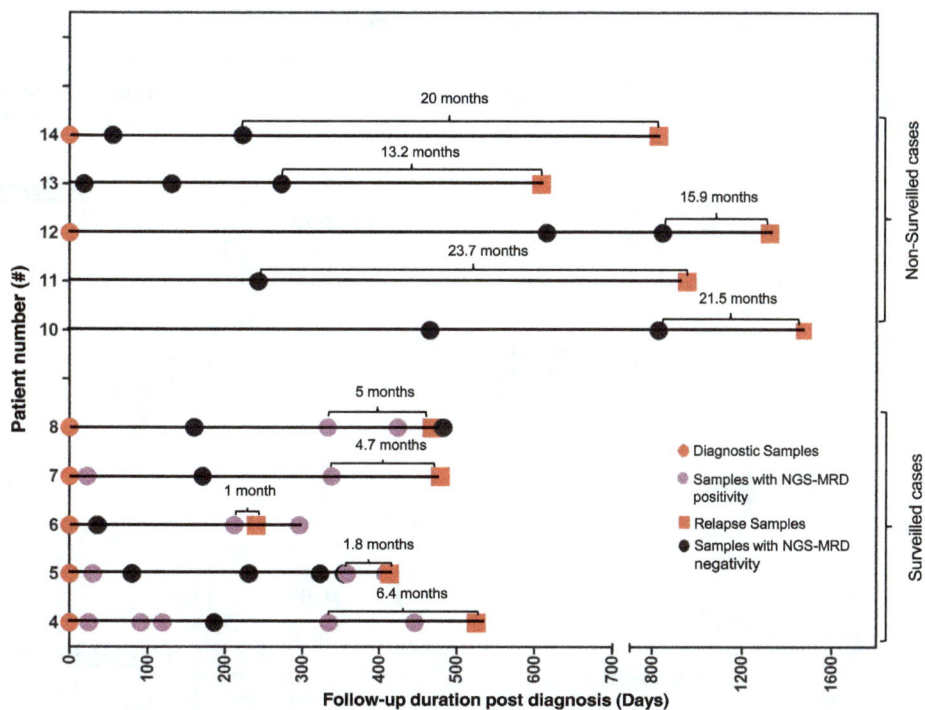

Fig. 5 Chronology of specimen collections in the surveilled and non-surveilled relapsed B-ALL cases. Each horizontal line represents one patient with B-ALL relapse. The mean time interval between the most recent follow-up sample and overt relapse (marked) in the non-surveilled cases is significantly longer compared to that between conversion to positive MRD (CPMRD) and overt relapse (marked) in surveilled cases (20 months vs 4.7 months, $p < 0.0001$). See Fig. 6 for treatment information

patients, CPMRD most likely has escaped detection in these patients because of the lack of sampling in the immediate months before clinical relapse. In line with this explanation, the median interval between the most recent post-treatment sample and clinical relapse in this group of patients was 20 months (13.2 to 23.7 months, Fig. 5), which was significantly longer compared to the interval between the detection of CPMRD and overt relapse in the surveilled patients (20 months vs 4.7 months, $p = 0.0001$) (Fig. 5). These findings suggest the utility of more frequent MRD surveillance based on *IGH* deep sequencing in a post-remission clinical setting for the detection of early relapse.

In addition to the surveilled cases with CPMRD, there are also some cases without CPMRD during the observation period ($n = 10$). For example, as shown in Fig. 4, patients #16 and #17 became MRD negative by both methods at day 87 and 96 post initial diagnosis and have remained MRD negative since then to date (days 885 and 810 post initial diagnosis, respectively). Their median intervals for serial bone marrow sampling were 2 and 3.1 months, respectively. All patients have not had any recurring disease to date.

Our findings support an association between CPMRD detection and eventual clinical relapse. Overall, these data demonstrated that post-remission MRD surveillance with

NGS is superior to conventional MFC and offers a highly sensitive method to capture positive MRD conversion at earlier time points. This approach potentially expands the time window for preemptive therapies.

Superior predictive power of post-remission CPMRD detected by NGS-based MRD surveillance for clinical relapse

As stated earlier, previous large studies have unambiguously demonstrated predictive power of MRD levels at the end of induction (day 29 or week 5–16) for B-ALL relapse, primarily based on qPCR or flow cytometry [2, 3, 6, 24–27]. However, using those methods, some of B-ALL patients with positive MRD at the end of induction were found to have no relapse, and 30–40% of adult B-ALL with negative MRD at the end of induction or after achieving CR clinically relapsed [8, 9, 28]. Along the same line, we would like to determine if detection of MRD by NGS at the end of induction has similar prognostic significance in our cohort. To test this, 16 evaluable B-ALL patients were classified into two groups, NGS-MRD negative ($n = 7$) and positive ($n = 9$), according to whether the patients achieved NGS-based MRD negativity at the end of induction (within initial 3–4 months of treatment). Analysis of relapse-free survival by Kaplan–Meier

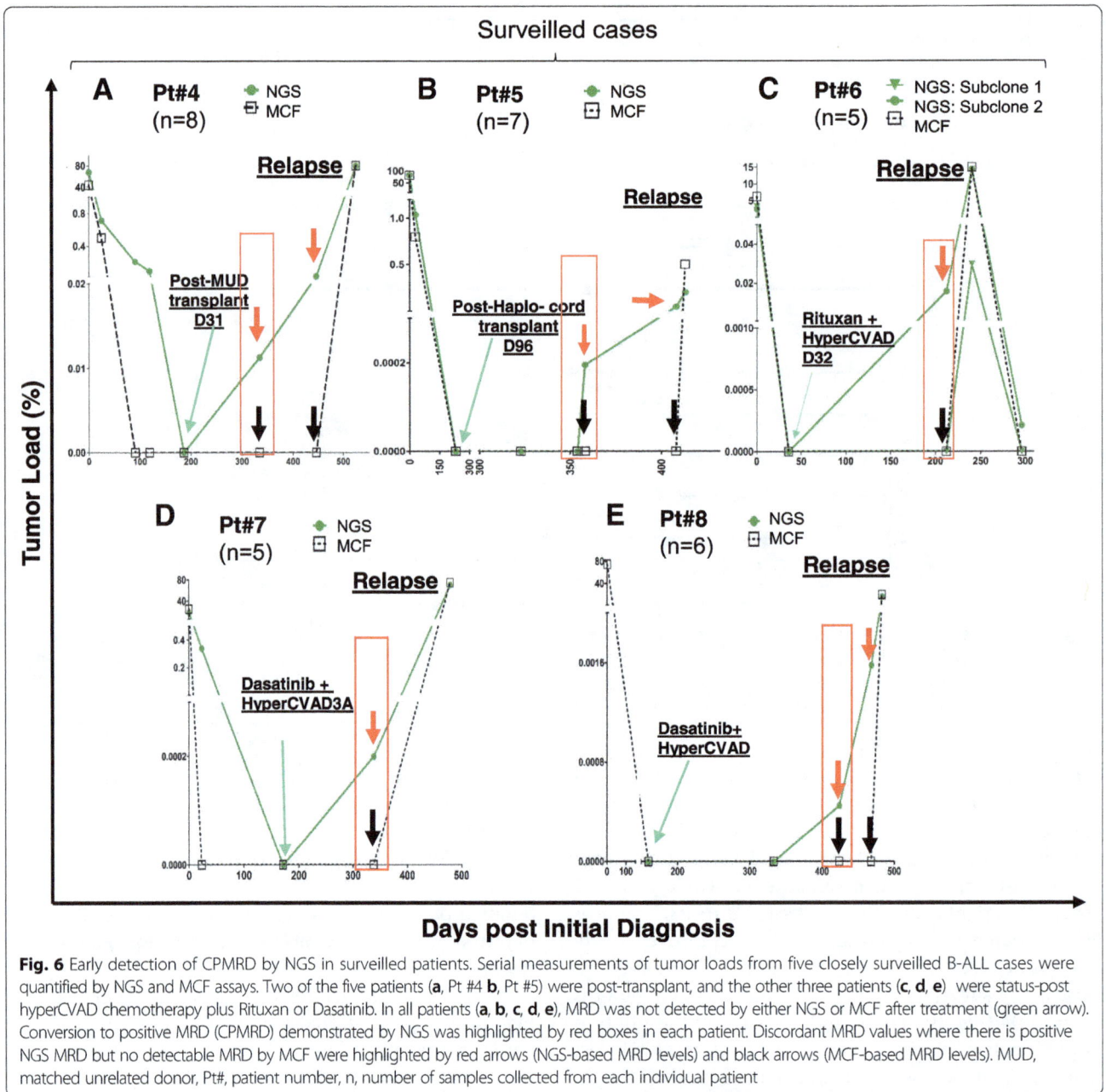

Fig. 6 Early detection of CPMRD by NGS in surveilled patients. Serial measurements of tumor loads from five closely surveilled B-ALL cases were quantified by NGS and MCF assays. Two of the five patients (**a**, Pt #4 **b**, Pt #5) were post-transplant, and the other three patients (**c**, **d**, **e**) were status-post hyperCVAD chemotherapy plus Rituxan or Dasatinib. In all patients (**a**, **b**, **c**, **d**, **e**), MRD was not detected by either NGS or MCF after treatment (green arrow). Conversion to positive MRD (CPMRD) demonstrated by NGS was highlighted by red boxes in each patient. Discordant MRD values where there is positive NGS MRD but no detectable MRD by MCF were highlighted by red arrows (NGS-based MRD levels) and black arrows (MCF-based MRD levels). MUD, matched unrelated donor, Pt#, patient number, n, number of samples collected from each individual patient

method showed that the patients with NGS-MRD positivity had a relatively but not statistically significant shorter time to relapse than the patients who achieved NGS-MRD negativity post-induction ($p = 0.224$ by the log-rank test, Fig. 7a). The relative risk of relapse in patients with NGS-MRD positivity was 2.84 times higher than in those with NGS-MRD negativity (95% CI, 0.4886 to 16.55). However, this difference was not significant ($p = 0.224$). It is conceivable that these results may be confounded by the small cohort size, but it is apparent from this limited study that about half of the patients with positive MRD by NGS did not relapse within the observation period.

We next investigated if CPMRD identified by NGS-based post-remission MRD surveillance could serve as a better marker to accurately predict clinical relapse. Eligible patients were classified into NMRDC or CPMRD groups according to the results of NGS-based serial MRD quantitative surveillance, and time to clinical relapse was calculated. NMRDC and CPMRD groups included 10 and 5 patients, respectively, and the time to clinical relapse (days) was defined as the duration from the day of diagnosis to the day of relapse or to the last available date if relapse has not occurred to Jan. 20, 2018. Kaplan-Meier analysis of relapse-free survival showed that the patients with CPMRD after CR1 had a significantly shorter time to relapse than

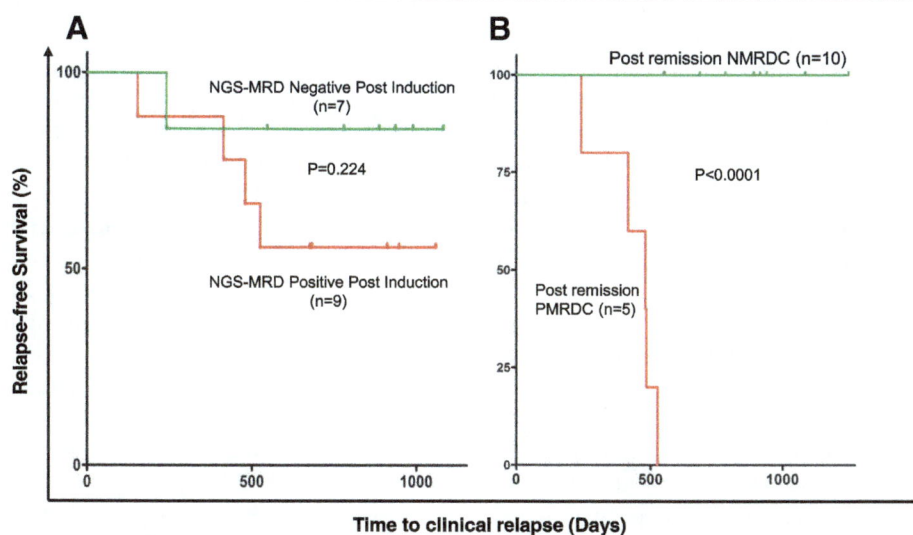

Fig. 7 Prediction of clinical relapse based on NGS-detected MRD status post-induction and post-remission CPMRD. **a** Kaplan-Meier relapse-free survival curves for patients with negative or positive NGS-MRD post induction (between days 30 and 90). **b** Kaplan-Meier relapse-free survival curves for patients with post remission conversion to positive MRD (CPMRD) or without conversion (NMRDC)

the patients with NMRDC (median time from diagnosis to relapse: 479 days vs not reached, $p < 0.0001$ by the log-rank test, Fig. 7b). CPMRD was associated with an impending clinical relapse in the near future (hazard ratio, 111.2, 95% confidence interval: 12.92 to 996.5) regardless of modality of treatment (chemotherapy or bone marrow transplantation), and none of the patients without CPMRD relapsed. CPMRD in our limited patient cohort had a clinical sensitivity of 100% and a clinical specificity of 100% with a positive predictive value (PPV) of 1 and a negative predictive value (NPV) of 1 for clinical relapse ($p = 0.0006$). These results suggest that CPMRD in post-remission MRD surveillance setting may serve as a reliable marker for clinical relapse prediction.

Discussion

We have evaluated and validated a simple and sensitive NGS-based MRD detection method for patients with B-ALL, which has an excellent potential to be adopted in clinical settings. Compared to the current NGS platform for B-ALL MRD qualification, which is proprietary and requires specimen send-out to a central commercial laboratory, the LIGV-Miseq method is simpler and can be easily implemented in a routine clinical molecular laboratory. We described a pilot proof-of-concept study to document its clinical utility in routine MRD surveillance and early detection of CPMRD in post-chemotherapy and post bone marrow transplantation settings. Detection of CPMRD reliably predicts impending clinical relapse, potentially expanding the time window for more effective preemptive therapies against impending relapsed B-ALL.

Several groups have explored the potential of NGS-based MRD detection assays and showed exceptional sensitivity and accuracy [10, 12–14, 17, 21, 29, 30]. However, platforms like LymphoSIGHT (Sequenta) were hardly applicable in a conventional clinical laboratory. In this study, evaluation of key analytical performance characteristics demonstrates that the LIGV-Miseq platform is an excellent alternative that is applicable in > 90% of B-ALL cases. The current method uses single rather than several rounds of multiplex PCR (as in LymphoSIGHT method) for sequencing library preparation, minimizing labor time and the potential for human error and contamination. The sensitivity of our method reaches 10^{-6} if adequate DNA input is available. This makes this approach superior to MCF [21] as evidenced by the observation that NGS detected MRD in 22 MCF-based MRD-negative samples (Fig. 3c), and it may be better or at least comparable to alternative, much more demanding, assays [10, 12–14, 17, 29, 30]. Our NGS method also demonstrates excellent intra-run and inter-run reproducibility near the established limit of detection. High concordance with MCF results is observed across a broad range of tumor load, demonstrating high accuracy of the LIGV-Miseq MRD testing platform. These findings support our NGS platform as a simple, sensitive, and reliable assay for MRD monitoring in B-ALL patients, and a practical option for a routine clinical laboratory.

The highly quantitative results generated with this assay from our retrospective cohort of B-ALL patients support the clinical utility of NGS-based post-remission MRD surveillance. As far as we know, the current study is the first that evaluates the clinical significance of NGS-based MRD surveillance during the period of complete remission by retrospectively analyzing serial post-treatment samples. There appears to be a strong correlation between CPMRD and clinical relapse, suggesting that CPMRD may signify impending relapse. Several previous investigations demonstrated the clinical potential and prognostic value of flow cytometry or qPCR-based MRD quantification in post-remission setting, producing the lead times from clinical relapse of 3.6 and 4.1 months, respectively [8, 28]. However, the accuracy of prediction of relapse for these MRD determinations was less than 100%. Some of the patients with MRD positivity by a flow cytometry method never underwent hematologic relapse, and a fraction of the patients with MRD negativity relapsed clinically (up to 30–40% for some studies) [7, 8, 28]. The occurrence of relapse with prior MRD negativity may be attributable to the limited sensitivity of the MFC or qPCR-based assays as suggested by our data (Figs. 3d and 6), or as seen in our non-surveilled cases, to insufficient surveillance since MRD surveillance is not routinely performed in many post remission settings. False positive readouts, i.e., positive MRD but no eventual relapse, might suggest stable or even decreasing MRD, which again could not have been detected unless periodic MRD measurements are made. As suggested by our results, it is possible that the determining predictive factor for relapse is not the presence or absence of MRD per se, but a rising trend of MRD, which, in the cases of prior molecular remission, is equivalent to CPMRD. Our results support the potential clinical relevance of NGS-based MRD surveillance involving periodic MRD measurements to detect CPMRD. Whether a continuous increase in MRD in cases without molecular remission has the same predictive value as CPMRD awaits further investigation.

The dynamic quantitative results generated by this assay during post treatment MRD surveillance may serve as a highly useful biomarker in patients with B-ALL for early detection of relapse disease. Early relapse detection widens the window for preemptive therapy against overt relapse. Implementation of preemptive therapies such as CAR T immunotherapy and allogenic stem cell transplantation has been associated with significant responses and prolonged survival with fewer side effects in relapsed patients with lower leukemia burdens [22, 31, 32]. A number of studies have shown that the efficacy of preemptive therapies, such as withdrawal of immunosuppression or infusion of donor lymphocyte, is closely correlated with low leukemia burdens [32, 33]. A long-term follow-up clinical trial showed that relapsed B-ALL patients with a low disease burden, who were treated with CD19 CAR T Therapy, had longer long-term survival and a lower incidence of the cytokine release syndrome and neurotoxic events than did patients with a higher tumor load [22], supporting critical role of early detection of CPMRD in effectively managing relapsed patients with preemptive therapy like CAR T immunotherapy. MRD surveillance should be taken into account in modern B-ALL management protocol and to guide personalized therapy decisions. The superb precision and analytic sensitivity of this test is particularly suited for generating highly quantitative results for determination of molecular remission and pre-clinical molecular relapse.

Since the size of our cohort is limited, the clinical utility of MRD surveillance needs to be further verified in a larger prospective clinical study. Confounding factors may limit the clinical utility/performance of the LIGV-Miseq platform. First, leukemia-specific clonotypes were not identified in a small subset of patients (2 of 32, ~ 6.25%). The reason is likely due to V gene deletion or incomplete DJ rearrangement during evolution of leukemia clones [33, 34]. To address this problem, integration of clonal *IgH* DJ rearrangement detection may be one of the options, potentially increasing the applicability of the test to more than 96% of B-ALL cases. The second limitation factor is availability of sufficient DNA material. Although most of the bone marrow samples produce substantial amount of DNA, those collected from B-ALL with severe BM fibrosis may be difficult to yield enough DNA for NGS-based MRD monitoring [35].

Conclusion

In summary, we have described and characterized a simple, reliable, and highly sensitive NGS platform that can be easily implemented in a routine molecular laboratory for MRD testing of B-ALL. Moreover, using this platform, we demonstrate the clinical utility of a dynamic NGS-based post-remission MRD surveillance method for better risk stratification and earlier preemptive therapies against impending relapse, thus potentially improving outcome for B-ALL patients. Besides B-ALL, the current NGS-based MRD testing platform should be readily applicable to MRD monitoring in other B-cell neoplasms, to assess response to therapies with innovative drugs and to design tailored protocols involving minimal disease detection in patients with B-cell lymphoproliferative disorders.

Additional files

Additional file 1: Overview of MRD measurement in B-ALL. (1) Genomic DNAs were extracted from evaluable pre-treatment and post-treatment B-ALL samples; (2) VDJ rearrangements were amplified with indicated indexed primer sets (FR3, FR1, or Leader with J$_H$) in a single multiplex PCR reaction to capture all immunoglobulin heavy-chain VDJ rearrangements. For the forward primers, we recommend using FR3 first. If no clonality were detected, FR1 or Leader may be used. The same sets of primer pairs were used for the initial diagnostic and corresponding follow-up specimens; (3) Resulting libraries were purified and quantified, followed by Miseq sequencing; (4) A customized algorithm was used to analyze NGS data to identify clonal *IGH* VDJ rearrangements for diagnostic specimens and to generate MRD values for post-treatment specimens. (DOCX 129 kb)

Additional file 2: Observed and expected MRD levels after serial dilution in representative B-ALL samples. (XLSX 15 kb)

Additional file 3: Intra-run reproducibility of LIGV-Miseq assay in MRD detection. (DOCX 13 kb)

Additional file 4: Inter-run reproducibility of LIGV-Miseq assay in MRD detection. (DOCX 12 kb)

Additional file 5: Patient characteristic. (DOCX 12 kb)

Additional file 6: Correlation between two NGS-based tumor load measurement methods. *X*-axis represents tumor load calculated by using B-cell fraction size in mononuclear cell populations measured by flow cytometry; *Y*-axis, tumor load based on the spike-in method. More details for the derivation of tumor load values based on these two methods are described in Material & Methods section. r, correlation coefficient, n, number of samples. (DOCX 63 kb)

Additional file 7: Tumor load measured by NGS vs MCF assays for all evaluable diagnostic and follow-up B-ALL samples. (XLSX 14 kb)

Additional file 8: Tumor load or MRD levels measured by NGS and MCF in patient related and unrelated samples. (XLSX 14 kb)

Abbreviations
ASO-PCR: Allele-specific oligonucleotide PCR; B-ALL: B acute lymphoblastic leukemia/lymphoma; CDR3: Complementary determining region 3; CPMRD: Conversion to positive MRD; CR: Complete remission; IGH: Immunoglobulin heavy chain; LIGV-Miseq: LymphoTrack® IGHV-based deep sequencing assay (Miseq platform); MCF: Multi-color flow cytometry; MRD: Minimal (measurable) residual disease; MUD: Matched unrelated donor; NGS: Next-generation sequencing; NMRDC: Negative MRD conversion; NPV: Negative predictive value; PPV: Positive predictive value

Authors' contributions
SHC designed the study, performed experiments, collected and analyzed data, interpreted the results, and wrote the manuscript; GI provided critical reagent and critically reviewed the manuscript; SC developed and coded the software for MRD detection; WT designed the study, analyzed data, interpreted the results, and wrote the manuscript; WT and SHC also contributed to the MRD software design and development. All authors reviewed and approved the final draft of the manuscript.

Consent for publication
Not applicable.

Competing interests
The authors declare that they have no competing interests.

Author details
[1]Department of Pathology and Laboratory Medicine, Weill Cornell Medicine, New York, NY 10021, USA. [2]Department of Computer Science, School of Engineering, Cornell University, Ithaca, New York, NY 14853, USA.

References

1. Ciudad J, San Miguel JF, Lopez-Berges MC, Vidriales B, Valverde B, Ocqueteau M, Mateos G, Caballero MD, Hernandez J, Moro MJ, et al. Prognostic value of immunophenotypic detection of minimal residual disease in acute lymphoblastic leukemia. J Clin Oncol. 1998;16:3774–81.

2. Cave H, van der Werff ten Bosch J, Suciu S, Guidal C, Waterkeyn C, Otten J, Bakkus M, Thielemans K, Grandchamp B, Vilmer E. Clinical significance of minimal residual disease in childhood acute lymphoblastic leukemia. European Organization for Research and Treatment of Cancer—Childhood Leukemia Cooperative Group. N Engl J Med. 1998;339:591–8.

3. Borowitz MJ, Devidas M, Hunger SP, Bowman WP, Carroll AJ, Carroll WL, Linda S, Martin PL, Pullen DJ, Viswanatha D, et al. Clinical significance of minimal residual disease in childhood acute lymphoblastic leukemia and its relationship to other prognostic factors: a children's oncology group study. Blood. 2008;111:5477–85.

4. Conter V, Bartram CR, Valsecchi MG, Schrauder A, Panzer-Grumayer R, Moricke A, Arico M, Zimmermann M, Mann G, De Rossi G, et al. Molecular response to treatment redefines all prognostic factors in children and adolescents with B-cell precursor acute lymphoblastic leukemia: results in 3184 patients of the AIEOP-BFM ALL 2000 study. Blood. 2010;115:3206–14.

5. Zugmaier G, Gokbuget N, Klinger M, Viardot A, Stelljes M, Neumann S, Horst HA, Marks R, Faul C, Diedrich H, et al. Long-term survival and T-cell kinetics in relapsed/refractory ALL patients who achieved MRD response after blinatumomab treatment. Blood. 2015;126:2578–84.

6. van Dongen JJ, van der Velden VH, Bruggemann M, Orfao A. Minimal residual disease diagnostics in acute lymphoblastic leukemia: need for sensitive, fast, and standardized technologies. Blood. 2015;125:3996–4009.

7. Dworzak MN, Froschl G, Printz D, Mann G, Potschger U, Muhlegger N, Fritsch G, Gadner H. Prognostic significance and modalities of flow cytometric minimal residual disease detection in childhood acute lymphoblastic leukemia. Blood. 2002;99:1952–8.

8. Raff T, Gokbuget N, Luschen S, Reutzel R, Ritgen M, Irmer S, Bottcher S, Horst HA, Kneba M, Hoelzer D, et al. Molecular relapse in adult standard-risk ALL patients detected by prospective MRD monitoring during and after maintenance treatment: data from the GMALL 06/99 and 07/03 trials. Blood. 2007;109:910–5.

9. Bruggemann M, Raff T, Flohr T, Gokbuget N, Nakao M, Droese J, Luschen S, Pott C, Ritgen M, Scheuring U, et al. Clinical significance of minimal residual disease quantification in adult patients with standard-risk acute lymphoblastic leukemia. Blood. 2006;107:1116–23.

10. Faham M, Zheng J, Moorhead M, Carlton VE, Stow P, Coustan-Smith E, Pui CH, Campana D. Deep-sequencing approach for minimal residual disease detection in acute lymphoblastic leukemia. Blood. 2012;120:5173–80.

11. Pulsipher MA, Carlson C, Langholz B, Wall DA, Schultz KR, Bunin N, Kirsch I, Gastier-Foster JM, Borowitz M, Desmarais C, et al. IgH-V(D)J NGS-MRD measurement pre- and early post-allotransplant defines very low- and very high-risk ALL patients. Blood. 2015;125:3501–8.

12. Boyd SD, Marshall EL, Merker JD, Maniar JM, Zhang LN, Sahaf B, Jones CD, Simen BB, Hanczaruk B, Nguyen KD, et al. Measurement and clinical monitoring of human lymphocyte clonality by massively parallel VDJ pyrosequencing. Sci Transl Med. 2009;1:12ra23.

13. Logan AC, Vashi N, Faham M, Carlton V, Kong K, Buno I, Zheng J, Moorhead M, Klinger M, Zhang B, et al. Immunoglobulin and T cell receptor gene high-throughput sequencing quantifies minimal residual disease in acute lymphoblastic leukemia and predicts post-transplantation relapse and survival. Biol Blood Marrow Transplant. 2014;20:1307–13.

14. Kotrova M, Muzikova K, Mejstrikova E, Novakova M, Bakardjieva-Mihaylova V, Fiser K, Stuchly J, Giraud M, Salson M, Pott C, et al. The predictive strength of next-generation sequencing MRD detection for relapse compared with current methods in childhood ALL. Blood. 2015;126:1045–7.

15. Wu J, Jia S, Wang C, Zhang W, Liu S, Zeng X, Mai H, Yuan X, Du Y, Wang X, et al. Minimal residual disease detection and evolved IGH clones analysis in acute B lymphoblastic leukemia using IGH deep sequencing. Front Immunol. 2016;7:403.

16. Wu D, Emerson RO, Sherwood A, Loh ML, Angiolillo A, Howie B, Vogt J, Rieder M, Kirsch I, Carlson C, et al. Detection of minimal residual disease in B lymphoblastic leukemia by high-throughput sequencing of IGH. Clin Cancer Res. 2014;20:4540–8.

17. Ladetto M, Bruggemann M, Monitillo L, Ferrero S, Pepin F, Drandi D, Barbero D, Palumbo A, Passera R, Boccadoro M, et al. Next-generation sequencing and real-time quantitative PCR for minimal residual disease detection in B-cell disorders. Leukemia. 2014;28:1299–307.

18. Meek K. Analysis of junctional diversity during B lymphocyte development. Science. 1990;250:820–3.

19. Komori T, Okada A, Stewart V, Alt FW. Lack of N regions in antigen receptor variable region genes of TdT-deficient lymphocytes. Science. 1993;261:1171–5.

20. Gilfillan S, Dierich A, Lemeur M, Benoist C, Mathis D. Mice lacking TdT: mature animals with an immature lymphocyte repertoire. Science. 1993; 261:1175–8.

21. Wood B, Wu D, Crossley B, Dai Y, Williamson D, Gawad C, Borowitz MJ, Devidas M, Maloney KW, Larsen E, et al. Measurable residual disease detection by high-throughput sequencing improves risk stratification for pediatric B-ALL. Blood. 2018;131:1350–9.

22. Park JH, Riviere I, Gonen M, Wang X, Senechal B, Curran KJ, Sauter C, Wang Y, Santomasso B, Mead E, et al. Long-term follow-up of CD19 CAR therapy in acute lymphoblastic leukemia. N Engl J Med. 2018;378: 449–59.

23. Sala Torra O, Othus M, Williamson DW, Wood B, Kirsch I, Robins H, Beppu L, O'Donnell MR, Forman SJ, Appelbaum FR, Radich JP. Next-generation sequencing in adult B cell acute lymphoblastic leukemia patients. Biol Blood Marrow Transplant. 2017;23:691–6.

24. Pieters R, de Groot-Kruseman H, Van der Velden V, Fiocco M, van den Berg H, de Bont E, Egeler RM, Hoogerbrugge P, Kaspers G, Van der Schoot E, et al. Successful therapy reduction and intensification for childhood acute lymphoblastic leukemia based on minimal residual disease monitoring: study ALL10 from the Dutch childhood oncology group. J Clin Oncol. 2016; 34:2591–601.

25. Paganin M, Fabbri G, Conter V, Barisone E, Polato K, Cazzaniga G, Giraldi E, Fagioli F, Arico M, Valsecchi MG, Basso G. Postinduction minimal residual disease monitoring by polymerase chain reaction in children with acute lymphoblastic leukemia. J Clin Oncol. 2014;32:3553–8.

26. Bassan R, Spinelli O, Oldani E, Intermesoli T, Tosi M, Peruta B, Rossi G, Borlenghi E, Pogliani EM, Terruzzi E, et al. Improved risk classification for risk-specific therapy based on the molecular study of minimal residual disease (MRD) in adult acute lymphoblastic leukemia (ALL). Blood. 2009;113:4153–62.

27. Bader P, Kreyenberg H, Henze GH, Eckert C, Reising M, Willasch A, Barth A, Borkhardt A, Peters C, Handgretinger R, et al. Prognostic value of minimal residual disease quantification before allogeneic stem-cell transplantation in relapsed childhood acute lymphoblastic leukemia: the ALL-REZ BFM study group. J Clin Oncol. 2009;27:377–84.

28. Pemmaraju N, Kantarjian H, Jorgensen JL, Jabbour E, Jain N, Thomas D, O'Brien S, Wang X, Huang X, Wang SA, et al. Significance of recurrence of minimal residual disease detected by multi-parameter flow cytometry in patients with acute lymphoblastic leukemia in morphological remission. Am J Hematol. 2017;92:279–85.

29. Salson M, Giraud M, Caillault A, Grardel N, Duployez N, Ferret Y, Duez M, Herbert R, Rocher T, Sebda S, et al. High-throughput sequencing in acute lymphoblastic leukemia: follow-up of minimal residual disease and emergence of new clones. Leuk Res. 2016;53:1–7.

30. Logan AC, Zhang B, Narasimhan B, Carlton V, Zheng J, Moorhead M, Krampf MR, Jones CD, Waqar AN, Faham M, et al. Minimal residual disease quantification using consensus primers and high-throughput IGH sequencing predicts post-transplant relapse in chronic lymphocytic leukemia. Leukemia. 2013;27:1659–65.

31. Liu J, Zhong JF, Zhang X, Zhang C. Allogeneic CD19-CAR-T cell infusion after allogeneic hematopoietic stem cell transplantation in B cell malignancies. J Hematol Oncol. 2017;10:35.

32. Nagafuji K, Miyamoto T, Eto T, Kamimura T, Taniguchi S, Okamura T, Ohtsuka E, Yoshida T, Higuchi M, Yoshimoto G, et al. Monitoring of minimal residual disease (MRD) is useful to predict prognosis of adult patients with Ph-negative ALL: results of a prospective study (ALL MRD2002 study). J Hematol Oncol. 2013;6:14.

33. Buckley SA, Appelbaum FR, Walter RB. Prognostic and therapeutic implications of minimal residual disease at the time of transplantation in acute leukemia. Bone Marrow Transplant. 2013;48:630–41.

34. Buccisano F, Maurillo L, Del Principe MI, Del Poeta G, Sconocchia G, Lo-Coco F, Arcese W, Amadori S, Venditti A. Prognostic and therapeutic implications of minimal residual disease detection in acute myeloid leukemia. Blood. 2012;119:332–41.

35. Noren-Nystrom U, Roos G, Bergh A, Botling J, Lonnerholm G, Porwit A, Heyman M, Forestier E. Bone marrow fibrosis in childhood acute lymphoblastic leukemia correlates to biological factors, treatment response and outcome. Leukemia. 2008;22:504–510.

9

Long non-coding RNAs in esophageal cancer: molecular mechanisms, functions, and potential applications

Min Su[1,2]* , Yuhang Xiao[3†], Junliang Ma[1†], Deliang Cao[1], Yong Zhou[1], Hui Wang[4], Qianjin Liao[2]* and Wenxiang Wang[1]*

Abstract

Esophageal cancer (EC) is the sixth leading cause of cancer-related death worldwide. The lack of early diagnostic biomarkers and effective prognostic indicators for metastasis and recurrence has resulted in the poor prognosis of EC. In addition, the underlying molecular mechanisms of EC development have yet to be elucidated. Accumulating evidence has demonstrated that lncRNAs play a vital role in the pathological progression of EC. LncRNAs may regulate gene expression through the recruitment of histone-modifying complexes to the chromatin and through interactions with RNAs or proteins. Recent evidence has demonstrated that the dysregulation of lncRNAs plays important roles in the proliferation, metastasis, invasion, angiogenesis, apoptosis, chemoradiotherapy resistance, and stemness of EC, which suggests potential clinical implications. In this review, we highlight the emerging roles and regulatory mechanisms of lncRNAs in the context of EC and discuss their potential clinical applications as diagnostic and prognostic biomarkers.

Keywords: Long non-coding RNA, Esophageal cancer, Mechanism, Application, Biomarker

Background

Esophageal carcinoma (EC), a serious malignant cancer, is the sixth leading cause of cancer-related death [1, 2]. Despite advances in multidisciplinary treatment, the 5-year relative survival rate remains less than 20% [3]. EC includes the following two primary pathological types: esophageal adenocarcinoma (EAC) and esophageal squamous cell carcinoma (ESCC) [2]. EAC is the leading histological type observed in patients from western countries, whereas ESCC has become the leading cause of EC in Asian countries and predominates over EAC worldwide [4, 5]. The pathogenesis of EC is complex and differs between EAC and ESCC. For EAC, the primary predisposing cause is metaplasia that is likely caused by chronic exposure to acid and bile reflux, such as in the case of Barrett's esophagus and chronic gastroesophageal reflux disease [6]. However, the origin of ESCC carcinogenesis is not fully understood. Early-stage EC can be effectively treated with curative surgery, but for advanced cases, the therapeutic strategies are limited [7]. Unfortunately, EC patients are usually diagnosed at an advanced stage accompanied with lymphatic metastasis, and therefore they are not eligible for surgical resection [8]. The current standard treatment for these patients is concurrent definitive chemo- or radiotherapy, or a combination of both [9]. However, therapy resistance and tumor recurrence are major obstacles for EC therapy and are critical issues leading to poor prognoses [10]. Within the EC, a small number of cells termed cancer stem-like cells (CSCs) are considered to account for the initiation, recurrence, and therapeutic resistance of EC [10]. In recent years, compelling evidence has demonstrated the crucial roles of long non-coding RNAs (lncRNAs) in the pathogenesis and progression of EC.

* Correspondence: sumin27@126.com; liaoqianjin@hnszlyy.com; hnchw11@163.com

†Yuhang Xiao and Junliang Ma contributed equally to this work.

[1]Department of the 2nd Department of Thoracic Surgery, Hunan Cancer Hospital and The Affiliated Cancer Hospital of Xiangya School of Medicine, Central South University, Changsha 410013, Hunan, People's Republic of China

[2]Department of the Central Laboratory, Hunan Cancer Hospital and The Affiliated Cancer Hospital of Xiangya School of Medicine, Central South University, Changsha 410013, Hunan, People's Republic of China

Full list of author information is available at the end of the article

LncRNAs, which are an emerging focus of current cancer research, are defined as endogenous cellular RNAs that are more than 200 nucleotides in length and are incapable of encoding protein [11, 12]. Initially, lncRNAs were considered as transcriptional "noise," given their relatively low expression levels compared with mRNAs and their lack of protein-coding capacity [13]. However, in-depth studies in recent years revealed that lncRNAs possess certain characteristics of mRNAs; for instance, lncRNAs are transcribed by RNA polymerase II, equipped with a 3′ polyA tail and a 5′ cap, and contain a promoter and structure consisting of multiple exons [14, 15]. Accumulating evidence suggests that the aberrant lncRNA expression is associated with oncogenesis and the development of various cancers [16, 17]. LncRNAs have been shown to interact directly with DNA, RNA, and proteins to regulate several mechanisms, including the following: chromatin modification, RNA transcription, pre-mRNA splicing, mRNA translation, and other mechanisms that influence gene expression [18, 19]. Moreover, several lncRNAs have been functionally well-characterized in cancer pathogenesis and development and may be potential novel biomarkers for cancer diagnosis and prognosis, as well as therapeutic targets.

In this review, we focused our efforts on the recent findings regarding the molecular mechanisms and functional roles of lncRNA in EC oncogenesis and development. In addition, we discussed the potential implications of lncRNAs as biomarkers for the diagnosis and prognosis of EC.

Mechanisms of lncRNAs in EC

LncRNAs may act as signals or guides for the recruitment of chromatin-modifying complexes to induce transcription, and they may even act as decoys that bind to transcription factors (TFs) to prevent the transcription factors from binding to target gene promoter regions, thereby suppressing transcription [20, 21]. In addition, lncRNAs can hybridize to pre-mRNAs, block the recognition of splice sites by spliceosomes, and regulate the alternative splicing of pre-mRNAs to produce alternate transcripts [17, 22]. An additional biological function of lncRNAs may include serving as "miRNA sponges" through interactions with miRNAs to inactivate these small regulatory RNAs and hence increase the expression of the miRNA target genes [23–25]. Finally, lncRNAs may be involved in the modulation of protein localization, activity, and function [26]. In this section, we highlight the molecular mechanisms of lncRNAs in EC via their interactions with chromatin, DNA, RNA, and regulatory proteins (Fig. 1 and Table 1).

LncRNAs localized to the chromatin

LncRNA-dependent chromatin regulation involves the recruitment and modulation of histone-modifying enzymes that induce chromatin modification at promoters and enhancers [27, 28]. In this manner, lncRNAs can regulate gene expression through histone modification, DNA methylation, and chromatin structure alteration [29, 30].

It has been demonstrated that many lncRNAs are associated with polycomb repressive complex 2 (PRC2), which is responsible for the trimethylation of lysine 27 on histone 3 (H3K27me3) and mediates the silencing of the target gene through local chromatin reorganization [31]. Enhancer of zeste homolog 2 (EZH2) and SUZ12 are subunits of the PRC2 complex. Wu et al. [32] demonstrated that cancer susceptibility candidate 9 (CASC9) downregulates the expression of PDCD4 via the recruitment of EZH2 to alter H3K27me3 levels at the promoter region of PDCD4. In addition, SET-binding factor 2 antisense RNA1 (SBF2-AS1) was demonstrated to bind to SUZ12 and guide PRC2 to the promoter of CDKN1A to decrease CDKN1A expression in ESCC [33].

The acetylation of histone H3 and H4 is another core mechanism through which chromatin structure and gene expression are altered [34]. In addition to recruiting EZH2, CASC9 also associates with the transcriptional coactivator CBP in the nucleus to increase the enrichment of CBP and H3K27 acetylation in the promoter region of LAMC2, thereby increasing LAMC2 expression [35].

DNA methylation is one of the most common and stable chromatin modification that is associated with gene inactivation [36, 37]. Lung cancer associated transcript 1 (LUCAT1) was originally identified in smoking-related lung cancer [38] and is also associated with colorectal cancer [39], clear cell renal cell carcinoma, and osteosarcoma [40]. A recent study demonstrated that LUCAT1 binds to DNMT1, the most abundant DNA methyltransferase in mammalian cells, and regulates its stability by inducing the ubiquitination of DNMT1 in ESCC [41]. The high levels of LUCAT1 in ESCC inhibit the expression of certain tumor suppressors through DNA methylation.

In addition, NMR, a novel lncRNA identified through microarray assays, was found to be upregulated in ESCC tissues and primarily located in the cell nucleus [42]. NMR interacts with the chromatin regulator BPTF [42], which was demonstrated to be involved in ATP-dependent chromatin remodeling and transcriptional regulation [43]. Hence, by recruiting BPTF to specific loci of chromatin, NMR upregulates the expression of MMP3 and MMP10 via ERK1/2 activation to promote ESCC tumorigenesis.

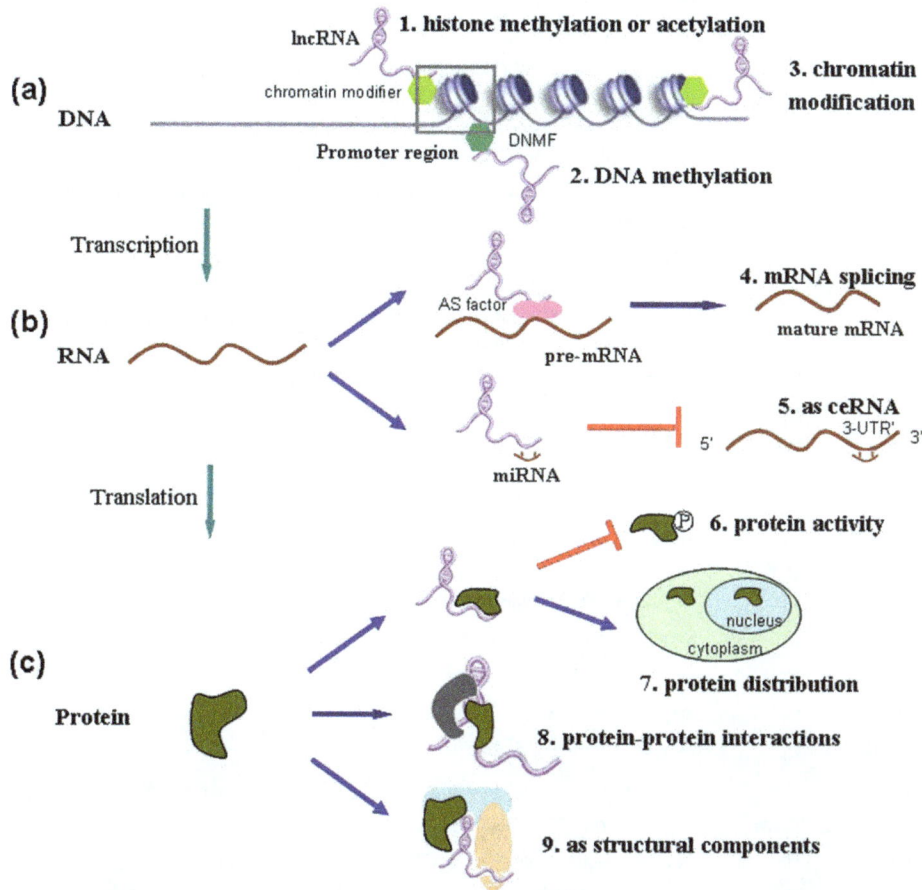

Fig. 1 The molecular mechanisms underlying esophageal cancer-related lncRNAs rely on interactions with cellular macromolecules. (a) LncRNAs localize to the chromatin. LncRNAs recruit chromatin modification complexes to the promoter region of chromatin and the results in (1) histone methylation or acetylation, (2) DNA methylation; lncRNAs recruit chromatin modification complexes to specific loci of chromatin and modulate gene expression through (3) chromatin modification. (b) LncRNAs interacts with RNA. (4) LncRNAs interacts with pre-mRNA, affect alternative splicing and help to produce mature mRNAs; (5) lncRNAs act as miRNA sponges or compete for endogenous RNAs (ceRNAs) and compete for miRNAs to inactivate these small regulatory RNAs, followed by relief of the repression of the target gene. (c) LncRNAs interact with proteins.(6) LncRNAs regulates protein dephosphorylation and activity; (7) lncRNAs regulate protein localization; (8) lncRNAs modulate protein–protein interactions; (9) lncRNAs directly localize within cellular compartments to serve as structural components

LncRNAs target RNA

Following the transcription of RNA in the nucleus, a series of conserved processes are essential for the production of mature mRNAs that can be translated into proteins. LncRNAs modulate gene expression at the RNA level through the regulation of alternative splicing and the stability of mRNAs; additionally, lncRNAs act as miRNA sponges or competing endogenous RNAs (ceRNAs) [17, 26].

mRNA splicing

Alternative splicing is a regulated process that produces different mRNA splice isoforms from a single mRNA precursor [44]. Alternative splicing produces different proteins that are translated from alternatively spliced mRNAs. This process results in proteins that have different biological functions and phenotypes [45, 46]. LincRNA-uc002yug.2, a

lncRNA principally localized to the nucleus, is increased significantly in ESCC tissues [47]. LincRNA-uc002yug.2 was shown to promote the recruitment of alternative splicing factors and RUNX1 to the nucleus to produce more RUNX1a (an inhibitor of RUNX1) relative to the other two isoforms (RUNX1b and RUNX1c) [48]. Moreover, decreased RUNX1 expression was shown to reduce the mRNA levels of CEBPα, which promotes cell proliferation [49]. Thus, LincRNA-uc002yug.2 may modulate cell proliferation and the tumor growth of ESCC through the alternative splicing of RUNX1.

CeRNA

The ceRNA hypothesis is a novel theory regarding the regulation of gene expression through post-transcriptional processes [50]. According to this hypothesis, ceRNA acts as a molecular sponge for common miRNAs through the

Table 1 Molecular mechanisms of deregulated lncRNAs in EC

Mode of mechanism	LncRNA	Expression	Molecular mechanisms	Ref.
Localizes to chromatin	CASC9	Up	Negatively regulates PDCD4 expression through recruiting EZH2 and altering H3K27me3 level	[32]
	SBF2-AS1	Up	Binds with PRC2 and guided PRC2 to the promoter of CDKN1A and decreased CDKN1A expression	[33]
	CASC9	Up	Activates the FAK-PI3K/Akt signaling pathways through upregulating LAMC2 expression by interacting with the CREB-binding protein	[35]
	LUCAT1		Binds to DNMT1 and regulates its stability, inhibits the expression of tumor suppressors through DNA methylation	[41]
	NMR,		Interacts with BPTF and recruits it to chromatin, upregulates expression of MMP3 and MMP10 via ERK1/2 activation	[42]
Interacts with RNA (mRNA splicing)	LincRNA-uc002yug.2	Up	Associates with alternative splicing of RUNX1	[48]
Interacts with RNA (ceRNA)	ATB	Up	Regulates miR-200b/Kindlin-2 axis	[51]
	SNHG16	Up	Regulates miR-140-5p/ZEB1 axis	[54]
	HOTAIR	Up	Regulates miR-125/HK2 and miR-143/HK2 axis, miR-148a/Snail2 axis, miR-1/CCND1 axis	[61] [64] [65]
	CCAT1	Up	Regulates miR-7/HOXB13 axis	[69]
	NEAT1	Up	Regulates miR-129/CTBP2 axis	[70]
	PVT1	Up	Regulates miR-203/LASP1 axis	[71]
	SNHG1	Up	Regulates miR-338/CST3 axis	[72]
	UCA1	Up	Regulates miR-204/ Sox4 axis	[73]
	XIST	Up	Regulates miR-101/EZH2 axis	[74]
	TUSC7	Down	Regulates miR-224/DESC1 axis	[75]
Interacts with protein	LINC01503	Up	Activates ERK signaling via MAPK and increases AKT signaling	[78]
	EZR-AS1	Up	Upregulates EZR expression by causing SMYD3 redistribution	[85]

miRNA response elements (MREs) to regulate the expression of the target genes of the miRNAs. Several lncRNAs have recently been found to act as ceRNAs by sponging miRNAs to reduce their inhibitory effect on their target protein-coding mRNAs.

There are numerous examples of lncRNAs functioning as sponges and therefore oncogenes in EC. Transforming growth factor β (ATB) may act as a ceRNA of miR-200b and thereby promote the expression of kindlin-2 in ESCC, as miR-200b potentially targets the 3′-untranslated region (3′-UTR) of kindlin-2 [51]. Kindlin-2 was reported to act as an oncogene by participating in cytoskeleton shaping via RhoA/FAK signaling to modulate cell migration [52, 53]. Moreover, ATB is overexpressed in ESCC. The knockdown of ATB resulted in the suppression of activated RhoA and phosphorylated FAK and the inhibition of ESCC cell proliferation, migration, and lung metastasis. Hence, the dysregulation of the lnc-ATB/miR-200b/kindlin-2 axis is involved in the development of ESCC. Small nucleolar RNA host gene 16 (SNHG16) is significantly upregulated in ESCC, and this lncRNA is primarily distributed within the cytoplasm [54]. SNHG16 promotes the progression of ESCC cells by binding with miR-140-5p to positively regulate the miR-140-5p target gene ZEB1. The

transcription factor ZEB1 has been reported to promote the epithelial-to-mesenchymal transition (EMT) in multiple tumors, including ESCC [55, 56]. Thus, SNHG16 functions as an oncogene by promoting tumor progression by competing with miR-140-5p to regulate ZEB1.

HOX transcript antisense RNA (HOTAIR) is a well-studied lncRNA that was shown to have multiple ceRNA regulatory roles in EC. HOTAIR is transcribed from the antisense strand of the HOXC gene cluster [57] and has been shown to be involved in reprogramming chromatin organization and promoting cancer cell proliferation and metastasis [58–60]. Ma et al. [61] reported that HOTAIR upregulates the expression of HK2 by functioning as a molecular sponge for miR-125 and miR-143, both of which modulate HK2 expression by targeting the 3′UTR of HK2. HK2 is overexpressed in a variety of cancers and is well-known to play a key role in tumor growth and metastasis [62, 63]. Hence, HOTAIR plays an oncogenic role in ESCC. Another study by Xu et al. [64] showed that HOTAIR promoted EC cell invasion and metastasis by promoting the EMT through the upregulation of Snail2, a transcription factor associated with the EMT. Mechanistically, HOTAIR positively regulates Snail2 by sponging miR-148a. HOTAIR has also been reported to bind directly to miR-1 and act as an endogenous sponge to inhibit miR-1 expression [65], thereby positively regulating CCND1 expression. CCND1 functions as an oncogene in various human cancers by promoting G1-S progression to regulate the cell cycle [66–68]. Thus, the HOTAIR/miR-1/CCND1 axis may promote ESCC tumorigenesis.

Several other lncRNAs have also been shown to function as oncogenes through sponging miRNAs and positively regulating their target tumor-promoting genes, including CCAT1 [69], NEAT1 [70], plasmacytoma variant translocation 1 (PVT1) [71], small nucleolar RNA host gene 1 (SNHG1) [72], UCA1 [73], and XIST [74].

In addition to these oncogenic lncRNAs sponges, there are also lncRNA sponges involved in tumor suppression. Tumor suppressor candidate 7 (TUSC7) is downregulated in ESCC tissues and is associated with shorter OS time in ESCC patients [75]. TUSC7 was shown to bind to and negatively regulate the expression of miR-224, which specifically binds to the 3′UTR region of DESC1 to negatively regulate DESC1 expression. DESC1 is an epithelial-specific enzyme and exerts tumor suppressive roles by promoting cell apoptosis via the downregulation of the EGFR/AKT pathway in ESCC [76, 77]. Thus, TUSC7 promotes cell apoptosis and suppresses the proliferation and chemotherapy resistance of ESCC cells by regulating the DESC1/EGFR/AKT pathway through miR-224. These findings indicate that TUSC7 may act as a tumor suppressor in ESCC.

LncRNAs interact with proteins

Several lncRNAs have been reported to interact with specific proteins to participate in global cellular processes in EC by regulating protein activity and function, modulating protein–protein interactions or directing the localization of proteins within cellular compartments to serve as structural components [26].

Through RNA pull-down assays and chromatin isolation by RNA purification (ChIRP), Xie and colleagues [78] demonstrated that LINC01503 could bind with both EBP-1 and ERK2 in the cytoplasm. Further analysis revealed that both basal and EGF- and IGF-induced phosphorylation of ERK1/2, Akt, p70S6K, and mTOR were significantly decreased following the knockdown of LINC01503. In addition, silencing LINC01503 expression increased the binding of EBP-1 to the PI3K subunit p85, suggesting that LINC01503 inhibits PI3K deubiquitination to activate the PI3K/Akt signaling pathway. Taken together, these findings suggest that LINC01503 contributes to ESCC cell proliferation, migration, and invasion through the activation of the ERK/MAPK and PI3K/Akt signaling pathways.

Snail, an important transcription factor influencing the EMT, binds to the E-box site in the promoter region of E-cad to suppress E-cad expression [79, 80].

This suppression triggers the EMT in a variety of cancer types, including ESCC [81, 82]. Thus, the nuclear localization of Snail is crucial for its role in the EMT progression [83]. A study by Zhang et al. [84] showed that Sprouty4-Intron 1 (SPRY4-IT1) directly increased the transcription and expression of Snail, as well as its nuclear localization, by directly binding with Snail in ESCC cells. SPRY4-IT1 is highly expressed in ESCC tissues, and overexpression of SPRY4-IT1 promotes the EMT in ESCC cells. This finding demonstrates that SPRY4-IT1 may act as an oncogene in ESCC progression via the regulation of Snail.

EZR-antisense 1 (EZR-AS1) interacts with and is part of the RNA polymerase II complex [85]. RIP assays have revealed that EZR-AS1 directly binds with SMYD3, a histone H3-lysine 4 (H3K4)-specific methyltransferase, causing SMYD3 redistribution and recruiting SMYD3 to the binding site in GC-rich regions downstream of the EZR promoter in ESCC cells. This recruitment results in the localized enrichment of SMYD3 and H3K4me3 in the EZR promoter. Lastly, EZR-AS1 was shown to promote ESCC cell migration via enhancing EZR transcription and expression.

Functions of lncRNAs in EC

Increasing evidence in the last decade indicates that lncRNAs function in a plethora of biological processes, including cell survival and apoptosis, cell cycle progression and proliferation, migration and invasion, stemness, and chemoradiotherapy (CRT) resistance (Table 2).

Involvement of lncRNAs in the hallmarks of cancer

Although cancer is a complex and heterogeneous disease, one of the common features of cancer is that abnormal cells grow beyond control. In 2000, Hanahan and Weinberg proposed six properties that are the hallmarks of cancer [86]. These basic hallmarks include sustaining growth signaling, evading growth inhibitors, uncontrolled replicative immortality, tissue invasion and metastasis, promoting angiogenesis, and resisting cell death.

Sustaining growth signaling

Tumor cells acquire the capability to sustain growth signaling through autocrine and paracrine growth factor pathways [87]. LncRNAs mediate tumor growth signals primarily by acting on the regulation of growth factors or receptors. Epidermal growth factor receptor (EGFR) is a crucial regulator in tumor growth [67]. LINC00152 has been reported to directly bind to EGFR and activate the downstream PI3K/AKT signaling pathway in gastric cancer [88]. Recently, Yang and colleagues [89] demonstrated that both LINC00152 and EGFR were highly

Table 2 Functions of deregulated lncRNAs in EC

Function	LncRNA	Expression	Targets	Ref.
Sustaining growth signaling	LINC00152	Up	EGFR	[89]
Evading growth inhibitors	AK001796	Up	MDM2/p53 signaling	[93]
	CASC2	Down	miR-18a-5p/PTEN axis	[99]
Uncontrolled replicative immortality	CDKN2B-AS1	Up	hTERT	[104]
	BC032469	Up	hTERT	[105]
Activating invasion and metastasis	PVT1	Up	–	[106]
	SNHG16	Up	miR-140-5p/ZEB1 axis	[54]
	HOTAIR	Up	miR-148a/Snail2 axis	[64]
	SNHG1	Up	Notch pathway	[112]
	MALAT1	Up	Ezh2-Notch1 signaling, miR-200a/ZEB1, and miR-200a/ZEB2 axis	[113] [114]
	CASC9	Up	–	[115]
	GHET1	Up	–	[116]
	TTN-AS1	Up	miR-133b/Snail1 axis, miR-133b/FSCN1 axis HuR	[117]
	HOTTIP	Up	miR-30b/HOXA13 axis	[118, 119]
Promoting angiogenesis	HNF1A-AS1	Up	VEGF	[123]
Resisting apoptosis	TP73-AS1	Up	BDH2	[126]
	POU6F2-AS2	Up	Ybx1	[127]
	AFAP1-AS1	Up	–	[128]
	LET	Down	–	[129]
Chemoradiotherapy resistance	AFAP1-AS1	Up	–	[132]
	LOC285194	Up	–	[136]
	BOKAS	Up	WISP1	[47]
	TUSC7	down	miR-224/DESC1	[75]
Regulation of EC stem cells	MALAT1	Up	OCT4 and Nanog	[147]

expressed in the subtype 1 of ESCC. By performing differential coexpression analysis (DCEA) and traditional differential expression analysis (DEA), the authors detected the "gain" of miRNA-mediated crosstalk between EGFR and LINC00152 in ESCC. However, the exact regulatory relationship between LINC00152 and EGFR needs further clarification.

Evading growth inhibitors
Several tumor suppressors that regulate the cell cycle and inhibit cellular growth have been discovered, such as p53 and PTEN [87]. Certain lncRNAs regulate EC cell growth through altering the expression of these tumor suppressors. P53 is a master "gatekeeper" of the cell and functions as a tumor suppressor gene [90]. P53 regulates the expression of numerous target genes, which leads to the suppression of tumor growth through the induction of cell cycle arrest and apoptosis. Mouse double minute 2 (MDM2), which acts as a primary regulator of p53, inhibits the transcription of p53 via promoting its ubiquitination and degradation [91, 92]. Thus, the MDM2/p53 axis is an important signaling pathway that regulates cell growth and the cell cycle. The expression of lncRNA

AK001796 was shown to be positively associated with MDM2 levels in ESCC tissues [93]. Knockdown of AK001796 downregulated the expression of MDM2 and upregulated the expression of p53 along with its target gene, p21. Taken together, these findings indicate that AK001796 mediates the cell cycle and cell proliferation by activating p53 signaling.

Another important tumor suppressor is PTEN, which is a crucial inhibitor of the PI3K/AKT/Mtor pathway [94, 95]. This signaling pathway is a well-known regulator of the cell cycle, proliferation, migration, and apoptosis [96–98]. Zhang et al. [99] reported that miR-18a-5p directly binds to the 3′UTR regions of PTEN, thereby inhibiting the expression of PTEN in EC cells. In addition, lncRNA cancer susceptibility candidate 2 (CASC2) was demonstrated to directly interact with miR-18a-5p and modulate the expression of PTEN by targeting miR-18a-5p. These data revealed that CASC2 may inhibit the proliferation of EC cells.

Uncontrolled replicative immortality
The telomeres, located at the chromosome ends, are important for limiting cell division cycles and replication.

Telomerase was shown to regulate the expression of a variety of growth-controlling genes and promote cell proliferation [100, 101]. As a catalytic subunit of telomerase, human telomerase reverse transcriptase (hTERT) maintains the telomere length and plays crucial roles in cell proliferation [102, 103]. Hu et al. [104] reported that hTERT expression is mediated by lncRNA cyclin-dependent kinase inhibitor 2B-antisense 1 (CDKN2B-AS1). Thus, the knockdown of CDKN2B-AS1 rescued the slow proliferation of EC109 cells induced by β-elemene, an anticancer drug. BC032469, another lncRNA that is overexpressed in ESCC tissues, was positively associated with a larger tumor size and shorter OS [105]. Silencing BC032469 expression in ESCC cells resulted in the inhibition of cell proliferation. Mechanical assays revealed that BC032469 induced cell cycle arrest in the G0/G1 phase by regulating the expression of hTERT.

Activating invasion and metastasis

The process of EMT has been confirmed to play a critical role in cell invasion in various types of cancer. This process transforms adherent and polarized epithelial cells into invasive and motile mesenchymal cells, accompanied with the loss of epithelial markers E-cadherin and the acquisition of mesenchymal markers N-cadherin and vimentin. Multiple lncRNAs have been demonstrated to be involved in EC development through the regulation of the EMT and metastasis. PVT1 has been identified as an oncogene, and high PVT1 expression was shown to be associated with the development of EC. Upregulation of PVT1 in EC cells resulted in increased N-cadherin and vimentin expression and decreased E-cadherin expression [106]. Thus, PVT1 induced the EMT and promoted the invasion of EC cells.

The EMT is also induced by several signaling pathways, such as the TGF-β and Notch signaling pathways [107–109]. The Notch signaling pathway is important for the development and progression of some tumors [110, 111]. The lncRNA SNHG1 was shown to be overexpressed in ESCC tissues and correlated with lymph node metastasis, depth of invasion, and shorter OS time in ESCC patients [112]. Silencing the expression of SNHG1 in ESCC cells was demonstrated to inhibit cell proliferation and cell invasion capacity, as well as the EMT phenomenon, through suppressing the Notch signaling pathway.

Additional lncRNAs involved in the EMT and invasion of EC include SNHG16 [54], HOTAIR [64], SNHG1 [112], metastasis associated in lung adenocarcinoma transcript 1 (MALAT1) [113, 114], CASC9 [115], gastric carcinoma highly expressed transcript 1 (GHET1) [116], TTN-antisense 1 (TTN-AS1) [117], and HOXA transcript at the distal tip (HOTTIP) [118, 119].

Promoting angiogenesis

Angiogenesis is a universal characteristic of EC progression, as it supplies the tumor with nutrients and oxygen and facilitates proliferation and migration [120, 121]. Vascular endothelial growth factor (VEGF) is the most potent activator of angiogenesis [122]. LncRNAs may regulate angiogenesis primarily by regulating VEGF. HNF1A-antisense 1 (HNF1A-AS1) is the sole lncRNA reported to modulate VEGF thus far. Recently, Wang reported that the knockdown of HAS1 suppressed the expression of VEGF in ESCC cells [123]. However, direct supporting evidence that HAS1 inhibits angiogenesis requires further studies.

Resisting cell death

The following three major pathways lead to cell death: apoptosis, autophagy, and necrosis [124]. Currently, few lncRNAs are known to be associated with the latter two pathways of cell death in EC, but several lncRNAs are involved in apoptosis via regulating the transcription of key apoptotic factors. For instance, BDH2, which functions as an anti-apoptotic factor, is regulated by survivin via the caspase-3-independent pathway [125]. P73 antisense RNA 1T (TP73-AS1), a lncRNA mapped to chromosome 1p36.32, was shown to mediate apoptosis via BDH2 [126]. The knockdown of TP73-AS1 suppressed BDH2 expression and induced the expression of pro-apoptotic proteins, which subsequently induced apoptosis in EC cells. POU6F2-antisense 2 (POU6-F2-AS2) is a lncRNA that is especially overexpressed in ESCC tissues and cells other than EAC [127]. POU6F2-AS2 knockdown induced prolonged DNA tails in ESCC cells following ionizing radiation (IR) and caused sensitivity to IR, indicating that POU6F2-AS2 is involved in the DNA damage response. Mechanical assays revealed that POU6F2-AS2 interacts with DNA repair-related protein Ybx1 and mediates the recruitment of Ybx1 to the promoter region of target genes, such as p53 and CCNB1. Finally, the dysregulation of POU6F2-AS2 expression in ESCC cell lines regulates cell survival after IR. However, the exact underlying mechanism of several other lncRNAs involved in apoptosis of EC cells, such as AFAP1-AS1 [128] and Low Expression in Tumor (LET) [129], warrants further investigation.

LncRNAs related to chemoradiotherapy resistance

Acquired CRT resistance is one of the major obstacles in the treatment of EC [130]. Studies have shown that less than 50% of patients benefit from CRT treatment, and the remaining half patients present resistance to CRT [131]. Recently, several lines of evidence have suggested that lncRNAs are likely to play vital roles in CRT resistance in EC. Zhou et al. [132] examined 18 lncRNAs that were previously reported to be dysregulated in EC or involved in CRT resistance in cisplatin-resistant ESCC cell lines and samples from patients treated with dCRT. The authors detected that three lncRNAs (AFAP1-AS1, UCA1, and HOTAIR) were dysregulated in cisplatin-resistant cells compared with the parent cell line. Moreover, AFAP1-AS1 was significantly overexpressed in tumor tissues compared to the adjacent paired tissues. Furthermore, the overexpression of AFAP1-AS1 was strongly related to the response to dCRT and to the shorter progression-free survival (PFS) and OS of ESCC patients. High AFAP1-AS1 expression could predict resistance to CRT in patients with ESCC. Another lncRNA, LOC285194, also known as LSAMP antisense RNA 3, has been reported to be downregulated in several cancers, including EC and was found to be closely associated with a poor patient prognosis [133–135]. Additionally, the low expression of LOC285194 could predict resistance to CRT [136]. As mentioned above, TUSC7 promotes cell apoptosis and inhibits chemotherapy resistance through the miR-224-dependent regulation of DESC1 [75].

Tumor radioresistance is very complex and heterogeneous. Although the mechanism underlying radioresistance is not well-understood, several signaling pathways have been demonstrated to be involved in radioresistance. The Wnt/β-catenin pathway is well-known to promote cell growth and survival and has been proven to modulate radioresistance in various cancers [137, 138]. WISP1, a Wnt- and β-catenin-responsive gene, mediates radioresistance primarily through suppressing irradiation-induced DNA damage and activating PI3K kinase [139]. Zhang and colleagues [47] reported that ESCC patients with high WISP1 expression had a significantly poorer prognosis compared with those with low WISP1 levels after radiotherapy. The authors further assayed the expression of 94 cancer-related lncRNAs in WISP1-overexpressed EC cells that received radiation, and they identified 14 upregulated lncRNAs and 5 downregulated lncRNAs. Among these lncRNAs, BOKAS was strongly associated with the irradiation-induced upregulation of WISP1. BOKAS is a natural antisense transcript of BOK, a member of the pro-apoptotic Bcl-2 family. Moreover, the downregulation of BOKAS decreased WISP1 expression and greatly enhanced irradiation-induced DNA damage in EC cells. Taken together, these findings indicate that BOKAS induces radioresistance via promoting the upregulation of WISP1.

LncRNAs in the regulation of cancer stem cells

CSCs only represent a small portion of cells within a given cancer, but they are believed to be responsible for self-renewal, metastatic ability, tumorigenicity, and therapeutic resistance [140–143]. Although ECSCs play

a critical role in EC, only a few lncRNAs have been discovered to be associated with the functions of these cells. As an example, MALAT1 has been demonstrated to be associated with tumor stem regulation in several cancer types [144–146]. A recent study by Wang et al. [147] reported that the downregulation of MALAT1 repressed the cancer stem cell-like traits of ECSS through decreasing the expression of tumor stem genes OCT4 and Nanog.

Clinical applications of lncRNAs in EC

It is recognized that the delayed diagnosis of EC results in metastasis and recurrence and is therefore a major obstacle for EC therapy. Recent studies have demonstrated that lncRNAs play a vital role in the pathological progression of EC. More importantly, lncRNAs have tissue and cell-type specificity. These patterns make lncRNAs attractive as potential biomarkers for the diagnosis and prognosis of EC (Table 3).

Tumor diagnosis

Emerging evidence has demonstrated that early diagnosis and effective intervention improves the survival of EC patients. LncRNAs are involved in EC oncogenesis and progression, and the presence of lncRNAs in the peripheral blood and body fluids of EC patients suggests that lncRNAs could serve as diagnostic biomarkers [89, 90]. Tong et al. [148] analyzed the levels of ten lncRNAs in 48 plasma samples and found that POU class 3 homeobox 3 (POU3F3), HNF1A-AS1, and SPRY4-IT1 were markedly higher in ESCC patients compared to healthy controls. In addition, in a cohort of 147 ESCC patients and 123 healthy volunteers, the receiver operating characteristics (ROC) curves demonstrated a strong separation between ESCC patients and healthy volunteers, with an area under the curve (AUC) of 0.842 (95% CI 0.794–0.890; $p < 0.001$) for POU3F3, with a 72.8% sensitivity and 89.4% specificity. In another study, Hu and colleagues [149] found that Linc00152, CASP8- and FADD-like apoptosis regulator-antisense 1 (CFLAR-AS1), and POU3F3 were significantly upregulated in a large cohort of 205 ESCC patients and 82 esophagus dysplasia patients compared to 210 healthy controls, with an AUC of 0.698, 0.651, and 0.584, respectively. The merged AUCs of the three lncRNAs were 0.765, while the AUC increased to 0.955 after merging the three factors with CEA. The circulating levels of the three lncRNAs were associated with poor postsurgery prognoses of ESCC patients in Kaplan–Meier curves. The authors also demonstrated the stability of the lncRNAs that were expressed in the human plasma, which is a crucial prerequisite for a biomarker. HOTAIR was shown to be significantly upregulated in ESCC tissues [150, 151]. A recent study demonstrated that the

Table 3 The potential clinical applications of deregulated lncRNAs in EC

Potential application	LncRNA	Expression	Clinical significance	Sample size	Ref.
Diagnostic biomarker	POU3F3	Up	–	Plasma of 147 ESCC patients and 123 healthy donors	[148]
	Linc00152, CFLAR-AS1, and POU3F3	Up	Poor post-surgery prognosis	Plasma of 205 ESCC patients, 82 esophagus dysplasia patients and 210 healthy donors	[149]
	MIR31HG	Down	TNM stage, lymphatic metastasis, and poorer OS	Plasma of 205 ESCC patients and 39 healthy donors	[153]
Prognostic biomarker	ATB	Up	TNM stage and poor DFS	150 paired ESCC tissues	[51]
	XIST	Up	Shorter DFS and OS	127 paired ESCC tissues	[74]
	AK001796	Up	TNM stages, lymph node metastasis, and shorter OS	50 paired ESCC tissues	[93]
	ZEB1-AS1	Up	Tumor grade, depth of invasion, lymph node metastasis, and shorter DFS and OS	87 paired ESCC tissues	[145]
	MALAT1	Up	Lymphatic invasion, distant metastasis, tumor differentiation, and shorter OS	106 paired ESCC tissues	[147]
	PCAT-1	Up	Lymph node metastasis, TNM stage, and poorer OS	130 paired ESCC tissues	[161]
	NKILA	Down	Tumor size, TNM stage, poor DFS, and OS	137 paired ESCC tissues	[162]
	SPRY4-IT1	Up	Clinical stage and shorter OS	92 paired ESCC tissues	[163]
	ZFAS1	Up	Poor OS	50 paired ESCC tissues	[164]

expression level of HOTAIR in the serum of ESCC patients ($n = 50$) was significantly higher compared to healthy controls ($n = 20$), with an AUC of 0.793 (95% CI 0.692 to 0.895, $P < 0.01$) and optimal cutoff values of 0.094 (sensitivity 56.0%, specificity 90.0%) [152]. In addition, the serum level of HOTAIR was positively correlated with the distant metastasis and TNM stage. MicroRNA-31 host gene (MIR31HG) is another EC-related lncRNA that is significantly upregulated in EC tissues compared to the adjacent normal tissues, as well as in ESCC plasma, compared to the healthy individuals [153]. In addition, plasma MIR31HG was found to differentiate between ESCC patients and healthy individuals by AUC analysis (95% CI 0.656 to 0.841, $P < 0.01$). These findings indicated that POU3F3, HOTAIR, and MIR31HG may be potential biomarkers for EC diagnosis. However, given that these lncRNAs have been shown to be dysregulated in cancers other than EC [154–160], they may best serve as effective diagnostic biomarkers in EC in combination with other variables.

Tumor prognosis

In recent years, great advances have been made in research into lncRNA-related prognostic biomarkers. The aberrant expression of several lncRNAs has been significantly associated with EC prognosis and may serve as potential prognostic predictors.

The expression of prostate cancer-associated ncRNA transcript 1 (PCAT-1) was markedly upregulated in 130 cancerous tissues compared to matched noncancerous

tissues in ESCC [161]. High expression levels of PCAT-1 have been correlated with the depth of tumor invasion, lymph node metastasis, and TNM stage. Kaplan–Meier analysis has revealed that patients in the high PCAT-1 group ($n = 65$) had shorter survival times compared with those in the low PCAT-1 group ($n = 39$). The expression of lncRNA ZEB1-AS1 (ZEB1 antisense 1) was significantly upregulated in 87 ESCC tissues compared to the adjacent noncancerous tissues and was significantly associated with the depth of invasion and lymph node metastasis [145]. In addition, from the Kaplan–Meier survival curves, it was observed that the 5-year overall survival (OS) and disease-free survival (DFS) of ESCC patients with high levels of ZEB1-AS1 were shorter compared with those with low levels of ZEB1-AS1.

Additionally, the dysregulation of lncRNAs ATB [51], XIST [74], AK001796 [93], MALAT1 [147], nuclear transcription factor NF-κB interacting lncRNA (NKILA) [162], SPRY4-IT1 [163], and zinc finger antisense 1 (ZFAS1) [164] has also been demonstrated to be markedly associated with advanced lymph node metastasis, aggressive TNM stage, and shorter survival time. These lncRNAs may also serve as potential prognostic biomarkers for EC.

Conclusions

EC is the eighth most frequently diagnosed malignancy worldwide. Due to typically late diagnoses at the advanced stage, combined with lymphatic metastasis, the prognosis of EC patients is poor. Despite advancements in surgery, chemo- and radiotherapy treatment over the past decades, few encouraging improvements in the 5-year OS rate of EC patients have been achieved. Moreover, the molecular mechanisms underlying EC tumorigenesis and development are still elusive. Hence, a comprehensive understanding of the molecular pathogenesis and identification of potential biomarkers of this disease are urgently needed. It is now recognized that aberrant expression of lncRNAs is a crucial determinant for human cancer. In this review, we have summarized the molecular mechanisms of lncRNAs and how they function in EC by localizing to the chromatin and interacting with proteins and RNAs. Uncovering the underlying mechanisms of lncRNAs may help us to understand the pathogenesis and progress of EC, including cell apoptosis, proliferation, migration, stemness, and therapy resistance. Furthermore, lncRNAs have the potential to serve as promising biomarkers for diagnosing EC and predicting prognosis and relapse, and they may even be novel attractive targets for clinical therapy of EC. However, there remain significant gaps in our understanding of the functions of lncRNAs in EC; these gaps must be bridged before lncRNAs can be used in clinical practice.

Abbreviations

3'-UTR: 3'-Untranslated regions; AFAP1-AS1: AFAP1-antisense 1; AS: Alternative splicing; ATB: Activated by transforming growth factor β; AUC: Area under the curve; CASC2: Cancer susceptibility candidate 2; CASC9: Cancer susceptibility candidate 9; CBP: CREB-binding protein; CCAT1: Colon cancer-associated transcript-1; CDKN2B-AS1: Cyclin-dependent kinase inhibitor 2B-antisense 1; ceRNAs: Competing endogenous RNAs; CFLAR-AS1: CASP8 and FADD-like apoptosis regulator-antisense 1; ChIRP: Chromatin isolation by RNA purification; DFS: Disease-free survival; EAC: Esophageal adenocarcinoma; EC: Esophageal cancer; EMT: Epithelial-mesenchymal transition; ESCC: Esophageal squamous cell carcinoma; EZR-AS1: EZR-antisense 1; GHET1: Gastric carcinoma highly expressed transcript 1; HNF1A-AS1: HNF1A-antisense 1; HOTAIR: HOX transcript antisense RNA; HOTTIP: HOXA transcript at the distal tip; LET: Low Expression in Tumor; lncRNAs: Long non-coding RNAs; LUCAT1: Lung cancer-associated transcript 1; MALAT1: Metastasis associated in lung adenocarcinoma transcript 1; MIR31HG: MicroRNA-31 host gene; MREs: miRNA response elements; NEAT1: Nuclear paraspeckle assembly transcript 1; NKILA: Nuclear transcription factor NF-κB interacting lncRNA; OS: Overall survival; PCAT-1: Prostate cancer-associated ncRNA transcript 1; POU3F3: POU class 3 homeobox 3; POU6F2-AS2: POU6F2-antisense 2; PVT1: Plasmacytoma variant translocation 1; ROC: Receiver operating characteristics; SBF2-AS1: SET-binding factor 2 antisense RNA 1; SNHG1: Small nucleolar RNA host gene 1; SNHG16: Small nucleolar RNA host gene 16; SPRY4-IT1: Sprouty4-Intron 1; TF: Transcription factor; TP73-AS1: P73 antisense RNA 1T; TTN-AS1: TTN-antisense 1; TUSC7: Tumor suppressor candidate 7; UCA1: Urothelial carcinoma associated 1; XIST: X-inactive specific transcript; ZEB1-AS: ZEB1 antisense 1; ZFAS1: Zinc finger antisense 1

Acknowledgements

We thank Dr. Kunjian Peng and Yuqin Zhang for the helpful discussion.

Funding

This work is supported by grants from the National Natural Scientific Foundation of China (81802947, 81472595, 81772842), Health and Family Planning Commission of Hunan Province (B20180545), and the Natural Science Foundation of Hunan Province (2017JJ2173), Changsha Science and Technology Board (kq1706045).

Authors' contributions

All authors have contributed to the preparation of this manuscript. All authors have read and approved the manuscript.

Consent for publication

Not applicable

Competing interests

The authors declare that they have no competing interests.

Author details

[1]Department of the 2nd Department of Thoracic Surgery, Hunan Cancer Hospital and The Affiliated Cancer Hospital of Xiangya School of Medicine, Central South University, Changsha 410013, Hunan, People's Republic of China. [2]Department of the Central Laboratory, Hunan Cancer Hospital and The Affiliated Cancer Hospital of Xiangya School of Medicine, Central South University, Changsha 410013, Hunan, People's Republic of China. [3]Department of Pharmacy, Xiangya Hospital of Xiangya School of Medicine, Central South University, Changsha 410001, Hunan, People's Republic of China. [4]Department of Thoracic Radiotherapy, Key laboratory of Translational Radiation Oncology, Department of Radiation Oncology, Hunan Cancer Hospital and The Affiliated Cancer Hospital of Xiangya School of Medicine, Central South University, Changsha 410013, Hunan, People's Republic of China.

References

1. Holmes RS, Vaughan TL. Epidemiology and pathogenesis of esophageal cancer. Semin Radiat Oncol. 2007;17(1):2–9.
2. Pennathur A, Gibson MK, Jobe BA, Luketich JD. Oesophageal carcinoma. Lancet. 2013;381(9864):400–12.
3. Ohashi S, Miyamoto S, Kikuchi O, Goto T, Amanuma Y, Muto M. Recent advances from basic and clinical studies of esophageal squamous cell carcinoma. Gastroenterology. 2015;149(7):1700–15.
4. Pohl H, Welch HG. The role of overdiagnosis and reclassification in the marked increase of esophageal adenocarcinoma incidence. J Natl Cancer Inst. 2005;97(2):142–6.
5. Rustgi AK, El-Serag HB. Esophageal carcinoma. N Engl J Med. 2014;371(26): 2499–509.
6. Reid BJ, Li X, Galipeau PC, Vaughan TL. Barrett's oesophagus and oesophageal adenocarcinoma: time for a new synthesis. Nat Rev Cancer. 2010;10(2):87–101.
7. Mocanu A, Barla R, Hoara P, Constantinoiu S. Current endoscopic methods of radical therapy in early esophageal cancer. J Med Life. 2015;8(2):150–6.
8. Zheng X, Xing S, Liu XM, Liu W, Liu D, Chi PD, Chen H, Dai SQ, Zhong Q, Zeng MS, et al. Establishment of using serum YKL-40 and SCCA in combination for the diagnosis of patients with esophageal squamous cell carcinoma. BMC Cancer. 2014;14:490.
9. Belkhiri A, El-Rifai W. Advances in targeted therapies and new promising targets in esophageal cancer. Oncotarget. 2015;6(3):1348–58.
10. Qian X, Tan C, Wang F, Yang B, Ge Y, Guan Z, Cai J. Esophageal cancer stem cells and implications for future therapeutics. Onco Targets Ther. 2016;9: 2247–54.
11. Iyer MK, Niknafs YS, Malik R, Singhal U, Sahu A, Hosono Y, Barrette TR, Prensner JR, Evans JR, Zhao S, et al. The landscape of long noncoding RNAs in the human transcriptome. Nat Genet. 2015;47(3):199–208.
12. Okazaki Y, Furuno M, Kasukawa T, Adachi J, Bono H, Kondo S, Nikaido I, Osato N, Saito R, Suzuki H, et al. Analysis of the mouse transcriptome based on functional annotation of 60,770 full-length cDNAs. Nature. 2002; 420(6915):563–73.

13. Ponjavic J, Ponting CP, Lunter G. Functionality or transcriptional noise? Evidence for selection within long noncoding RNAs. Genome Res. 2007; 17(5):556–65.

14. Ma L, Bajic VB, Zhang Z. On the classification of long non-coding RNAs. RNA Biol. 2013;10(6):925–33.

15. Devaux Y, Zangrando J, Schroen B, Creemers EE, Pedrazzini T, Chang CP, Dorn GW 2nd, Thum T, Heymans S. Long noncoding RNAs in cardiac development and ageing. Nat Rev Cardiol. 2015;12(7):415–25.

16. Batista PJ, Chang HY. Long noncoding RNAs: cellular address codes in development and disease. Cell. 2013;152(6):1298–307.

17. Mercer TR, Dinger ME, Mattick JS. Long non-coding RNAs: insights into functions. Nat Rev Genet. 2009;10(3):155–9.

18. Ponting CP, Oliver PL, Reik W. Evolution and functions of long noncoding RNAs. Cell. 2009;136(4):629–41.

19. Geisler S, Coller J. RNA in unexpected places: long non-coding RNA functions in diverse cellular contexts. Nat Rev Mol Cell Biol. 2013;14(11):699–712.

20. Wang KC, Chang HY. Molecular mechanisms of long noncoding RNAs. Mol Cell. 2011;43(6):904–14.

21. Hung T, Wang Y, Lin MF, Koegel AK, Kotake Y, Grant GD, Horlings HM, Shah N, Umbricht C, Wang P, et al. Extensive and coordinated transcription of noncoding RNAs within cell-cycle promoters. Nat Genet. 2011;43(7):621–9.

22. Tripathi V, Ellis JD, Shen Z, Song DY, Pan Q, Watt AT, Freier SM, Bennett CF, Sharma A, Bubulya PA, et al. The nuclear-retained noncoding RNA MALAT1 regulates alternative splicing by modulating SR splicing factor phosphorylation. Mol Cell. 2010;39(6):925–38.

23. Xie C, Yuan J, Li H, Li M, Zhao G, Bu D, Zhu W, Wu W, Chen R, Zhao Y. NONCODEv4: exploring the world of long non-coding RNA genes. Nucleic Acids Res. 2014;42(Database issue):D98–103.

24. Yan B, Yao J, Liu JY, Li XM, Wang XQ, Li YJ, Tao ZF, Song YC, Chen Q, Jiang Q. lncRNA-MIAT regulates microvascular dysfunction by functioning as a competing endogenous RNA. Circ Res. 2015;116(7):1143–56.

25. Qu J, Li M, Zhong W, Hu C. Competing endogenous RNA in cancer: a new pattern of gene expression regulation. Int J Clin Exp Med. 2015;8(10): 17110–6.

26. Schmitt AM, Chang HY. Long noncoding RNAs in cancer pathways. Cancer Cell. 2016;29(4):452–63.

27. Yang L, Lin C, Jin C, Yang JC, Tanasa B, Li W, Merkurjev D, Ohgi KA, Meng D, Zhang J, et al. lncRNA-dependent mechanisms of androgen-receptor-regulated gene activation programs. Nature. 2013;500(7464):598–602.

28. Wang KC, Yang YW, Liu B, Sanyal A, Corces-Zimmerman R, Chen Y, Lajoie BR, Protacio A, Flynn RA, Gupta RA, et al. A long noncoding RNA maintains active chromatin to coordinate homeotic gene expression. Nature. 2011; 472(7341):120–4.

29. Morlando M, Fatica A. Alteration of epigenetic regulation by long noncoding RNAs in cancer. Int J Mol Sci. 2018;19(2).

30. Langevin SM, Kratzke RA, Kelsey KT. Epigenetics of lung cancer. Transl Res. 2015;165(1):74–90.

31. Davidovich C, Zheng L, Goodrich KJ, Cech TR. Promiscuous RNA. Binding by polycomb repressive complex 2. Nat Struct Mol Biol. 2013;20(11):1250–7.

32. Wu Y, Hu L, Liang Y, Li J, Wang K, Chen X, Meng H, Guan X, Yang K, Bai Y. Up-regulation of lncRNA CASC9 promotes esophageal squamous cell carcinoma growth by negatively regulating PDCD4 expression through EZH2. Mol Cancer. 2017;16(1):150.

33. Chen R, Xia W, Wang X, Qiu M, Yin R, Wang S, Xi X, Wang J, Xu Y, Dong G, et al. Upregulated long non-coding RNA SBF2-AS1 promotes proliferation in esophageal squamous cell carcinoma. Oncol Lett. 2018;15(4):5071–80.

34. Penney J, Tsai LH. Histone deacetylases in memory and cognition. Sci Signal. 2014;7(355):re12.

35. Liang Y, Chen X, Wu Y, Li J, Zhang S, Wang K, Guan X, Yang K, Bai Y. LncRNA CASC9 promotes esophageal squamous cell carcinoma metastasis through upregulating LAMC2 expression by interacting with the CREB-binding protein. Cell Death Differ. 2018.

36. Sayols-Baixeras S, Irvin MR, Arnett DK, Elosua R, Aslibekyan SW. Epigenetics of lipid phenotypes. Curr Cardiovasc Risk Rep. 2016;10(10).

37. Ghaznavi H, Mahmoodi K, Soltanpour MS. A preliminary study of the association between the ABCA1 gene promoter DNA methylation and coronary artery disease risk. Mol Biol Res Commun. 2018;7(2):59–65.

38. Thai P, Statt S, Chen CH, Liang E, Campbell C, Wu R. Characterization of a novel long noncoding RNA, SCAL1, induced by cigarette smoke and elevated in lung cancer cell lines. Am J Respir Cell Mol Biol. 2013; 49(2):204–11.

39. Chen Y, Yu X, Xu Y, Shen H. Identification of dysregulated lncRNAs profiling and metastasis-associated lncRNAs in colorectal cancer by genome-wide analysis. Cancer Med. 2017;6(10):2321–30.

40. Han Z, Shi L. Long non-coding RNA LUCAT1 modulates methotrexate resistance in osteosarcoma via miR-200c/ABCB1 axis. Biochem Biophys Res Commun. 2018;495(1):947–53.

41. Yoon JH, You BH, Park CH, Kim YJ, Nam JW, Lee SK. The long noncoding RNA LUCAT1 promotes tumorigenesis by controlling ubiquitination and stability of DNA methyltransferase 1 in esophageal squamous cell carcinoma. Cancer Lett. 2018;417:47–57.

42. Li Y, Li J, Luo M, Zhou C, Shi X, Yang W, Lu Z, Chen Z, Sun N, He J. Novel long noncoding RNA NMR promotes tumor progression via NSUN2 and BPTF in esophageal squamous cell carcinoma. Cancer Lett. 2018;430:57–66.

43. Dar AA, Nosrati M, Bezrookove V, de Semir D, Majid S, Thummala S, Sun V, Tong S, Leong SP, Minor D, et al. The role of BPTF in melanoma progression and in response to BRAF-targeted therapy. J Natl Cancer Inst. 2015;107(5).

44. Modrek B, Lee C. A genomic view of alternative splicing. Nat Genet. 2002; 30(1):13–9.

45. Gaur S, Shively JE, Yen Y, Gaur RK. Altered splicing of CEACAM1 in breast cancer: identification of regulatory sequences that control splicing of CEACAM1 into long or short cytoplasmic domain isoforms. Mol Cancer. 2008;7:46.

46. Gu Z, Xia J, Xu H, Frech I, Tricot G, Zhan F. NEK2 promotes aerobic glycolysis in multiple myeloma through regulating splicing of pyruvate kinase. J Hematol Oncol. 2017;10(1):17.

47. Zhang H, Luo H, Hu Z, Peng J, Jiang Z, Song T, Wu B, Yue J, Zhou R, Xie R, et al. Targeting WISP1 to sensitize esophageal squamous cell carcinoma to irradiation. Oncotarget. 2015;6(8):6218–34.

48. Wu H, Zheng J, Deng J, Zhang L, Li N, Li W, Li F, Lu J, Zhou Y. LincRNA-uc002yug.2 involves in alternative splicing of RUNX1 and serves as a predictor for esophageal cancer and prognosis. Oncogene. 2015;34(36): 4723–34.

49. Wang H, Iakova P, Wilde M, Welm A, Goode T, Roesler WJ, Timchenko NA. C/EBPalpha arrests cell proliferation through direct inhibition of Cdk2 and Cdk4. Mol Cell. 2001;8(4):817–28.

50. Salmena L, Poliseno L, Tay Y, Kats L, Pandolfi PP. A ceRNA hypothesis: the Rosetta stone of a hidden RNA language? Cell. 2011;146(3):353–8.

51. Li Z, Wu X, Gu L, Shen Q, Luo W, Deng C, Zhou Q, Chen X, Li Y, Lim Z, et al. Long non-coding RNA ATB promotes malignancy of esophageal squamous cell carcinoma by regulating miR-200b/Kindlin-2 axis. Cell Death Dis. 2017; 8(6):e2888.

52. Ren Y, Jin H, Xue Z, Xu Q, Wang S, Zhao G, Huang J, Huang H. Kindlin-2 inhibited the growth and migration of colorectal cancer cells. Tumour Biol. 2015;36(6):4107–14.

53. Guo B, Gao J, Zhan J, Zhang H. Kindlin-2 interacts with and stabilizes EGFR and is required for EGF-induced breast cancer cell migration. Cancer Lett. 2015;361(2):271–81.

54. Zhang K, Chen J, Song H, Chen LB. SNHG16/miR-140-5p axis promotes esophagus cancer cell proliferation, migration and EMT formation through regulating ZEB1. Oncotarget. 2018;9(1):1028–40.

55. Ma J, Zhan Y, Xu Z, Li Y, Luo A, Ding F, Cao X, Chen H, Liu Z. ZEB1 induced miR-99b/let-7e/miR-125a cluster promotes invasion and metastasis in esophageal squamous cell carcinoma. Cancer Lett. 2017;398:37–45.

56. Yokobori T, Suzuki S, Tanaka N, Inose T, Sohda M, Sano A, Sakai M, Nakajima M, Miyazaki T, Kato H, et al. MiR-150 is associated with poor prognosis in esophageal squamous cell carcinoma via targeting the EMT inducer ZEB1. Cancer Sci. 2013;104(1):48–54.

57. Woo CJ, Kingston RE. HOTAIR lifts noncoding RNAs to new levels. Cell. 2007; 129(7):1257–9.

58. Spizzo R, Almeida MI, Colombatti A, Calin GA. Long non-coding RNAs and cancer: a new frontier of translational research? Oncogene. 2012;31(43): 4577–87.

59. Wu Y, Zhang L, Wang Y, Li H, Ren X, Wei F, Yu W, Wang X, Yu J, Hao X. Long noncoding RNA HOTAIR involvement in cancer. Tumour Biol. 2014; 35(10):9531–8.

60. Loewen G, Jayawickramarajah J, Zhuo Y, Shan B. Functions of lncRNA HOTAIR in lung cancer. J Hematol Oncol. 2014;7:90.

61. Ma J, Fan Y, Feng T, Chen F, Xu Z, Li S, Lin Q, He X, Shi W, Liu Y, et al. HOTAIR regulates HK2 expression by binding endogenous miR-125 and miR-143 in oesophageal squamous cell carcinoma progression. Oncotarget. 2017;8(49):86410–22.

62. Pedersen PL. Warburg, me and hexokinase 2: multiple discoveries of key molecular events underlying one of cancers' most common phenotypes, the "Warburg effect", i.e., elevated glycolysis in the presence of oxygen. J Bioenerg Biomembr. 2007;39(3):211–22.

63. Wolf A, Agnihotri S, Micallef J, Mukherjee J, Sabha N, Cairns R, Hawkins C, Guha A. Hexokinase 2 is a key mediator of aerobic glycolysis and promotes tumor growth in human glioblastoma multiforme. J Exp Med. 2011;208(2):313–26.

64. Xu F, Zhang J. Long non-coding RNA HOTAIR functions as miRNA sponge to promote the epithelial to mesenchymal transition in esophageal cancer. Biomed Pharmacother. 2017;90:888–96.

65. Ren K, Li Y, Lu H, Li Z, Wu K, Han X. Long noncoding RNA HOTAIR controls cell cycle by functioning as a competing endogenous RNA in esophageal squamous cell carcinoma. Transl Oncol. 2016;9(6):489–97.

66. Buschges R, Weber RG, Actor B, Lichter P, Collins VP, Reifenberger G. Amplification and expression of cyclin D genes (CCND1, CCND2 and CCND3) in human malignant gliomas. Brain Pathol. 1999;9(3):435–42 discussion 432-3.

67. Sunpaweravong P, Sunpaweravong S, Puttawibul P, Mitarnun W, Zeng C, Baron AE, Franklin W, Said S, Varella-Garcia M. Epidermal growth factor receptor and cyclin D1 are independently amplified and overexpressed in esophageal squamous cell carcinoma. J Cancer Res Clin Oncol. 2005;131(2):111–9.

68. Tashiro E, Tsuchiya A, Imoto M. Functions of cyclin D1 as an oncogene and regulation of cyclin D1 expression. Cancer Sci. 2007;98(5):629–35.

69. Zhang E, Han L, Yin D, He X, Hong L, Si X, Qiu M, Xu T, De W, Xu L, et al. H3K27 acetylation activated-long non-coding RNA CCAT1 affects cell proliferation and migration by regulating SPRY4 and HOXB13 expression in esophageal squamous cell carcinoma. Nucleic Acids Res. 2017;45(6):3086–101.

70. Li Y, Chen D, Gao X, Li X, Shi G. LncRNA NEAT1 regulates cell viability and invasion in esophageal squamous cell carcinoma through the miR-129/CTBP2 Axis. Dis Markers. 2017;2017:5314649.

71. Li PD, Hu JL, Ma C, Ma H, Yao J, Chen LL, Chen J, Cheng TT, Yang KY, Wu G, et al. Upregulation of the long non-coding RNA PVT1 promotes esophageal squamous cell carcinoma progression by acting as a molecular sponge of miR-203 and LASP1. Oncotarget. 2017;8(21):34164–76.

72. Yan Y, Fan Q, Wang L, Zhou Y, Li J, Zhou K. LncRNA Snhg1, a non-degradable sponge for miR-338, promotes expression of proto-oncogene CST3 in primary esophageal cancer cells. Oncotarget. 2017;8(22):35750–60.

73. Jiao C, Song Z, Chen J, Zhong J, Cai W, Tian S, Chen S, Yi Y, Xiao Y. lncRNA-UCA1 enhances cell proliferation through functioning as a ceRNA of Sox4 in esophageal cancer. Oncol Rep. 2016;36(5):2960–6.

74. Wu X, Dinglin X, Wang X, Luo W, Shen Q, Li Y, Gu L, Zhou Q, Zhu H, Tan C, et al. Long noncoding RNA XIST promotes malignancies of esophageal squamous cell carcinoma via regulation of miR-101/EZH2. Oncotarget. 2017;8(44):76015–28.

75. Chang ZW, Jia YX, Zhang WJ, Song LJ, Gao M, Li MJ, Zhao RH, Li J, Zhong YL, Sun QZ, et al. LncRNA-TUSC7/miR-224 affected chemotherapy resistance of esophageal squamous cell carcinoma by competitively regulating DESC1. J Exp Clin Cancer Res. 2018;37(1):56.

76. Kyrieleis OJ, Huber R, Ong E, Oehler R, Hunter M, Madison EL, Jacob U. Crystal structure of the catalytic domain of DESC1, a new member of the type II transmembrane serine proteinase family. FEBS J. 2007;274(8):2148–60.

77. Ng HY, Ko JM, Yu VZ, Ip JC, Dai W, Cal S, Lung ML. DESC1, a novel tumor suppressor, sensitizes cells to apoptosis by downregulating the EGFR/AKT pathway in esophageal squamous cell carcinoma. Int J Cancer. 2016;138(12):2940–51.

78. Xie JJ, Jiang YY, Jiang Y, Li CQ, Lim MC, An O, Mayakonda A, Ding LW, Long L, Sun C, et al. Super-enhancer-driven long non-coding RNA LINC01503, regulated by TP63, is over-expressed and oncogenic in squamous cell carcinoma. Gastroenterology. 2018;154(8):2137–2151 e1.

79. Thiery JP, Acloque H, Huang RY, Nieto MA. Epithelial-mesenchymal transitions in development and disease. Cell. 2009;139(5):871–90.

80. Kudo-Saito C, Shirako H, Takeuchi T, Kawakami Y. Cancer metastasis is accelerated through immunosuppression during Snail-induced EMT of cancer cells. Cancer Cell. 2009;15(3):195–206.

81. Kuo KT, Chou TY, Hsu HS, Chen WL, Wang LS. Prognostic significance of NBS1 and Snail expression in esophageal squamous cell carcinoma. Ann Surg Oncol. 2012;19(Suppl 3):S549–57.

82. Natsugoe S, Uchikado Y, Okumura H, Matsumoto M, Setoyama T, Tamotsu K, Kita Y, Sakamoto A, Owaki T, Ishigami S, et al. Snail plays a key role in E-cadherin-preserved esophageal squamous cell carcinoma. Oncol Rep. 2007;17(3):517–23.

83. Papiewska-Pajak I, Kowalska MA, Boncela J. Expression and activity of SNAIL transcription factor during epithelial to mesenchymal transition (EMT) in cancer progression. Postepy Hig Med Dosw (Online). 2016;70(0):968–80.

84. Zhang CY, Li RK, Qi Y, Li XN, Yang Y, Liu DL, Zhao J, Zhu DY, Wu K, Zhou XD, et al. Upregulation of long noncoding RNA SPRY4-IT1 promotes metastasis of esophageal squamous cell carcinoma via induction of epithelial-mesenchymal transition. Cell Biol Toxicol. 2016;32(5):391–401.

85. Zhang XD, Huang GW, Xie YH, He JZ, Guo JC, Xu XE, Liao LD, Xie YM, Song YM, Li EM, et al. The interaction of lncRNA EZR-AS1 with SMYD3 maintains overexpression of EZR in ESCC cells. Nucleic Acids Res. 2018;46(4):1793–809.

86. Hanahan D, Weinberg RA. The hallmarks of cancer. Cell. 2000;100(1):57–70.

87. Gutschner T, Diederichs S. The hallmarks of cancer: a long non-coding RNA point of view. RNA Biol. 2012;9(6):703–19.

88. Zhou J, Zhi X, Wang L, Wang W, Li Z, Tang J, Wang J, Zhang Q, Xu Z. Linc00152 promotes proliferation in gastric cancer through the EGFR-dependent pathway. J Exp Clin Cancer Res. 2015;34:135.

89. Yang S, Ning Q, Zhang G, Sun H, Wang Z, Li Y. Construction of differential mRNA-lncRNA crosstalk networks based on ceRNA hypothesis uncover key roles of lncRNAs implicated in esophageal squamous cell carcinoma. Oncotarget. 2016;7(52):85728–40.

90. Levine AJ, Oren M. The first 30 years of p53: growing ever more complex. Nat Rev Cancer. 2009;9(10):749–58.

91. Xie N, Ma L, Zhu F, Zhao W, Tian F, Yuan F, Fu J, Huang D, Lv C, Tong T. Regulation of the MDM2-p53 pathway by the nucleolar protein CSIG in response to nucleolar stress. Sci Rep. 2016;6:36171.

92. Brooks CL, Gu W. p53 ubiquitination: Mdm2 and beyond. Mol Cell. 2006;21(3):307–15.

93. Liu B, Pan CF, Yao GL, Wei K, Xia Y, Chen YJ. The long non-coding RNA AK001796 contributes to tumor growth via regulating expression of p53 in esophageal squamous cell carcinoma. Cancer Cell Int. 2018;18:38.

94. Yin Y, Shen WH. PTEN: a new guardian of the genome. Oncogene. 2008;27(41):5443–53.

95. Khalid A, Hussain T, Manzoor S, Saalim M, Khaliq S. PTEN: a potential prognostic marker in virus-induced hepatocellular carcinoma. Tumour Biol. 2017;39(6):1010428317705754.

96. Chalhoub N, Baker SJ. PTEN and the PI3-kinase pathway in cancer. Annu Rev Pathol. 2009;4:127–50.

97. Tamura M, Gu J, Matsumoto K, Aota S, Parsons R, Yamada KM. Inhibition of cell migration, spreading, and focal adhesions by tumor suppressor PTEN. Science. 1998;280(5369):1614–7.

98. Choi BH, Xie S, Dai W. PTEN is a negative regulator of mitotic checkpoint complex during the cell cycle. Exp Hematol Oncol. 2017;6:19.

99. Wang D, Gao ZM, Han LG, Xu F, Liu K, Shen Y. Long noncoding RNA CASC2 inhibits metastasis and epithelial to mesenchymal transition of lung adenocarcinoma via suppressing SOX4. Eur Rev Med Pharmacol Sci. 2017;21(20):4584–90.

100. Smith LL, Coller HA, Roberts JM. Telomerase modulates expression of growth-controlling genes and enhances cell proliferation. Nat Cell Biol. 2003;5(5):474–9.

101. Masutomi K, Yu EY, Khurts S, Ben-Porath I, Currier JL, Metz GB, Brooks MW, Kaneko S, Murakami S, DeCaprio JA, et al. Telomerase maintains telomere structure in normal human cells. Cell. 2003;114(2):241–53.

102. Horikawa I, Barrett JC. Transcriptional regulation of the telomerase hTERT gene as a target for cellular and viral oncogenic mechanisms. Carcinogenesis. 2003;24(7):1167–76.

103. Cao Y, Li H, Deb S, Liu JP. TERT regulates cell survival independent of telomerase enzymatic activity. Oncogene. 2002;21(20):3130–8.

104. Hu Z, Wu H, Li Y, Hou Q, Wang Y, Li S, Xia B, Wu S. Beta-Elemene inhibits the proliferation of esophageal squamous cell carcinoma by regulating long noncoding RNA-mediated inhibition of hTERT expression. Anti-Cancer Drugs. 2015;26(5):531–9.

105. Lu C, Yang L, Chen H, Shan Z. Upregulated long non-coding RNA BC032469 enhances carcinogenesis and metastasis of esophageal squamous cell carcinoma through regulating hTERT expression. Tumour Biol. 2016.

106. Zheng X, Hu H, Li S. High expression of lncRNA PVT1 promotes invasion by inducing epithelial-to-mesenchymal transition in esophageal cancer. Oncol Lett. 2016;12(4):2357–62.

107. Ungefroren H, Witte D, Lehnert H. The role of small GTPases of the rho/Rac family in TGF-beta-induced EMT and cell motility in cancer. Dev Dyn. 2018; 247(3):451–61.

108. Li Y, Ma J, Qian X, Wu Q, Xia J, Miele L, Sarkar FH, Wang Z. Regulation of EMT by notch signaling pathway in tumor progression. Curr Cancer Drug Targets. 2013;13(9):957–62.

109. Wang Z, Li Y, Kong D, Sarkar FH. The role of Notch signaling pathway in epithelial-mesenchymal transition (EMT) during development and tumor aggressiveness. Curr Drug Targets. 2010;11(6):745–51.

110. Venkatesh V, Nataraj R, Thangaraj GS, Karthikeyan M, Gnanasekaran A, Kaginelli SB, Kuppanna G, Kallappa CG, Basalingappa KM. Targeting Notch signalling pathway of cancer stem cells. Stem Cell Investig. 2018;5:5.

111. Tamagnone L, Zacchigna S, Rehman M. Taming the Notch transcriptional regulator for cancer therapy. Molecules. 2018;23(2).

112. Zhang Y, Jin X, Wang Z, Zhang X, Liu S, Liu G. Downregulation of SNHG1 suppresses cell proliferation and invasion by regulating Notch signaling pathway in esophageal squamous cell cancer. Cancer Biomark. 2017; 21(1):89–96.

113. Chen M, Xia Z, Chen C, Hu W, Yuan Y. LncRNA MALAT1 promotes epithelial-to-mesenchymal transition of esophageal cancer through Ezh2-Notch1 signaling pathway. Anti-Cancer Drugs. 2018;29(8):767–73.

114. Zhang QQ, Cui YH, Wang Y, Kou WZ, Cao F, Cao XJ, Miao ZH, Kang XH. Mechanism of long non-coding RNA-metastasis associated lung adenocarcinoma transcript 1 induced invasion and metastasis of esophageal cancer cell EC-109. Zhonghua Zhong Liu Za Zhi. 2017; 39(6):405–11.

115. Gao GD, Liu XY, Lin Y, Liu HF, Zhang GJ. LncRNA CASC9 promotes tumorigenesis by affecting EMT and predicts poor prognosis in esophageal squamous cell cancer. Eur Rev Med Pharmacol Sci. 2018;22(2):422–9.

116. Xia Y, Yan Z, Wan Y, Wei S, Bi Y, Zhao J, Liu J, Liao DJ, Huang H. Knockdown of long noncoding RNA GHET1 inhibits cell-cycle progression and invasion of gastric cancer cells. Mol Med Rep. 2018;18(3):3375–81.

117. Lin C, Zhang S, Wang Y, Nice E, Guo C, Zhang E, Yu L, Li M, Liu C, Hu L, et al. Functional role of a novel long noncoding RNA TTN-AS1 in esophageal squamous cell carcinoma progression and metastasis. Clin Cancer Res. 2018;24(2):486–98.

118. Chen X, Han H, Li Y, Zhang Q, Mo K, Chen S. Upregulation of long noncoding RNA HOTTIP promotes metastasis of esophageal squamous cell carcinoma via induction of EMT. Oncotarget. 2016;7(51):84480–5.

119. Lin C, Wang Y, Zhang S, Yu L, Guo C, Xu H. Transcriptional and posttranscriptional regulation of HOXA13 by lncRNA HOTTIP facilitates tumorigenesis and metastasis in esophageal squamous carcinoma cells. Oncogene. 2017;36(38):5392–406.

120. Barzi A, Lenz HJ. Angiogenesis-related agents in esophageal cancer. Expert Opin Biol Ther. 2012;12(10):1335–45.

121. Barzi A, Thara E. Angiogenesis in esophageal and gastric cancer: a paradigm shift in treatment. Expert Opin Biol Ther. 2014;14(9):1319–32.

122. Fantozzi A, Gruber DC, Pisarsky L, Heck C, Kunita A, Yilmaz M, Meyer-Schaller N, Cornille K, Hopfer U, Bentires-Alj M, et al. VEGF-mediated angiogenesis links EMT-induced cancer stemness to tumor initiation. Cancer Res. 2014; 74(5):1566–75.

123. Wang G, Zhao W, Gao X, Zhang D, Li Y, Zhang Y, Li W. HNF1AAS1 promotes growth and metastasis of esophageal squamous cell carcinoma by sponging miR214 to upregulate the expression of SOX-4. Int J Oncol. 2017; 51(2):657–67.

124. Chen Q, Kang J, Fu C. The independence of and associations among apoptosis, autophagy, and necrosis. Signal Transduct Target Ther. 2018;3:18.

125. Yang WC, Tsai WC, Lin PM, Yang MY, Liu YC, Chang CS, Yu WH, Lin SF. Human BDH2, an anti-apoptosis factor, is a novel poor prognostic factor for de novo cytogenetically normal acute myeloid leukemia. J Biomed Sci. 2013;20:58.

126. Zang W, Wang T, Wang Y, Chen X, Du Y, Sun Q, Li M, Dong Z, Zhao G. Knockdown of long non-coding RNA TP73-AS1 inhibits cell proliferation and induces apoptosis in esophageal squamous cell carcinoma. Oncotarget. 2016;7(15):19960–74.

127. Liu J, Sun X, Zhu H, Qin Q, Yang X. Long noncoding RNA POU6F2-AS2 is associated with oesophageal squamous cell carcinoma. J Biochem. 2016; 160(4):195–204.

128. Luo HL, Huang MD, Guo JN, Fan RH, Xia XT, He JD, Chen XF. AFAP1-AS1 is upregulated and promotes esophageal squamous cell carcinoma cell proliferation and inhibits cell apoptosis. Cancer Med. 2016;5(10):2879–85.

129. Wang PL, Liu B, Xia Y, Pan CF, Ma T, Chen YJ. Long non-coding RNA-low expression in tumor inhibits the invasion and metastasis of esophageal squamous cell carcinoma by regulating p53 expression. Mol Med Rep. 2016; 13(4):3074–82.

130. Akutsu Y, Hanari N, Yusup G, Komatsu-Akimoto A, Ikeda N, Mori M, Yoneyama Y, Endo S, Miyazawa Y, Matsubara H. COX2 expression predicts resistance to chemoradiotherapy in esophageal squamous cell carcinoma. Ann Surg Oncol. 2011;18(10):2946–51.

131. Courrech Staal EF, Aleman BM, Boot H, van Velthuysen ML, van Tinteren H, van Sandick JW. Systematic review of the benefits and risks of neoadjuvant chemoradiation for oesophageal cancer. Br J Surg. 2010;97(10):1482–96.

132. Zhou XL, Wang WW, Zhu WG, Yu CH, Tao GZ, Wu QQ, Song YQ, Pan P, Tong YS. High expression of long non-coding RNA AFAP1-AS1 predicts chemoradioresistance and poor prognosis in patients with esophageal squamous cell carcinoma treated with definitive chemoradiotherapy. Mol Carcinog. 2016;55(12):2095–105.

133. Pasic I, Shlien A, Durbin AD, Stavropoulos DJ, Baskin B, Ray PN, Novokmet A, Malkin D. Recurrent focal copy-number changes and loss of heterozygosity implicate two noncoding RNAs and one tumor suppressor gene at chromosome 3q13.31 in osteosarcoma. Cancer Res. 2010;70(1):160–71.

134. Liu Q, Huang J, Zhou N, Zhang Z, Zhang A, Lu Z, Wu F, Mo YY. LncRNA loc285194 is a p53-regulated tumor suppressor. Nucleic Acids Res. 2013; 41(9):4976–87.

135. Qi P, Xu MD, Ni SJ, Huang D, Wei P, Tan C, Zhou XY, Du X. Low expression of LOC285194 is associated with poor prognosis in colorectal cancer. J Transl Med. 2013;11:122.

136. Tong YS, Zhou XL, Wang XW, Wu QQ, Yang TX, Lv J, Yang JS, Zhu B, Cao XF. Association of decreased expression of long non-coding RNA LOC285194 with chemoradiotherapy resistance and poor prognosis in esophageal squamous cell carcinoma. J Transl Med. 2014;12:233.

137. Chen MS, Woodward WA, Behbod F, Peddibhotla S, Alfaro MP, Buchholz TA, Rosen JM. Wnt/beta-catenin mediates radiation resistance of Sca1+ progenitors in an immortalized mammary gland cell line. J Cell Sci. 2007; 120(Pt 3):468–77.

138. Chang HW, Roh JL, Jeong EJ, Lee SW, Kim SW, Choi SH, Park SK, Kim SY. Wnt signaling controls radiosensitivity via cyclooxygenase-2-mediated Ku expression in head and neck cancer. Int J Cancer. 2008;122(1):100–7.

139. Clevers H. Wnt/beta-catenin signaling in development and disease. Cell. 2006;127(3):469–80.

140. Dalerba P, Clarke MF. Cancer stem cells and tumor metastasis: first steps into uncharted territory. Cell Stem Cell. 2007;1(3):241–2.

141. Dean M, Fojo T, Bates S. Tumour stem cells and drug resistance. Nat Rev Cancer. 2005;5(4):275–84.

142. Islam F, Gopalan V, Lam AK. Identification of cancer stem cells in esophageal adenocarcinoma. Methods Mol Biol. 2018;1756:165–76.

143. Huang X, Xiao R, Pan S, Yang X, Yuan W, Tu Z, Xu M, Zhu Y, Yin Q, Wu Y, et al. Uncovering the roles of long non-coding RNAs in cancer stem cells. J Hematol Oncol. 2017;10(1):62.

144. Yang MH, Hu ZY, Xu C, Xie LY, Wang XY, Chen SY, Li ZG. MALAT1 promotes colorectal cancer cell proliferation/migration/invasion via PRKA kinase anchor protein 9. Biochim Biophys Acta. 2015;1852(1):166–74.

145. Zhang J, Zhang B, Wang T, Wang H. LncRNA MALAT1 overexpression is an unfavorable prognostic factor in human cancer: evidence from a meta-analysis. Int J Clin Exp Med. 2015;8(4):5499–505.

146. Michalik KM, You X, Manavski Y, Doddaballapur A, Zornig M, Braun T, John D, Ponomareva Y, Chen W, Uchida S, et al. Long noncoding RNA MALAT1 regulates endothelial cell function and vessel growth. Circ Res. 2014;114(9):1389–97.

147. Wang W, Zhu Y, Li S, Chen X, Jiang G, Shen Z, Qiao Y, Wang L, Zheng P, Zhang Y. Long noncoding RNA MALAT1 promotes malignant development of esophageal squamous cell carcinoma by targeting beta-catenin via Ezh2. Oncotarget. 2016;7(18):25668–82.

148. Tong YS, Wang XW, Zhou XL, Liu ZH, Yang TX, Shi WH, Xie HW, Lv J, Wu QQ, Cao XF. Identification of the long non-coding RNA POU3F3 in plasma as a novel biomarker for diagnosis of esophageal squamous cell carcinoma. Mol Cancer. 2015;14:3.

149. Hu HB, Jie HY, Zheng XX. Three circulating LncRNA predict early progress of esophageal squamous cell carcinoma. Cell Physiol Biochem. 2016;40(1–2):117–25.

150. Ge XS, Ma HJ, Zheng XH, Ruan HL, Liao XY, Xue WQ, Chen YB, Zhang Y, Jia WH. HOTAIR, a prognostic factor in esophageal squamous cell carcinoma,

inhibits WIF-1 expression and activates Wnt pathway. Cancer Sci. 2013; 104(12):1675–82.

151. Da C, Zhan Y, Li Y, Tan Y, Li R, Wang R. The expression and significance of HOX transcript antisense RNA and epithelial-mesenchymal transition-related factors in esophageal squamous cell carcinoma. Mol Med Rep. 2017;15(4):1853–62.

152. Wang W, He X, Zheng Z, Ma X, Hu X, Wu D, Wang M, Serum HOTAIR. As a novel diagnostic biomarker for esophageal squamous cell carcinoma. Mol Cancer. 2017;16(1):75.

153. Sun K, Zhao X, Wan J, Yang L, Chu J, Dong S, Yin H, Ming L, He F. The diagnostic value of long non-coding RNA MIR31HG and its role in esophageal squamous cell carcinoma. Life Sci. 2018;202:124–30.

154. Li Y, Wang D, Meng Q. Linc-POU3F3 is overexpressed in hepatocellular carcinoma and regulates cell proliferation, migration and invasion. Biomed Pharmacother. 2018;105:683–9.

155. Xiong G, Yang L, Chen Y, Fan Z. Linc-POU3F3 promotes cell proliferation in gastric cancer via increasing T-reg distribution. Am J Transl Res. 2015; 7(11):2262–9.

156. Shan TD, Xu JH, Yu T, Li JY, Zhao LN, Ouyang H, Luo S, Lu XJ, Huang CZ, Lan QS, et al. Knockdown of linc-POU3F3 suppresses the proliferation, apoptosis, and migration resistance of colorectal cancer. Oncotarget. 2016; 7(1):961–75.

157. Li J, Wang J, Zhong Y, Guo R, Chu D, Qiu H, Yuan Z. HOTAIR: a key regulator in gynecologic cancers. Cancer Cell Int. 2017;17:65.

158. Miao Z, Ding J, Chen B, Yang Y, Chen Y. HOTAIR overexpression correlated with worse survival in patients with solid tumors. Minerva Med. 2016; 107(6):392–400.

159. Qin J, Ning H, Zhou Y, Hu Y, Yang L, Huang R. LncRNA MIR31HG overexpression serves as poor prognostic biomarker and promotes cells proliferation in lung adenocarcinoma. Biomed Pharmacother. 2018;99:363–8.

160. He A, Chen Z, Mei H, Liu Y. Decreased expression of LncRNA MIR31HG in human bladder cancer. Cancer Biomark. 2016;17(2):231–6.

161. Shi WH, Wu QQ, Li SQ, Yang TX, Liu ZH, Tong YS, Tuo L, Wang S, Cao XF. Upregulation of the long noncoding RNA PCAT-1 correlates with advanced clinical stage and poor prognosis in esophageal squamous carcinoma. Tumour Biol. 2015;36(4):2501–7.

162. Ke S, Li RC, Meng FK, Fang MH. NKILA inhibits NF-kappaB signaling and suppresses tumor metastasis. Aging (Albany NY). 2018;10(1):56–71.

163. Xie HW, Wu QQ, Zhu B, Chen FJ, Ji L, Li SQ, Wang CM, Tong YS, Tuo L, Wu M, et al. Long noncoding RNA SPRY4-IT1 is upregulated in esophageal squamous cell carcinoma and associated with poor prognosis. Tumour Biol. 2014;35(8):7743–54.

164. Shi H, Liu Z, Pei D, Jiang Y, Zhu H, Chen B. Development and validation of nomogram based on lncRNA ZFAS1 for predicting survival in lymph node-negative esophageal squamous cell carcinoma patients. Oncotarget. 2017; 8(35):59048–57.

10

Targeting the IDO1 pathway in cancer: from bench to bedside

Ming Liu[1,2*], Xu Wang[2], Lei Wang[2,3], Xiaodong Ma[3], Zhaojian Gong[2,4], Shanshan Zhang[2,5] and Yong Li[2*] (iD)

Abstract

Indoleamine 2, 3-dioxygenases (IDO1 and IDO2) and tryptophan 2, 3-dioxygenase (TDO) are tryptophan catabolic enzymes that catalyze the conversion of tryptophan into kynurenine. The depletion of tryptophan and the increase in kynurenine exert important immunosuppressive functions by activating T regulatory cells and myeloid-derived suppressor cells, suppressing the functions of effector T and natural killer cells, and promoting neovascularization of solid tumors. Targeting IDO1 represents a therapeutic opportunity in cancer immunotherapy beyond checkpoint blockade or adoptive transfer of chimeric antigen receptor T cells. In this review, we discuss the function of the IDO1 pathway in tumor progression and immune surveillance. We highlight recent preclinical and clinical progress in targeting the IDO1 pathway in cancer therapeutics, including peptide vaccines, expression inhibitors, enzymatic inhibitors, and effector inhibitors.

Keywords: Indoleamine 2, 3-dioxygenases, IDO1, Immunosuppression, Immunotherapy, Clinical trial

Background

The tryptophan (Trp) catabolism pathway plays an important role in tumor cell evasion of the innate and adaptive immune systems [1, 2]. Trp is generally utilized in three major metabolic pathways: incorporation into proteins, production of serotonin, and breakdown into kynurenine (Kyn). Kyn is generated via two major routes: in peripheral tissues, controlled by the rate-limiting enzymes indoleamine 2, 3-dioxygenase 1 (IDO1) and indoleamine 2, 3-dioxygenase 2 (IDO2), and the hepatic route, in which tryptophan 2, 3-dioxygenase (TDO) is the rate-limiting enzyme [3] (Fig. 1). Discovered in the 1950s, IDO1 is the most fully characterized enzyme in the Kyn biosynthesis pathway. In healthy post-natal individuals, IDO1 facilitates tolerance by dampening the immune response, whereas during gestation, IDO1 helps protect the fetus from maternal T lymphocytes [4]. On the other hand, IDO1 is a crucial innate immunity regulator that acts by depleting Trp in both the inflammatory and tumor microenvironments [1, 5, 6]. IDO1 is involved in the suppression of effector T and NK cells and differentiation and activation of regulatory T (Treg) cells and myeloid-derived suppressor cells (MDSCs) [7–9]. In addition, IDO1 plays a key role in promoting tumor neovascularization by modulating the expression of interferon-γ (IFN-γ) and interleukin-6 (IL-6) [10, 11]. In prostate cancer cells, IFN-γ and TNF-α-treatment induce IDO1 and IL-6 gene expression [12]. Furthermore, IDO1 is involved in the formation of resistance to immune checkpoint inhibitors [13], and the combination of an IDO1 inhibitor with checkpoint inhibitors represents an alternative strategy in cancer immunotherapy [14].

IDO1 is overexpressed in the vast majority of cancers (Fig. 2, data are summarized from The Cancer Genome Atlas, https://cancergenome.nih.gov/). Several strategies for targeting IDO1 have been assessed in multiple clinical trials and have produced encouraging results. Blockade of IDO1 activity decreased tumor proliferation in a T-lymphocyte-mediated manner and enhanced the efficacy of chemotherapy, radiotherapy, targeted therapy, and immunotherapy [15–19]. In this review, we will first discuss the complex role of IDO1 in regulating the innate and adaptive immune responses. We will then highlight the role of IDO1-related signaling pathways in the tumor microenvironment. Finally, we summarize the current preclinical and clinical studies of IDO-targeting interventions.

* Correspondence: mingliu128@hotmail.com; liy2@ccf.org
[1]State Key Laboratory of Respiratory Diseases, Guangzhou Institute of Respiratory Diseases, The First Affiliated Hospital of Guangzhou Medical University, Guangzhou Medical University, Guangzhou, China
[2]Department of Cancer Biology, Lerner Research Institute, Cleveland Clinic, Cleveland, OH, USA
Full list of author information is available at the end of the article

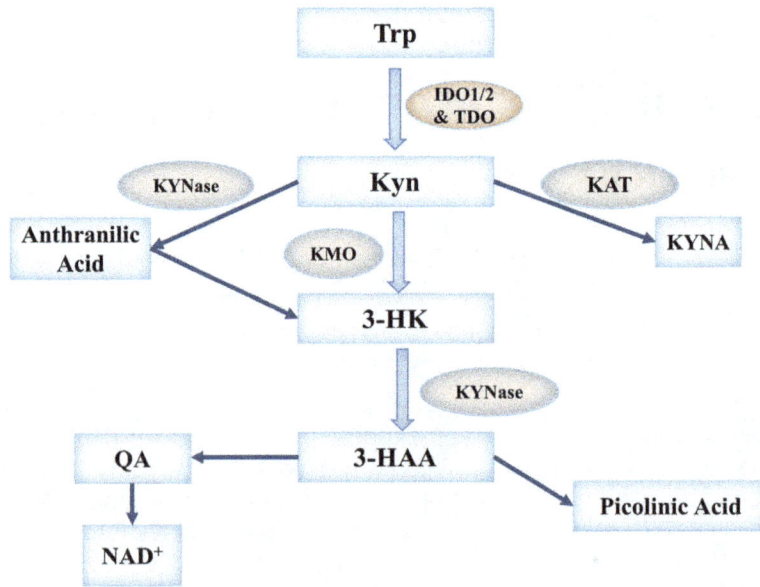

Fig. 1 Overview of the IDO metabolic pathway. Approximately 95% of L-tryptophan (Trp) is catabolized into kynurenine (Kyn) through three rate-limiting enzymes: tryptophan 2,3-dioxygenase (TDO) in the liver and indoleamine 2, 3-dioxygenase 1/2 (IDO1/2) in peripheral tissues. Kyn is converted to 3-hydroxykynurenine (3-HK) by kynurenine 3-monooxygenase (KMO), to anthranilic acid (AA) by kynureninase (KYNase), or to kynurenic acid (KYNA) by kynurenine aminotransferase (KAT). Next, catalyzed by KYNase, 3-HK is converted to 3-hydroxyanthranilic acid (3-HAA), which is further converted to quinolinic acid (QA), picolinic acid, nicotinamide adenine dinucleotide (NAD$^+$), and other molecules

IDO regulatory and effector signaling pathways

Multiple upstream pathways regulate IDO1 expression and function, including the Janus kinase–signal transducer and activator of transcription (JAK–STAT), RAS–protein kinase C (RAS–PKC), nuclear factor kappa-light-chain enhancer of activated B cells (NF-κB), and Kit signaling pathways [20–22]. Downstream of IDO1 are three effector pathways that transduce the effects of IDO1 activity: general control over nonderepressible 2 (GCN2) is activated, mammalian target of rapamycin (mTOR) is inhibited,

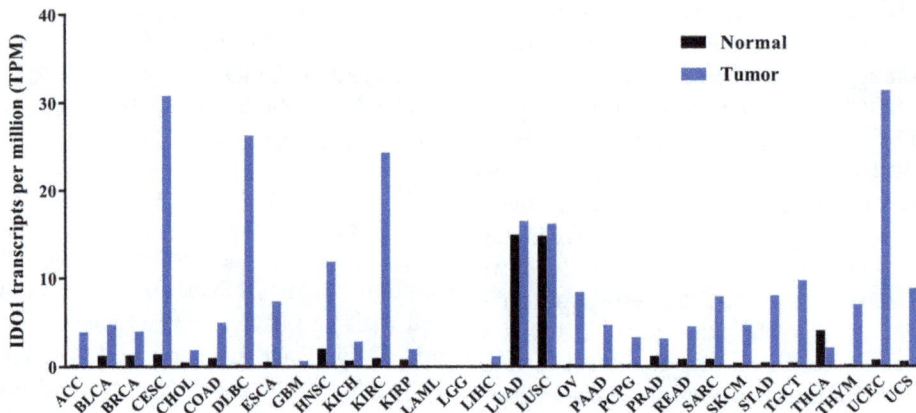

Fig. 2 The IDO1 gene transcripts across tumor samples and paired normal tissues. Data are summarized from The Cancer Genome Atlas, https://cancergenome.nih.gov/. The Y axis denotes the number of IDO1 transcripts per million of total RNA reads. Abbreviations: ACC, adrenocortical carcinoma; BLCA, bladder urothelial carcinoma; BRCA, breast invasive carcinoma; CESC, cervical squamous cell carcinoma and endocervical adenocarcinoma; CHOL, cholangiocarcinoma; COAD, colon adenocarcinoma; DLBC, lymphoid neoplasm diffuse large B-cell lymphoma; ESCA, esophageal carcinoma; GBM, glioblastoma multiforme; HNSC, head and neck squamous cell carcinoma; KICH, kidney chromophobe; KIRC, kidney renal clear cell carcinoma; KIRP, kidney renal papillary cell carcinoma; LAML, acute myeloid leukemia; LGG, brain lower grade glioma; LIHC, liver hepatocellular carcinoma; LUAD, lung adenocarcinoma; LUSC, lung squamous cell carcinoma; OV, ovarian serous cystadenocarcinoma; PAAD, pancreatic adenocarcinoma; PCPG, pheochromocytoma and paraganglioma; PRAD, prostate adenocarcinoma; READ, rectum adenocarcinoma; SARC, sarcoma; SKCM, skin cutaneous melanoma; STAD, stomach adenocarcinoma; TGCT, testicular germ cell tumors; THCA, thyroid carcinoma; THYM, thymoma; UCS, uterine carcinosarcoma; UCEC, uterine corpus endometrial carcinoma

which is related to Trp deprivation, and the aryl hydrocarbon receptor (AhR) pathway is activated with Kyn as an endogenous AhR ligand [23–25]. These regulatory and effector pathways mediate immunosuppression and neovascularization in the tumor microenvironment.

Upstream regulators

IDO1 is not expressed in most tissues in adult humans under physiological conditions but is constitutively expressed in many types of cancer cells, stromal cells, and immune cells in the tumor microenvironment (Fig. 3a). IDO1 is activated by diverse inflammatory molecules, such as IFN-γ, tumor necrosis factor α (TNF-α), transforming growth factor β (TGF-β), pathogen-associated molecular patterns (PAMPs), damage-associated molecular patterns (DAMPs), and prostaglandin E2 (PGE2), through canonical and non-canonical NF-κB and JAK–STAT pathways [21, 23, 25–27]. Constitutive IDO1 expression in human cancers is driven by cyclooxygenase 2 (COX-2) and PGE2 via the PKC and PI3K pathways [28]. Moreover, autocrine TGF-β sustains the activation of IDO1 in a tolerogenic subpopulation of CD8$^+$ dendritic cells (DCs), while exogenous TGF-β converts immunogenic CD8$^-$ DCs into tolerogenic cells in conjunction with induction of IDO1 [29]. IDO1 is under genetic control of the cancer-suppression gene *bridging integrator 1* (Bin1), and *Bin1* knockout results in tumor growth and immune suppression in mice by upregulating STAT1- and NF-κB-dependent expression of IDO1 [20]. Ras and Kit also upregulate IDO1 expression in cancer cells [22, 27]. Importantly, several immune checkpoints (e.g., PD-1 and CTLA4) on the T cell surface modulate IDO1 expression in antigen-presenting cells. Recently, Wang et al. [30] demonstrated that the IL-6-inducible proto-oncogene protein intestine-specific homeobox (ISX) gene induces IDO1 and TDO expression, which increases Kyn and AhR and thereby promotes the tumorigenic potential and immunosuppression of hepatocellular carcinoma cells expressing CD86 and PD-L1. Others report that hypoxia enhances IDO1 production in monocyte-derived dendritic cells, yet the underlying mechanisms remain elusive [31].

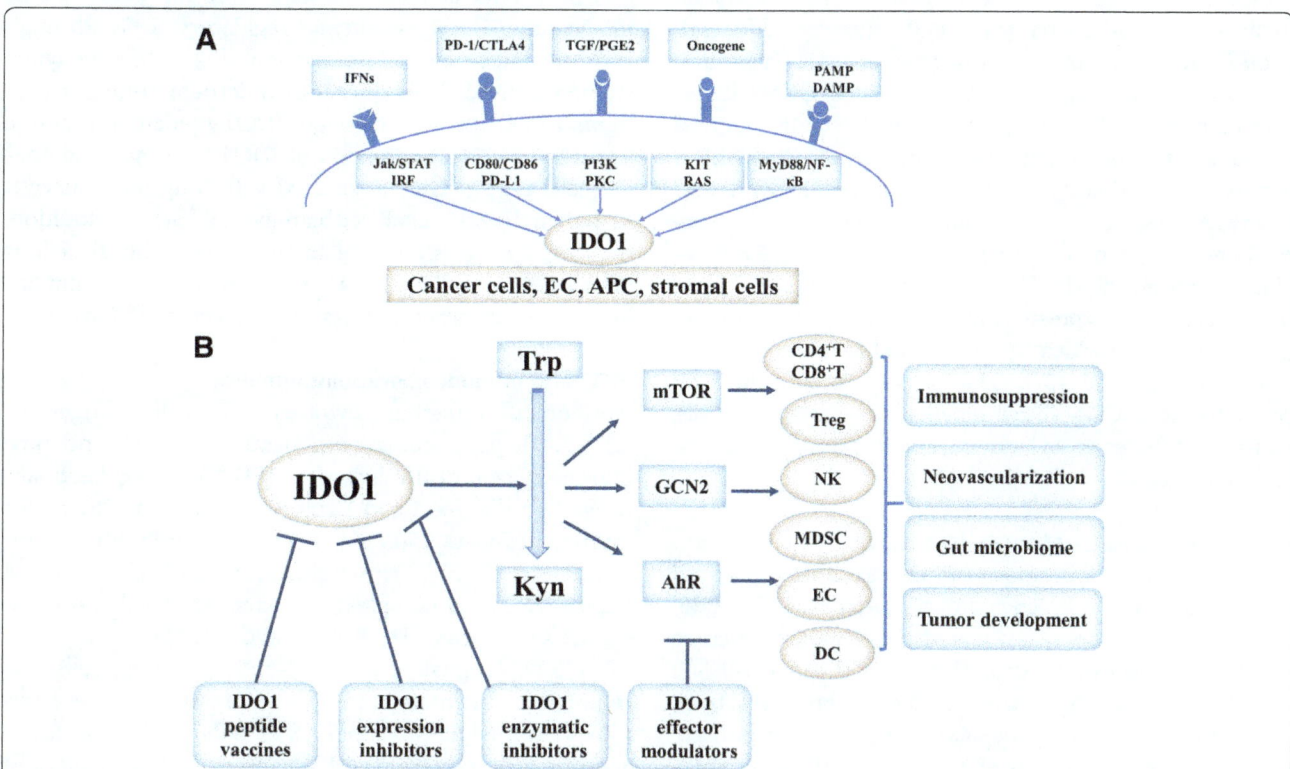

Fig. 3 Regulation, function, and targeting of IDO1 in cancer. **a** The upstream regulators of IDO1. IDO1 is expressed in cancer cells, endothelial cells, antigen-presenting cells, and stromal cells. IDO1 expression is regulated by IFNs, PD-1, oncogene activation (KIT or RAS), PAMPs, and DAMPs through relevant signaling pathways like IFN-γ/JAK/STAT, PI3K/PKC, and NF-κB. **b** The downstream effectors of IDO1 and IDO1 targeting. Three effector pathways (mTOR, GCN2, and AhR) mediate the effects of IDO1 activities in various types of cells in regard to immunosuppression, neovascularization, interactions with the gut microbiome, and the tumor microenvironment. Four strategies have been developed to target the IDO1 pathway in preclinical and clinical studies. IDO1, indoleamine 2, 3-dioxygenase 1; Trp, tryptophan; Kyn, kynurenine; IFN, interferon; PD-1, programmed death receptor 1; PAMP, pathogen-associated molecular pattern; DAMP, damage-associated molecular pattern; GCN2, general control over nonderepressible 2; mTOR, mammalian target of rapamycin; AhR, aryl hydrocarbon receptor; NK, natural killer cell; Treg, regulatory T cell; MDSC, myeloid-derived suppressor cell; EC, endothelial cell; DC, dendritic cell

Downstream effectors

IDO1 transduces signaling through three major effectors: GCN2, mTOR, and AhR. The depletion of Trp by IDO1 leads to the accumulation of uncharged Trp–tRNA, which binds and activates GCN2, a stress-response kinase. Activated GCN2 phosphorylates and inhibits eukaryotic initiation factor 2α kinase, resulting in attenuation of RNA transcription and protein translation. Specific to T effector cells, GCN2 activation mediated by Trp deprivation leads to cell cycle arrest and/or apoptosis [25, 32]. Another signaling molecule inhibited by Trp deprivation is the mammalian target of rapamycin (mTOR) [23]. IDO1-mediated suppression through mTORC1 triggers autophagy, leading to anergy in T cells in the tumor microenvironment [23, 33]. Most relevant publications report that mTOR inhibition suppresses effector T cell function and promotes Treg cell function although others dispute these findings [34], and the precise role of IDO1 in mTOR signaling and immune regulation continues to be debated. Both GCN2 kinase activation and mTOR inhibition are immunosuppressive. During CD4+ T-cell differentiation, GCN2 kinase activation suppresses only Th2 differentiation, whereas mTOR inhibition induces Treg cell differentiation and suppresses differentiation of the Th1, Th2, and Th17 lineages [35]. These findings suggest that Trp deprivation-mediated GCN2 kinase activation and mTOR inhibition have differential impacts on the function of distinct CD4+ T cell populations. AhR is a cytosolic ligand-activated transcription factor involved in embryogenesis, adaptive immunity, mucosal barrier function, and malignancy. Its most potent ligand, 2,3,7,8-tetrachlorodibenzo-p-dioxin (TCDD), activates AhR signaling to upregulate IDO1 expression [36]. A breakthrough was reported in 2011 in which Kyn was found to be an endogenous ligand of AhR [37]. The binding of Kyn to AhR promotes naive CD4+ T cell differentiation into Treg cells, which contributes to an immunosuppressive tumor microenvironment [38].

Role of the IDO1 pathway in cancers

IDO1 is expressed by various cancer and cancer-associated cells in the tumor microenvironment, including DCs, endothelial cells, tumor-associated macrophages, tumor-associated fibroblasts, mesenchymal stromal cells (MSCs), and MDSCs [2, 39]. Most cancer types have high IDO1 expression (Fig. 2), which is correlated with poor survival and prognosis [40–42]. Besides its role in immunosuppression, IDO1 also contributes to cancer development by promoting inflammatory neovascularization [27], interacting with checkpoint inhibitors, and modulating gut microbiota [43].

IDO1 ablates T effector cells and promotes the induction of Treg cells and MDSCs in the tumor microenvironment

Increased IDO1 and accumulating Trp metabolites prevent the activation of CD8+ and CD4+ effector T cells, inhibit NK cell function, stimulate the activation of Treg cells, and promote the expansion and activation of DCs and MDSCs [25, 44–46]. Treg cells are a major suppressive cell type in the tumor microenvironment, as their recruitment is induced by high IDO1 levels and correlates with poor prognosis in several tumor types [47]. Furthermore, IDO1 presence leads to activation of the phosphatase and tensin homolog (PTEN) pathway in Treg cells to maintain their immunosuppressive phenotype in vitro [48].

IDO1 is also essential for the recruitment and sustenance of MDSCs through a Treg-dependent mechanism [49]. MDSCs can suppress antitumor immune responses through STAT3-dependent IDO1 expression in breast cancer [50]. Increased STAT3 activation in MDSCs was found to be correlated with activation of the non-canonical NF-κB pathway, in which RelB–p52 dimers directly bind to the IDO1 promoter, leading to IDO1 expression in MDSCs [51]. In a Kras mutant lung cancer model, Ido1-deficient mice had impaired MDSC function [27].

Cancer-associated fibroblasts recruit and educate DCs to become IDO1-producing regulatory DCs through IL-6-mediated STAT3 activation [52]. Mesenchymal stem/stromal cells in the tumor microenvironment promote tumor growth through IDO1-mediated immune suppression [53]. Expression of IDO1 in tumor endothelial cells is negatively associated with long-term survival in patients with renal cell carcinoma [54]. In addition, the IDO1 expression level in tumor endothelial cells is associated with the tumor's response to checkpoint inhibitor treatment in metastatic renal cell carcinoma [55].

IDO1 and immune checkpoint inhibitors

Antibodies targeting cytotoxic T cell antigen 4 (CTLA-4), programmed cell death 1 (PD-1), and programmed cell death ligand 1 (PD-L1) have been approved by the Food and Drug Administration (FDA) for multiple cancers [56, 57]. Recent research further revealed that IDO1 is closely linked to both CTLA-4 and PD-1–PD-L1 via complex pathways. Treg cell-expressed CTLA-4 induced IDO1 expression in DCs [46], and PD-1/PTEN signaling in IDO1-activated Treg cells was required to maintain immune suppression of the Tregs [58]. IDO1 expression in DCs is induced by the interaction of PD-1 with PD-L1 on the surface of mast cells and/or with PD-L2 on the surface of DCs [59]. Moreover, IDO1 participates in the intracellular signaling events responsible for long-term tolerance by DCs [29]. Based on its upstream effects on DCs, this IDO1 activity is non-redundant with that of the more distal T cell checkpoints, and combined therapy with IDO1 inhibitors and CTLA-4 or PD-1 inhibitors should confer additional benefit.

IDO1 has also been reported to participate in a resistance mechanism to checkpoint inhibitors, and the combination of CTLA-4 blockade and an IDO1 inhibitor resulted in more effective antitumor immunity in a melanoma mouse model [13]. In a phase 2 trial, excessive infiltration of IDO1$^+$ macrophages and a significant increase in the kynurenine-to-Trp ratio were observed in the majority of patients who had poor response to metronomic cyclophosphamide and pembrolizumab combination treatment [60]. In addition, Liu and colleagues identified a Kyn–AhR pathway-dependent mechanism that promoted tumor-repopulating cell immune escape by increasing PD-1 binding to CD8$^+$ T cells. Local IFN-γ produced by tumor-infiltrating CD8$^+$ T cells stimulates tumor-repopulating cell release at high levels of Kyn, which then activates AhR on the T cell surface to promote PD-1 upregulation. Thus, targeting the Kyn–AhR pathway (such as by inhibiting IDO1 in tumor-repopulating cell or AhR in CD8$^+$ T cells) may enhance the efficacy of adoptive T cell therapy. Taken together, these results suggest that combination strategies targeting multiple immune checkpoints might be the preferred weapon of the future.

Tumor neovascularization

Neovascularization, characterized by excessive and disorganized growth of blood vessels, is critical for tumor development, progression, and metastasis. In mice, *Ido1* deficiency inhibited lung tumor growth and improved animal survival with reduced density of the underlying pulmonary blood vessels [27]. Recent work also showed a new role for IDO1 in supporting pathologic neovascularization [11]. In 4T1 breast cancer pulmonary metastases and oxygen-induced retinopathy mouse models, IDO1 ablation was sufficient to reduce pathological neovascularization in both lung metastases and reinopathy. IL-6 is regarded as a pro-angiogenic cytokine potentiated by IDO1, and IL-6 deletion results in IFN-γ-dependent reduction in neovascularization and increases resistance to metastasis [11]. Administration of the IDO1 inhibitor epacodostat (INCB024360) in mice with tumors or vascularized metastases significantly reduced neovascularization [11]. High IDO1 expression positively correlates with microvessel density and poor prognosis in breast cancer patients [61]. In summary, IDO1-mediated effects on neovascular development and established neovascular networks broaden the potential effectiveness of IDO1 inhibitors in clinical trials and in practice.

IDO1 and the gut microbiome

The gut microbiome has been found to regulate cancer initiation, progression, and response to therapies [62]. Preclinical mouse models suggest that resistance in melanoma patients to anti-PD-1 immunotherapy can be attributed to abnormal gut microbiome composition [63]. Bacteria, including *Bifidobacterium longum, Collinsella aerofaciens, and Enterococcus faecium*, are more abundant in treatment responders, whereas the efficacy of immune checkpoint blockade therapies is diminished with administration of antibiotics [64–66]. As an essential nutrient in mammals, Trp and its IDO1-catalyzed endogenous metabolites play a key role in the gut microbiota and immune homeostasis. Recent discoveries have underscored the modulation of host immune systems by changes in the microbiota that affect Trp metabolism [43]. Activation of toll-like receptors by microbial components has been identified as a key factor in initiating Kyn metabolism and gut microbial homeostasis, as reduced toll-like receptor stimulation in germ-free mice resulted in decreased Trp metabolism [53, 67].

IDO1 inhibitors in preclinical development and clinical trials

Based on the important role of IDO1 in cancer immune tolerance and development, targeting IDO1 is becoming an attractive approach in cancer therapeutic development (Fig. 3b). Unlike cell-surface checkpoint receptor molecules that can be effectively targeted by antibody-based therapeutics, IDO1 and its downstream effector molecules are intracellular targets that are still best addressed by small molecule drugs. An increasing number of IDO1 inhibitors are being tested in preclinical development or clinical trials [15, 16] (Table 1).

The effector inhibitor indoximod

Indoximod (1-methyl-D-tryptophan, 1MT, NLG-8189) is the most-studied IDO1 inhibitor and has been granted orphan-drug designation by the US FDA for the indication of stage IIb to stage IV melanoma. Recent results suggest that indoximod is not only a valid inhibitor of IDO1 enzymatic activity but also acts as a high-potency Trp mimetic in reversing mTORC1 inhibition [23]. mTORC1 is a central integrator of cell growth signals that monitors levels of essential amino acids that are needed to activate cell growth [68]. Clinical results indicated that indoximod exerted little antitumor efficacy as a single agent, but efficacy was markedly enhanced when it was combined with other therapies, such as PD-1 checkpoint inhibitors (in advanced melanoma), cancer vaccines (in metastatic prostate cancer), and chemotherapy (in pancreatic cancer and acute myeloid leukemia). A phase 1 dose-escalation trial aiming to evaluate the safety, dosing, pharmacokinetics, and immunologic effects of indoximod found indoximod to be safe at doses up to 2000 mg orally twice daily [69]. Another phase 1 dose-escalation trial designed to study co-administration of docetaxel and indoximod reported that this combination is well tolerated, with no increase in expected toxicities in patients

Table 1 IDO1 inhibitors in clinical trials

Drug	Strategies	Tumor type	Phase	Clinical efficacy	Safety (% patients)	Trial number	Status
Indoximod	Single agent	Metastatic or refractory solid tumors	I	NR	NR	NCT00739609	Terminated
		Metastatic or refractory solid tumors	I	ORR 10% (5/48)	Fatigue (56.3%), anemia (37.5%), anorexia (37.5%) dyspnea (35.4%) cough (33.3%) nausea (29.2%)	NCT00567931	Completed
	Docetaxel	Metastatic solid tumors	I	4/22PRs, 9/22 SD, and 9/22 PD	Fatigue (58.6%) anemia (51.7%) hyperglycemia (48.3%), infection (44.8%), nausea (41.4%)	NCT01191216	Completed
	Temozolomide/ bevacizumab	Primary malignant brain tumors	I/II	NR	NR	NCT02052648	Recruiting
	Temozolomide	Progressive primary malignant brain tumors	I			NCT02502708	Recruiting
	Docetaxel/ paclitaxel	Metastatic breast cancer	II			NCT01792050	Unknown
	Nab-Paclitaxel/ gemcitabine	Metastatic pancreatic cancer	I/II	ORR 11/30 (37%)	1/30 (colitis)	NCT02077881	Recruiting
	Idarubicin/ cytarabine	Acute myeloid leukemia	I/II			NCT02835729	Recruiting
	Adenovirus-p53 transduced dendritic cell (DC) vaccine	Metastatic breast cancer	I/II	Chemosensitization effect, median PFS 13.3 weeks and median OS 20.71 weeks. 9/22 patients benefitted from chemotherapy after vaccination.	Most common grade 1–2 (fatigue, anemia, transient lymphopenia, nausea, anorexia)	NCT01042535	Completed
	Sipuleucel-T	Refractory metastatic prostate cancer	II	NR	NR	NCT01560923	Active, not recruiting
	Tergenpumatucel-L/docetaxel	Advanced previously treated non-small cell lung cancer	I/II			NCT02460367	Unknown
	Ipilimumab/ nivolumab/ pembrolizumab	Metastatic melanoma	II/ III			NCT03301636	Recruiting
Epacadostat	Single agent	Advanced malignancy	I/II	NR	Fatigue, nausea, decreased appetite, vomiting, constipation, abdominal pain, diarrhea, dyspnea, back pain, cough	NCT01195311	Completed
		Solid tumor	I			NCT03471286	Not yet recruiting
		Myelodysplastic syndromes	II			NCT01822691	Completed
	Fludarabine/ cyclophosphamide/ NK cells/IL-2	Recurrent ovarian, fallopian tube, and primary peritoneal cancer	I			NCT02118285	Completed
	Tamoxifen	Ovarian cancer genitourinary tumors	II	Median PFS, 3.75 months	Fatigue (36.4%) rash (18.2%) pruritus (9.1%)	NCT01685255	Terminated
	Azacitidine + pembrolizumab	Advanced solid tumors	I/II	NR	NR	NCT02959437	Recruiting

Table 1 IDO1 inhibitors in clinical trials *(Continued)*

Drug	Strategies	Tumor type	Phase	Clinical efficacy	Safety (% patients)	Trial number	Status
	MELITAC 12.1 peptide vaccine	Stage III-IV melanoma	II	NR	NR	NCT01961115	Active, not recruiting
	DPX-survivac/ cyclophosphamide	Ovarian cancer	I	NR	NR	NCT02785250	Recruiting
	ALVAC(2)-NY-ESO-1 (M)/TRICOM vaccine	Ovarian, fallopian tube, or primary peritoneal cancer	I/II	NR	NR	NCT01982487	Withdrawn
	DEC-205/NY-ESO-1 fusion protein CDX-1401/poly ICLC	Ovarian, fallopian tube, or primary peritoneal cancer	I/II	NR	NR	NCT02166905	Recruiting
	CRS-207/ pembrolizumab	Metastatic pancreas cancer, platinum-resistant ovarian, fallopian, or peri-toneal cancer	II,I/II	NR	NR	NCT03006302 / NCT02575807	Recruiting / active, not recruiting
	Atezolizumab	Non-small cell lung cancer and urothelial carcinoma	I	NR	NR	NCT02298153	Terminated
	Durvalumab	Advanced solid tumor	I/II	NR	NR	NCT02318277	Recruiting
	Ipilimumab	Melanoma	I/II			NCT01604889	Terminated
	Nivolumab/ ipilimumab/ lirilumab	Solid tumors	I/II			NCT03347123	Recruiting
	Nivolumab/ chemotherapy	Advanced cancers	I/II	ORR 75%(melanoma) 11% (ovarian) 4% (colorectal)	Rash (10% and 12% in epacadostat 100 and 300 mg subgroups)	NCT02327078	Recruiting
	Pembrolizumab/ chemotherapy	Advanced solid tumors	I, I/II	NR	NR	NCT02862457 / NCT03085914	Recruiting / Recruiting
	pembrolizumab	Solid tumors, thymic carcinoma, sarcoma, junction or gastric cancer, lung cancer, urothelial cancer, metastatic melanoma, and others.	I, I/II, III	Melanoma (ORR 57% and DCR 86%), Renal cell carcinoma (ORR 40% and DCR 80%)	Fatigue, diarrhea, rash, arthralgia, and nausea	NCT02178722 / NCT02364076 / NCT03414229 / NCT03196232 / NCT03322540 / NCT03361865	Recruiting / Recruiting / Recruiting / Recruiting / Recruiting / Recruiting
	Pembrolizumab	Melanoma	III			NCT02752074	Halted
Navoximod	Single agent	Advanced solid tumors	I	NR	NR	NCT02048709	Completed
	Atezolizumab	Solid tumors	I			NCT02471846	Active, not recruiting
PF-06840003	Single agent	Malignant gliomas	I			NCT02764151	Active, not recruiting
BMS-986205	Nivolumab	Melanoma advanced cancers	III, I/II	NR	3/42 patients with grade 3 autoimmune hepatitis	NCT03329846 / NCT03192943	Recruiting / Recruiting
	Nivolumab/ ipilimumab	Advanced cancer melanoma non-small cell lung cancer	I/II	ORR 32%(bladder cancer) 14%(cervical cancer) PD-L1 > 1%: 46% (bladder cancer)and 25% (cervical cancer)	Fatigue (18.2% nausea (18.2%) decreased appetite (13.6%) vomiting (6.8%)	NCT02658890	Recruiting
	Nivolumab/ ipilimumab/ relatlimab	Advanced gastric cancer, advanced renal cell carcinoma, advanced cancer	II, I/II	NR	NR	NCT02935634 / NCT02996110 / NCT03459222	Recruiting / Recruiting / Not yet recruiting

Table 1 IDO1 inhibitors in clinical trials *(Continued)*

Drug	Strategies	Tumor type	Phase	Clinical efficacy	Safety (% patients)	Trial number	Status
						NCT03335540	Recruiting
	Nivolumab/ cetuximab/ chemotherapy	Head and neck cancer	III	NR	NR	NCT03386838	Halted
	Nivolumab/ chemotherapy	Lung cancer	III			NCT03417037	Halted

with metastatic solid tumors [70]. Administering indoximod with the PD-1 antibody pembrolizumab (Keytruda) led to a 61% overall response rate, including 10 complete responses (20%) and 21 partial responses (41%), in patients with advanced melanoma. The median progression-free survival under combinatorial treatment was 12.9 months, with a 1-year rate of 56%, suggesting a synergistic antitumor therapeutic effect [71].

IDO1 enzymatic inhibitors
Epacadostat (INCB024360)
Epacadostat is a Trp competitive inhibitor that has been widely investigated in clinical trials. With an IC50 of 72 nM, it has a > 1000-fold selectivity for the IDO1 enzyme relative to IDO2 or TDO [72]. In vitro studies found that epacadostat promoted T cell and NK cell proliferation, increased the number of $CD86^{high}$ DCs, and reduced Treg cells [73], and its administration to tumor-bearing syngeneic mice inhibited plasma and tumor Kyn levels by approximately 90% and reduced tumor growth in immunocompetent but not immunocompromised mice.

In a phase 1 clinical study, epacadostat was well tolerated at doses of 100 mg twice daily. No objective responses were detected although stable disease was observed in 7 of 52 patients over 16 weeks of observation [74]. A randomized phase 2 study compared epacadostat with tamoxifen treatment in 42 patients with biochemically recurrent epithelial ovarian cancer, primary peritoneal carcinoma, or fallopian tube cancer, found that epacadostat was well tolerated but its efficacy was no better than tamoxifen [75]. Based on encouraging results from its combination with immune checkpoint inhibitors, epacadostat was propelled into three clinical trials [76]. In melanoma, anti-PD-1 antibody combinations (either pembrolizumab or nivolumab) showed rates of overall response and disease control similar to those produced by the approved combination of anti-PD-1 and anti-CTLA-4 antibodies (ipilimumab) without the significant side effects of the latter. In head and neck cancer, an interim report on 38 patients who were previously treated suggested that epacadostat increased rates of overall response and disease control without any notable increase in side effects when administered with an anti-PD-1 antibody. Epacadostat is

currently being tested in clinical trials in 14 tumor types (including the above cancers) with co-administration of anti-PD-1 antibodies (nivolumab or pembrolizumab) or anti-PD-L1 antibodies (atezolizumab and durvalumab).

Navoximod (NLG-919, GDC-0919)
Navoximod was initially developed as an orally bioavailable IDO1 and TDO inhibitor with a superior pharmacokinetic and toxicity profile based on 4-phenylimidazole, a compound that binds the heme iron at the IDO1-active site [77]. In preclinical studies, navoximod inhibited IDO1-induced T cell suppression and restored robust T cell responses (EC50 = 80 nM). Kyn levels in plasma were reduced by approximately 50% in mice treated with navoximod [78]. In a syngeneic murine B16-F10 melanoma model, navoximod potentiated the antitumor efficacy of paclitaxel without increasing side effects [79]. A combination of navoximod, anti-PD1/PD-L1/PD-L2 antibodies, and indoximod with chemotherapy and a glycoprotein 100 (gp100) peptide vaccine achieved a significant synergistic antitumor effect [80]. In a phase 1b clinical trial, the combination of navoximod and atezolizumab was well tolerated [81]; preliminary efficacy data from 45 patients with over 1 on-treatment tumor assessments included 4 patients (9%) with partial response and 11 (24%) patients with stable disease.

BMS-986205
BMS-986205 is an irreversible IDO1 inhibitor. In preclinical studies, BMS-986205 was found to specifically target and bind to IDO1 but not IDO2 or TDO [15]. By inhibiting IDO1 and decreasing Kyn levels in tumor cells, BMS-986205 reversed immunosuppression in cancer patients. In a phase 1/2a study, BMS-986205 was administered alone or in combination with nivolumab in multiple advanced malignancies. It was well tolerated, with no grade 3 events in BMS-986205 monotherapy and no grade 4 or 5 events in the combination group. In a dose escalation and expansion study (NCT02658890), an encouraging response was observed for BMS-986205 plus nivolumab. The maximum tolerated dose of BMS-986205 in combination with nivolumab was 200 mg, and the recommended dose for further study was 100 mg. Objective response rates in the bladder and cervical cancer cohorts were 32% and 14%, respectively,

which improved to 46% and 25%, respectively, in tumors where over 1% of tumor cells expressed PD-L1. An increase in tumor-infiltrating CD8$^+$ T cells and a decrease in Kyn were also observed [82]. Based on this potent effect and encouraging results overall, about 10 ongoing trials are investigating the effect of BMS-986205 combined with nivolumab as compared with nivolumab alone in patients with advanced melanoma, non-small cell lung cancer, head and neck cancer, advanced gastric cancer, and other types of cancer.

PF-06840003 and other inhibitors

PF-06840003 is an orally bioavailable, highly selective IDO1 inhibitor that can cross the blood–brain barrier. In vitro, it reverses IDO1-induced T-cell anergy. In preclinical syngeneic mouse tumor models, PF-06840003 reduced Kyn levels in mice by > 80% and enhanced the antitumor efficacy of anti-PD-1 or anti-PD-L1 antibodies. This compound has favorable human pharmacokinetic characteristics, with a prolonged half-life that enables single-dose daily administration. More importantly, its central nerve system (CNS) penetration properties allow its application in brain metastases [83]. An ongoing multi-center clinical trial aims to assess the safety, pharmacokinetic, and pharmacodynamic activity of PF-06840003 in malignant glioma and to validate its CNS penetration and effectiveness in combination with other drugs. Recently, BGB-5777, a potent CNS-penetrating IDO1 inhibitor, when combined with nivolumab and radiation therapy, achieved a durable survival benefit in patients with advanced glioblastoma [17]. A few other IDO1 inhibitors are in preclinical development, including Trp analogs, imidazoles, phenyl benzenesulfonylhydrazides, N-hydroxyamidines, and tryptanthrin derivatives [84]. These compounds offer novel scaffolds for central nerve system (CNS) optimization, providing abundant possibilities for developing highly specific IDO1 inhibitors.

IDO1 peptide vaccines

Previous studies have found that IDO1 peptides elicit specific CD8$^+$ T cells that recognize and kill IDO1-expressing tumor cells and DCs and simultaneously enhance other T-cell responses [85]. In a phase 1 trial to evaluate the efficacy and safety of IDO1 vaccines, 15 patients with advanced NSCLC were injected with an IDO1-derived human leukocyte antigen A2-restricted epitope. The median overall survival was 25.9 months with no grade 3 or 4 toxicities. Furthermore, all treated patients had a significantly reduced Treg cell population after the sixth dose of vaccine [86]. Based on these promising results and distinct mechanisms of action, an additional phase 1 trial combining IDO1 vaccines with CTLA-4 inhibitor ipilimumab (Yervoy) for stage III or

IV melanoma patients and a phase 1/2 clinical trial that tests a combination treatment with a PD-1 monoclonal antibody (nivolumab) and a PD-L1–IDO1 peptide vaccine, have been initiated. Other potential strategies, such as combining IDO1 inhibitors with IDO1 vaccines may also produce synergistic anti-tumor effects [87].

IDO1 expression inhibitors

Gene expression is often repressed by microRNAs. Our group analyzed IDO1 downregulation by microRNA-153 (miR-153) in colon cancer cells and the association of IDO1 and miR-153 expression with colorectal patient survival [18]. We found that IDO1 is highly expressed in colorectal tumors and is inversely associated with patient survival. miR-153 directly inhibits IDO1 expression by targeting its 3′ untranslated region in colon cancer cells, yet miR-153 overexpression does not affect colon cancer cell survival, apoptosis, or colony formation. When colon cancer cells are targeted by chimeric antigen receptor (CAR) T cells, miR-153 overexpression within tumor cells significantly enhances T cell killing in vitro and suppresses xenograft tumor growth in mice. These findings indicate that miR-153 is a tumor-suppressive miRNA that enhances CAR T cell immunotherapy and supports the combinatorial use of IDO1 inhibitors and CAR T cells in treating solid tumors [18].

Conclusions

IDO1 has diverse biological roles in immune suppression and tumor progression, rendering it an attractive target in cancer therapeutic development. IDO1 inhibitors may serve as an "immunometabolic" adjuvant to enhance systemic immune responses and turn immunologically "cold" tumors "hot." Targeting IDO1 represents a therapeutic opportunity in cancer immunotherapy beyond checkpoint blockade [88–90] or adoptive transfer of CAR T cells [91–95]. Although IDO1 inhibitor monotherapies have shown disappointing efficacy, combinations of IDO1 inhibitors with conventional treatments show satisfactory efficacy in several trials. We note that IDO1 inhibitors suffered major setbacks in recent clinical trials. For the pivotal phase 3 ECHO-301/KEYNOTE-252 clinical trial (NCT02752074) that evaluated epacadostat in combination with pembrolizumab in patients with unresectable or metastatic melanoma, the study did not meet the primary endpoint of improving progression-free survival in the overall population compared with pembrolizumab monotherapy [96]. Two phase 3 trials (NCT03386838 and NCT03417037) evaluating the IDO1 inhibitor BMS-986205 in combination with nivolumab were also halted after re-evaluation. These negative results underscore that much about IDO1's role in immune suppression remains unresolved. Further studies on the basic biology of IDO1/2 and

TDO are essential to guide clinicians in identifying drug combinations that are more effective and selecting patients who are most likely to benefit from them. IDO1's role in neovascular development suggests that when clinical results of IDO1 inhibitors are assessed, the impact on tumor vasculature should be examined. Targeting IDO2 and TDO in addition to IDO1 may open new windows for cancer immunotherapy.

Abbreviations
AhR: Aryl hydrocarbon receptor; CAF: Cancer-associated fibroblast; CAR: Chimeric antigen receptor; CNS: Central nerve system; CTLA-4: Cytotoxic T cell antigen 4; DAMP: Damage-associated molecular pattern; DC: Dendritic cell; DCR: Disease control rate; GCN2: General control over nonderepressible 2; IDO: Indoleamine 2, 3-dioxygenase; IFN-γ: Interferon-γ; JAK: Janus kinase; Kyn: Kynurenine; MDSC: Myeloid-derived suppressor cell; MSC: Mesenchymal stromal cell; mTOR: Mammalian target of rapamycin; NF-κB: Nuclear factor kappa-light-chain-enhancer of activated B cells; NR: Not reported; ORR: Objective response rate; OS: Overall survival; PAMP: Pathogen-associated molecular pattern; PD: Progressive disease; PD-1: Programmed death receptor 1; PD-L1: Programmed death receptor ligand 1; PFS: Progression-free survival; PGE2: Prostaglandin E2; PKC: Protein kinase C; PR: Partial response; SD: Stable disease; STAT: Signal transducer and activator of transcription; TAM: Tumor-associated macrophage; TDO: Tryptophan 2,3-dioxygenase; TGF-β: Transforming growth factor β; TNF-α: Tumor necrosis factor α; Treg: Regulatory T cell; Trp: Tryptophan

Acknowledgements
The authors are grateful to Dr. Cassandra Talerico for editing the manuscript and providing critical comments.

Funding
This study was supported in part by an NIH R01 grant (CA177810 to YL); Natural Science Foundation of Guangdong Province grants (no. 2014A030313505 to ML, no. 2015A030315372 and no. 2017A030311004 to XM); and Science and Technology Program of Guangdong Province grants (no. 2015A020212034 to ML and no. 2014A050503062 to XM).

Authors' contributions
ML and YL designed the study and wrote the manuscript. All authors contributed to data analyses and interpretation, and read and approved the final manuscript.

Consent for publication
Not applicable.

Competing interests
The authors declare that they have no competing interests.

Author details
[1]State Key Laboratory of Respiratory Diseases, Guangzhou Institute of Respiratory Diseases, The First Affiliated Hospital of Guangzhou Medical University, Guangzhou Medical University, Guangzhou, China. [2]Department of Cancer Biology, Lerner Research Institute, Cleveland Clinic, Cleveland, OH, USA. [3]Institute for Brain Research and Rehabilitation, South China Normal University, Guangzhou, China. [4]Department of Stomatology, The Second Xiangya Hospital, Central South University, Changsha, China. [5]Department of Stomatology, Xiangya Hospital, Central South University, Changsha, China.

References
1. Prendergast GC, Smith C, Thomas S, Mandik-Nayak L, Laury-Kleintop L, Metz R, Muller AJ. Indoleamine 2,3-dioxygenase pathways of pathogenic inflammation and immune escape in cancer. Cancer Immunol Immunother. 2014;63(7):721–35.
2. Munn DH, Mellor AL. IDO in the tumor microenvironment: inflammation, counter-regulation, and tolerance. Trends Immunol. 2016;37(3):193–207.
3. Cheong JE, Sun L. Targeting the IDO1/TDO2-KYN-AhR pathway for cancer immunotherapy - challenges and opportunities. Trends Pharmacol Sci. 2018; 39(3):307–25.
4. Yeung AW, Terentis AC, King NJ, Thomas SR. Role of indoleamine 2,3-dioxygenase in health and disease. Clin Sci (Lond). 2015;129(7):601–72.
5. Yoshida R, Urade Y, Tokuda M, Hayaishi O. Induction of indoleamine 2,3-dioxygenase in mouse lung during virus infection. Proc Natl Acad Sci USA. 1979;76(8):4084–6.
6. Munn DH, Mellor AL. Indoleamine 2,3-dioxygenase and tumor-induced tolerance. J Clin Invest. 2007;117(5):1147–54.
7. Munn DH, Shafizadeh E, Attwood JT, Bondarev I, Pashine A, Mellor AL. Inhibition of T cell proliferation by macrophage tryptophan catabolism. J Exp Med. 1999;189(9):1363–72.
8. Hwu P, Du MX, Lapointe R, Do M, Taylor MW, Young HA. Indoleamine 2,3-dioxygenase production by human dendritic cells results in the inhibition of T cell proliferation. J Immunol. 2000;164(7):3596–9.
9. Chung DJ, Rossi M, Romano E, Ghith J, Yuan J, Munn DH, Young JW. Indoleamine 2,3-dioxygenase-expressing mature human monocyte-derived dendritic cells expand potent autologous regulatory T cells. Blood. 2009; 114(3):555–63.
10. Munn DH, Mellor AL. Indoleamine 2,3 dioxygenase and metabolic control of immune responses. Trends Immunol. 2013;34(3):137–43.
11. Mondal A, Smith C, DuHadaway JB, Sutanto-Ward E, Prendergast GC, Bravo-Nuevo A, Muller AJ. IDO1 is an integral mediator of inflammatory neovascularization. EBioMedicine. 2016;14:74–82.
12. Banzola I, Mengus C, Wyler S, Hudolin T, Manzella G, Chiarugi A, Boldorini R, Sais G, Schmidli TS, Chiffi G, et al. Expression of indoleamine 2,3-dioxygenase induced by IFN-gamma and TNF-alpha as potential biomarker of prostate cancer progression. Front Immunol. 2018;9:1051.
13. Holmgaard RB, Zamarin D, Munn DH, Wolchok JD, Allison JP. Indoleamine 2,3-dioxygenase is a critical resistance mechanism in antitumor T cell immunotherapy targeting CTLA-4. J Exp Med. 2013;210(7):1389–402.
14. Marin-Acevedo JA, Dholaria B, Soyano AE, Knutson KL, Chumsri S, Lou Y. Next generation of immune checkpoint therapy in cancer: new developments and challenges. J Hematol Oncol. 2018;11(1):39.
15. Prendergast GC, Malachowski WP, DuHadaway JB, Muller AJ. Discovery of IDO1 Inhibitors: From Bench to Bedside. Cancer Res. 2017;77(24):6795–811.
16. Rohrig UF, Majjigapu SR, Vogel P, Zoete V, Michielin O. Challenges in the discovery of indoleamine 2,3-dioxygenase 1 (IDO1) inhibitors. J Med Chem. 2015;58(24):9421–37.
17. Ladomersky E, Zhai L, Lenzen A, Lauing KL, Qian J, Scholtens DM, Gritsina G, Sun X, Liu Y, Yu F, et al. IDO1 inhibition synergizes with radiation and PD-1 blockade to durably increase survival against advanced glioblastoma. Clin Cancer Res. 2018;
18. Huang Q, Xia J, Wang L, Wang X, Ma X, Deng Q, Lu Y, Kumar M, Zhou Z, Li L, et al. miR-153 suppresses IDO1 expression and enhances CAR T cell immunotherapy. J Hematol Oncol. 2018;11(1):58.
19. Ninomiya S, Narala N, Huye L, Yagyu S, Savoldo B, Dotti G, Heslop HE, Brenner MK, Rooney CM, Ramos CA. Tumor indoleamine 2,3-dioxygenase (IDO) inhibits CD19-CAR T cells and is downregulated by lymphodepleting drugs. Blood. 2015;125(25):3905–16.
20. Muller AJ, DuHadaway JB, Donover PS, Sutanto-Ward E, Prendergast GC. Inhibition of indoleamine 2,3-dioxygenase, an immunoregulatory target of the cancer suppression gene Bin1, potentiates cancer chemotherapy. Nat Med. 2005;11(3):312–9.
21. Muller AJ, Sharma MD, Chandler PR, Duhadaway JB, Everhart ME, Johnson BA 3rd, Kahler DJ, Pihkala J, Soler AP, Munn DH, et al. Chronic inflammation that facilitates tumor progression creates local immune suppression by inducing indoleamine 2,3 dioxygenase. Proc Natl Acad Sci USA. 2008; 105(44):17073–8.
22. Balachandran VP, Cavnar MJ, Zeng S, Bamboat ZM, Ocuin LM, Obaid H, Sorenson EC, Popow R, Ariyan C, Rossi F, et al. Imatinib potentiates

antitumor T cell responses in gastrointestinal stromal tumor through the inhibition of Ido. Nat Med. 2011;17(9):1094–100.

23. Metz R, Rust S, Duhadaway JB, Mautino MR, Munn DH, Vahanian NN, Link CJ, Prendergast GC. IDO inhibits a tryptophan sufficiency signal that stimulates mTOR: A novel IDO effector pathway targeted by D-1-methyl-tryptophan. Oncoimmunology. 2012;1(9):1460–8.

24. Li Q, Harden JL, Anderson CD, Egilmez NK. Tolerogenic phenotype of IFN-gamma-induced IDO+ dendritic cells is maintained via an autocrine IDO-kynurenine/AhR-IDO loop. J Immunol. 2016;197(3):962–70.

25. Munn DH, Sharma MD, Baban B, Harding HP, Zhang Y, Ron D, Mellor AL. GCN2 kinase in T cells mediates proliferative arrest and anergy induction in response to indoleamine 2,3-dioxygenase. Immunity. 2005;22(5):633–42.

26. Prendergast GC, Mondal A, Dey S, Laury-Kleintop LD, Muller AJ. Inflammatory reprogramming with IDO1 inhibitors: turning immunologically unresponsive 'cold' tumors 'hot'. Trends Cancer. 2018;4(1):38–58.

27. Smith C, Chang MY, Parker KH, Beury DW, DuHadaway JB, Flick HE, Boulden J, Sutanto-Ward E, Soler AP, Laury-Kleintop LD, et al. IDO is a nodal pathogenic driver of lung cancer and metastasis development. Cancer Discov. 2012;2(8):722–35.

28. Hennequart M, Pilotte L, Cane S, Hoffmann D, Stroobant V, Plaen E, Van den Eynde BJ. Constitutive IDO1 expression in human tumors is driven by cyclooxygenase-2 and mediates intrinsic immune resistance. Cancer Immunol Res. 2017;5(8):695–709.

29. Pallotta MT, Orabona C, Volpi C, Vacca C, Belladonna ML, Bianchi R, Servillo G, Brunacci C, Calvitti M, Bicciato S, et al. Indoleamine 2,3-dioxygenase is a signaling protein in long-term tolerance by dendritic cells. Nat Immunol. 2011;12(9):870–8.

30. Wang LT, Chiou SS, Chai CY, Hsi E, Yokoyama KK, Wang SN, Huang SK, Hsu SH. Intestine-specific homeobox gene ISX integrates IL6 signaling, tryptophan catabolism, and immune suppression. Cancer Res. 2017;77(15):4065–77.

31. Song X, Zhang Y, Zhang L, Song W, Shi L. Hypoxia enhances indoleamine 2,3-dioxygenase production in dendritic cells. Oncotarget. 2018;9(14):11572–80.

32. Ravishankar B, Liu H, Shinde R, Chaudhary K, Xiao W, Bradley J, Koritzinsky M, Madaio MP, McGaha TL. The amino acid sensor GCN2 inhibits inflammatory responses to apoptotic cells promoting tolerance and suppressing systemic autoimmunity. Proc Natl Acad Sci USA. 2015;112(34):10774–9.

33. Xie DL, Wu J, Lou YL, Zhong XP. Tumor suppressor TSC1 is critical for T-cell anergy. Proc Natl Acad Sci USA. 2012;109(35):14152–7.

34. Pollizzi KN, Powell JD. Regulation of T cells by mTOR: the known knowns and the known unknowns. Trends Immunol. 2015;36(1):13–20.

35. Eleftheriadis T, Pissas G, Antoniadi G, Liakopoulos V, Tsogka K, Sounidaki M, Stefanidis I. Differential effects of the two amino acid sensing systems, the GCN2 kinase and the mTOR complex 1, on primary human alloreactive CD4(+) T-cells. Int J Mol Med. 2016;37(5):1412–20.

36. Vogel CF, Goth SR, Dong B, Pessah IN, Matsumura F. Aryl hydrocarbon receptor signaling mediates expression of indoleamine 2,3-dioxygenase. Biochem Biophys Res Commun. 2008;375(3):331–5.

37. Opitz CA, Litzenburger UM, Sahm F, Ott M, Tritschler I, Trump S, Schumacher T, Jestaedt L, Schrenk D, Weller M, et al. An endogenous tumour-promoting ligand of the human aryl hydrocarbon receptor. Nature. 2011;478(7368):197–203.

38. Grohmann U, Puccetti P. The coevolution of IDO1 and AhR in the emergence of regulatory T-cells in mammals. Front Immunol. 2015;6:58.

39. Godin-Ethier J, Hanafi LA, Piccirillo CA, Lapointe R. Indoleamine 2,3-dioxygenase expression in human cancers: clinical and immunologic perspectives. Clin Cancer Res. 2011;17(22):6985–91.

40. Ferdinande L, Decaestecker C, Verset L, Mathieu A, Moles Lopez X, Negulescu AM, Van Maerken T, Salmon I, Cuvelier CA, Demetter P. Clinicopathological significance of indoleamine 2,3-dioxygenase 1 expression in colorectal cancer. Br J Cancer. 2012;106(1):141–7.

41. Hornyak L, Dobos N, Koncz G, Karanyi Z, Pall D, Szabo Z, Halmos G, Szekvolgyi L. The role of indoleamine-2,3-dioxygenase in cancer development, diagnostics, and therapy. Front Immunol. 2018;9:151.

42. Vigneron N, van Baren N, Van den Eynde BJ. Expression profile of the human IDO1 protein, a cancer drug target involved in tumoral immune resistance. Oncoimmunology. 2015;4(5):e1003012.

43. Gao J, Xu K, Liu H, Liu G, Bai M, Peng C, Li T, Yin Y. Impact of the gut microbiota on intestinal immunity mediated by tryptophan metabolism. Front Cell Infect Microbiol. 2018;8:13.

44. Fallarino F, Grohmann U, You S, McGrath BC, Cavener DR, Vacca C, Orabona C, Bianchi R, Belladonna ML, Volpi C, et al. The combined effects of tryptophan starvation and tryptophan catabolites down-regulate T cell receptor zeta-chain and induce a regulatory phenotype in naive T cells. J Immunol. 2006;176(11):6752–61.

45. Frumento G, Rotondo R, Tonetti M, Damonte G, Benatti U, Ferrara GB. Tryptophan-derived catabolites are responsible for inhibition of T and natural killer cell proliferation induced by indoleamine 2,3-dioxygenase. J Exp Med. 2002;196(4):459–68.

46. Fallarino F, Grohmann U, Hwang KW, Orabona C, Vacca C, Bianchi R, Belladonna ML, Fioretti MC, Alegre ML, Puccetti P. Modulation of tryptophan catabolism by regulatory T cells. Nat Immunol. 2003;4(12):1206–12.

47. Wainwright DA, Balyasnikova IV, Chang AL, Ahmed AU, Moon KS, Auffinger B, Tobias AL, Han Y, Lesniak MS. IDO expression in brain tumors increases the recruitment of regulatory T cells and negatively impacts survival. Clin Cancer Res. 2012;18(22):6110–21.

48. Munn DH, Sharma MD, Johnson TS, Rodriguez P. IDO, PTEN-expressing Tregs and control of antigen-presentation in the murine tumor microenvironment. Cancer Immunol Immunother. 2017;66(8):1049–58.

49. Holmgaard RB, Zamarin D, Li Y, Gasmi B, Munn DH, Allison JP, Merghoub T, Wolchok JD. Tumor-Expressed IDO Recruits and Activates MDSCs in a Treg-Dependent Manner. Cell Rep. 2015;13(2):412–24.

50. Yu J, Du W, Yan F, Wang Y, Li H, Cao S, Yu W, Shen C, Liu J, Ren X. Myeloid-derived suppressor cells suppress antitumor immune responses through IDO expression and correlate with lymph node metastasis in patients with breast cancer. J Immunol. 2013;190(7):3783–97.

51. Yu J, Wang Y, Yan F, Zhang P, Li H, Zhao H, Yan C, Yan F, Ren X. Noncanonical NF-kappaB activation mediates STAT3-stimulated IDO upregulation in myeloid-derived suppressor cells in breast cancer. J Immunol. 2014;193(5):2574–86.

52. Cheng JT, Deng YN, Yi HM, Wang GY, Fu BS, Chen WJ, Liu W, Tai Y, Peng YW, Zhang Q. Hepatic carcinoma-associated fibroblasts induce IDO-producing regulatory dendritic cells through IL-6-mediated STAT3 activation. Oncogenesis. 2016;5:e198.

53. Ling W, Zhang J, Yuan Z, Ren G, Zhang L, Chen X, Rabson AB, Roberts AI, Wang Y, Shi Y. Mesenchymal stem cells use IDO to regulate immunity in tumor microenvironment. Cancer Res. 2014;74(5):1576–87.

54. Riesenberg R, Weiler C, Spring O, Eder M, Buchner A, Popp T, Castro M, Kammerer R, Takikawa O, Hatz RA, et al. Expression of indoleamine 2,3-dioxygenase in tumor endothelial cells correlates with long-term survival of patients with renal cell carcinoma. Clin Cancer Res. 2007; 13(23):6993–7002.

55. Seeber A, Klinglmair G, Fritz J, Steinkohl F, Zimmer KC, Aigner F, Horninger W, Gastl G, Zelger B, Brunner A, et al. High IDO-1 expression in tumor endothelial cells is associated with response to immunotherapy in metastatic renal cell carcinoma. Cancer Sci. 2018;109(5):1583–91.

56. Patel SA, Minn AJ. Combination cancer therapy with immune checkpoint blockade: mechanisms and strategies. Immunity. 2018;48(3):417–33.

57. Marin-Acevedo JA, Soyano AE, Dholaria B, Knutson KL, Lou Y. Cancer immunotherapy beyond immune checkpoint inhibitors. J Hematol Oncol. 2018;11(1):8.

58. Sharma MD, Shinde R, McGaha TL, Huang L, Holmgaard RB, Wolchok JD, Mautino MR, Celis E, Sharpe AH, Francisco LM, et al. The PTEN pathway in Tregs is a critical driver of the suppressive tumor microenvironment. Sci Adv. 2015;1(10):e1500845.

59. Rodrigues CP, Ferreira AC, Pinho MP, de Moraes CJ, Bergami-Santos PC, Barbuto JA. Tolerogenic IDO(+) dendritic cells are induced by PD-1-expressing mast cells. Front Immunol. 2016;7:9.

60. Toulmonde M, Penel N, Adam J, Chevreau C, Blay JY, Le Cesne A, Bompas E, Piperno-Neumann S, Cousin S, Grellety T, et al. Use of PD-1 targeting, macrophage infiltration, and IDO pathway activation in sarcomas: a phase 2 clinical trial. JAMA Oncol. 2018;4(1):93–7.

61. Wei L, Zhu S, Li M, Li F, Wei F, Liu J, Ren X. High indoleamine 2,3-dioxygenase is correlated with microvessel density and worse prognosis in breast cancer. Front Immunol. 2018;9:724.

62. York A. Microbiome: Gut microbiota sways response to cancer immunotherapy. Nat Rev Microbiol. 2018;16(3):121.

63. Yi M, Yu S, Qin S, Liu Q, Xu H, Zhao W, Chu Q, Wu K. Gut microbiome modulates efficacy of immune checkpoint inhibitors. J Hematol Oncol. 2018;11(1):47.

64. Gopalakrishnan V, Spencer CN, Nezi L, Reuben A, Andrews MC, Karpinets TV, Prieto PA, Vicente D, Hoffman K, Wei SC, et al. Gut microbiome modulates response to anti-PD-1 immunotherapy in melanoma patients. Science. 2018; 359(6371):97–103.

65. Routy B, Le Chatelier E, Derosa L, Duong CPM, Alou MT, Daillere R, Fluckiger A, Messaoudene M, Rauber C, Roberti MP, et al. Gut microbiome influences efficacy of PD-1-based immunotherapy against epithelial tumors. Science. 2018;359(6371):91–7.

66. Pushalkar S, Hundeyin M, Daley D, Zambirinis CP, Kurz E, Mishra A, Mohan N, Aykut B, Usyk M, Torres LE, et al. The pancreatic cancer microbiome promotes oncogenesis by induction of innate and adaptive immune suppression. Cancer Discov. 2018;

67. Pavlova T, Vidova V, Bienertova-Vasku J, Janku P, Almasi M, Klanova J, Spacil Z. Urinary intermediates of tryptophan as indicators of the gut microbial metabolism. Anal Chim Acta. 2017;987:72–80.

68. Saxton RA, Sabatini DM. mTOR signaling in growth, metabolism, and disease. Cell. 2017;169(2):361–71.

69. Soliman HH, Minton SE, Han HS, Ismail-Khan R, Neuger A, Khambati F, Noyes D, Lush R, Chiappori AA, Roberts JD, et al. A phase I study of indoximod in patients with advanced malignancies. Oncotarget. 2016;7(16): 22928–38.

70. Soliman HH, Jackson E, Neuger T, Dees EC, Harvey RD, Han H, Ismail-Khan R, Minton S, Vahanian NN, Link C, et al. A first in man phase I trial of the oral immunomodulator, indoximod, combined with docetaxel in patients with metastatic solid tumors. Oncotarget. 2014;5(18):8136–46.

71. Berrong Z, Mkrtichyan M, Ahmad S, Webb M, Mohamed E, Okoev G, Matevosyan A, Shrimali R, Eid RA, Hammond S, et al. Antigen-specific antitumor responses induced by OX40 agonist are enhanced by the IDO inhibitor indoximod. Cancer Immunol Res. 2018;6(2):201–8.

72. Dhiman V, Giri KK, SP S, Zainuddin M, Rajagopal S, Mullangi R. Determination of epacadostat, a novel IDO1 inhibitor in mouse plasma by LC-MS/MS and its application to a pharmacokinetic study in mice. Biomed Chromatogr. 2017;31(2) https://doi.org/10.1002/bmc.3794.

73. Jochems C, Fantini M, Fernando RI, Kwilas AR, Donahue RN, Lepone LM, Grenga I, Kim YS, Brechbiel MW, Gulley JL, et al. The IDO1 selective inhibitor epacadostat enhances dendritic cell immunogenicity and lytic ability of tumor antigen-specific T cells. Oncotarget. 2016;7(25):37762–72.

74. Beatty GL, O'Dwyer PJ, Clark J, Shi JG, Bowman KJ, Scherle PA, Newton RC, Schaub R, Maleski J, Leopold L, et al. First-in-human phase I study of the oral inhibitor of indoleamine 2,3-dioxygenase-1 epacadostat (INCB024360) in patients with advanced solid malignancies. Clin Cancer Res. 2017;23(13): 3269–76.

75. Kristeleit R, Davidenko I, Shirinkin V, El-Khouly F, Bondarenko I, Goodheart MJ, Gorbunova V, Penning CA, Shi JG, Liu X, et al. A randomised, open-label, phase 2 study of the IDO1 inhibitor epacadostat (INCB024360) versus tamoxifen as therapy for biochemically recurrent (CA-125 relapse)-only epithelial ovarian cancer, primary peritoneal carcinoma, or fallopian tube cancer. Gynecol Oncol. 2017;146(3):484–90.

76. Yue EW, Sparks R, Polam P, Modi D, Douty B, Wayland B, Glass B, Takvorian A, Glenn J, Zhu W, et al. INCB24360 (Epacadostat), a highly potent and selective indoleamine-2,3-dioxygenase 1 (IDO1) inhibitor for immuno-oncology. ACS Med Chem Lett. 2017;8(5):486–91.

77. Yan D, Lin YW, Tan X. Heme-containing enzymes and inhibitors for tryptophan metabolism. Metallomics. 2017;9(9):1230–40.

78. Mautino MR, Jaipuri FA, Waldo J, Kumar S, Adams J, Van Allen C, Marcinowicz-Flick A, Munn D, Vahanian N, Link CJ. Abstract 491: NLG919, a novel indoleamine-2,3-dioxygenase (IDO)-pathway inhibitor drug candidate for cancer therapy. Cancer Res. 2013;73(8 Supplement):491.

79. Meng X, Du G, Ye L, Sun S, Liu Q, Wang H, Wang W, Wu Z, Tian J. Combinatorial antitumor effects of indoleamine 2,3-dioxygenase inhibitor NLG919 and paclitaxel in a murine B16-F10 melanoma model. Int J Immunopathol Pharmacol. 2017;30(3):215–26.

80. Mautino MR, Link CJ, Vahanian NN, Adams JT, Allen CV, Sharma MD, Johnson TS, Munn D. Abstract 5023: Synergistic antitumor effects of combinatorial immune checkpoint inhibition with anti-PD-1/PD-L antibodies and the IDO pathway inhibitors NLG-919 and indoximod in the context of active immunotherapy. Cancer Res. 2014;74(19 Supplement):5023.

81. Burris HA, Gordon MS, Hellmann MD, LoRusso P, Emens LA, Hodi FS, Lieu CH, Infante JR, Tsai FY-C, Eder JP, et al. A phase Ib dose escalation study of combined inhibition of IDO1 (GDC-0919) and PD-L1 (atezolizumab) in patients with locally advanced or metastatic solid tumors. J Clin Oncol. 2017;35(15_suppl):105.

82. Siu LL, Gelmon K, Chu Q, Pachynski R, Alese O, Basciano P, Walker J, Mitra P, Zhu L, Phillips P, et al. Abstract CT116: BMS-986205, an optimized indoleamine 2,3-dioxygenase 1 (IDO1) inhibitor, is well tolerated with potent pharmacodynamic (PD) activity, alone and in combination with nivolumab (nivo) in advanced cancers in a phase 1/2a trial. Cancer Res. 2017;77(13 Supplement):CT116.

83. Tumang J, Gomes B, Wythes M, Crosignani S, Bingham P, Bottemanne P, Cannelle H, Cauwenberghs S, Chaplin J, Dalvie D, et al. Abstract 4863: PF-06840003: a highly selective IDO-1 inhibitor that shows good in vivo efficacy in combination with immune checkpoint inhibitors. Cancer Res. 2016;76(14 Supplement):4863.

84. Dounay AB, Tuttle JB, Verhoest PR. Challenges and opportunities in the discovery of new therapeutics targeting the kynurenine pathway. J Med Chem. 2015;58(22):8762–82.

85. Andersen MH, Svane IM. Indoleamine 2,3-dioxygenase vaccination. Oncoimmunology. 2015;4(1):e983770.

86. Iversen TZ, Engell-Noerregaard L, Ellebaek E, Andersen R, Larsen SK, Bjoern J, Zeyher C, Gouttefangeas C, Thomsen BM, Holm B, et al. Long-lasting disease stabilization in the absence of toxicity in metastatic lung cancer patients vaccinated with an epitope derived from indoleamine 2,3 dioxygenase. Clin Cancer Res. 2014;20(1):221–32.

87. Vilgelm AE, Johnson DB, Richmond A. Combinatorial approach to cancer immunotherapy: strength in numbers. J Leukoc Biol. 2016;100(2):275–90.

88. Diggs LP, Hsueh EC. Utility of PD-L1 immunohistochemistry assays for predicting PD-1/PD-L1 inhibitor response. Biomark Res. 2017;5:12.

89. Liu B, Song Y, Liu D. Recent development in clinical applications of PD-1 and PD-L1 antibodies for cancer immunotherapy. J Hematol Oncol. 2017; 10(1):174.

90. Zhang X, Yang Y, Fan D, Xiong D. The development of bispecific antibodies and their applications in tumor immune escape. Exp Hematol Oncol. 2017;6:12.

91. Fan M, Li M, Gao L, Geng S, Wang J, Wang Y, Yan Z, Yu L. Chimeric antigen receptors for adoptive T cell therapy in acute myeloid leukemia. J Hematol Oncol. 2017;10(1):151.

92. Liu B, Song Y, Liu D. Clinical trials of CAR-T cells in China. J Hematol Oncol. 2017;10(1):166.

93. Qin L, Zhao R, Li P. Incorporation of functional elements enhances the antitumor capacity of CAR T cells. Exp Hematol Oncol. 2017;6:28.

94. Wei G, Ding L, Wang J, Hu Y, Huang H. Advances of CD19-directed chimeric antigen receptor-modified T cells in refractory/relapsed acute lymphoblastic leukemia. Exp Hematol Oncol. 2017;6:10.

95. Zhang C, Liu J, Zhong JF, Zhang X. Engineering CAR-T cells. Biomark Res. 2017;5:22.

96. Mullard A. IDO takes a blow. Nature Rev Drug Disc. 2018;17(5):307.

11

Combating head and neck cancer metastases by targeting Src using multifunctional nanoparticle-based saracatinib

Liwei Lang[1], Chloe Shay[2], Yuanping Xiong[1], Parth Thakkar[3], Ron Chemmalakuzhy[3], Xuli Wang[4*] and Yong Teng[1,5,6*] (iD)

Abstract

Background: Inhibition of metastasis of head and neck squamous cell carcinoma (HNSCC) is one of the most important challenges in cancer treatment. Src, a non-receptor tyrosine kinase, has been implicated as a key promoter in tumor progression and metastasis of HNSCC. However, Src therapy for HNSCC is limited by lack of efficient in vivo delivery and underlying mechanisms remain elusive.

Methods: Src knockdown cells were achieved by lentiviral-mediated interference. Cell migration and invasion were examined by wound healing and Transwell assays. Protein levels were determined by Western blot and/or immunohistochemistry. The Src inhibitor saracatinib was loaded into self-assembling nanoparticles by the solvent evaporation method. An experimental metastasis mouse model was generated to investigate the drug efficacy in metastasis.

Results: Blockade of Src kinase activity by saracatinib effectively suppressed invasion and metastasis of HNSCC. Mechanistic assessment of the drug effects in HNSCC cells showed that saracatinib induced suppression of Src-dependent invasion/metastasis through downregulating the expression levels of Vimentin and Snail proteins. In tests in mice, saracatinib loaded into the novel multifunctional nanoparticles exhibited superior effects on suppression of HNSCC metastasis compared with the free drug, which is mainly attributed to highly specific and efficient tumor-targeted drug delivery system.

Conclusions: These findings and advances are of great importance to the development of Src-targeted nanomedicine as a more effective therapy for metastatic HNSCC.

Keywords: Src, Saracatinib, Nanoparticles, HNSCC, Metastasis

Background

More than 90% of tumors in the head and neck are squamous carcinomas (HNSCC) that arise in the paranasal sinuses, nasal cavity, oral cavity, pharynx, and larynx [1]. About two-thirds of patients with HNSCC present with advanced-stage disease (stages III and IV), and the high rate of metastasis is highly associated with

a poor 5-year survival rate [2, 3]. Despite significant improvements in multiple-modality therapy with surgery, chemotherapy, and radiation, long-term survival rates in patients with advanced-stage HNSCC have not increased significantly in the past few decades [4]. The poor clinical outcomes reveal an obvious and urgent need to develop more effective and tolerated treatments against HNSCC, especially for aggressive tumors.

Modern research is now focusing on seeking specific molecular targets involved in the development and procession of cancer in an attempt to develop more officious and selective treatments. Src, a member of Src

* Correspondence: xuli.wang@utah.edu; yteng@augusta.edu
[4]Department of Radiology and Imaging Sciences, School of Medicine, University of Utah, 201 Presidents Cir, Salt Lake City, UT 84112, USA
[1]Department of Oral Biology, Dental College of Georgia, Augusta University, Augusta, GA, USA
Full list of author information is available at the end of the article

family of non-receptor tyrosine kinases (SFKs), is often activated by direct or indirect interaction with receptor tyrosine kinases (RTK), such as epidermal growth factor receptor (EGFR), platelet-derived growth factor receptor (PDGFR), fibroblast growth factor receptor (FGFR), and insulin-like growth factor 1 receptor (IGF-1R), as well as G-protein-coupled receptors (GPCRs), cytokines, integrins, and others [5]. It appears that Src acts as a critical molecular switch in regulating signal transduction for many fundamental cellular processes by a diverse set of cell surface receptors in the context of a variety of cellular environments. Overexpression and hyperactivation of Src have been found in a wide variety of human cancers, including HNSCC [5, 6]. Additionally, the extent of increased Src activity often correlates with malignant potential and patient survival [7]. Multiple signaling pathways converge on Src activation to epithelial-mesenchymal transition (EMT) phenotypic features to promote tumor cell metastasis [8]. In mice models of breast cancer, inhibition of Src kinase activity can improve survival through suppressing metastasis [9]. In HNSCC, Src is activated following EGF stimulation and decreases cell migration and invasion in treatment with Src inhibitors [10, 11]. The involvement of Src in tumor progression and metastasis has generated considerable interest in Src as a therapeutic strategy to treat metastatic disease.

Src-targeting agents, including dasatinib and saracatinib (AZD0530), are currently in clinical development for patients with solid tumors. Dasatinib, a potent oral tyrosine kinase inhibitor which targets Src and other several kinases [7], has shown a marked efficacy in patients with chronic myeloid leukemia (CML) as first-line treatment [12]. The capacity of dasatinib to block migration and invasion without affecting proliferation and survival is demonstrated in human melanoma cells [13]. Dasatinib is also reported to suppress migration and invasion of HNSCC cells, coupled with the inhibition of Src and downstream mediators of cell adhesion, such as focal adhesion kinase (FAK) [11]. Dasatinib as a single agent has modest clinical activity with liver failure on many types of solid tumors, including non-small cell lung cancer, prostate cancer, and breast cancer [14]. Saracatinib, originally developed by AstraZeneca, is a novel anilinoquinazoline inhibiting deregulated elevated Src kinase activity in a wide range of cancer cells, such as colorectal, ovary, prostate, and breast cancer [7, 15–17]. Several preclinical reports suggest that saracatinib has potent anti-migratory and anti-invasive effects in endocrine-resistant breast cancer cells [18] and significantly suppressed the metastatic nature of bladder cancer in a murine model [19]. Although saracatinib was evaluated in phase I/II clinical trials for advanced stage HNSCC and other various types of cancer [20], the anti-cancer efficacy was not sufficiently promising to justify

continued accrual to active trials. Therefore, developing a novel saracatinib-based strategy would open a new avenue for Src-targeted therapy.

Physicochemical and pharmacokinetic profiles of anti-cancer drugs render optimal delivery challenging. Moreover, distribution, biotransformation, and clearance of anticancer drugs in the body must be overcome to deliver therapeutic agents to tumor cells in vivo [21]. Nanoparticles (NPs) have shown promise as both drug delivery vehicles and direct anticancer systems, based on the quantum properties and the ability to carry and absorption [22]. Most solid tumors possess unique pathophysiological characteristics that are not observed in normal tissues or organs (e.g., extensive angiogenesis, low pH and hypoxia), which greatly increase production of a number of the tumor site-specific delivery of NPs. Numerous studies have shown that both tissue and cell distribution profiles of anticancer drugs can be controlled by their entrapment in NPs [23, 24].

In the present study, we show that Src is one of the most targetable molecules involved in invasion and metastasis of HNSCC, and saracatinib can significantly suppress the invasive and metastatic phenotype through inhibiting Src kinase activity and its mediated metastatic signaling in HNSCC cells. We also designed and synthesized novel multifunctional NPs for selective release of saracatinib into head and neck tumor cells and evaluated the anti-tumor efficacy and efficiency of saracatinib-loaded NPs (Nano-sar) in mice. Our studies reveal that Nano-sar has superior anticancer effects than the free drug through suppressing head and neck tumor metastasis more efficiently. The tumor site-specific delivery of NPs, especially with the use of saracatinib, would be straightforwardly extended from HNSCC to other types of solid tumors.

Methods

Cell lines and standard assays

HNSCC cell lines HN6, HN8, and HN12 were maintained in Dulbecco's Modified Eagle's Medium (DMEM) containing 10% fetal bovine serum as previously described [25, 26]. HN6 was derived from tongue squamous cell carcinoma. HN8 and HN12 were derived from the metastatic lymph node site from oral cavity and tongue squamous cell carcinoma, respectively. The cell passage number less than 10 was used for experiments. Cell proliferation was determined by CellTiter 96® AQueous One Solution Cell Proliferation Assay (MTS) (Promega, Madison, WI), and invasion was determined by Transwells (BD biosciences, San Jose, CA) with 8-μm pore size filters covered with Matrigel. Transfection and infection, colony formation, and scratch-wound healing were carried out as previously described [7, 27–29].

Constructs, reagents, and antibodies

pLKO.1 lentiviral vectors harboring short hairpin RNAs (shRNAs) targeting Src or green fluorescent protein (GFP) were obtained from Open Biosystems (Huntsville, AL). Saracatinib and dasatinib were purchased from Selleckchem (Houston, TX). For Western blot, antibodies that recognize p-Src (Tyr416) and Src were purchased from Cell Signaling Technology (Beverly, MA). β-Actin antibody was purchased from Sigma-Aldrich (St Louis, MO). Epithelial-Mesenchymal Transition (EMT) Antibody Sampler Kit (#9782) and Tight Junction Antibody Sampler Kit (#8683) were purchased from Cell Signaling Technology (Beverly, MA).

Western blot assay

The protein levels for the biomarkers were semi-quantified by Western blot analysis as previously described [29, 30]. Electrophoresis was performed on 10% SDS-PAGE gel, and the proteins were transferred to nitrocellulose membrane. The membranes were incubated with the primary antibodies overnight at 4 °C and with secondary antibody for 1 h at room temperature. The antigen-antibody complexes were then visualized using Clarity™ Western ECL Substrate (Bio-Rad, Hercules, CA). The protein bands were quantified by densitometry analysis.

Solid-phase peptide synthesis

Synthesis of the peptide was carried out using the Fmoc strategy manually in a glass reaction vessel fitted with a sintered glass frit using 2-chlorotritylchloride. Coupling reactions were performed manually by using 2 equiv. of N-Fmoc-protected amino acid (relative to the resin loading) activated in situ with 2 equiv. of PyBOP and 4 equiv. of diisopropylethylamine (DIPEA) in DMF (10 mL/g resin). The coupling efficiency was assessed by Kaiser test. N-Fmoc protecting groups were removed by treatment with a piperidine/DMF solution (1:4) for 10 min (10 mL/g resin). The process was repeated three times and the completeness of deprotection verified by UV absorption of the piperidine washings at 301 nm. Synthetic linear peptides were recovered directly upon acid cleavage. Before cleavage, the resin was washed thoroughly with methylene chloride. The linear peptides were then released from the resin by treatments with a solution of acetic acid/trifluoroethanol/methylene chloride (1:1:8, 10 mL/mg resin, 2 × 30 min). Hexane (5–10 volumes) was added to the collected filtrates, and the crude peptides were isolated after concentration as white solids. The residue was dissolved in the minimum of methylene chloride, and diethyl ether was added to precipitate peptides. Then, they were triturated and washed three times with diethyl ether to obtain crude materials. Peptide was further purified by preparative high-performance liquid chromatography (HPLC) prior to conjugation.

Synthesis of the polymeric drug carrier

Linear-dendritic mPEG-BMA4 was synthesized according to a method in literature [31, 32]. Under a nitrogen atmosphere, branched mPEG-BMA4 (1 equv. based on amino group), peptide (Ac-K(Boc) GFLG-OH, 1 equv.), HBTU (1 equv.), and HOBT (1 equv.) were added into a round flask and dissolved in anhydrous DMF. Then, DIPEA (2 equv.) was added dropwise under ice bath. The solution was stirred in ice bath for 30 min and at room temperature for 48 h. The solution was dialyzed against deionized water using dialysis membrane (MWCO = 2000). The final product was obtained via lyophilization.

Saracatinib-loading into NPs

Hydrophobic saracatinib was loaded into the NPs by the solvent evaporation method as described in literature [33, 34]. Briefly, drug (1.0 mg) and amphiphilic polymer (10 mg) were first dissolved in anhydrous chloroform/methanol (1/1) in a 10 mL round bottom flask. The solvent mixture was evaporated under vacuum to form a thin film. PBS buffer (1 mL) was added to re-hydrate the thin film, followed by 30 min of sonication. The unloaded drug was removed by running the NP solutions through centrifugal filter devices (MWCO: 3.5 kDa, Microcon®). The saracatinib-loaded formulation on the filters were recovered with PBS.

Characterization of NPs

The amount of drug loaded in the NPs was analyzed on a HPLC system (Agilent 1200 LC, Santa Clara, CA). The drug loading was calculated according to the calibration curve between the HPLC area values and concentrations of drug standard. The loading efficiency was defined as the ratio of drug loaded into NPs to the initial drug content. The size and size distribution of Nano-sar were measured by dynamic light scattering (DLS) instrument for three times with an acquisition time of 30 s at room temperature.

Drug release study

The drug release from Nano-sar was carried out in the solution with or without cathepsin B (CTSB). Cysteine solution in McIlvaine's buffer (10 mm) was added in equal volume of enzyme stock solution and pre-incubated at 37 °C for 5 min. NPs were incubated in the buffer at 37 °C for 48 h in the presence or absence of CTSB (100 nM, pH = 5.4). A drug release control study at physiological condition (without enzyme, pH 7.4) was also performed. At pre-determined time points, the samples were withdrawn and analyzed by reversed-phase HPLC (RP HPLC) with gradient elution.

Three-dimensional (3D) tumor spheroid invasion assay

The experiment was modified and carried out as previously described [35, 36]. Briefly, 2×10^4 HN12 cells were incubated overnight to form 3D spheroid in hanging droplet in a well of an inverted round bottom 96-well plate. Then, 150 µl mixture of Matrigel: DMEM without serum (1:1 ratio) was added in the well and solidified at 37 °C, followed by adding 150 µl complete culture medium containing double doses of drugs. After 3 days, spheroids from different treatments were imaged under a microscope.

Animal study

Six-week-old NOD.Cg-*Prkdcscid Il2rgtm1Wjl/SzJ* (NSG) mice were purchased from the Jackson Laboratory (Bar Harbor, ME, USA), and all animal experiments were approved by the Institutional Animal Care and Use Committee (IACUC) of Augusta University. To generate a metastasis model in NSG mice, 5×10^5 HN12 with a luciferase reporter gene were suspended in 100 µl of PBS/Matrigel (3:1) and injected into the right flank. When mean tumor volumes reached approximately 100 mm^3, mice were randomized to receive equal volume treatment of vehicle (sterile saline), the free drug saracatinib (20 mg/kg), or Nano-sar (at dose 10 mg/kg) by tail vein administration every other day for a total of 12 days. Tumor growth was measured externally every 4 days using vernier calipers as length × width^2 × 0.52. Mice were imaged for bioluminescent luciferase signal by an intraperitoneal injection of D-luciferin bioluminescent substrate (Sigma-Aldrich, St Louis, MO) using a Xenogen IVIS-200 In Vivo Imaging System (PerkinElmer, Waltham, MA). When the experiment was terminated, blood was collected via ocular vein for determination of serum Alanine Transaminase (ALT/GPT), Aspartate Transaminase (AST/GOP), and creatinine. ALT and AST were measured by EnzyChrom™ Alanine Transaminase Assay Kit and Aspartate Transaminase Assay kits (Bio-Assay System, Hayward, CA), respectively. Serum creatinine was measured by Creatinine Assay Kit (Cayman chemical, Ann Arbor, MI). The mice were then sacrificed, and the xenografts and the major organs (heart, intestine, liver, spleen, lung, and kidney) were removed for histopathological analysis with hematoxylin-and-eosin (H&E) staining.

Immunohistochemistry (IHC)

Paraffin-embedded xenografts were cut into 3 µm sections and mounted on slides, and IHC was performed as described previously [7, 37]. Briefly, tissue sections were blocked in 10% of normal goat serum after antigen retrieval in hot citrate buffer and were incubated with the primary antibodies against p-Src, Vimentin, and Snail, respectively. Immuno-reactivity was visualized by using

the DAB Kit (Vector Laboratories, Burlingame, CA, USA) according to the manufacturers' procedure, and images were reviewed and analyzed by a CCD camera (Olympus, Center Valley, PA). At least nine random microscopic fields were captured, and signal intensity was quantified using the Image pro-Plus6.0 software.

Statistical analysis

Treatment effects were evaluated using one-way ANOVA at each measurement time-point. To assess the longitudinal effect of treatment, a mixed model was employed to test the overall difference across all groups as well as between each pair of groups during the whole study period. Experiments shown are the means of multiple individual points from multiple experiments (± S.D.), and $p < 0.05$ was considered as statistically significant.

Results

Saracatinib strongly inhibits Src kinase activity and migration in HNSCC cells

To study the role of Src in cell movement, we depleted Src in high-invasive HNSCC cells (HN6, HN8, and HN12) by shRNAs. Lentivirus-mediated knockdown of Src remarkably reduced Src expression levels, leading to decreased migration compared with the control cells transfected with a shRNA against GFP (Fig. 1a, b). These results showed that loss of Src reduced migratory potential in HNSCC cells. We then treated HN6, HN8, and HN12 cells with dasatinib and saracatinib, which showed increased protein levels of Src upon drug treatment (Fig. 1c). However, dramatically decreased Src phosphorylation was observed in cells either treated with dasatinib or saracatinib (Fig. 1c). Saracatinib-induced Src inactivation was in a dose-dependent manner, and this inhibitory effect was more efficient than dasatinib at the same dosage (Fig. 1c). Moreover, a clear reduction in scratch-wound healing capability was noted in cells exposed to dasatinib or saracatinib (Fig. 1d), which was consistent with the observations in Src knockdown cells (Fig. 1b).

Saracatinib suppresses migration of mesenchymal-like HNSCC cells by inactivating Src-dependent Vimentin/Snail signaling

Src has been shown to play an important role in promoting EMT [8], which often contributes to cancer cell migration and invasion. We thus assessed whether loss of Src led to a reversal of EMT in HNSCC cells. HN6, HN8, and HN12 cell lines examined in this study were mesenchymal-like cells, and they switched to epithelial-like shape when loss of Src expression (Additional file 1: Figure S1A). Similar to the observations from Src knockdown cells, cells

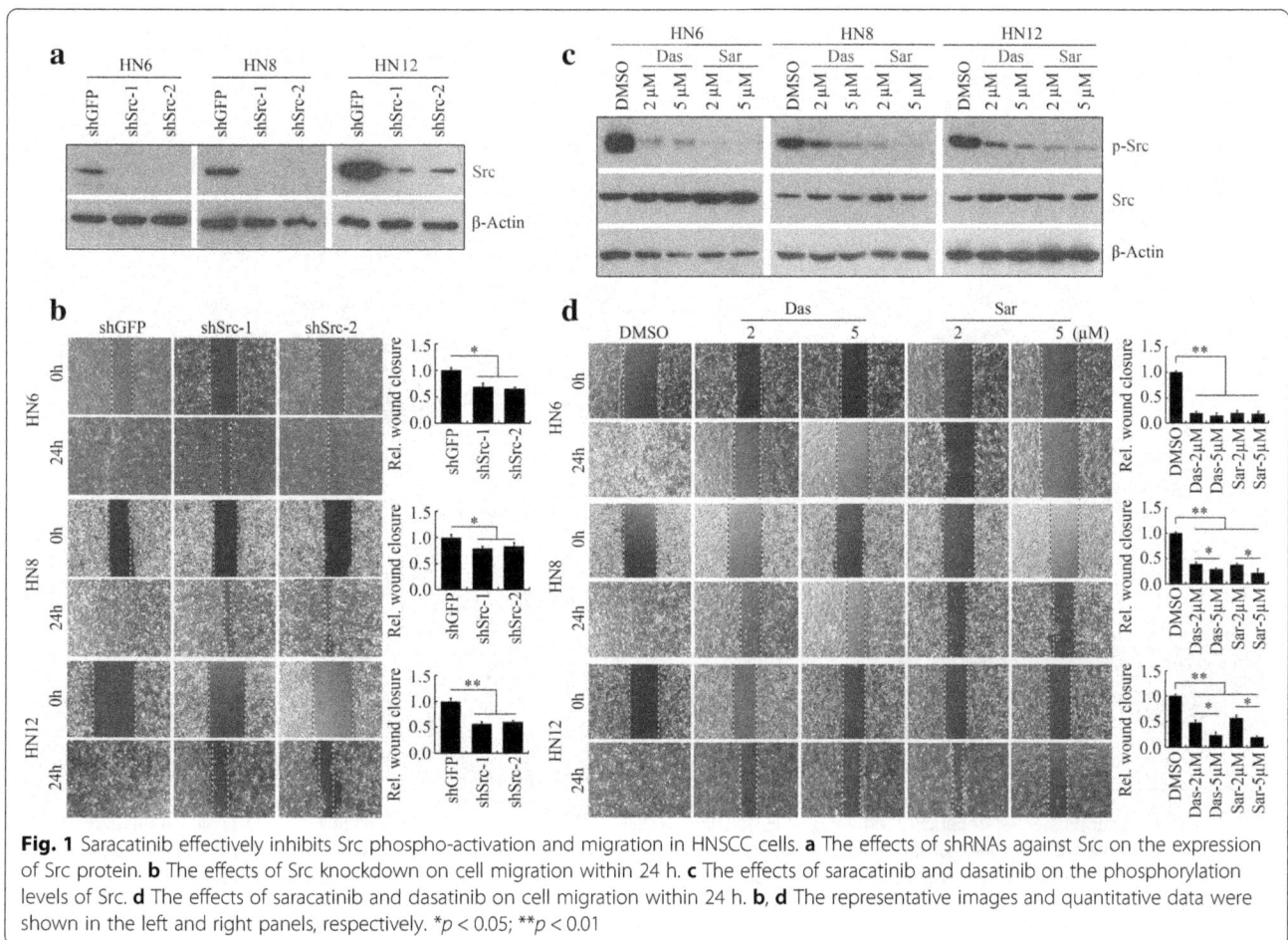

Fig. 1 Saracatinib effectively inhibits Src phospho-activation and migration in HNSCC cells. **a** The effects of shRNAs against Src on the expression of Src protein. **b** The effects of Src knockdown on cell migration within 24 h. **c** The effects of saracatinib and dasatinib on the phosphorylation levels of Src. **d** The effects of saracatinib and dasatinib on cell migration within 24 h. **b, d** The representative images and quantitative data were shown in the left and right panels, respectively. *$p < 0.05$; **$p < 0.01$

appeared to clump together with the Src inhibitor treatment (Additional file 1: Figure S1B). To understand the mechanism involved, we determined the molecules that were mostly involved in EMT process. This analysis showed a sharp decrease in protein levels of mesenchymal marker Vimentin in the presence of Src inhibitors, which was accompanied by downregulation of Snail (Fig. 2a, d). There were no significant changes in the protein levels of epithelial marker E-cadherin protein, indicating that E-cadherin does not contribute to HNSCC cell MET induced by Src inactivation (Fig. 2a). No consistent tendency of other EMT-related proteins (N-cadherin, β-catenin, Slug, and ZEB1) was observed in three cell lines in the presence and absence of Src inhibitors, excluding their common functions in drug-induced diminishment of EMT traits in mesenchymal-like HNSCC cells (Fig. 2a). We also examined tight junction-related proteins (Caludin1, CD2AP, ZO-1, ZO-2, and Afadin), which showed cell content-dependent changes in the treatment with Src inhibitors (Fig. 2b). To study whether saracatinib and dasatinib share a common mechanism to regulate cell motility through downregulation of Src-dependent Vimentin and

Snail expression, we determined these molecules in Src knockdown cells. Consistently, knockdown of Src was associated with decreased Vimentin and Snail levels (Fig. 2c, d).

Synthesis and characterization of Nano-sar

Saracatinib suppressed Src kinase activity more efficiently than dasatinib in HNSCC cells (Fig. 1b). Therefore, saracatinib was dissolved and encapsulated into nano-matrix with a CTSB-sensitive amphiphilic polymer. A short peptide of GFLG linker was used as hydrophobic tails, which not only facilitated to load saracatinib to obtain stable NPs but also subjected to CTSB cleavage so as to release saracatinib in tumor tissues with acidic extracellular pH feature (Fig. 3a–d). DLS study demonstrated that saracatinib was facilely encapsulated into NPs with a nanoscale size approximately 60 nm (Fig. 3e). Most importantly, Nano-sar exhibited enzyme-response drug release profile with an accelerate drug release from NPs (over 90% drug release in 48 h) in the presence of CTSB at pH 5.4, which was the active condition for CTSB (Fig. 3f). In contrast, less than 15% saracatinib was released in the absence of enzyme or at pH 7.4

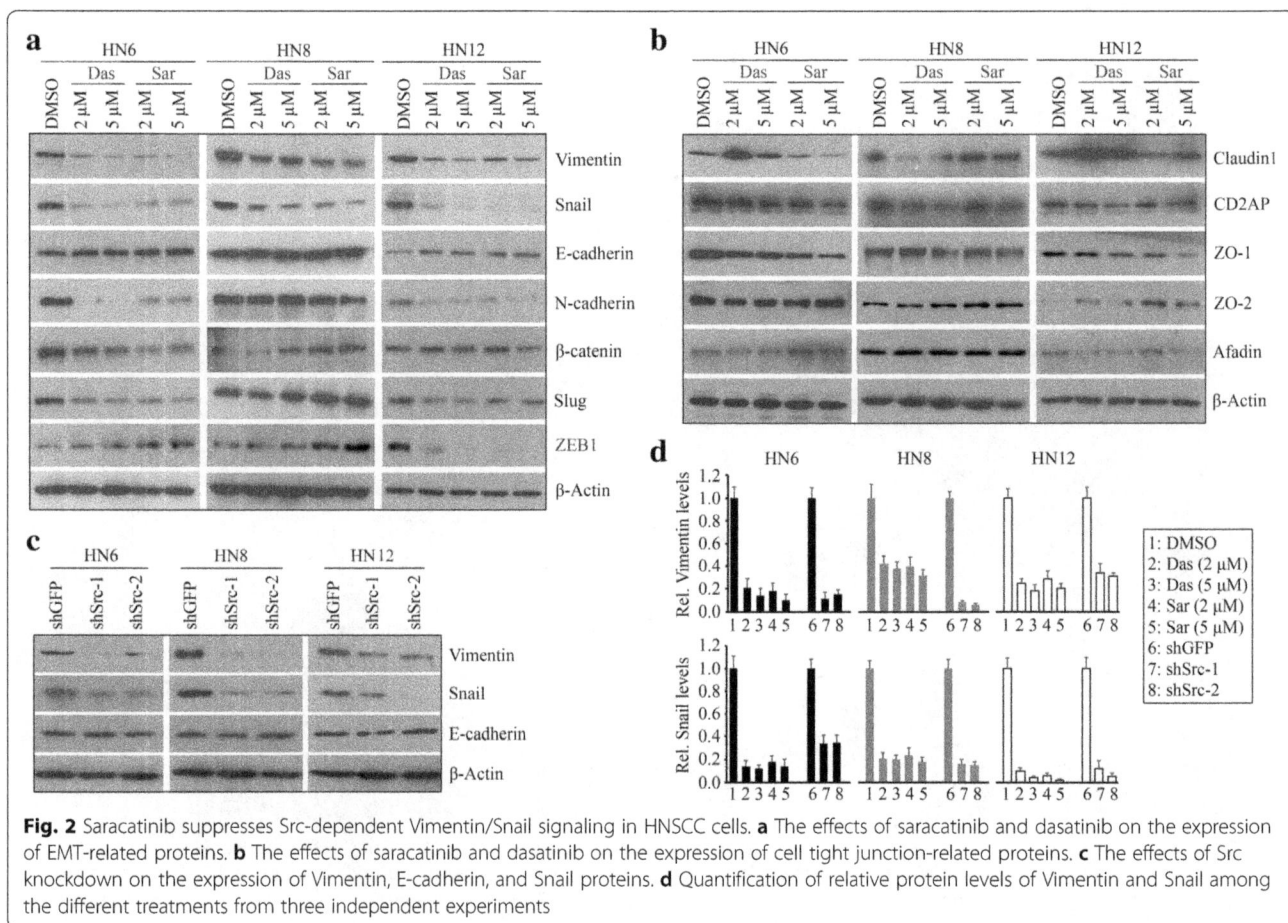

Fig. 2 Saracatinib suppresses Src-dependent Vimentin/Snail signaling in HNSCC cells. **a** The effects of saracatinib and dasatinib on the expression of EMT-related proteins. **b** The effects of saracatinib and dasatinib on the expression of cell tight junction-related proteins. **c** The effects of Src knockdown on the expression of Vimentin, E-cadherin, and Snail proteins. **d** Quantification of relative protein levels of Vimentin and Snail among the different treatments from three independent experiments

(Fig. 3f). These findings suggest that Nano-sar can be stable during circulation, and saracatinib can be selectively released with the cleavage of CTSB in tumor cells.

Nano-sar effectively inactivates Src and inhibits migration and invasion of HNSCC cells

We first determined the effects of Nano-sar on Src inactivation. HN6, HN8, and HN12 cells were treated with DMSO, saracatinib, and Nano-sar, respectively. Similar to saracatinib, Nano-sar markedly inhibited the phosphorylation levels of Src, coupled with downregulation of Vimentin and Snail in HNSCC cells (Fig. 4a). Given that HN12 cells are derived from metastatic HNSCC, we further determined the anticancer effects of NP-based saracatinib in this cell line. MTS assays revealed that either the free drug or Nano-sar at the concentration of 5 μM did not exhibit the inhibitory effects on cell proliferation within 48 h after treatment, but the anti-proliferative effects of these drugs were observed from 72-h post treatment (Additional file 2: Figure S2). To confirm the long-term drug effects on cell self-renewal capability, we performed colony formation assays, which showed that the cells treated with either saracatinib or Nano-sar had lower colony forming ability

than control cells (Fig. 4b). Migratory and invasive potential of HN12 cells were also significantly reduced in the presence of saracatinib, which were consistently observed in Nano-sar-treated cells (Fig. 4c, d). Next, 3D tumor spheroid invasion was assessed to confirm the results from Transwell-based assays. The process was followed over a period of 72 h as shown in Fig. 4e for HN12 spheroids, when treated with saracatinib or Nano-sar, invasion was much less pronounced compared with DMSO treatment. Nano-sar appears not to achieve obvious enhancement effects compared with the free drug in these in vitro assays, which may be resulted from quick internalization and removal of saracatinib through passive diffusion by cancer cells.

Nano-sar exhibits superior effects on suppression of head and neck tumor metastasis than the free drug in mice

The encouraging in vitro data prompted us to evaluate the efficacy of Nano-sar in mice. We have demonstrated that the subcutaneous injection of invasive cancer cells in NSG mice leads to coincident development of primary and metastatic tumors [7, 27, 38]. We then carried out the in vivo study using this cancer model. After 12 days of treatment, a reduced xenograft size and

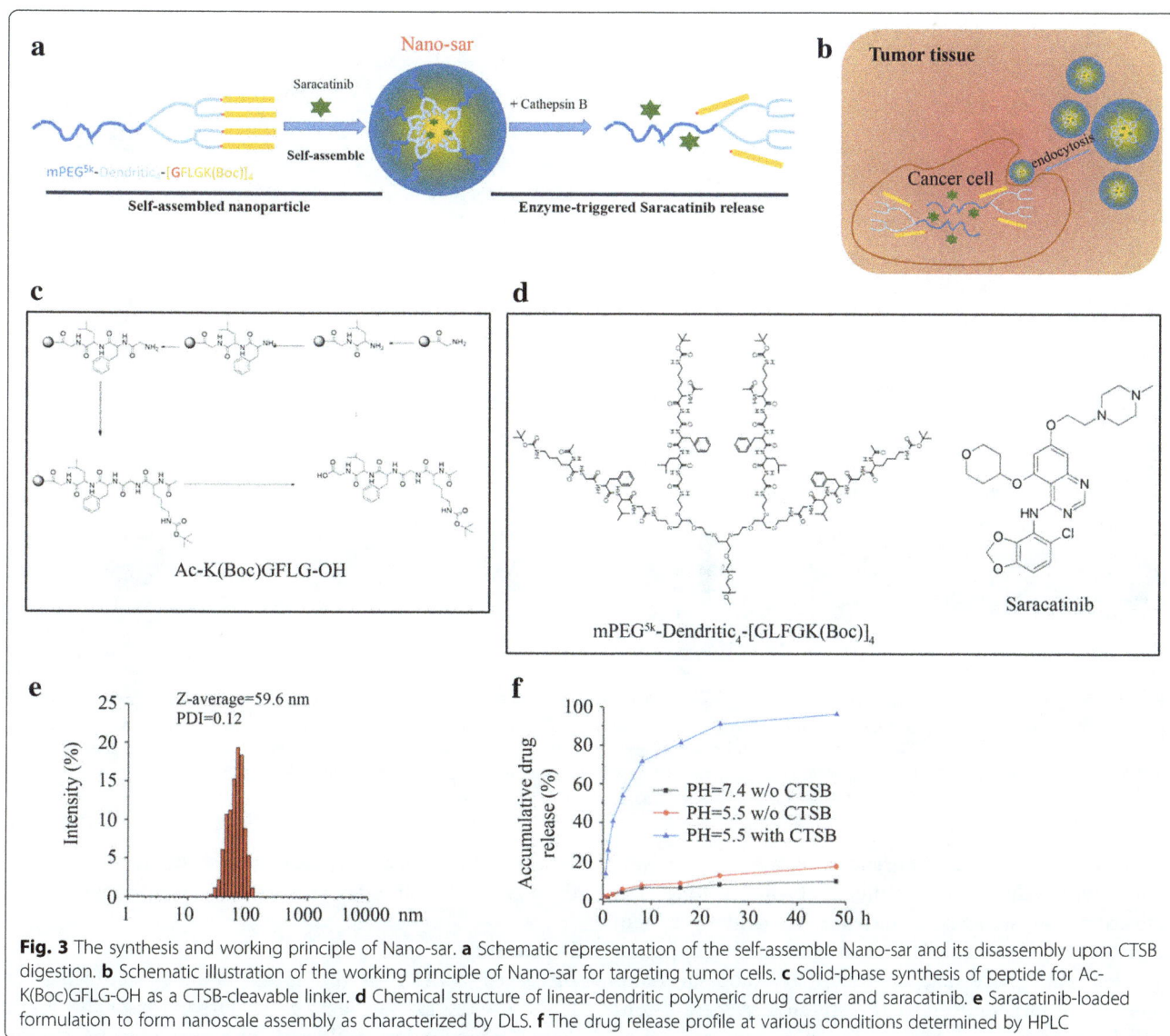

Fig. 3 The synthesis and working principle of Nano-sar. **a** Schematic representation of the self-assemble Nano-sar and its disassembly upon CTSB digestion. **b** Schematic illustration of the working principle of Nano-sar for targeting tumor cells. **c** Solid-phase synthesis of peptide for Ac-K(Boc)GFLG-OH as a CTSB-cleavable linker. **d** Chemical structure of linear-dendritic polymeric drug carrier and saracatinib. **e** Saracatinib-loaded formulation to form nanoscale assembly as characterized by DLS. **f** The drug release profile at various conditions determined by HPLC

weight were observed from mice receiving saracatinib and Nano-sar, compared with those receiving vehicle (Fig. 5a, b). Saracatinib has not been shown to reduce body weight during the treatment (Fig. 5c), suggesting that this drug has no significant effects on the general well-being of the host. There was no remarkable difference in tumor growth between the mice treated with saracatinib and the mice treated with Nano-sar (Fig. 5a, b and Additional file 3: Figure S3A). However, Nano-sar suppressed tumor metastasis more efficiently compared with saracatinib as evidenced by reduced bioluminescence signal at distant sites (Fig. 5d and Additional file 3: Figure S3B) and decreased number of nodules on the mouse lung surface (Fig. 5e). Histopathological analysis further showed that treatment with Nano-sar resulted in fewer and smaller tumor foci in the lung section compared with the free drug treatment (Fig. 5f).

The promise of using Nano-sar to suppress metastasis of HNSCC encouraged us to determine the potential dose toxicity to the host. To evaluate hepatotoxicity and nephrotoxicity after drug administration, serum ALT, AST, and creatinine were measured at the endpoint of experiment. Saracatinib led to increased AST and ALT levels, but not creatinine, on mice (Additional file 4: Figure S4), which is similar to the findings from dasatinib treatment [14, 39]. Whereas, mice treated with Nano-sar did not render significant changes in all these blood biochemical indexes over a period of 12 days (Additional file 4: Figure S4), suggesting that Nano-sar at this dose does not induce notable systemic toxicity. We also collected major organs including the heart, intestine, kidney, liver, lung, and spleen from the mice receiving different treatments. Histology examinations with H&E staining on these organs did not show

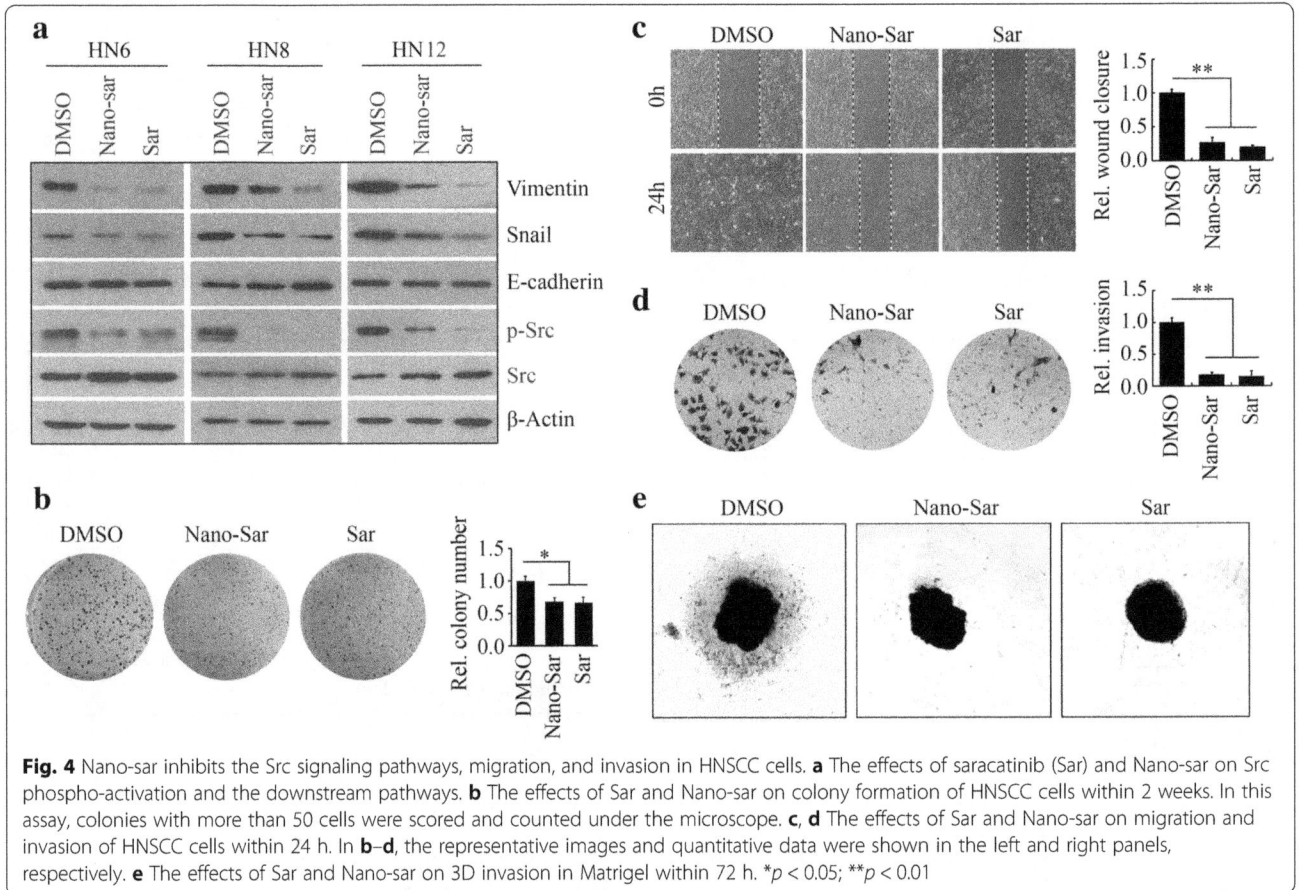

Fig. 4 Nano-sar inhibits the Src signaling pathways, migration, and invasion in HNSCC cells. **a** The effects of saracatinib (Sar) and Nano-sar on Src phospho-activation and the downstream pathways. **b** The effects of Sar and Nano-sar on colony formation of HNSCC cells within 2 weeks. In this assay, colonies with more than 50 cells were scored and counted under the microscope. **c, d** The effects of Sar and Nano-sar on migration and invasion of HNSCC cells within 24 h. In **b–d**, the representative images and quantitative data were shown in the left and right panels, respectively. **e** The effects of Sar and Nano-sar on 3D invasion in Matrigel within 72 h. *$p < 0.05$; **$p < 0.01$

obviously histological difference among the groups treated with vehicle, saracatinib, or Nano-sar (Fig. 5g), indicating that saracatinib and the NP delivery system do not cause detectable systematic toxicities at pathological levels. These data suggest that Nano-sar holds potential for targeted cancer therapy in a triggered, controlled manner.

Nano-sar suppresses metastasis through inhibiting Src-mediated EMT signaling in head and neck tumors

To confirm that the effects of saracatinib on suppression of metastasis were beneficial from inactivation of Src in head and neck tumors, the xenografts from mice were immune-stained with the antibodies against p-Src, Vimentin, and Snail. Consistent with in vitro data, significantly reduced phosphorylation levels of Src were observed in tumor tissues from the mice either receiving the free drug or Nano-sar, compared with vehicle-treated mice (Fig. 6a and Additional file 5: Figure S5). Loss of protein expression of Vimentin and Snail following drug treatment was also demonstrated by IHC analysis (Fig. 6b, c). Additionally, this analysis revealed that Nano-sar suppressed Src activation and EMT-related proteins, Vimentin and Snail, more efficiently than the free drug in these head and neck tumor xenografts (Fig. 6). These observations indicate that

saracatinib suppresses HNSCC metastasis, at least in part, through inhibition of Src-mediated EMT pathways.

Discussion

Increased activity of Src is a frequent occurrence in HNSCC [10, 11]. Src acts as an integrator of divergent signal transduction pathways and promotes numerous tumor-promoting activities, including tumorigenesis, invasion, and metastasis. Therefore, inhibitors targeting Src are considered as promising drugs for cancer therapy. In this study, we demonstrate that saracatinib can effectively suppress invasion and metastasis of HNSCC, at least in part, through blocking Src-dependent Vimentin/Snail signaling. Our findings also show, for the first time, that the efficiency of tumor-responsive nano-based drug delivery system largely improves effectiveness of saracatinib in suppressing metastasis of HNSCC without systemic toxicity.

EMT is a dynamic process that endows the incipient cancer cell with invasive and metastatic properties [30]. Loss of E-cadherin-mediated cell-cell adhesion leading to detachment from neighbor epithelial cells and/or acquisition of some mesenchymal characteristics are key events of EMT [30, 40]. Src is frequently hyperactivated in cancer cells, resulting in facilitating tumor progression

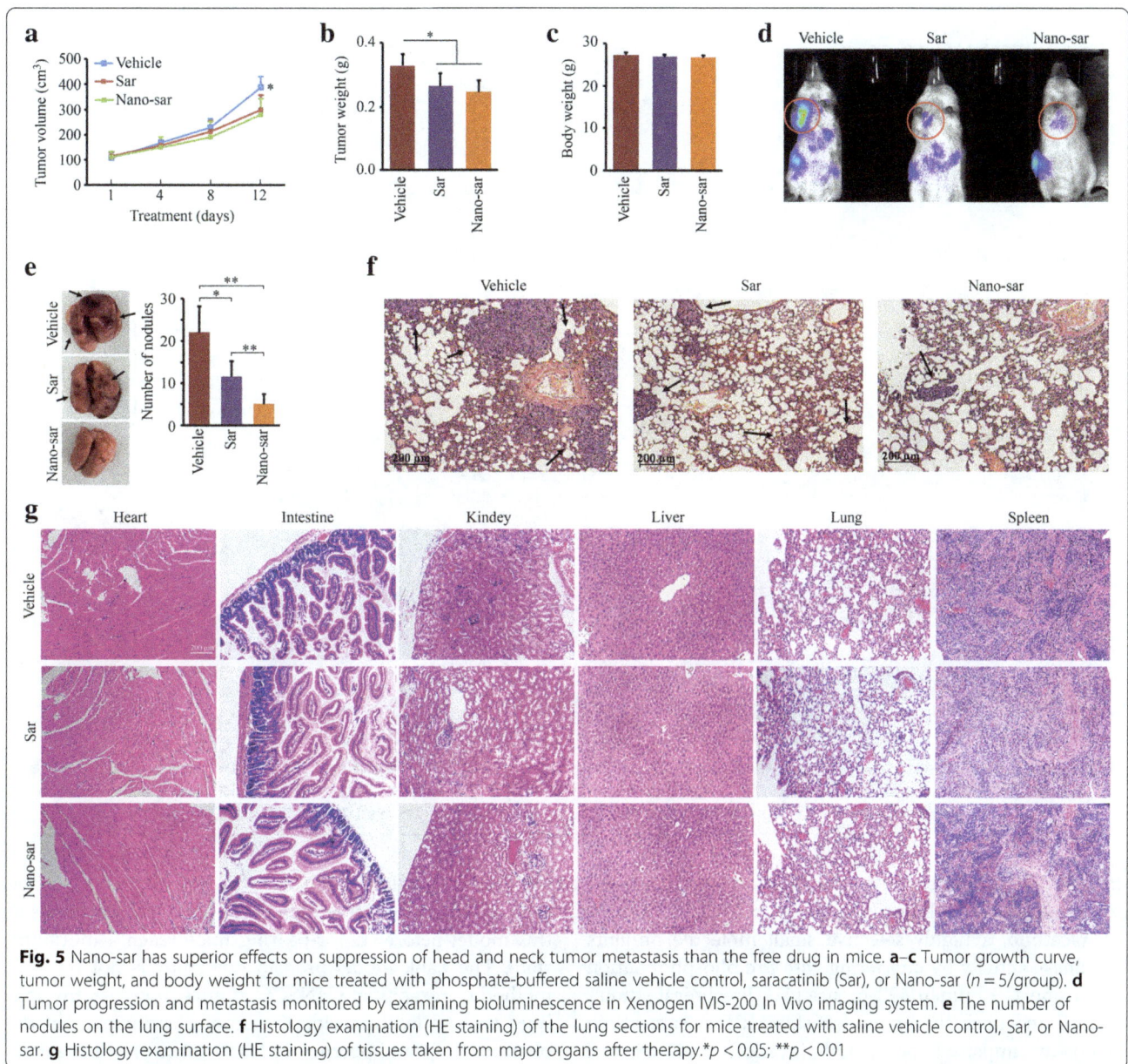

Fig. 5 Nano-sar has superior effects on suppression of head and neck tumor metastasis than the free drug in mice. **a–c** Tumor growth curve, tumor weight, and body weight for mice treated with phosphate-buffered saline vehicle control, saracatinib (Sar), or Nano-sar ($n = 5$/group). **d** Tumor progression and metastasis monitored by examining bioluminescence in Xenogen IVIS-200 In Vivo imaging system. **e** The number of nodules on the lung surface. **f** Histology examination (HE staining) of the lung sections for mice treated with saline vehicle control, Sar, or Nano-sar. **g** Histology examination (HE staining) of tissues taken from major organs after therapy.*$p < 0.05$; **$p < 0.01$

towards metastasis by promoting EMT [8]. For example, Src signaling has been shown to regulate E-cadherin associated EMT in pancreatic cancer cells [41]. In contrast to these studies, knockdown of Src by shRNAs or inactivation of it by small molecule inhibitors in HNSCC cells cannot affect E-cadherin levels. Instead of this, it appears that invasion repression induced by loss of Src function is resulted from downregulation of mesenchymal markers Vimentin and Snail proteins. Interestingly, all three cell lines used in this study express E-cadherin, although they show mesenchymal morphology. The possible reason is that HNSCC involves transformation of the squamous epithelial lineage, which is histologically similar to the epidermis [42]. Consistently, there were

no changes in E-cadherin levels in epidermoid carcinoma A431 cells in the presence or absence of dasatinib [43]. Nevertheless, Src-mediated EMT in HNSCC cells remains to be better defined.

Surprisingly, the protein levels of total Src were increased in HNSCC cells treated with Src inhibitors, dasatinib or saracatinib, although its phosphorylation was markedly inhibited. The similar results were also observed in other studies when HNSCC cells and other types of cancer cells were treated with Src inhibitors [44–46]. Our data and previous studies suggest an unrecognized feedback mechanism for compensation of Src kinase inhibition with increased levels of Src protein expression, which maybe through downregulation of Src

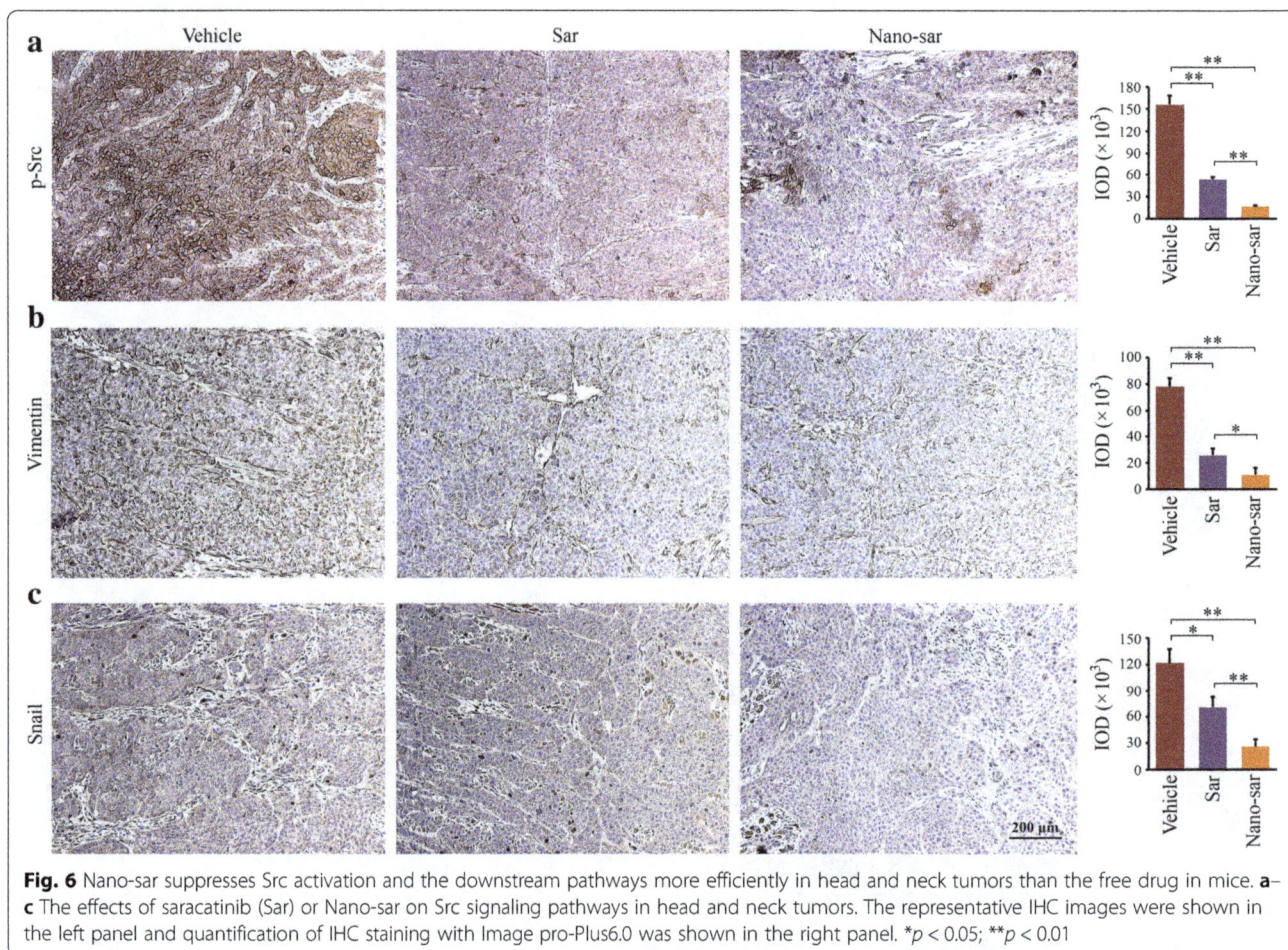

Fig. 6 Nano-sar suppresses Src activation and the downstream pathways more efficiently in head and neck tumors than the free drug in mice. **a–c** The effects of saracatinib (Sar) or Nano-sar on Src signaling pathways in head and neck tumors. The representative IHC images were shown in the left panel and quantification of IHC staining with Image pro-Plus6.0 was shown in the right panel. *$p < 0.05$; **$p < 0.01$

degradation or increase its transcription. However, the exact mechanism still needs to be deciphered.

Saracatinib, a highly selective small molecule, inhibits Src kinase activity by interfering with Src phosphorylation at tyrosine 419-human/423-mouse [47]. Preclinical studies of head and neck tumor models showed that saracatinib treatment impaired perineural invasion and cervical lymph node metastasis [48]. Here, we show a higher inhibitory rate of nano-based saracatinib in HNSCC metastasis compared with the free drug. The efficacy of Nano-sar seems to be on metastasis, which may be due to drug administration of a fixed dose within a short period of experimental time. Expansion of the time window for treatment of Nano-sar may achieve better therapeutic outcomes either on tumorigenesis or metastasis, resulting from the combined influence of Src inactivation and the tumor site-specific delivery of NPs. One of the major challenges for new therapeutics to enter the clinic remains improving their translational value to the clinical situation. We are aware that HNSCC rarely displays distant metastasis; rather, it invades and colonizes cervical lymph nodes in the clinical setting. The orthotopic mouse model of tongue tumors has been established in our group by

sublingual injection of HN12 cells, but we are still facing the challenge to observe high rate of cervical metastasis in this model before tumor-bearing mice reach a moribund state. The flank model used in our study is not the best method to recapitulate HNSCC in mice; however, the analyses on it at least provide the proof of principle that the pharmacology and potency of Nano-sar is promising. Further exploration of this novel treatment in highly preclinical animal models of HNSCC is warranted.

Biocompatible and amphiphilic polymers are able to self-assemble to nanoscale formulations that possess ideal features for drug delivery, including prolonged blood circulation, high stability, and high accumulation in tumor tissues [49, 50]. As such, NPs have been explored as one of the most promising drug vehicles in the development of drug delivery system to enhance drug efficacy as well as reduce systematic toxicity. Particularly, stimuli-responsive NPs that are sensitive to biological stimuli such as pH, temperature, redox potential, and enzymes have been extensively exploited for triggered drug release. Enzymes that express at relatively low level in normal tissue but frequently overexpressed in pathological tissues appear to be an ideal stimulus. Lysosomal enzyme of CTSB, an overexpressed and secreted enzyme in tumor endothelial and epithelial cells, is one of targets that are frequently used in the development of enzyme-triggered nanomedicine. The expression of CTSB has been reported to be increased along with the cancerization in oral squamous cell carcinoma [38, 51], which is also positively associated with highly invasive and metastatic phenotypes [52]. We collected 19 primary HNSCC tissues with paired adjacent normal tissues and determined the expression levels of CTSB by real-time RT-PCR. More than tenfold higher levels of CTSB were observed in HNSCC tissues compared with paired adjacent normal tissues (data not shown), providing a strong rational basis for the design of CTSB-sensitive NP for saracatinib delivery. Given that solid tumors have an acidic extracellular environment and an altered pH gradient across their cell compartments [53, 54], the formulations of Nano-sar were designed to exploit the pH gradients that exist in tumor microenvironments. Therefore, Nano-sar can be selectively activated and release the loaded saracatinib into head and neck tumors in order to maintain effective drug levels at tumor tissues.

Conclusion

Taking the obtained findings together, this work unveils that inactivation of Src by saracatinib can suppress invasion and metastasis of HNSCC. Several Src inhibitors have been FDA approved for the treatment of solid tumors including HNSCC. The present study provides favorable data for possible clinical application of the nano-based Src-targeting therapeutic strategy. We are convinced that with our novel drug delivery system, innovative and smart saracatinib nanomedicine can be developed for safe, efficient, and targeted cancer therapy.

Additional files

Additional file 1: Figure S1. Either knockdown of Src by shRNA (A) or inhibition of Src phosphorylation by saracatinib or dasatinib (B) promotes reversible EMT in mesenchymal-like HNSCC cells. (DOCX 715 kb)

Additional file 2: Figure S2. MTS analysis of HN12 cell proliferation in the treatment of saracatinib and Nano-sar within 96 h. (DOCX 23 kb)

Additional file 3: Figure S3. Quantitative analysis of bioluminescence intensity from primary (A) and metastatic tumors (B). The representative bioluminescent images were illustrated in Fig. 5d. *$p < 0.05$; **$p < 0.01$. (DOCX 71 kb)

Additional file 4: Figure S4. Blood biochemical indexes of NSG mice following injection of vehicle, Sar, or Nano-sar. AST (A) and ALT (B) levels reflect hepatic functions, and creatinine (C) levels reflect nephron functions. *$p < 0.05$. (DOCX 33 kb)

Additional file 5: Figure S5. Mice were sacrificed on day 12 after treatment, and xenografts were dissected and removed for Western blot with the indicated antibodies. The representative image of Western blot was shown in the left panel, and quantitative data of p-Src levels were shown in the right panel ($n = 5$). 1, 2, and 3 indicate the tumor samples from three different mice. **$p < 0.01$. (DOCX 40 kb)

Abbreviations

ALT: Alanine transaminase; AST: Aspartate transaminase; CML: Chronic myeloid leukemia; DMEM: Dulbecco's Modified Eagle's Medium; EGFR: Epidermal growth factor receptor; EMT: Epithelial-mesenchymal transition; FAK: Focal adhesion kinase; FGFR: Fibroblast growth factor receptor; GFP: Green fluorescent protein; GPCRs: G-protein-coupled receptors; HNSCC: Head and neck squamous cell carcinomas; HPLC: High-performance liquid chromatography; IGF-1R: Insulin-like growth factor 1 receptor; IHC: Immunohistochemistry; MET: Mesenchymal-epithelial transition; NP: Nanoparticle; NSG: NOD.Cg-$Prkdc^{scid}$ $Il2rg^{tm1Wjl}$/SzJ; PDGFR: Platelet-derived growth factor receptor; RTK: Receptor tyrosine kinases; SFKs: Src family of non-receptor tyrosine kinases; shRNA: Short hairpin RNA

Acknowledgements
The authors are grateful to Dr. W. Andrew Yeudall for providing us the cell lines and support that are essential for this work.

Funding
This work was supported in part by the Dental College of Georgia Special Funding Initiative and Augusta University Center for Undergraduate Research and Scholarship (CURS).

Authors' contributions
LL, CS, YX, PT, and RC performed research and analyzed results. CS and XW discussed results and edited the paper. YT designed research, wrote the paper, and supervised the study. All authors read and approved the final manuscript.

Consent for publication
All authors have reviewed and approved the manuscript for submission.

Competing interests
The authors declare that they have no competing interests.

Author details
[1]Department of Oral Biology, Dental College of Georgia, Augusta University, Augusta, GA, USA. [2]Department of Pediatrics, Emory Children's Center, Emory University, Atlanta, GA, USA. [3]Department of Biology, College of Science and Mathematics, Augusta University, Augusta, GA, USA. [4]Department of Radiology and Imaging Sciences, School of Medicine, University of Utah, 201 Presidents Cir, Salt Lake City, UT 84112, USA. [5]Georgia Cancer Center, Department of Biochemistry and Molecular Biology, Medical College of Georgia, Augusta University, Augusta, GA, USA. [6]Department of Medical Laboratory, Imaging and Radiologic Sciences, College of Allied Health, Augusta University, 1120 15th Street, Augusta, GA 30912, USA.

References
1. Argiris A, Karamouzis MV, Raben D, Ferris RL. Head and neck cancer. Lancet. 2008;371(9625):1695–709.
2. Noguti J, De Moura CFG, De Jesus GPP, Da Silva VHP, Hossaka TA, Oshima CTF, Ribeiro DA. Metastasis from oral cancer: an overview. Cancer Genomics-Proteomics. 2012;9(5):329–35.
3. Woolgar JA, Scott J, Vaughan E, Brown J, West C, Rogers S. Survival, metastasis and recurrence of oral cancer in relation to pathological features. Ann R Coll Surg Engl. 1995;77(5):325–31.
4. Price KA, Cohen EE. Current treatment options for metastatic head and neck cancer. Curr Treat Options in Oncol. 2012;13(1):35–46.
5. Irby RB, Yeatman TJ. Role of Src expression and activation in human cancer. Oncogene. 2000;19(49):5636–42.
6. Finn R. Targeting Src in breast cancer. Ann Oncol. 2008;19(8):1379–86.

7. Teng Y, Cai Y, Pi W, Gao L, Shay C. Augmentation of the anticancer activity of CYT997 in human prostate cancer by inhibiting Src activity. J Hematol Oncol. 2017;10(1):118–27.

8. Summy JM, Gallick GE. Src family kinases in tumor progression and metastasis. Cancer Metastasis Rev. 2003;22(4):337–58.

9. Jallal H, Valentino M-L, Chen G, Boschelli F, Ali S, Rabbani SA. A Src/Abl kinase inhibitor, SKI-606, blocks breast cancer invasion, growth, and metastasis in vitro and in vivo. Cancer Res. 2007;67(4):1580–8.

10. Yang Z, Bagheri-Yarmand R, Wang R-A, Adam L, Papadimitrakopoulou VV, Clayman GL, El-Naggar A, Lotan R, Barnes CJ, Hong WK. The epidermal growth factor receptor tyrosine kinase inhibitor ZD1839 (Iressa) suppresses c-Src and Pak1 pathways and invasiveness of human cancer cells. Clin Cancer Res. 2004;10(2):658–67.

11. Johnson FM, Saigal B, Talpaz M, Donato NJ. Dasatinib (BMS-354825) tyrosine kinase inhibitor suppresses invasion and induces cell cycle arrest and apoptosis of head and neck squamous cell carcinoma and non–small cell lung cancer cells. Clin Cancer Res. 2005;11(19):6924–32.

12. Kantarjian H, Shah NP, Hochhaus A, Cortes J, Shah S, Ayala M, Moiraghi B, Shen Z, Mayer J, Pasquini R. Dasatinib versus imatinib in newly diagnosed chronic-phase chronic myeloid leukemia. N Engl J Med. 2010;362(24):2260–70.

13. Buettner R, Mesa T, Vultur A, Lee F, Jove R. Inhibition of Src family kinases with dasatinib blocks migration and invasion of human melanoma cells. Mol Cancer Res. 2008;6(11):1766–74.

14. Johnson FM, Bekele BN, Feng L, Wistuba I, Tang XM, Tran HT, Erasmus JJ, Hwang L-L, Takebe N, Blumenschein GR. Phase II study of dasatinib in patients with advanced non–small-cell lung cancer. J Clin Oncol. 2010; 28(30):4609–15.

15. Morrow CJ, Ghattas M, Smith C, Bönisch H, Bryce RA, Hickinson DM, Green TP, Dive C. Src family kinase inhibitor Saracatinib (AZD0530) impairs oxaliplatin uptake in colorectal cancer cells and blocks organic cation transporters. Cancer Res. 2010;70(14):5931–41.

16. Posadas EM, Ahmed RS, Karrison T, Szmulewitz RZ, O'donnell PH, Wade JL, Shen J, Gururajan M, Sievert M, Stadler WM. Saracatinib as a metastasis inhibitor in metastatic castration-resistant prostate cancer: a University of Chicago Phase 2 Consortium and DOD/PCF Prostate Cancer Clinical Trials Consortium Study. Prostate. 2016;76(3):286–93.

17. Gucalp A, Sparano JA, Caravelli J, Santamauro J, Patil S, Abbruzzi A, Pellegrino C, Bromberg J, Dang C, Theodoulou M. Phase II trial of saracatinib (AZD0530), an oral SRC-inhibitor for the treatment of patients with hormone receptor-negative metastatic breast cancer. Clin Breast Cancer. 2011;11(5):306–11.

18. Hiscox S, Morgan L, Green TP, Barrow D, Gee J, Nicholson RI. Elevated Src activity promotes cellular invasion and motility in tamoxifen resistant breast cancer cells. Breast Cancer Res Treat. 2006;97(3):263–74.

19. Green TP, Fennell M, Whittaker R, Curwen J, Jacobs V, Allen J, Logie A, Hargreaves J, Hickinson DM, Wilkinson RW. Preclinical anticancer activity of the potent, oral Src inhibitor AZD0530. Mol Oncol. 2009;3(3):248–61.

20. Kopetz S, Shah AN, Gallick GE. Src continues aging: current and future clinical directions. Clin Cancer Res. 2007;13(24):7232–6.

21. Gao W, Chan JM, Farokhzad OC. pH-responsive nanoparticles for drug delivery. Mol Pharm. 2010;7(6):1913–20.

22. Blanco E, Shen H, Ferrari M. Principles of nanoparticle design for overcoming biological barriers to drug delivery. Nat Biotechnol. 2015; 33(9):941–51.

23. Ryu JH, Koo H, Sun I-C, Yuk SH, Choi K, Kim K, Kwon IC. Tumor-targeting multi-functional nanoparticles for theragnosis: new paradigm for cancer therapy. Adv Drug Deliv Rev. 2012;64(13):1447–58.

24. Brigger I, Dubernet C, Couvreur P. Nanoparticles in cancer therapy and diagnosis. Adv Drug Deliv Rev. 2012;64:24–36.

25. Yeudall WA, Crawford RY, Ensley J, Robbins K. MTS1/CDK4I is altered in cell lines derived from primary and metastatic oral squamous cell carcinoma. Carcinogenesis. 1994;15(12):2683–6.

26. Cardinali M, Pietraszkiewicz H, Ensley JF, Robbins KC. Tyrosine phosphorylation as a marker for aberrantly regulated growth-promoting pathways in cell lines derived from head and neck malignancies. Int J Cancer. 1995;61(1):98–103.

27. Zhao H, Lv F, Liang G, Huang X, Wu G, Zhang W, Yu L, Shi L, Teng Y. FGF19 promotes epithelial-mesenchymal transition in hepatocellular carcinoma cells by modulating the GSK3β/β-catenin signaling cascade via FGFR4 activation. Oncotarget. 2016;7(12):13575–86.

28. Gao L, Wang X, Tang Y, Huang S, Hu C-AA, Teng Y. FGF19/FGFR4 signaling contributes to the resistance of hepatocellular carcinoma to sorafenib. J Exp Clin Cancer Res. 2017;36(1):8–17.

29. Teng Y, Zhao H, Gao L, Zhang W, Shull AY, Shay C. FGF19 protects hepatocellular carcinoma cells against endoplasmic reticulum stress via activation of FGFR4–GSK3β–Nrf2 signaling. Cancer Res. 2017;77(22):6215–25.

30. Teng Y, Mei Y, Hawthorn L, Cowell JK. WASF3 regulates miR-200 inactivation by ZEB1 through suppression of KISS1 leading to increased invasiveness in breast cancer cells. Oncogene. 2014;33(2):203–11.

31. Cheng C, Convertine AJ, Stayton PS, Bryers JD. Multifunctional triblock copolymers for intracellular messenger RNA delivery. Biomaterials. 2012; 33(28):6868–76.

32. Lee SB, Russell AJ, Matyjaszewski K. ATRP synthesis of amphiphilic random, gradient, and block copolymers of 2-(dimethylamino) ethyl methacrylate and n-butyl methacrylate in aqueous media. Biomacromolecules. 2003;4(5):1386–93.

33. Wang X, Yang Y, Jia H, Jia W, Miller S, Bowman B, Feng J, Zhan F. Peptide decoration of nanovehicles to achieve active targeting and pathology-responsive cellular uptake for bone metastasis chemotherapy. Biomater Sci. 2014;2(7):961–71.

34. Zhu J-Y, Lei Q, Yang B, Jia H-Z, Qiu W-X, Wang X, Zeng X, Zhuo R-X, Feng J, Zhang X-Z. Efficient nuclear drug translocation and improved drug efficacy mediated by acidity-responsive boronate-linked dextran/cholesterol nanoassembly. Biomaterials. 2015;52:281–90.

35. Olsen CJ, Moreira J, Lukanidin EM, Ambartsumian NS. Human mammary fibroblasts stimulate invasion of breast cancer cells in a three-dimensional culture and increase stroma development in mouse xenografts. BMC Cancer. 2010;10(1):444.

36. Vinci M, Box C, Eccles SA. Three-dimensional (3D) tumor spheroid invasion assay. J Vis Exp. 2015;(99):e52686.

37. Cai Y, Li J, Zhang Z, Chen J, Zhu Y, Li R, Chen J, Gao L, Liu R, Teng Y. Zbtb38 is a novel target for spinal cord injury. Oncotarget. 2017; 8(28):45356–66.

38. Xie X, Tang S-C, Cai Y, Pi W, Deng L, Wu G, Chavanieu A, Teng Y. Suppression of breast cancer metastasis through the inactivation of ADP-ribosylation factor 1. Oncotarget. 2016;7(36):58111–20.

39. Yang X, Wang J, Dai J, Shao J, Ma J, Chen C, Ma S, He Q, Luo P, Yang B. Autophagy protects against dasatinib-induced hepatotoxicity via p38 signaling. Oncotarget. 2015;6(8):6203.

40. Guarino M, Rubino B, Ballabio G. The role of epithelial-mesenchymal transition in cancer pathology. Pathology. 2007;39(3):305–18.

41. Nagathihalli NS, Merchant NB. Src-mediated regulation of E-cadherin and EMT in pancreatic cancer. Front Biosci (Landmark edition). 2012;17:2059–69.

42. Pai SI, Westra WH. Molecular pathology of head and neck cancer: implications for diagnosis, prognosis, and treatment. Annu Rev Pathol Mech Dis. 2009;4:49–70.

43. Serrels A, Timpson P, Canel M, Schwarz JP, Carragher NO, Frame MC, Brunton VG, Anderson KI. Real-time study of E-cadherin and membrane dynamics in living animals: implications for disease modeling and drug development. Cancer Res. 2009;69(7):2714–9.

44. Lin Y-C, Wu M-H, Wei T-T, Chung S-H, Chen K-F, Cheng A-L, Chen C-C. Degradation of epidermal growth factor receptor mediates dasatinib-induced apoptosis in head and neck squamous cell carcinoma cells. Neoplasia. 2012;14(6):463–75.

45. Shor AC, Keschman EA, Lee FY, Muro-Cacho C, Letson GD, Trent JC, Pledger WJ, Jove R. Dasatinib inhibits migration and invasion in diverse human sarcoma cell lines and induces apoptosis in bone sarcoma cells dependent on SRC kinase for survival. Cancer Res. 2007;67(6):2800–8.

46. Schweppe RE, Kerege AA, French JD, Sharma V, Grzywa RL, Haugen BR. Inhibition of Src with AZD0530 reveals the Src-focal adhesion kinase complex as a novel therapeutic target in papillary and anaplastic thyroid cancer. J Clin Endocrinol Metab. 2009;94(6):2199–203.

47. Hennequin LF, Allen J, Breed J, Curwen J, Fennell M, Green TP, Lambert-van der Brempt C, Morgentin R, Norman RA, Olivier A. N-(5-Chloro-1, 3-benzodioxol-4-yl)-7-[2-(4-methylpiperazin-1-yl) ethoxy]-5-(tetrahydro-2 H-pyran-4-yloxy) quinazolin-4-amine, a novel, highly selective, orally available, dual-specific c-Src/Abl kinase inhibitor. J Med Chem. 2006;49(22):6465–88.

48. Ammer AG, Kelley LC, Hayes KE, Evans JV, Lopez-Skinner LA, Martin KH, Frederick B, Rothschild BL, Raben D, Elvin P. Saracatinib impairs head and neck squamous cell carcinoma invasion by disrupting invadopodia function. J Cancer Sci Ther. 2009;1(2):052–69.

49. Singh R, Lillard JW. Nanoparticle-based targeted drug delivery. Exp Mol Pathol. 2009;86(3):215–23.

50. Yin J, Lang T, Cun D, Zheng Z, Huang Y, Yin Q, Yu H, Li Y. pH-sensitive nano-complexes overcome drug resistance and inhibit metastasis of breast cancer by silencing Akt expression. Theranostics. 2017;7(17):4204–16.

51. Yang X, K-j W, Zhang L, H-y P, Li J, L-p Z, Z-y Z. Increased expression of Cathepsin B in oral squamous cell carcinoma. Int J Oral Maxillofac Surg. 2010;39(2):174–81.

52. Vigneswaran N, Zhao W, Dassanayake A, Muller S, Miller DM, Zacharias W. Variable expression of cathepsin B and D correlates with highly invasive and metastatic phenotype of oral cancer. Hum Pathol. 2000;31(8):931–7.

53. Shen Y, Tang H, Radosz M, Van Kirk E, Murdoch WJ. pH-responsive nanoparticles for cancer drug delivery. Methods Mol Biol. 2008;437:183–216.

54. Zhou Q, Hou Y, Zhang L, Wang J, Qiao Y, Guo S, Fan L, Yang T, Zhu L, Wu H. Dual-pH sensitive charge-reversal nanocomplex for tumor-targeted drug delivery with enhanced anticancer activity. Theranostics. 2017;7(7):1806–19.

12

JAG1 overexpression contributes to Notch1 signaling and the migration of HTLV-1-transformed ATL cells

Marcia Bellon, Ramona Moles, Hassiba Chaib-Mezrag, Joanna Pancewicz and Christophe Nicot[*]

Abstract

Background: HTLV-1 is a retrovirus that infects over 20 million people worldwide and is responsible for the hematopoietic malignancy adult T cell leukemia (ATL). We previously demonstrated that Notch is constitutively activated in ATL cells. Activating genetic mutations were found in Notch; however, Notch signaling was also activated in the absence of genetic mutations suggesting the existence of other mechanisms.

Methods: We analyzed the expression of Notch receptor ligands in HTLV-I-transformed cells, ATL patient-derived cell lines, and fresh uncultured ATL samples by RT-PCR, FACS, and immunohistochemistry. We then investigated viral and cellular molecular mechanisms regulating expression of JAG1. Finally, using shRNA knock-down and neutralizing antibodies, we investigated the function of JAG1 in ATL cells.

Results: Here, we report the overexpression of the Notch ligand, JAG1, in freshly uncultured ATL patient samples compared to normal PBMCs. We found that in ATL cells, JAG1 overexpression relies upon the viral protein Tax and cellular miR-124a, STAT3, and NFATc1. Interestingly, our data show that blockade of JAG1 signaling dampens Notch1 downstream signaling and limits cell migration of transformed ATL cells.

Conclusions: Our results suggest that targeting JAG1 can block Notch1 activation in HTLV-I-transformed cells and represents a new target for immunotherapy in ATL patients.

Keywords: HTLV-I, ATL, Notch, JAG1, NF-κB, miR-124, STAT3, NFATc1

Background

The Notch pathway is one of the most frequently activated signaling pathways in human malignancies. Activating mutations or amplification of the Notch pathway is commonly reported in various types of human cancer. T cell and glial cell cancers are especially prone to having an oncogenic Notch pathway, since Notch plays a key role in differentiation and development in these cell types [1]. Activated Notch1 has also been shown to play important roles in virus-associated cancers such as Kaposi's sarcoma (KSHV) [2] and HCV- or EBV-associated lymphoma [3, 4]. The human Notch family includes four receptors, Notch 1–4, and five ligands, delta-like ligand 1 (DLL1), delta-like ligand 3 (DLL3), delta-like ligand 4 (DLL4), Jagged-1 (JAG1), and Jagged-2 (JAG2) [5]. In physiological conditions, interactions between these ligands and the extracellular domain of the Notch receptor, which is located on the cellular surface of neighboring cells, lead to the proteolytic cleavage and release of the Notch intracellular domain (NICD). NICD then translocates to the nucleus where it interacts with DNA-binding proteins and activates target genes. Termination of Notch1 signaling can occur at, or downstream of, the Notch receptor through ubiquitin ligases Itch/AIP4 (itchy E3 ubiquitin protein ligase) or Nedd4 (neural precursor cell-expressed developmentally downregulated protein 4) [6, 7]. NICD can also be phosphorylated by glycogen synthase kinase 3 beta (GSK3β), which regulates its interaction with the E3 ubiquitin ligase, FBXW7 (F-box and WD repeat domain containing 7). This promotes ubiquitination and proteasome-mediated degradation of NICD [8].

* Correspondence: cnicot@kumc.edu
Department of Pathology and Laboratory Medicine, Center for Viral Pathogenesis, University of Kansas Medical Center, 3901 Rainbow Boulevard, MS 3046, Kansas City, KS 66160, USA

The average life expectancy for HTLV-I-associated acute adult T cell leukemia (ATL) is less than 12 months, and since there is no cure for the disease and treatment options are very limited, new therapeutic targets are greatly needed [9]. Although the etiologic agent has been well characterized, a mechanistic understanding of the initiation and progression of this disease has been elusive. The low incidence and long latency of HTLV-I-associated ATL suggest that in addition to viral infection, accumulation of genetic mutations and genomic alterations is required for cellular transformation [10]. In the early stages of the transformation process, the viral transcriptional activator protein Tax plays an essential role by disrupting the normal state of many cellular signaling pathways, inactivating tumor suppressors, increasing the mutation rate, and inhibiting DNA repair pathways [11, 12]. We have previously demonstrated that HTLV-I-transformed cells and ATL cells display constitutive activation of Notch1 signaling [13]. We further demonstrated that inhibition of Notch1 signaling by a gamma-secretase inhibitor (GSI) reduced ATL tumor cell proliferation and tumor formation in a xenograft mouse model of ATL [13].

Notch1 activating mutations have been reported in various cancers [14]. Genetic aberrations in hematological malignancies frequently involve Notch receptors or its regulators, such as FBXW7. In T cell acute lymphocytic leukemia (T-ALL) patients, these mutations usually cluster at the hetero-dimerization (HD) and proline-glutamate -serine-threonine-rich (PEST) domains of Notch [15]. HD domain mutations are characterized by ligand-independent constitutive cleavage of the Notch1 receptor, resulting in increased expression of NICD. In contrast, mutations in ATL patients do not occur in the HD domain, but instead occur solely in the PEST domain of NICD. Mutations in the PEST domain have been shown to increase the stability of NICD. As much as 30% of ATL patients harbor mutations within the PEST domain of NICD, thereby preventing proper ubiquitination and NICD proteasome degradation [13]. These observations and the lack of mutations within the HD domain of NICD in ATL patients suggests that interaction between the Notch receptor and one of its ligands is required for activation of Notch signaling in ATL cells.

To better understand the regulation of the Notch signaling pathway in ATL, we investigated the expression of Notch receptor ligands. Here, we show that HTLV-I-transformed and fresh uncultured ATL cells overexpress JAG1 and to a lesser extent DLL4. We further demonstrate that the viral Tax protein, but not HBZ, stimulates expression of JAG1 in part through activation of the nuclear factor kappa B (NF-κB) pathway. In ATL cells, the expression of JAG1 is also correlated with the transcriptional regulators, STAT3 (signal transducer and activator of transcription 3) and NFATc1 (nuclear factor of activated T cells 1). We also show that miR-124 expression can target STAT3 and NFATc1 to lower JAG1 expression in ATL cells. Finally, we found that blockade of JAG1 signaling by shRNA or neutralizing antibodies dampened Notch signaling and limited cell migration of transformed ATL cells. Our results suggest that JAG1 may represent a new target for immunotherapy in ATL patients.

Methods
Cell cultures and ATL patient samples
The HTLV-I-transformed (IL-2 independent) cell lines (MT2, MT4, C8166, and C91PL), ATL-like cell lines (ATLT, ATL25, ED-40515(−), and TL-Om1), and ALL cell lines (Jurkat and Molt4) were grown in RPMI 1640 with 10% fetal bovine serum. The HTLV-I-immortalized (IL-2 dependent) cell lines (LAF and 1185) and the ATL-like cell lines (ATL43T, ATL55T, KOB, KK1, SO4, and LM-Y1) were grown in media with 20% serum and 50 U/mL IL-2. The ATL patient samples used in this study were previously described in another publication [13, 16]. Samples were obtained after informed consent after internal institutional review board approval, respecting the regulations for the protection of human subjects. The present study control samples consist of isolated peripheral blood mononuclear cells (PBMCs) from healthy HTLV-1-negative donors that have been previously reported [16]. Pharmacological inhibitors used to treat cells include STAT3 inhibitor, S3I-201 (Calbiochem), and NFAT inhibitor (Cayman Chemical Company).

RNA extraction and RT-PCR
RNA was extracted using TRIzol (Invitrogen) followed by DNase I treatment and reverse transcription with an RNA-to-cDNA synthesis kit (Applied Biosystems). The StepOnePlus Real-time PCR System (Applied Biosystems) was used in the study to quantify the expression of the genes of interest. The following primers were used in this study with iTaq Universal SYBR green (Bio-Rad): GAPDH (S-GAAGGTGAAGGTCGGAGTC and AS-GAAGATGGTGATGGGATTTC), STAT3 (S-GATTGACCAGCAGTATAGCCGCTTC and AS-CTGCAGTCTGTAGAAGGCGTG), pre-miR-124a (S-AGGCCTCTCTCTCCGTGTTC and AS-CAGCCCCATTCTTGGCATTC), JAG1 (S-ATCGTGCTGCCTTTCAGTTT and AS-GATCATGCCCGAGTGAGAA), JAG2 (S-GTCGTCATCCCCTTCCAGT and AS-CTCCTCATTCGGGGTGGTAT), DLL4 (S-AGGCCTGTTTTGTGACCAAG and AS-GTGCAGGTGTAGCTTCGCT), IL-8 (S-CTGATTTCTGCAGCTCTGTGTG and AS-CAGACAGAGCTCTCTTCCATCAG), RelA (S-CTCTGCTTCCAGGTGACAGT and AS-TCCTCTTTCTGCACCTTGTC), Hes1 (S-CTGGAAATGACAGTGAAGCACCT and AS-ATTGATCTGGGTCATGCAGTTG), Hey1 (S-CCGAGATCCTG

CAGATGACC and AS-CCCGAAATCCCAAACTCCG A), and VEGF (S-TCTACCTCCACCATGCCAAGT and AS- GATGATTCTGCCCTCCTCCTT). NFATc1 was detected using iTaq Universal Probes (Bio-Rad) with the following primers: NFATc1 (S-CCATCCTCTCCAAC ACCAAA, AS-GTCTCTCCTTTCCGAAGTTCAA, and probe-ACTGTGCCGGAATCCTGAAACTCA).

Antibody staining and fluorescence-activated cell sorting (FACS)

Cells were collected, washed twice with PBS, and stained with the antibodies according to the manufacturer's instructions. The samples were then washed twice with PBS before analysis with a LSR II flow cytometer. Fixation with PFA 4% was included for JAG1 antibody staining before incubation with the antibody. The following antibodies were used: FITC anti-human JAG1 (Sino Biological Inc.), FITC Mouse IgG2a isotype control (BD PharMingen), and PE anti-Human DLL4 (Biolegend).

Immunohistochemistry

Cells were grown on a coverslip slide coated with poly-Lysine or cytospined onto a coverslip. Cells were then fixed with 4% PFA. Immunohistochemistry (IHC) was performed using an EXPOSE HRP/DAB Detection IHC Kit (Abcam), with JAG1 (R&D Systems) and DLL4 (Abcam) antibodies, counterstaining with Mayer's hematoxylin (Lillie's modification) and Bluing reagent (ScyTek). Images were taken with a Nikon Eclipse 80i microscope (Nikon Instruments, Inc., Melville, NY) with a × 60 objective lens and a Nikon DSFI1 camera.

Plasmids

The HTLV-1 Tax gene was cloned into the pTRIPZ, lentiviral inducible vector, engineered to become Tet-On. The pTRIPZ vector contains puromycin resistance, which was used to select a stable cell line. The stable cell lines were incubated in the absence or presence of doxycycline to induce the expression of the viral protein Tax. Tax and HBZ genes were also cloned in the pSIH1-green fluorescent protein (GFP) lentiviral vector. A shRNA against JAG1 was cloned into the pSIH1-GFP vector. The pTRIPZ and miR-124a/pTRIPZ stable lines and the miR-124a/pCDNA construct are previously described [16]. Luciferase assays were performed using the Dual-Luciferase Reporter System (Promega). The wild-type 3′UTR of NFATc1 was cloned into a modified pGL3-Promoter luciferase vector (Promega) with the primers S-GGTCTAGATTGCCACATTGGAGCACTC AGTTCAGC and AS-CCGAATTCCGGCTTTATTG GATCTATTTCCTAACTAC. Mutant NFATC1 3′UTR sites were generated using the site-directed mutagenesis kit (Stratagene).

Western blotting

Cell lysates were separated on SDS-PAGE gels followed by electroblotting to polyvinylidene difluoride membranes and probed with Actin (sc-1615), NFATC1 (7A6), and a Tax mouse monoclonal antibody from the NIH AIDS Reagent Program, HTLV-I Tax Hybridoma (168B17), and with appropriate secondary antibodies from Santa Cruz Biotechnology.

XTT proliferation assays

Cell viability and proliferation were measured by Cell Proliferation Kit II (XTT) (Roche) according to the manufacturer's instructions. One hundred microliters of cells were seeded in a 96-well plate, and 50 μL of XTT labeling mixture was added to each well and incubated for 4–6 h. Spectrophotometry was used to measure the absorbance at 450 and 620 nm. The results were plotted as mean, and the standard deviation is shown from at least two independent experiments.

Scratch-wound assays

Cells were plated in a 12-well plate, and when the cells reached confluence, they were treated with 3 μg/ml of JAG1-neutralizing antibody. After 3 days, the media was removed and replaced with fresh media with 3 μg/ml of JAG1-neutralizing antibody. After 3 days, the p1000 tip was used to scratch the plate. The plate was then washed twice with PBS, and fresh media with neutralizing antibody (3 μg/ml) was added. After 48 h, the cells were fixed with cold methanol (MeOH) and then stained with crystal violet dye (0.5% MeOH) for 20 min at room temperature. Images were taken with an Olympus 1x71 Inverted Microscope with a × 40 objective lens.

Statistical analysis

Experiments in figures were performed multiple times in duplicate. Representative results were shown in the final figures. P values were calculated by using paired and two-tailed Student's t test. In the figures, asterisk indicates p value $< .05$, two asterisks indicate p value $< .01$, and three asterisks indicate p value $< .001$. Correlation analysis was performed by using Pearson's correlation. The Pearson's correlation coefficient, coefficient of determination, and p values are reported in the figures.

Results

Overexpression of JAG1 in HTLV-I-transformed and ATL-derived patient cell lines

We used RT-PCR to test the expression of Notch receptor ligands JAG1, JAG2, DLL1, and DLL4 in HTLV-I-infected immortalized (IL-2-dependent) and transformed (IL-2-independent) cell lines compared to the HTLV-I-uninfected T cell line, Jurkat, and PBMCs isolated from healthy donors. Generally, Notch receptor ligands JAG2 and DLL1 were downregulated when compared to normal PBMCs (Fig. 1c, d). Overexpression of the Notch receptor ligand JAG1 was detected in five of six HTLV-I cell lines tested when compared to HTLV-I-negative cells. Only HTLV-I-immortalized 1185 cells did not significantly overexpress JAG1 (Fig. 1a). To confirm that the JAG1 ligand was overexpressed on the cell surface of HTLV-I-infected cells, we used JAG1 antibody staining followed by FACS analysis. Our analysis confirmed high cell surface expression of JAG1 (Fig. 1b), suggesting that it may play a role in the constitutive activation of Notch signaling in HTLV-I-infected cells.

Finally, expression of the Notch receptor ligand DLL4 was variable in HTLV-I-infected cell lines compared to HTLV-I-negative cells, but was overexpressed on the cell surface of MT4 and C8166 transformed cells (Fig. 1e, f). We next investigated the expression of Notch receptor ligands JAG1 and DLL4 in a series of ATL patient-derived cell lines. These cell lines are of ATL origin and display varying levels of the HTLV-I oncoprotein, Tax (Fig. 2a). Overexpression of JAG1 was detected in seven out of ten ATL cell lines tested (Fig. 2b), and cell surface expression was confirmed by FACS and IHC analysis (Fig. 2c, d). In contrast, DLL4 was found to be

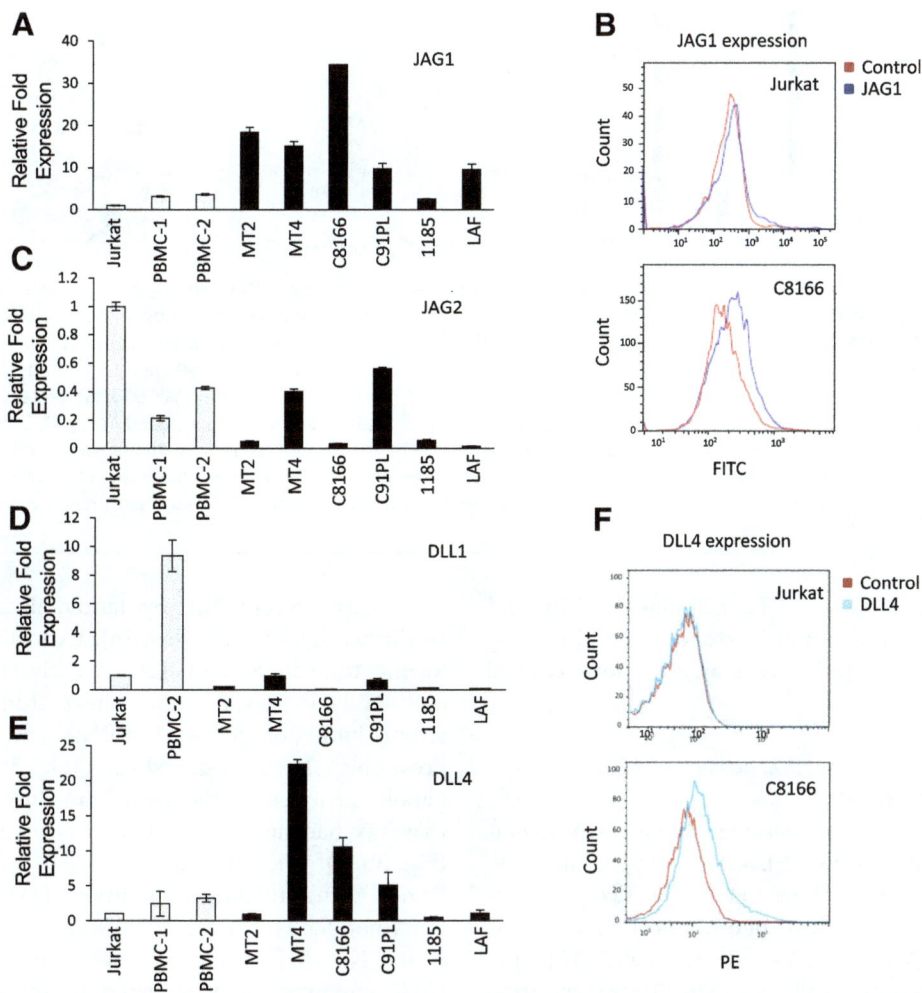

Fig. 1 Expression of Notch ligands in HTLV-I cell lines. **a** Real-time PCR was performed on JAG1 from cDNA derived from HTLV-I-immortalized and transformed cells (MT2, MT4, C8166, C91PL, 1185, and LAF). The non-HTLV-I Jurkat T cell line and normal PBMCs isolated from HTLV-1-negative donors were used as controls. Real-time PCR was performed in duplicate, and samples were normalized to GAPDH expression. Fold change was calculated by comparing values with Jurkat normalized JAG1 expression. **b** Antibody staining of JAG1 surface expression was performed on the HTLV-I-transformed cell line C8166 and negative control Jurkat cells. Cells stained with FITC Mouse IgG2a isotype were used as a control. Red peaks indicate the isotype control, while blue peaks indicate the JAG1 antibody. Bar diagrams representing the FACS results are provided. **c** Same as **a** for JAG2 (**d**). Same as **a** for DLL1. **e** Same as **a** for DLL4. **f** Antibody staining for cell surface expression of DLL4 was performed on the HTLV-1-transformed cell line C8166 and negative control Jurkat with an antibody against DLL4. Unstained cells were used as a control. Red peaks indicate the control, while blue peaks indicate the DLL4 antibody

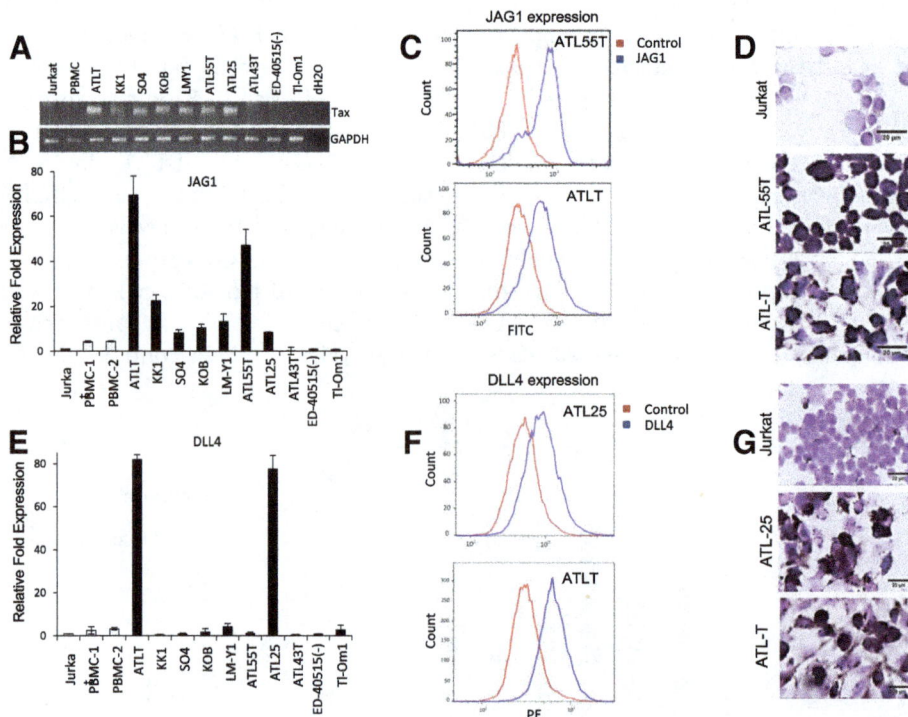

Fig. 2 Expression of notch ligands in ATL cell lines. **a** PCR on Tax and GADPH expression from cDNA derived from ATL-derived cell lines and negative controls, Jurkat and PBMCs. GAPDH expression was used as an internal control. Real-time PCR was performed on JAG1 (**b**) or DLL4 (**e**) using cDNA from ATL-derived cell lines (ATLT, KK1, SO4, KOB, LM-Y1, ATL55T, ATL-5, ATL43T, ED-40515(−), and Tl-Om1). HTLV-I-negative Jurkat T cell line and normal PBMCs isolated from HTLV-1-negative donors were used as controls. Real-time PCR was performed in duplicate, and samples were normalized to GAPDH expression. Fold change was calculated by comparing values with Jurkat normalized JAG1 expression. Antibody staining of JAG1 (**c**) or DLL4 (**f**) was performed on the ATL cell lines, ATL55T and ATLT, and Jurkat (data included in Fig. 1). Cells were stained with the antibody against JAG1 and analyzed via a flow cytometer. FITC Mouse IgG2a isotype was used as an internal control. Red peaks indicate the control, while blue peaks indicate JAG1 or DLL4 antibodies. Bar diagrams representing the FACS results are provided. Immunohistochemistry of JAG1 on ATL55T and ATLT (**d**) or DLL4 on ATL25 and ATLT (**g**) and Jurkat as a negative control was performed. Images were taken with a ×60 objective lens

overexpressed in only two ATL cell lines, ATLT and ATL25 (Fig. 2e). These results were validated by using FACS and IHC, using Jurkat cells as a negative control (Fig. 2f, g).

Virus-encoded Tax, but not HBZ, activates JAG1 expression through NF-κB

We next investigated the molecular mechanism associated with increased JAG1 expression in HTLV-I-transformed cell lines. The viral Tax gene encodes for a 40-kDa nuclear phosphoprotein that has pleiotropic effects on HTLV-I-infected cells [17]. Tax has been shown to positively regulate the transcription of many cellular genes. Furthermore, JAG1 expression was elevated in all ATL lines that had detectable Tax expression (Fig. 2a). JAG1 expression was lower in ED-40515(−), ATL43T, and Tl-Om1, where Tax expression from cDNA was undetectable by PCR analysis. To test whether Tax can activate JAG1 expression, we transiently expressed Tax in Molt4, an HTLV-I-negative T cell line, where Tax is not expressed. Successful delivery

and expression of Tax by lentiviral transduction was confirmed by RT-PCR (Fig. 3a). Expression of JAG1 following transduction of Tax was investigated by FACS and RT-PCR. Results from these studies confirmed a strong induction of JAG1 mRNA and cell surface expression in Tax-transduced cells (Fig. 3b, c). In contrast, parallel analyses on the same transduced cells indicated that Tax had no significant effects on DLL4 expression (Fig. 3b, c). These results were also independently confirmed using an inducible Jurkat Tax Tet-On cell line (data not shown). Since HTLV-I Tax is a potent inducer of the NF-κB pathway, we investigated if Tax-mediated JAG1 overexpression occurred in an NF-κB-dependent manner. To this end, we constructed and transduced Tax-expressing MT4 cells with an IκBα (NF-κB inhibitor alpha) dominant negative mutant lentivirus able to suppress Tax-mediated NF-κB canonical activation [18]. As expected, transduction with IκBα-DN resulted in significant suppression of interleukin-8 (IL-8) mRNA expression (Fig. 3g), a well-known NF-κB target gene [19]. Consistent with a role for Tax-mediated NF-κB

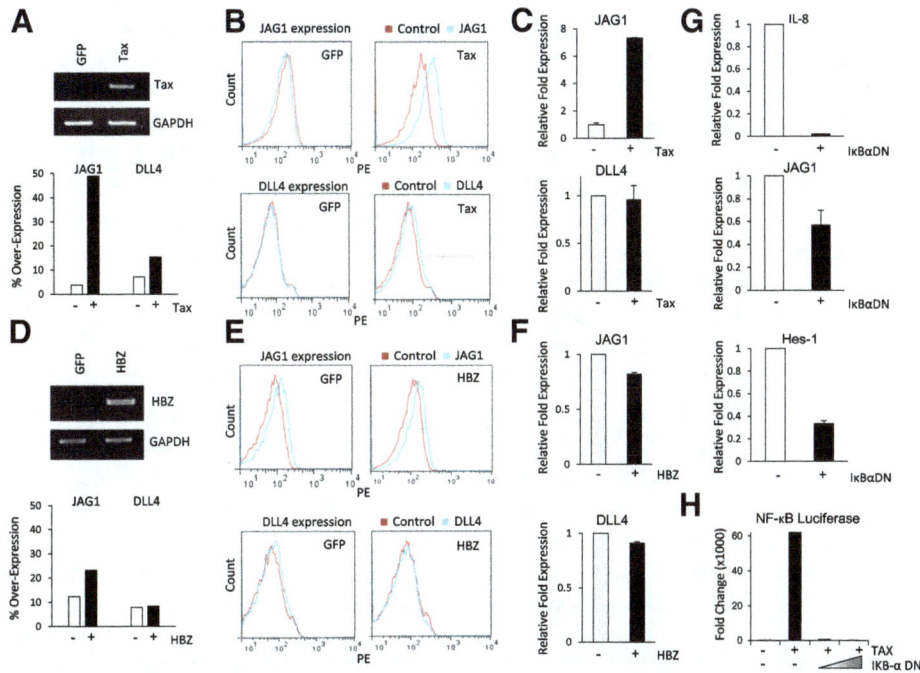

Fig. 3 HTLV-I, Tax, induces expression of JAG1 through NF-κB. **a** PCR was performed to detect Tax expression on cDNA derived from the ALL cell line, Molt4, infected with the lentivirus pSIH1-Tax. Cells infected with the empty vector pSIH1. **b** Antibody staining of JAG1 and DLL4 was performed on Molt4 cells infected with pSIH1-Tax and pSIH1-GFP. Red peaks indicate the control, while blue peaks indicate the JAG1 or DLL4 antibodies. Bar diagrams representing the FACS results are provided. **c** Real-time PCR of JAG1 and DLL4 expression on cDNA derived from Molt4 infected with pSIH1-Tax. Cells infected with the empty vector expressing pSIH1-GFP were used as a control. The expression of JAG1 and DLL4 were normalized to GAPDH expression. Results were plotted as mean ± standard deviation from at least two independent experiments. **d** PCR was performed to detect HBZ expression on cDNA derived from Molt4 infected with a lentivirus pSIH1-HBZ. Cells infected with the empty vector expressing pSIH1-GFP were used as a control. GAPDH expression was used as an internal control. **e** Antibody staining of JAG1 and DLL4 was performed on the Molt4 cells infected pSIH1-HBZ and pSIH1-GFP. Red peaks indicate the control, while blue peaks indicate the JAG1 or DLL4 antibodies. Bar diagrams representing the FACS results are provided. **f** Real-time PCR to detect JAG1 and DLL4 expression on cDNA extracted from Molt4 cells infected with pSIH1-HBZ. Cells infected with the empty vector expressing pSIH1-GFP were used as a control. Real-time PCR was performed in duplicate, and samples were normalized to GAPDH expression. Results were plotted as mean ± standard deviation from at least two independent experiments. **g** Real-time PCR analysis of IL-8, JAG1, and Hes-1 expression on cDNA from Molt4 cells infected with pSIHI-GFP and a lentivirus vector expressing IκB-α-DN mutant. Cells infected with the empty vector expressing pSIH1-GFP were used as a control. Extracts were analyzed 48 h after infection and normalized to GAPDH expression. Real-time PCR was performed in duplicate. Results were plotted as mean ± standard deviation from two independent experiments. **h** NF-κB luciferase was performed on 293T cells transfected with Tax and/or IκBα-DN plasmids

activation in controlling JAG1 expression, JAG1 mRNA expression was also downregulated following transduction of the IκBα dominant negative mutant (Fig. 3g). Notably, the Notch1 target gene, hairy and enhancer of split 1 (Hes1), was also significantly suppressed (Fig. 3g), suggesting that Tax-mediated JAG1 expression partly contributes to Notch signaling. In order to confirm that the IκBα-DN plasmid used could indeed block Tax transactivation of NF-κB, we transfected cells with NF-κB luciferase (Fig. 3h). Tax expression increased NF-κB luciferase, but was blocked in the presence of increasing IκBα-DN plasmid. The HTLV-I HBZ gene is reportedly expressed at the mRNA level in most ATL cells, although its expression seems quite variable among samples and laboratories [20]. We tested if HBZ might be involved in the activation of JAG1 or DLL4 expression in ATL cells. Transduction of Molt4 cells with an HBZ lentiviral vector was performed, and both JAG1 and DLL4 expression were analyzed by RT-PCR and immunostaining. Our data suggests that HBZ does not play any significant role in the expression of JAG1 and/or DLL4 in ATL cells (Fig. 3d–f).

Regulation of JAG1 expression through direct and indirect mechanisms involving miR-124a, STAT3, and NFATc1 in ATL cells

Since Tax expression is retained in only 30% of ATL cells and HBZ did not play a significant role in activation of JAG1, we next investigated alternative pathways that could explain the high levels of JAG1 in ATL cells [21]. MicroRNAs (miRNAs) are transcriptional and post-transcriptional regulators of gene expression that are involved in many pathological conditions, including cancer [22]. A previous study identified JAG1 as a direct target of miRNA-124a [23]. Interestingly, our laboratory has shown that miR-124a is significantly downregulated in transformed cell lines and in primary ATL patient samples [16]. In addition to its direct effects on JAG1, miR-124a can also target STAT3 and NFATc1, two transcription factors known to regulate JAG1 gene expression (Fig. 4a). We have previously shown that STAT3 is a direct target of miR-124a [16]. In order to demonstrate a role for miR-124a inhibition of NFATc1, we first confirmed that NFATc1 is a direct target of miR-124a by 3′ UTR luciferase assays. We cloned the full-length NFATc1 3′UTR into a pGL3-luciferase vector and showed that miR-124a overexpression led to a statistically significant loss in NFATc1 3′UTR activity (Fig. 4b). The NFATc1 3′UTR contains three miR-124a binding sites. Mutation of individual miR-124a binding sites within the NFATc1 3′UTR led to a loss of miR-124a inhibition to varying degrees (Fig. 4c). However, loss of all three miR-124a binding sites led to complete loss of miR-124a inhibition (Fig. 4c). In addition, mutated

miR-124a lost the ability to inhibit NFATc1 3′UTR luciferase activity compared to wild-type miR-124a (Fig. 4b). To confirm that miR-124a can target NFATc1 protein levels, we generated miR-124a/pTRIPZ inducible 293T cells. Induction of miR-124a expression led to a loss of NFATc1 protein levels (Fig. 4d), whereas no loss was found in control, pTRIPZ, inducible cells. Since miRNA regulation of a target gene is context-dependent, we next investigated the role of miR-124a in the overexpression of JAG1 in the context of ATL cells. To this end, we used three TET-ON inducible cell lines expressing miR-124a under the control of an inducible promoter. The addition of doxycycline to the culture media efficiently induced expression of miR-124a (Fig. 4e), which was associated with a significant decrease in JAG1 levels of expression, in two out of three ATL lines (Fig. 4f). Expression of miR-124a in ATLT still led to a decrease in JAG1 expression; however, the level was not significant, possibly due to varying degrees of miR-124a expression after doxycycline induction. Finally, we found that

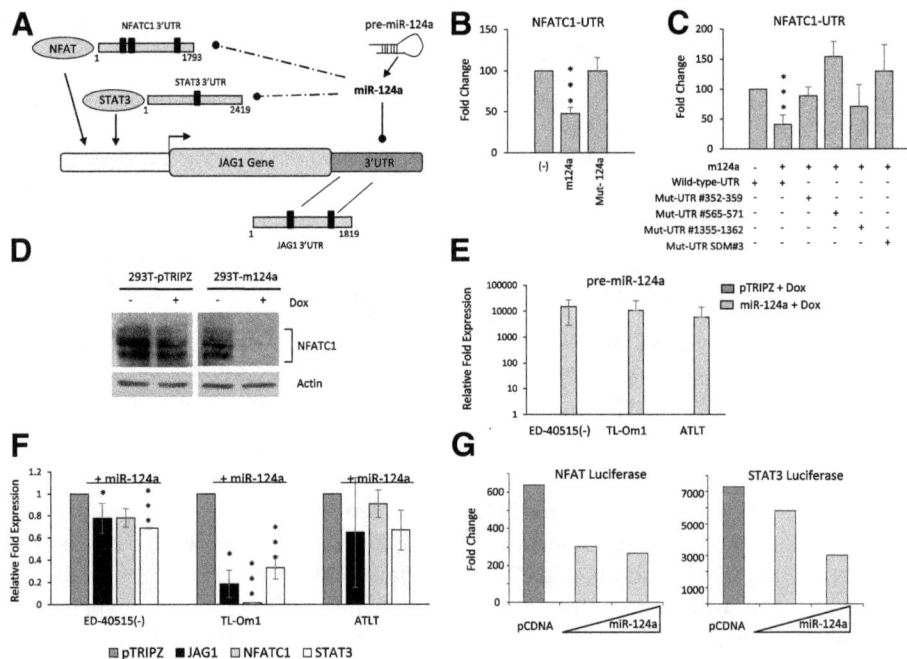

Fig. 4 miR-124a inhibits JAG1 expression directly and indirectly through STAT3 and NFATc1. **a** Schematic representation of the JAG1 transcript and its interplay with NFAT, STAT3, and miR-124. Solid black marks represent miR-124a binding sites within the 3′UTR of JAG1 (2 sites), STAT3 (1 site), and NFATc1 (3 sites). **b**, **c** pCDNA, miR-124a/pCDNA, or mutant miR-124a/pCDNA (**b**) (mutated miR-124a sequence) were transfected into 293T cells along with wild-type or mutant (**c**) NFATC1-UTR-pGL3 and the RL-TK plasmid. For mutant NFATC1-UTR, mutations were made at single miR-124a binding sites (#352-359, #565-571, or #1355-1362) or at all three mir-124a binding sites (Mut-UTR SDM#3). Forty-eight hours after transfection, cell lysates were measured for firefly (NFATC1 3′UTR) and renilla (RL-TK, internal control) activity. All luciferase was performed at least twice, and standard deviation is shown. Fold change was calculated compared to cells transfected with empty vector. **d** Detection of NFATC1 in stable 293T-pTRIPZ or –miR-124a cells induced 72 h with 2 μg/ml Dox. **e** Pre-miR-124a expression was detected by RT-PCR on ED-40515(–)-, Tl-Om1-, and ATLT-pTRIPZ and miR-124-pTRIPZ Tet-On inducible lines. **f** STAT3, NFATc1, and JAG1 expression were detected by RT-PCR on ED-40515(–)-, Tl-Om1-, and ATLT-pTRIPZ and miR-124-pTRIPZ Tet-On inducible lines. For **e** and **f**, 2 μg/ml Dox was added every day for 72 h. Post-induction, RT-PCR was performed and samples were normalized to GAPDH expression. Results are plotted as the average fold change from pTRIPZ-induced lines from at least two independent experiments. **g** 293T cells were transfected with pCDNA control or miR-124a/pCDNA, along with NFAT and STAT3 reporter luciferase vectors. Results are represented as a fold change compared to pCDNA transfected cells

miR-124a could not only suppress the expression of the STAT3 gene in ATL cell lines, but could also suppress NFATc1 mRNA (Fig. 4f). Consistent with these observations, miR-124a was able to inhibit both STAT3- and NFAT-dependent signaling as demonstrated by reduced luciferase activity from promoter reporter assays (Fig. 4g).

Overexpression of JAG1 in vivo in freshly isolated uncultured ATL patient RNA samples

We next investigated the expression of JAG1 mRNA in freshly isolated uncultured PBMCs from acute ATL patients. Our analysis shows that DLL4 was not consistently overexpressed in patient samples (data not shown). In contrast, JAG1 was significantly overexpressed in 12/17 ATL samples (70.6%) when compared to a healthy donor PBMC (Fig. 5a). Since Tax expression is variable to undetectable in ATL patients and NF-κB can induce JAG1 expression, we then tested whether the elevated JAG1 levels in ATL patients were due to an activated NF-κB pathway. Expression of the p65 subunit of NF-κB, RelA, is one of several markers used to test for NF-κB activity. The analysis of RT-PCR expression data for RelA and JAG1 showed no correlation between RelA expression and

JAG1 in ATL patients (Fig. 5b). This was in contrast to IL-8, a known downstream target of NF-κB, which strongly correlated with RelA expression in ATL patient samples ($r = 0.5997$). This indicates that NF-κB regulation of JAG1 in HTLV lines occurs through Tax expression and suggests that a Tax-independent mechanism elevates JAG1 RNA in ATL patients. Our previous work demonstrated that over half of ATL patients have high gene expression of STAT3 [16]. We found that NFATc1 gene expression was also high in a majority of ATL patients (data not shown). We then tested the expression of STAT3 and NFATc1 by RT-PCR and found both genes were positively correlated with JAG1 expression in ATL patients (STAT3, $r = 0.433$, and NFATc1, $r = 0.479$) (Fig. 5b). This suggests that STAT3 and NFATc1, which are at least partially regulated by miR-124a, could transcriptionally upregulate JAG1 expression in ATL patients. To further test this hypothesis, we treated an ATL line (ED-40515(−)) with specific pharmacological inhibitors to STAT3 (S3I-201) and NFAT (NFAT inhibitor, inNFAT). RT-PCR confirmed that inhibition of either the STAT3 or the NFAT pathway leads to loss of JAG1 expression in ATL lines; however, the result was only statistically significant for S3I-201 (Fig. 5c, d). The inNFAT prevents

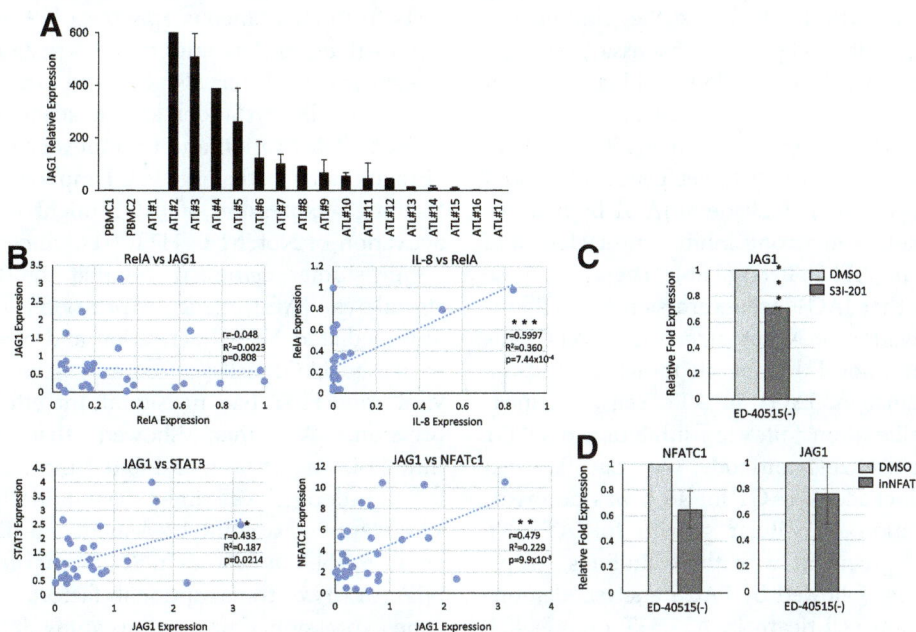

Fig. 5 Primary ATL patients overexpress JAG1, which correlates with STAT3 and NFATc1. **a** Real-time PCR analysis of JAG1 expression from cDNA derived from uncultured PBMCs of ATL patients and HTLV-1-negative donors. Samples were normalized to GAPDH expression, and the fold change was calculated by comparing values to healthy donor(s) normalized gene expression. **b** Real-time PCR analysis of JAG1, IL-8, RelA, STAT3, and NFATc1 expression from cDNA derived from PBMCs of patients with ATL and HTLV-1-negative donors. Samples were normalized to GAPDH expression, and the fold change was calculated by comparing values to healthy donor normalized gene expression. Correlation analysis was performed on JAG1 versus RelA, IL-8 versus RelA, JAG1 versus STAT3, and JAG1 versus NFATC1 in ATL patients. The Pearson's correlation coefficient (r), coefficient of determination (R^2), and p value of the Pearson's correlation coefficient are reported. **c, d** ED-40515(−) cells were treated 24 h with 50 μM S3I-201 (**c**) or 48 h with 100 μM NFAT inhibitor (inNFAT) (**d**). RT-PCR was performed on JAG1 expression, normalized to GAPDH control. For inNFAT, expression of NFATC1 was also noted. Experiments were performed at least twice, and fold change was calculated from the average repression compared to DMSO control samples

dephosphorylation of calcineurin-mediated dephosphorylation of NFAT, thereby preventing calcineurin binding. To test if the inhibitor was working, we performed RT-PCR on NFATc1 levels, since NFATc1 can auto-amplify its own transcription [24]. We found only a 40% loss in NFATc1 transcription following the addition of inNFAT to ED-40515(−) (Fig. 5d). It is possible that higher concentrations of drug are needed in order to fully downregulate the NFAT pathway in ATL cells.

Inhibition of JAG1 signaling dampened Notch1 signaling and migration of ATL cells

In order to validate the significance of JAG1 overexpression in the activation of Notch1 signaling in HTLV-I-transformed cells, we interrupted JAG1 signaling in ATL cells. Efficient downregulation of JAG1 was obtained by lentiviral delivery of JAG1 shRNA into the ATL line, ATL55T (Fig. 6a). Suppression of JAG1 expression was associated with downregulation of the Notch target genes VEGF (vascular endothelial growth factor), Hes1, and Hey1 (hairy-related transcription factor 1) (Fig. 6a). These results confirm that in ATL cells, JAG1 signaling is involved in the activation of the Notch1 pathway. To confirm these results, we then exposed HTLV-I-transformed cells to a JAG1-neutralizing antibody, which can selectively block the binding between the ligand and its receptor. In this assay, we used Jurkat and ATL55T, which display low and high levels of JAG1 expression, respectively. Exposure of Jurkat cells to a JAG1-neutralizing antibody had no significant effect on the expression of the Notch target genes, Hes1 and Hey1 (Fig. 6b). In contrast, blockade of JAG1 by neutralizing antibody resulted in strong inhibition of Hes1 and Hey1 expression in ATL55T (Fig. 6b). Together, these results confirmed that JAG1 overexpression is partly involved in the activation of Notch signaling in ATL cells and may represent a novel therapeutic target. To test the biological significance of JAG1 in ATL cells, we measured cellular proliferation following inhibition of JAG1 signaling by a neutralizing antibody. Our data showed that short-term blockade of JAG1 for 48 h was not associated with inhibition of cellular growth for ATL55T cells (Fig. 6c). In agreement with these findings, propidium iodide staining followed by FACS analysis demonstrated no significant cell death in ATL55T or ATL43T cells following transient inhibition of JAG1 (Fig. 6d). It is possible that JAG1 was not sufficiently inhibited or that alternative pathways are used. It is also possible that inhibition for longer periods are required to significantly halt ATL cell proliferation and survival. Additional studies may be warranted to answer these questions. Since JAG1 overexpression has been implicated in metastasis, we then investigated the role of JAG1 in ATL tumor cell migration by wound assays in vitro [25]. Results

presented in Fig. 6e demonstrate a reduction in wound healing 48 h after inhibition of JAG1, suggesting that in ATL cells, high JAG1 expression may contribute to tumor cell migration in vitro.

Discussion

In the present study, we investigated the molecular mechanisms that lead to constitutive Notch activation in HTLV-I-transformed and ATL cells. Among the Notch ligands, JAG1 was found to be significantly overexpressed both in virus-transformed cell lines and PBMCs isolated from acute ATL patients. Other Notch receptors, including JAG2, DLL1, and DLL4, were not significantly increased across all cells tested. JAG1 induction has been reported to affect both tumor cells and multiple components of the neoplastic microenvironment, including the vasculature and immune cells [26, 27]. Interestingly, several pieces of evidence demonstrate that JAG1 plays a role in some hematopoietic malignancies. For instance, in multiple myelomas, JAG1 is highly expressed and induces Notch activation, which in turn drives myeloma cell proliferation [28]. JAG1 also induces Notch over-activation in B cell chronic lymphocytic leukemia, and JAG1 stimulation in ex vivo cultures protects from spontaneous apoptosis [29, 30]. This demonstrates that JAG1 is important in sustaining the survival of cancer cells. It has also been reported that JAG1 overexpression by bystander and adjacent tumor cells leads to Notch1 activation and promotes cell growth in Hodgkin's and anaplastic large cell lymphoma [31], suggesting that high expression of JAG1 might have a role in the activation of Notch1 in HTLV-1-induced leukemia.

Our studies demonstrated that the Tax viral protein stimulates JAG1 gene expression in part through Tax-mediated NF-κB activation and was associated with increased JAG1 cell surface expression. In contrast, the viral gene HBZ had no significant effects on JAG1 expression. We then showed that the microRNA, miR-124a, significantly inhibited the expression of JAG1 in ATL-derived cell lines. The underlying mechanism was identified as miR-124a-mediated direct targeting of JAG1 mRNA as well as miR-124a-targeting STAT3 and NFATc1, two transcriptional factors controlling JAG1 gene expression. Our previous study described decreased expression of miR-124a in an HTLV-I context [16], suggesting that the absence of a negative regulator might contribute to JAG1 overexpression both in cell lines and ATL patients even in the absence of Tax expression. Consistent with this notion, the expression of STAT3 and NFATc1 were directly correlated to that of JAG1 in primary ATL patients, and pharmacological inhibition of either STAT3 or NFATc1 was associated with decreased JAG1 expression in ATL cell lines.

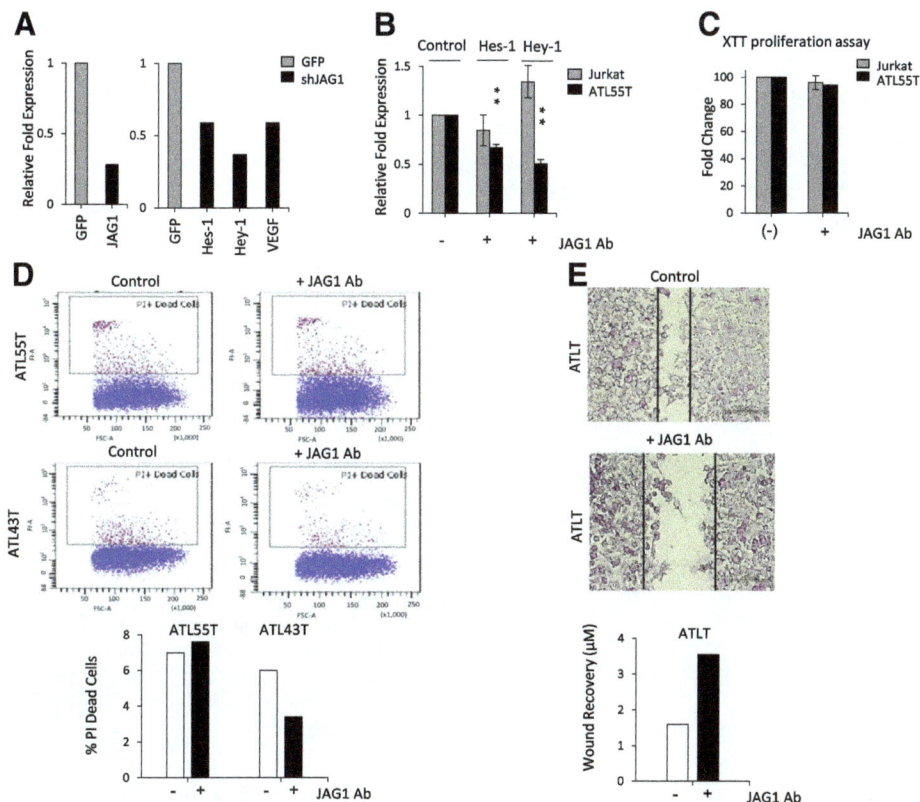

Fig. 6 Repression of JAG1 alters Notch signaling and wound healing in ATL lines. **a** RT-PCR was performed on JAG1 from cDNA derived from ATL cell line ATL55T infected with a lentivirus pSIH1-shRNA against JAG1. Cells infected with the empty vector expressing pSIH1-GFP were used as a control. The expression of JAG1 was normalized to GAPDH expression. RT-PCR was then performed on Hes-1, Hey-1, and VEGF from cDNA derived from ATL55T cells infected with pSIH1-shRNA against JAG1. Cells infected with the empty vector expressing pSIH1-GFP were used as a control. Real-time PCR was performed in duplicate, and samples were normalized to GAPDH expression. **b** Real-time PCR was performed on Hes-1 and Hey-1 on cDNA extracted from ATL55T and Jurkat cells incubated for 6 days with neutralizing antibody against JAG1 (3 µg/ml). Real-time PCR was performed in duplicate, and samples were normalized to GAPDH expression. **c** Cell proliferation was measured using XTT assay in ATL55T and Jurkat cells incubated for 6 days with neutralizing antibody against JAG1 (3 µg/ml). Results were plotted as mean ± standard deviation from at least two independent experiments. **d** PI staining was performed to study cell death in ATL55T and ATL43T cells incubated for 6 days with neutralizing antibody against JAG1 (3 µg/ml). Media with antibody was replaced every 3 days, and fresh antibody was added (3 µg/ml). Cells were analyzed for apoptosis by FACS analysis. Bar diagrams representing the FACS results are provided. **e** Wound healing was performed on confluent ATLT cells treated with 3 µg/ml of JAG1-neutralizing antibody for 72 h. After 72 h, the p1000 tip was used to scratch the plate. The plate was then washed, and fresh media with neutralizing antibody was added. After 48 h, the cells were fixed and images were taken with a ×40 objective lens. Bar diagrams representing the wound healing results are provided

Activation of the Notch signaling pathway is particularly relevant in HTLV-1-infected cells because its prolonged pharmacological inhibition significantly reduces tumor size in an engrafted ATL mouse model [13]. High expression of JAG1 has been associated with increased migration and invasion of tumor cells and metastasis and poor prognosis in non-small cell lung cancer (NSCLC) [25]. JAG1 is also highly expressed in medulloblastoma and colorectal cancer, and JAG1 causes poorer overall survival in breast cancer [32–34]. Studies have demonstrated that JAG1 signaling in cancer cells can activate downstream pathways such as AP-1 (activator protein 1), MAPK (mitogen-activated protein kinases), EGFR (epidermal growth factor receptor), and NF-κB [27, 35–37]. Along these lines, AP-1, MAPK, and NF-κB have also been shown to be activated in ATL cells. Whether JAG1 overexpression is involved in these processes warrants additional investigation. We also found that inhibition of JAG1 signaling by using a neutralizing antibody or shRNA does not affect the short-term proliferation or survival of ATL cells. It is possible that JAG1 inhibition is not sufficient to completely abrogate Notch1 activation. This notion is supported by the fact that blocking JAG1 reduced expression of Notch1 downstream targets (Hes-1, Hey-1, and VEGF) by 50%. However, our data suggest that inhibition of JAG1 even transiently is sufficient to significantly affect ATL tumor cell migration, which may be a function of JAG1 independent of Notch signaling and warrants additional studies.

Conclusions

Our study demonstrates a significant overexpression of the Notch ligand JAG1 in ATL cells versus normal PBMCs. This overexpression was linked to viral Tax, miR-124a, STAT3, and NFATc1. JAG1 overexpression was associated with Notch1 signaling in ATL cells. Our data further suggests JAG1 as a possible candidate for the development of immunotherapy against ATL cells.

Acknowledgements
The authors would like to thank Brandi Miller for the editorial assistance.

Funding
This work was supported by grant AI103851 and CA141386 to Christophe Nicot.

Authors' contributions
MB, RM, HC, and JP conducted the experiments. CN designed the study, interpreted the data, and wrote the manuscript. All authors read and approved the final manuscript.

Consent for publication
Not applicable

Competing interests
The authors declare that they have no competing interests.

References
1. Purow B. Notch inhibition as a promising new approach to cancer therapy. Adv Exp Med Biol. 2012;727:305–19.
2. Cheng F, Pekkonen P, Ojala PM. Instigation of Notch signaling in the pathogenesis of Kaposi's sarcoma-associated herpesvirus and other human tumor viruses. Future Microbiol. 2012;7(10):1191–205.
3. Arcaini L, Rossi D, Lucioni M, Nicola M, Bruscaggin A, Fiaccadori V, Riboni R, Ramponi A, Ferretti W, Cresta S, et al. The NOTCH pathway is recurrently mutated in diffuse large B-cell lymphoma associated with hepatitis C virus infection. Haematologica. 2015;100(2):246–52.
4. Hofelmayr H, Strobl LJ, Marschall G, Bornkamm GW, Zimber-Strobl U. Activated Notch1 can transiently substitute for EBNA2 in the maintenance of proliferation of LMP1-expressing immortalized B cells. J Virol. 2001;75(5):2033–40.
5. Pancewicz J, Nicot C. Current views on the role of Notch signaling and the pathogenesis of human leukemia. BMC Cancer. 2011;11:502.
6. Chastagner P, Israel A, Brou C. AIP4/Itch regulates Notch receptor degradation in the absence of ligand. PLoS One. 2008;3(7):e2735.
7. Kandachar V, Roegiers F. Endocytosis and control of Notch signaling. Curr Opin Cell Biol. 2012;24(4):534–40.
8. Welcker M, Clurman BE. FBW7 ubiquitin ligase: a tumour suppressor at the crossroads of cell division, growth and differentiation. Nat Rev Cancer. 2008;8(2):83–93.
9. Nasr R, Marcais A, Hermine O, Bazarbachi A. Overview of targeted therapies for adult T-cell leukemia/lymphoma. Methods Mol Biol. 2017;1582:197–216.
10. Nicot C. HTLV-I Tax-mediated inactivation of cell cycle checkpoints and DNA repair pathways contribute to cellular transformation: "a random mutagenesis model". J Cancer Sci. 2015;2(2).
11. Bellon M, Baydoun HH, Yao Y, Nicot C. HTLV-I Tax-dependent and -independent events associated with immortalization of human primary T lymphocytes. Blood. 2010;115(12):2441–8.
12. Giam CZ, Semmes OJ. HTLV-1 infection and adult T-cell leukemia/lymphoma-a tale of two proteins: tax and HBZ. Viruses. 2016;8(6).
13. Pancewicz J, Taylor JM, Datta A, Baydoun HH, Waldmann TA, Hermine O, Nicot C. Notch signaling contributes to proliferation and tumor formation of human T-cell leukemia virus type 1-associated adult T-cell leukemia. Proc Natl Acad Sci U S A. 2010;107(38):16619–24.
14. Weng AP, Ferrando AA, Lee W, Morris JP, Silverman LB, Sanchez-Irizarry C, Blacklow SC, Look AT, Aster JC. Activating mutations of NOTCH1 in human T cell acute lymphoblastic leukemia. Science. 2004;306(5694):269–71.
15. Lobry C, Oh P, Aifantis I. Oncogenic and tumor suppressor functions of Notch in cancer: it's NOTCH what you think. J Exp Med. 2011;208(10):1931–5.
16. Bellon M, Lu L, Nicot C. Constitutive activation of Pim1 kinase is a therapeutic target for adult T-cell leukemia. Blood. 2016;127(20):2439–50.
17. Chevalier SA, Durand S, Dasgupta A, Radonovich M, Cimarelli A, Brady JN, Mahieux R, Pise-Masison CA. The transcription profile of Tax-3 is more similar to Tax-1 than Tax-2: insights into HTLV-3 potential leukemogenic properties. PLoS One. 2012;7(7):e41003.
18. Gasparian AV, Yao YJ, Kowalczyk D, Lyakh LA, Karseladze A, Slaga TJ, Budunova IV. The role of IKK in constitutive activation of NF-kappaB transcription factor in prostate carcinoma cells. J Cell Sci. 2002;115(Pt 1):141–51.
19. Hoesel B, Schmid JA. The complexity of NF-kappaB signaling in inflammation and cancer. Mol Cancer. 2013;12:86.
20. Billman MR, Rueda D, Bangham CRM. Single-cell heterogeneity and cell-cycle-related viral gene bursts in the human leukaemia virus HTLV-1. Wellcome Open Res. 2017;2:87.
21. Takeda S, Maeda M, Morikawa S, Taniguchi Y, Yasunaga J, Nosaka K, Tanaka Y, Matsuoka M. Genetic and epigenetic inactivation of tax gene in adult T-cell leukemia cells. Int J Cancer. 2004;109(4):559–67.
22. Yeh CH, Moles R, Nicot C. Clinical significance of microRNAs in chronic and acute human leukemia. Mol Cancer. 2016;15(1):37.
23. Akerblom M, Sachdeva R, Barde I, Verp S, Gentner B, Trono D, Jakobsson J. MicroRNA-124 is a subventricular zone neuronal fate determinant. J Neurosci. 2012;32(26):8879–89.
24. Pan MG, Xiong Y, Chen F. NFAT gene family in inflammation and cancer. Curr Mol Med. 2013;13(4):543–54.
25. Chang WH, Ho BC, Hsiao YJ, Chen JS, Yeh CH, Chen HY, Chang GC, Su KY, Yu SL. JAG1 is associated with poor survival through inducing metastasis in lung cancer. PLoS One. 2016;11(3):e0150355.
26. Pedrosa AR, Trindade A, Fernandes AC, Carvalho C, Gigante J, Tavares AT, Dieguez-Hurtado R, Yagita H, Adams RH, Duarte A. Endothelial Jagged1 antagonizes Dll4 regulation of endothelial branching and promotes vascular maturation downstream of Dll4/Notch1. Arterioscler Thromb Vasc Biol. 2015;35(5):1134–46.
27. Choi K, Ahn YH, Gibbons DL, Tran HT, Creighton CJ, Girard L, Minna JD, Qin FX, Kurie JM. Distinct biological roles for the notch ligands Jagged-1 and Jagged-2. J Biol Chem. 2009;284(26):17766–74.
28. Jundt F, Probsting KS, Anagnostopoulos I, Muehlinghaus G, Chatterjee M, Mathas S, Bargou RC, Manz R, Stein H, Dorken B. Jagged1-induced Notch signaling drives proliferation of multiple myeloma cells. Blood. 2004;103(9):3511–5.
29. Li D, Masiero M, Banham AH, Harris AL. The notch ligand JAGGED1 as a target for anti-tumor therapy. Front Oncol. 2014;4:254.
30. Rosati E, Sabatini R, Rampino G, Tabilio A, Di Ianni M, Fettucciari K, Bartoli A, Coaccioli S, Screpanti I, Marconi P. Constitutively activated Notch signaling is involved in survival and apoptosis resistance of B-CLL cells. Blood. 2009;113(4):856–65.
31. Jundt F, Anagnostopoulos I, Forster R, Mathas S, Stein H, Dorken B. Activated Notch1 signaling promotes tumor cell proliferation and survival in Hodgkin and anaplastic large cell lymphoma. Blood. 2002;99(9):3398–403.
32. Fiaschetti G, Schroeder C, Castelletti D, Arcaro A, Westermann F, Baumgartner M, Shalaby T, Grotzer MA. NOTCH ligands JAG1 and JAG2 as critical pro-survival factors in childhood medulloblastoma. Acta Neuropathol Commun. 2014;2:39.
33. Dai Y, Wilson G, Huang B, Peng M, Teng G, Zhang D, Zhang R, Ebert MP, Chen J, Wong BC, et al. Silencing of Jagged1 inhibits cell growth and invasion in colorectal cancer. Cell Death Dis. 2014;5:e1170.
34. Reedijk M, Odorcic S, Chang L, Zhang H, Miller N, McCready DR, Lockwood G, Egan SE. High-level coexpression of JAG1 and NOTCH1 is observed in human breast cancer and is associated with poor overall survival. Cancer Res. 2005;65(18):8530 7.

35. LaVoie MJ, Selkoe DJ. The Notch ligands, Jagged and Delta, are sequentially processed by alpha-secretase and presenilin/gamma-secretase and release signaling fragments. J Biol Chem. 2003;278(36):34427–37.

36. Zeng Q, Li S, Chepeha DB, Giordano TJ, Li J, Zhang H, Polverini PJ, Nor J, Kitajewski J, Wang CY. Crosstalk between tumor and endothelial cells promotes tumor angiogenesis by MAPK activation of Notch signaling. Cancer Cell. 2005;8(1):13–23.

37. Nickoloff BJ, Qin JZ, Chaturvedi V, Denning MF, Bonish B, Miele L. Jagged-1 mediated activation of notch signaling induces complete maturation of human keratinocytes through NF-kappaB and PPARgamma. Cell Death Differ. 2002;9(8):842–55.

The roles of metallothioneins in carcinogenesis

Manfei Si and Jinghe Lang[*]

Abstract

Metallothioneins (MTs) are small cysteine-rich proteins that play important roles in metal homeostasis and protection against heavy metal toxicity, DNA damage, and oxidative stress. In humans, MTs have four main isoforms (MT1, MT2, MT3, and MT4) that are encoded by genes located on chromosome 16q13. MT1 comprises eight known functional (sub)isoforms (MT1A, MT1B, MT1E, MT1F, MT1G, MT1H, MT1M, and MT1X). Emerging evidence shows that MTs play a pivotal role in tumor formation, progression, and drug resistance. However, the expression of MTs is not universal in all human tumors and may depend on the type and differentiation status of tumors, as well as other environmental stimuli or gene mutations. More importantly, the differential expression of particular MT isoforms can be utilized for tumor diagnosis and therapy. This review summarizes the recent knowledge on the functions and mechanisms of MTs in carcinogenesis and describes the differential expression and regulation of MT isoforms in various malignant tumors. The roles of MTs in tumor growth, differentiation, angiogenesis, metastasis, microenvironment remodeling, immune escape, and drug resistance are also discussed. Finally, this review highlights the potential of MTs as biomarkers for cancer diagnosis and prognosis and introduces some current applications of targeting MT isoforms in cancer therapy. The knowledge on the MTs may provide new insights for treating cancer and bring hope for the elimination of cancer.

Keywords: Metallothionein, Metal homeostasis, Cancer, Carcinogenesis, Biomarker

Background

Metallothioneins (MTs) are a family of low molecular weight (ranging from 6 to 7 kDa), cysteine-rich cytosolic proteins that play a vital role in metal ion homeostasis and detoxification [1, 2]. MT was first isolated by Margoshes and Vallee from horse kidney cortex as a low molecular weight protein containing cadmium in 1957 [3]. MTs are involved in metalloregulatory processes by binding to heavy metals through the thiol group of their cysteine residues. MTs have a high affinity for heavy metals, which means that they can bind to xenobiotic heavy metals to provide protection against metal toxicity, especially cadmium toxicity [4]. When MTs bind to physiological heavy metals, such as zinc and copper, they can participate in regulating cell growth and proliferation and protecting the body against oxidative stress [5]. Recently, many studies have shown that MT expression varies in different tumors, suggesting that MTs may play a vital role in carcinogenesis

[6–10]. The elucidation of possible functions and mechanisms of MTs in tumor progression may provide potential promising markers for cancer. This review was conducted to summarize the latest data on the role of MTs in carcinogenesis and to provide diagnostic or therapeutic information to help oncologists in their clinical decision-making.

Structure and classification

MTs are highly conserved, low molecular weight proteins that are present in a broad range of taxonomic groups and display a high level of sequence heterogeneity, which results in varying molecular weights and number and distribution of cysteine residues [1, 11]. Mammalian MTs constitute a superfamily of nonenzymatic polypeptides of 61–68 amino acids, characterized by high cysteine content (30%), lack of aromatic amino acids, and few or no histidine residues but with abundant thiol groups to bind to heavy metals [9, 11, 12].

In humans, MTs are encoded by a family of genes located on chromosome 16q13 and include at least 11 functional members: MT1 (MT1A, MT1B, MT1E, MT1F, MT1G,

* Correspondence: langjh@hotmail.com
Department of Obstetrics and Gynecology, Peking Union Medical College Hospital, Peking Union Medical College, Chinese Academy of Medical Sciences, No. 1 Shuaifuyuan, Dongcheng District, Beijing 100730, China

MT1H, MT1M, and MT1X; MT1C, MT1D, MT1I, MT1J, and MT1L are pseudogenes that cannot encode MT proteins), MT2 (also known as MT2A), MT3, and MT4 [13, 14]. A summary of MT genes, isoforms, and location is shown in Table 1.

Roles of MTs in cancer

The well-known biological functions of MTs are related to their high affinity for heavy metals. MTs can control cellular homeostasis of zinc/copper, which is essential for cell proliferation and differentiation, and act as antioxidants to protect cells against free radicals and oxidative stress generated by mutagens, antineoplastic drugs, and radiation [15, 16]. MTs can also bind to cadmium, mercury, platinum, or other similar heavy metals to protect cells and tissues against heavy metal toxicity [4]. In addition, MTs play a protective role against DNA damage and apoptosis [17–19]. Accumulating evidence indicates that MTs play important roles in carcinogenesis and cancer therapy. MTs participate in the process of carcinogenesis and play critical roles in tumor growth, progression, metastasis, and drug resistance (Fig. 1). To provide a comprehensive insight into the complicated relation between MTs and cancer, we summarized the dysregulated expression and functions of MT isoforms in various tumor tissues in Table 2.

Expression of MT isoforms in various types of cancers

Numerous studies have demonstrated that changes in MT expression are associated with the process of carcinogenesis and cancer progression. However, the expression of MTs is not universal in all human cancers. Previous studies have shown that MT expression is upregulated in breast cancer, nasopharyngeal cancer, ovarian cancer, urinary bladder cancer, and melanoma [20–24], while in other cancers, such as hepatocellular carcinoma, prostate cancer, and papillary thyroid carcinoma, MT expression is

downregulated [7, 25, 26]. Theocharis et al. also observed that among lung cancer subtypes, MT expression was prominent in squamous cell lung carcinoma and adenocarcinoma but absent in small cell lung cancer [27]. The differential expression of MTs depends on the type and differentiation status of tumors, as well as other environmental stimuli and/or gene mutations [17, 28, 29]. Nevertheless, a better understanding of the changes in the expression of particular MT isoforms in various cancers can help identify specific therapeutic targets and reverse tumor progression.

In humans, MTs have four main isoforms: MT1, MT2, MT3, and MT4. Of these four isoforms, MT1 and MT2 are ubiquitously expressed in various tissues, while MT3 and MT4 are minor isoforms with restricted expression in specialized cells and tissues, such as the brain, reproductive organs, and stratified squamous epithelium [7, 17]. MT3 was first purified and characterized as a growth inhibitory factor (GIF) in the human brain [30] and was later designated as a third member of the MT family [31]. MT4 was discovered in the stratified squamous epithelium in the skin, esophagus, and tongue [32]. Furthermore, MT1 and MT2 are basally expressed and highly induced by a variety of stimuli including metals, hormones, cytokines, growth factors, oxidants, stress, and irradiation, while MT3 and MT4 are constitutively expressed despite signal changes in vitro or in vivo [33].

Krizkova et al. have provided a comprehensive summary of the expression and regulation of individual MT isoforms in various types of malignancies [34]. In Fig. 2, the transcript levels of MT isoforms in cancers are compared with those in normal samples by using Oncomine databases (threshold setting: p value, 0.01; fold change, 2; gene rank, top 10%). The figure shows that the mRNA levels of MT isoforms are significantly up/downregulated in various types of cancers (Fig. 2). These data clearly indicate that MT isoforms can be targeted to treat cancer and

Table 1 Genetic information related to functional MT isoforms obtained from the National Center of Biotechnology Information (NCBI)

MT isoforms	Gene ID	Location	GenBank accession number	References
MT1A	4489	Chromosome 16, NC_000016.10 (56638666..56640087)	NM_005946.2	[170, 171]
MT1B	4490	Chromosome 16, NC_000016.10 (56651899..56653204)	NM_005947.2	[172, 173]
MT1E	4493	Chromosome 16, NC_000016.10 (56625673..56627112)	NM_175617.3	[143, 172]
MT1F	4494	Chromosome 16, NC_000016.10 (56657943..56659303)	NM_005949.3	[131, 174]
MT1G	4495	Chromosome 16, NC_000016.10 (56666735..56668065, complement)	NM_005950.2	[172, 175]
MT1H	4496	Chromosome 16, NC_000016.10 (56669814..56671129)	NM_005951.2	[8, 176]
MT1M	4499	Chromosome 16, NC_000016.10 (56632622..56633986)	NM_176870.2	[142, 172]
MT1X	4501	Chromosome 16, NC_000016.10 (56682470..56684196)	NM_005952.3	[176, 177]
MT2A	4502	Chromosome 16, NC_000016.10 (56608566..56609497)	NM_005953.4	[178, 179]
MT3	4504	Chromosome 16, NC_000016.10 (56589355..56591088)	NM_005954.3	[31, 180]
MT4	84560	Chromosome 16, NC_000016.10 (56565049..56568957)	NM_032935.2	[32, 181]

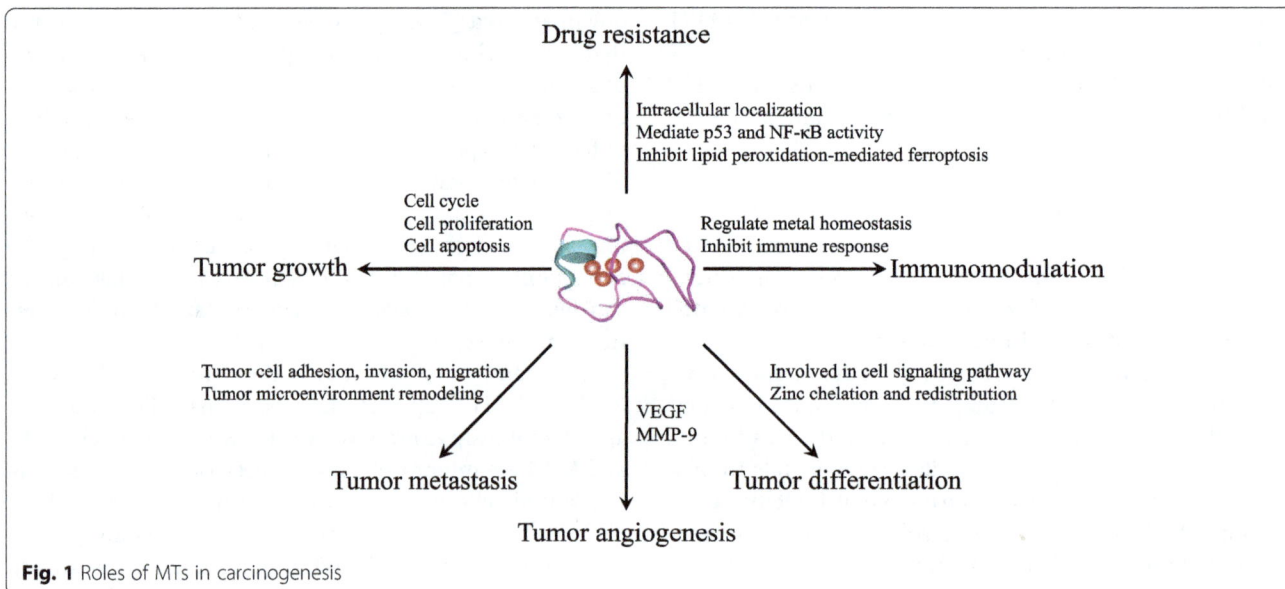

Fig. 1 Roles of MTs in carcinogenesis

enhance the efficiency of anticancer therapy due to their important roles and altered expression in various cancers. Therefore, knowledge on the expression of MT isoforms could be fully utilized for tumor diagnosis and anticancer therapy.

Tumorigenesis

Tumorigenesis, also called carcinogenesis or oncogenesis, refers to the formation of a tumor in which normal cells are transformed into cancer cells. Any changes at the cellular, genetic, and epigenetic levels that disrupt the balance between proliferation and programmed cell death, in the form of apoptosis, such as DNA mutations and epimutations, can contribute to the development of cancer. MTs have been shown to play an important role in carcinogenesis. To better understand the roles of MTs in cancer, the National Cancer Institute held a workshop that focused on three topics: the role of zinc in tumor cell pathobiology, the role of MTs in metal carcinogenesis, and the role of MTs in tumor cells and potential in cancer chemotherapy [35]. Since then, a large number of studies have been conducted to investigate the roles of MTs in carcinogenesis.

Tumor growth

The tumor growth-promoting effects of MTs involve the following potential mechanisms. Nagel et al. demonstrated that cytoplasmic MTs reached a maximum level during the G1/S cell cycle transition, a period when cells prepare for DNA synthesis, thereby demonstrating a physiological role of MTs in tumor cell proliferation [36]. Studies have shown that zinc is required for G1/S phase transition [37, 38]. Thus, it can be hypothesized that MTs regulate the supply of zinc for proteins and the

activity of zinc-dependent transcription factors to modulate tumor cell growth and proliferation. Later, Lim et al. observed that the downregulation of MT2A expression in breast cancer cells could induce cell cycle arrest at the G1 phase to inhibit cancer cell growth, and the underlying molecular mechanisms involved the regulation of cell cycle-related genes including ataxia telangiectasia mutated (ATM) and cell division cycle 25A (cdc25A) [39].

MTs also participate in cell proliferation. Ki-67 is one of the most sensitive markers of cell proliferation. Werynska and colleagues have shown a positive correlation between the expression of MT1/2 and that of the proliferation markers Ki-67 and minichromosome maintenance protein 2 (MCM-2) in non-small cell lung cancer [40]. A similar positive correlation between MTs and Ki-67 expression had also been confirmed in breast cancer [20, 41], nasopharyngeal carcinoma [21], large intestine adenocarcinoma [42], basal cell carcinoma [43], and soft tissue sarcomas such as malignant fibrous histiocytoma, liposarcoma, and synovial sarcoma [44].

MTs have also been shown to inhibit apoptosis [19]. MTs can act as zinc donors for transcription factors such as hypoxia-inducible factor-1α (HIF-1α) and tumor suppressors such as P53 to influence cell growth [17, 45]. P53 is a zinc-binding transcription factor that can inhibit cell cycle progression and induce apoptosis in response to DNA damage. MTs can remove zinc ions from P53 protein molecules, thus leading to the changes in the spatial structure of P53, leading to its inactivation and thus result in uncontrolled cell proliferation [20, 46]. Moreover, MTs have been demonstrated to interact with nuclear factor-κB (NF-κB) and mediate its antiapoptotic effects [47], probably because zinc is an essential component for the

Table 2 Overview of the dysregulated expression and functions of MT isoforms in cancer

Cancer type	MT isoforms	Expression	Functions	References
Acute nonlymphoblastic leukemia	MT	Positive	Resistance-related proteins	[182]
Acute myeloid leukemia	MT1G, MT1A	Positive	Inversely correlated with PU.1 expression	[183]
	MT3	Down	Promoter hypermethylation	[154]
Adenoid cystic carcinomas of the salivary glands	MT	Up	Myoepithelial differentiation	[184]
Basal cell carcinoma	MT	Up	Infiltrative growth	[185]
	MT1, MT2	Up	Promote proliferation: Ki-67 antigen expression	[43]
	MT3	Down	Possibly based on DNA methylation	[186]
	MT3	Low to moderate expression	Carcinogenesis	[187]
Bladder carcinoma	MT	Up	Drug resistance	[188]
	MT2	Up	Cisplatin resistance	[99]
	MT3	Up	Carcinogenesis and increase tumor grade	[189]
	MT1X	Up	Correlated with tumor grade	[190]
	MT	Up	Poor survival and cisplatin resistance	[23]
Breast cancer	MT3	Up	Poor prognosis	[130]
	MT2A	Up	Increase invasiveness	[191]
	MT1E	Present in estrogen receptor (ER)-negative breast cancer	Myoepithelial differentiation and tumor invasiveness	[191]
	MT2A	Up	Modulate cell cycle via the ATM/Chk2/cdc25A signaling pathway	[39]
	MT2A	Up	Upregulation of matrix metalloproteinase (MMP)-9; enhance cell invasion and migration	[82]
	MT3	Up	Increase invasiveness	[83]
Cholangiocarcinoma	MT	Partly positive	Poor prognosis	[128]
Colonic cancer	MT	Up	Promote proliferation	[36]
	MT1F	Down	Loss of heterozygosity	[52]
	MT1G, MT1X, MT2A	Down	Associated with the depth of tumor invasion, lymph node metastasis, and tumor stage	[52]
Colorectal cancer	MT2A, MT1B, MT1F, MT1G, MT1H, MT1B, MT1F, MT1G, MT1H, MT2A	Down	Poor clinical outcome	[192]
	MT1E, MT1F, MT1G, MT1H, MT1M, MT1X MT2A	Down	Epigenetic mechanisms	[6]
	MT2A	Up	Interact with Fas-associated death domain (FADD) in NF-κB pathway to promote cell proliferation	[49]
	MT1G	Down	Colorectal cancer cell differentiation	[67]
Ductal breast cancer	MT1E	High in ER-negative cancer tissues	Mediate effector genes downstream of ER	[193]
	MT1F	Up	Influence histological differentiation	[58]
	MT2A	Up	Cell proliferation	[41]
	MT2A	Up	Chemoresistance (doxorubicin)	[59]
	MT1, MT2	Up	Increased proliferative potential	[20]
	MT3	Down	Epigenetic changes	[88]
Endometrial carcinoma	MT1, MT2	Up	Modify p53 expression	[141]

Table 2 Overview of the dysregulated expression and functions of MT isoforms in cancer *(Continued)*

Cancer type	MT isoforms	Expression	Functions	References
	MT1E	Down	Promoter hypermethylation	[143]
Esophageal adenocarcinoma	MT3	Down	DNA methylation	[152]
Esophageal squamous cell carcinoma	MT	Up	Chemoresistance to cisplatin; poor prognosis	[194]
	MT3	Down	DNA methylation	[153]
	MT1G	Down	Gene methylation	[145]
	MT1G	Down	Promoter hypermethylation	[146]
	MT1M	Down	DNA methylation; correlated with smoking duration	[195]
Gallbladder carcinoma	MT	Up	Histological dedifferentiation	[63]
Gastric carcinoma	MT3	Down	Hypermethylation	[151]
	MT1G	Up	Cisplatin resistance	[196]
	MT1X	Up	Irinotecan resistance	[103]
	MT	Up	Poor survival and high recurrence rate	[81]
	MT2A	Down	Inhibit the activation of the NF-κB pathway	[135]
	MT2A	Down	Be a potential target of miR-23a	[197]
	MT1D (MTM)	Down	Enhance migration and invasion	[198]
	MT1M, MT1JP	Down	Associated with tumor diameter, differentiation, lymphatic metastasis, distal metastasis, invasion, and tumor node metastasis (TNM) stage	[199]
Glioma	MT1E	In proportion to the motility of glioma cell	Enhance tumor proliferation, invasion, and migration through regulation of activation and expression of MMPs	[84, 85]
Hepatoblastoma	MT1G	Down	Promoter hypermethylation	[147]
Hepatocellular carcinoma	MT1F	Down	Cell growth	[200]
	MT1G	Down	Allelic loss on chromosome 16q12.1-q23.1	[155]
	MT1, MT2A	Down	Transcriptional repression: dephosphorylation of the transcription factor CCAAT/enhancer-binding protein (C/EBP) α through phosphatidylinositol 3-kinase (PI3K)/AKT signaling pathway	[25]
	MT1X, MT2A	Down	Malignant transformation of hepatocytes; local invasion; hepatitis B virus infection	[201]
	MT1G	Down	Tumor suppressor gene; promoter hypermethylation	[148]
	MT1M	Down	Increase NF-κB activity	[142]
	MT1, MT2	Down	Promoter hypermethylation and transcriptional repression; prognostic marker	[133]
	MT1M, MT1G	Down	Promoter methylation	[136]
	MT1M	Down	Poor prognosis	[134]
	MT1, MT2	Down	Associated with the disruption of circadian clock genes	[202]
	MT1H	Down	Regulate the Wnt/β-catenin signaling pathway	[8]
	MT1M	Down	Inhibit tumorigenesis	[203]
Intrahepatic cholangiocarcinoma	MT1A, MT1E, MT1F, MT1G, MT1H, MT1IP, MT1X	Down	Hypermethylation	[204]
Lung cancer	MT1A, MT2A, MT1E, MT1G	Down	Gene methylation	[205]
Large cell lung cancer	MT1F, MT1G, MT1M, MT1X	Up	Poor prognosis	[206]
Melanoma	MT	Up	Poor prognosis	[24, 125]
	MT1E	Down	DNA methylation	[144]

Table 2 Overview of the dysregulated expression and functions of MT isoforms in cancer *(Continued)*

Cancer type	MT isoforms	Expression	Functions	References
	MT1, MT2	Up	Intratumoural macrophage infiltration to defect host immune response and metastasis formation	[77]
Nasopharyngeal cancer	MT	Up	Cell proliferation	[21]
Non-small cell lung cancer	MT	Up	Tumor cell proliferation and short survival	[122]
	MT1H	Up	Drug resistance (cisplatin)	[207]
	MT1, MT2	Up	Promote proliferation: expressions of Ki-67 and minichromosome maintenance protein-2 (MCM-2) (positive correlation)	[40]
	MT3	Up	Pathogenesis	[208]
	MT1B, MT1F, MT1G, MT1H, MT1X	Up	Pathogenesis	[131]
	MT1F, MT2A	Up	Poor outcome	[131]
	MT1E	Down	Cell differentiation	[131]
Oral squamous cell carcinoma	MT	Up	Poor prognosis	[127]
	MT1A, MT1X, MT3, MT4	Down	Possible markers for oral carcinogenesis	[209]
	MT1G	Down	Poor survival	[209]
	MT1F	Up	Associated with tobacco use	[209]
Osteosarcoma	MT1E, MT1H, MT1X, MT2A, MT1B, MT1G, MT1L	Up	Drug resistance	[210]
Ovarian cancer	MT1, MT2	Up	Mutant p53; histological grade	[22]
	MT2A	Up	Inhibit cell death	[211]
	MT1L, MT1X, MT2A	Up	Low malignant potential or early cancer onset	[212]
Pancreatic carcinoma	MT	Partly positive	Metastasis, poor prognosis, and poor histological grade	[62]
Papillary thyroid carcinoma	MT1G	Down	Promoter hypermethylation	[149]
	MT1E, MT1G, MT1X, MT2A	Down	Promoter methylation and transcriptional repression	[7]
	MT1G	Down	Modulate the activity of the PI3K/AKT and Rb/E2F pathways	[89]
Prostate cancer	MT3	Highly variable increase	Control prostate epithelial cell growth	[213]
	MT1X	Down	Advanced prostate cancer	[214]
	MT2A	Up	Inhibit cell death	[211]
	MT3	Up	Inhibit cell growth and increase drug resistance	[53]
	MT1G	Down	Promoter hypermethylation	[150]
	MT1F, MT1M	Down	Associated with perineural invasion	[215]
	MT1H	Down	Enhance the histone methyltransferase activity of euchromatin histone methyltransferase 1 (EHMT1)	[26]
	MT2A	Down	Single nucleotide polymorphism (SNP); metal accumulation	[14]
	MT3	Depend on cell type	Increase cell proliferation, invasion, and tumorigenic activities	[104]
	MT1E	Down	DNA methylation	[10]
Renal cell cancer	MT	Up	Tumor grade	[64]
	MT2A	Up	Stimulate cellular proliferation	[216]
	MT1A, MT1G	Down	Growth arrest and induction of apoptosis	[216]
	MT1A, MT1E, MT1G,	Down	Tumorigenesis	[217]

Table 2 Overview of the dysregulated expression and functions of MT isoforms in cancer *(Continued)*

Cancer type	MT isoforms	Expression	Functions	References
	MT1H, MT1L			
	MT1H, MT1G, MT2A	Down	Promoter methylation	[45]
Salivary gland adenocarcinoma	MT	Up	High immunoreactivity and microenvironment remodeling	[90]
Serous ovarian cancer	MT	Up	Diagnosis of malignancy and worse prognosis	[218]
Small cell lung cancer	MT	45% positive	P53 expression and short-term survival	[121]
Soft tissue sarcoma	MT	Up	Ki-67 expression, grade of malignancy, and prognostic appraisal	[44]
	MT2A, MT1X, MT1F, MT1H	Up	Metastasis	[219]
Squamous cell carcinoma of the tongue	MT	Positive	Delay cells entering apoptosis	[220]
	MT	Positive	Correlated with depth of invasion, vascular invasion, and lymph node metastasis	[221]
Testicular cancer	MT	Up	Chemoresistance	[222]
	MT	Up	Early diagnosis	[115]
Transitional cell carcinoma of the bladder	MT	Up	Poor survival	[126]

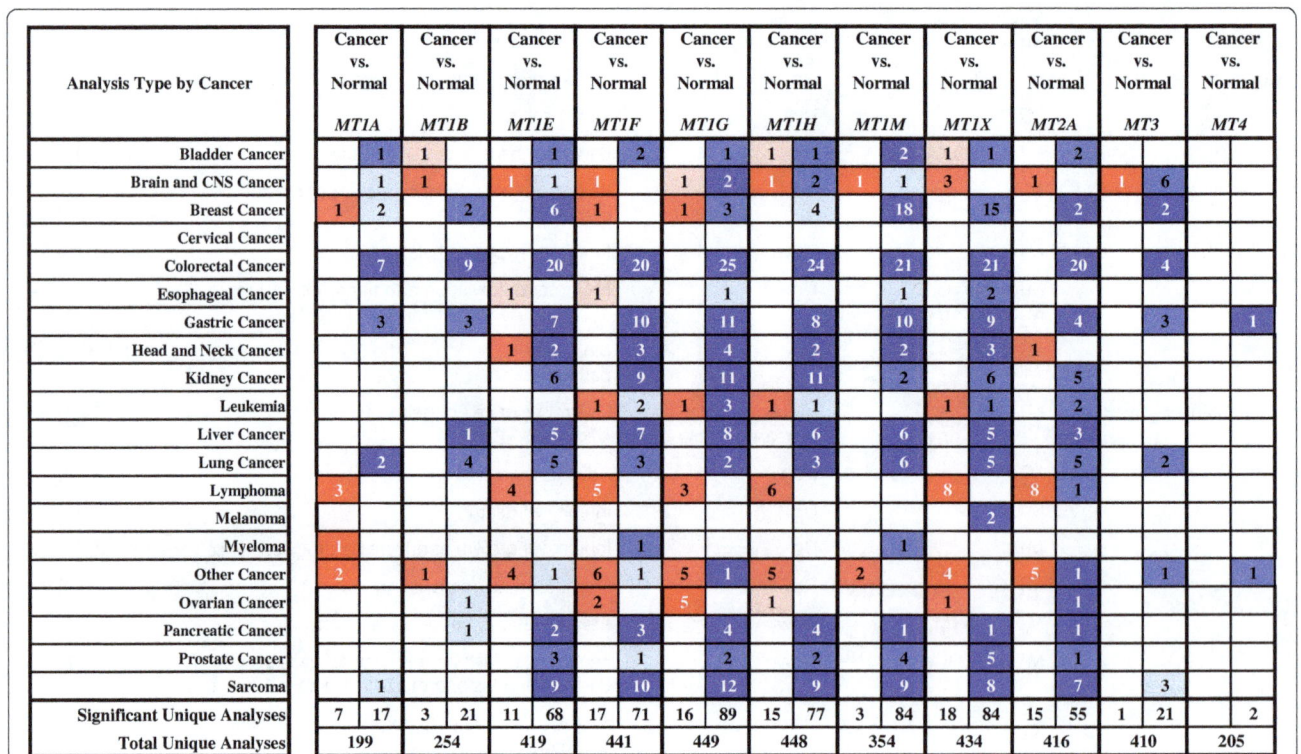

Fig. 2 — Transcript levels of MT isoforms in different types of cancers (each column: Cancer vs. Normal). The number in each colored cell represents the number of datasets meeting the threshold.

Analysis Type by Cancer	MT1A	MT1B	MT1E	MT1F	MT1G	MT1H	MT1M	MT1X	MT2A	MT3	MT4
Bladder Cancer	1	1		1	2	1	2	1 1	2		
Brain and CNS Cancer	1	1	1 1	1	1 2	1 2	1 1	3	1	1 6	
Breast Cancer	1 2	2	6	1	1 3	4	18	15	2	2	
Cervical Cancer											
Colorectal Cancer		7	9	20	20	25	24	21	21	20	4
Esophageal Cancer			1	1		1		1	2		
Gastric Cancer		3	3	7	10	11	8	10	9	4	1
Head and Neck Cancer			1	2	3	4	2	2	3	1	
Kidney Cancer				6	9	11	11	2	6	5	
Leukemia			1	2	1 3	1 1		1 1	2		
Liver Cancer			1	5	7	8	6	6	5	3	
Lung Cancer		2	4	5	3	2	3	6	5	5	2
Lymphoma	3		4	5	3	6		8	8 1		
Melanoma								2			
Myeloma	1			1			1				
Other Cancer	2	1	4 1	6 1	5 1	5	2	4	5 1	1	1
Ovarian Cancer		1		2	5	1		1	1		
Pancreatic Cancer		1	2	3	4	4	1	1	1		
Prostate Cancer			3	1	2	2	4	5	1		
Sarcoma		1	9	10	12	9	9	8	7	3	
Significant Unique Analyses	7 / 17	3 / 21	11 / 68	17 / 71	16 / 89	15 / 77	3 / 84	18 / 84	15 / 55	1 / 21	/ 2
Total Unique Analyses	199	254	419	441	449	448	354	434	416	410	205

Legend: 1   5   10   10   5   1   ← % →   Cell color is determined by the best gene rank percentile for the analyses within the cell.

Fig. 2 Transcript levels of MT isoforms in different types of cancers. This figure was generated from Oncomine, indicating the numbers of datasets with statistically significant MT mRNA upregulation (red) or downregulation (blue) (different types of cancer vs. corresponding normal tissues) (threshold setting: *p* value, 0.01; fold change, 2; gene rank, top 10%). The number in the colored cell represents the number of datasets meeting the threshold

DNA-binding function of NF-κB [48]. Marikar et al. revealed a new phenomenon that the interaction of the phosphorylated Fas-associated death domain (FADD) with MT2A was involved in the increase in cell proliferation and inhibition of cell apoptosis in colorectal cancer via the NF-κB pathway [49]. MT expression can protect cells from a variety of apoptotic stimuli, including oxidative stress, heavy metals, and chemotherapeutic agents (doxorubicin, etoposide, etc.) [18, 50, 51].

Intriguingly, in vitro experiments have confirmed that MT1F transfection into colon cancer cells could decrease cell proliferation and colony formation and increase cell apoptosis rates to inhibit cell growth. The authors also obtained similar results with in vivo experiments in which compared with those in empty vector-expressing mice, the tumor growth rate and average tumor size and weight were reduced in MT1F-expressing mice. These results highlighted MT1F as a tumor suppressor that can inhibit tumor growth in vivo [52]. Similarly, low expression and tumor suppressor activity of MT1H were identified in prostate cancer. In detail, the induced expression of MT1H reduced the colony formation and decreased the entry of prostate cells into the S and M phases to suppress cell growth [26]. A similar suppressive role of MT1H was also reported in hepatocellular carcinoma [8]. Dutta et al. demonstrated that the stable transfection of PC-3 cells to overexpress the MT3 gene significantly reduced the cell growth relative to both nontransfected PC-3 cells and blank vector-transfected control cells [53].

Altogether, these findings indicate that MTs may contribute to tumor growth by regulating cell cycle arrest, cell proliferation, and apoptosis. However, whether MTs play an oncogenic or tumor-suppressive role depends on their isoforms and the type of tumors.

Tumor differentiation

Cellular differentiation is the process by which a cell changes from one type to another. The "grade" of histological differentiation or the grade of malignancy is used as a measure of cancer progression and includes the ability to form glandular structures, cellular polymorphism, and evident mitotic activity. Many studies have reported that MTs participate in cell differentiation. Aikins and fellow researchers investigated the influence of extremely low-frequency electromagnetic fields (ELFEMFs) on zinc-MT3 interactions during the neural differentiation of human bone marrow-derived mesenchymal cells. Their study found that during this interaction, MT3 expression was downregulated, and the formation of zinc-MT3 complexes was enhanced to maintain zinc homeostasis. A new homeostatic regulatory mechanism was thus discovered, which involved the zinc-MT3 complex and other MT3-interacting proteins to drive neural differentiation, thereby highlighting the potential

diagnostic and clinical applications for MT3 in neurodegenerative diseases [54]. Moreover, Wu et al. demonstrated MTs as negative regulators for interleukin (IL)-27-induced type 1 regulatory T cell differentiation [55]. Hirako et al. uncovered that the overexpression of MT1G could inhibit the differentiation of all-trans retinoic acid (ATRA)-induced NB4 acute promyelocytic leukemia cells [56]. MT2A expression was reported to influence the osteosarcoma cell differentiation toward the osteogenic lineage. In other words, MT2A overexpression could the enhance cell differentiation [57]. Additionally, numerous studies have revealed a relationship between MT expression and tumor differentiation. Jin et al. found that the expression of MT1F and MT2A in histological grade 3 breast cancer was significantly higher than that in histological grades 1 and 2 in breast cancer [41, 58]. Similar results were recently demonstrated by other authors [20, 59–61]. The relationship between MT expression and tumor histological grade was also demonstrated in pancreatic ductal carcinoma [62], gallbladder carcinoma [63], renal cancer [64], ovarian adenocarcinoma [22, 65], and endometrial carcinoma [66]. All of the mentioned studies demonstrated a strong positive correlation between MT expression and tumor grade, showing that MT expression was enhanced with increasing tumor grade. To investigate the role of MT1G in the differentiation of colorectal cancer cells, Arriaga et al. transfected MT1G-myc expression plasmids into H29 cells, which stably overexpress MT1G. The authors uncovered that MT1G was involved in the process of tumor cell differentiation mainly through the Notch signaling pathway and labile zinc chelation and redistribution [67].

Cell differentiation is necessary for normal development. Undifferentiated and poorly differentiated cells have a high likelihood to form tumors. As mentioned above, MTs have been reported to participate in cell differentiation and have been found to be positively correlated with histological tumor grade. These findings may provide a new approach for treating cancers in which tumor cells are prompted to differentiate into more mature cells by using MT-related pharmacological agents.

Tumor angiogenesis

The formation of new blood vessels is a required step for tumorigenesis because tumors need a network of blood vessels to obtain sufficient oxygen and essential nutrients for their growth, progression, and metastasis [68]. Several studies have demonstrated that MTs play an important role in tumor angiogenesis. Miyashita and Sato showed that MT1 was expressed in vascular endothelial cells (ECs) at the site of angiogenesis, and the downregulation of MT1 expression inECs resulted in the inhibition of cell proliferation, migration, and angiogenesis in vivo, which indicated that MT1 was involved in the regulation of angiogenesis [69]. Penkowa et al. observed that decreased levels of the growth factors b-fibroblast growth factor (b-FGF), transforming growth factor β1 (TGFβ1), and vascular endothelial growth factor (VEGF) could mediate the reduction in angiogenesis and regeneration in MT1 +2-deficient mice after a cortical freeze injury in the central nervous system. Furthermore, the authors found that MT1+2-deficient transgenic mice expressing IL-6 displayed a dramatic reduction in IL-6-induced angiogenesis. These results suggested that MT1+2 participate in the angiogenic process possibly by regulating the expression of angiogenesis-promoting factors [70].

VEGF is a major contributor to angiogenic processes such as EC proliferation, migration, and sprouting. Wierzowiecka et al. carried out a study in three breast cancer cell lines, in which an increased expression of selected MT isoforms was induced by zinc ions to various degrees. The expression of VEGF was slightly increased after the stimulation with zinc ions, which suggested a correlation between MT expression and VEGF expression in breast cell lines [71]. Another study showed that MT3 could significantly induce the expression of VEGF through a HIF-1α-dependent mechanism in brain ECs [72]. Schuermann and colleagues also confirmed that MT2 acts upstream of VEGF expression in regulating EC proliferation, migration, and angiogenesis [73].

Matrix metallopeptidase (MMP)-9, also known as gelatinase B, is widely associated with tumor progression because of its role in extracellular matrix (ECM) remodeling, angiogenesis, and neovascularization [74]. MMP-9 is a member of the zinc-dependent metalloproteinase family that has been demonstrated to interact with MTs [75]. Hence, it can be hypothesized that MTs participate in angiogenesis via MMP-9. Zbinden et al. identified MTs as a participant in collaterogenesis and angiogenesis and observed combined dysfunction of ECs, smooth muscle cells (SMCs), and macrophages in MT knockout (KO) mice. MMP-9, platelet-derived growth factor (PDGF) receptor, and VEGF were significantly downregulated in SMCs isolated from MT KO animals, which contributed to SMC dysfunction [76].

In conclusion, MTs can induce the upregulation of angiogenesis-related genes, such as VEGF and MMP-9; act on ECs, SMCs, and macrophages; and result in the formation of new blood vessels to promote tumor growth, progression, and metastasis (Fig. 3). Therefore, further investigation of MTs may provide therapeutic targets for inhibiting angiogenesis and tumor progression.

Tumor metastasis

Metastasis is a complex, multistep process by which cancers spread from the primary site to a secondary site within the body. MT overexpression has been demonstrated as a marker of aggressive tumor behavior in many kinds of cancers. Emri et al. showed that MT1+2 overexpression was significantly more frequent in metastatic primary cutaneous malignant melanoma (CMM) ($p = 0.018$), which suggested the predictive value of MT overexpression in the metastatic ability of CMM [77]. In primary colorectal cancer, MT expression was significantly associated with lymph node metastasis, suggesting that MTs may modulate the tumor metastatic process [78]. A similar result has been reported in the lymph node metastasis

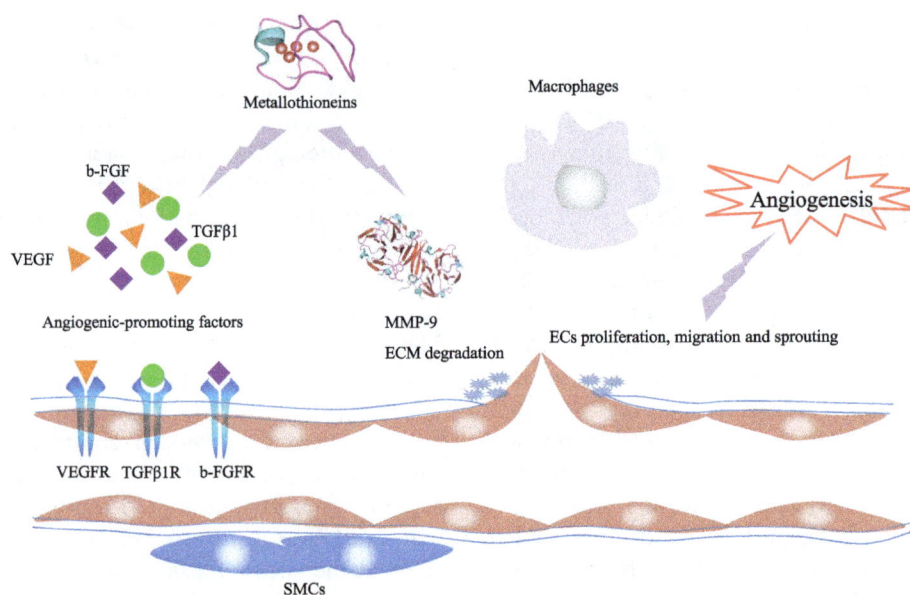

Fig. 3 Roles of MTs in tumor angiogenesis. ECM, extracellular matrix; ECs, endothelial cells; SMCs, smooth muscle cells

of breast cancers [79]. In esophageal squamous cell carcinoma, MT expression was indicative of metastatic potential and was associated with the lymph node metastasis ($p = 0.0343$) and distant metastasis ($p = 0.0452$) [80]. In gastric cancer patients, MT overexpression was significantly correlated with lymph node and distant metastasis, as well as the number of metastatic lymph nodes [81]. Clinical studies have demonstrated that MT2A overexpression enhanced breast cancer cell invasion and migration via the upregulation of MMP-9 induced by the activation of the AP-1 and NF-κB signaling pathways [82]. In addition, studies have suggested that MT3 overexpression can increase the invasiveness of breast cancer cell by modulating MMP-3 expression [83]. Similarly, Ryu et al. verified the expression of MT1E in relation to the motility of glioma cell lines, and MT1E enhanced the invasion and migration of malignant glioma cells by modulating the activity of MMPs and NF-κB/p50 [84, 85].

Interestingly, Yan et al. conducted an in vitro study to assess the effect of MT1F expression on colon cancer cells and found that migration, invasion, and adhesion were significantly inhibited in MT1F-expressing colon cancer cells [52]. Ramaswamy et al. have shown that the downregulation of MT3 was one of the 17-gene signature associated with metastasis in primary solid tumors [86]. A decrease in MT3 expression was observed in pituitary adenocarcinoma with spinal cord metastasis [87]. Likewise, Gomulkiewicz et al. showed that the MT3 expression was significantly lower in patients with ductal breast cancer with lymph node metastasis than in patients without metastasis [88]. Furthermore, Fu et al. demonstrated a significant positive association of MT1G hypermethylation with lymph node metastasis in 178 papillary thyroid cancer patients [89].

Studies have also demonstrated that MTs are involved in tumor microenvironment remodeling to facilitate tumor spread, invasion, and metastasis [90–92].

Collectively, these data suggest that MTs contribute to tumor metastasis by enhancing the invasion and migration of tumor cells and tumor microenvironment remodeling. However, the up/downregulation of MTs depends on their isoforms and the type of tumors, as well as other environmental stimuli or gene mutations.

Tumor microenvironment remodeling and immune escape
Subramanian Vignesh and Deepe elucidated the immunomodulatory role of MTs and demonstrated MTs as an important component of the innate and adaptive immune systems regulating metal homeostasis, particularly zinc and thus impacting the immune cell redox status, enzyme function, and cell signaling [93]. Emri et al. observed that metastatic CMM cases were associated with the presence of tumor-infiltrating CD68+ ($p = 0.001$) and CD163+ ($p < 0.001$) macrophages. Furthermore, MT

overexpression was found to be related to the presence of tumor-infiltrating CD68+ macrophages ($p = 0.003$). Hence, MTs might play an immunomodulatory role to contribute to melanoma progression [77]. MT expression has also been associated with the number and activity of immune cells during immune responses in breast cancer [94].

MTs can be released into the extracellular environment in response to cellular stress. Furthermore, extracellular MTs can bind to the plasma membrane of lymphocytes and influence their immunomodulatory activities [95]. MTs have been found to be able to suppress murine cytotoxic lymphocyte activity, reduce the level of detectable major histocompatibility complex class I and CD8 molecules on lymphocytes, and increase IL-2 receptor expression, indicating that MTs are involved in cell-mediated immunosuppression functions and contribute to antitumor immunity [96].

Studies have shown that MTs can inhibit immune responses and are involved in the microenvironment remodeling to control and accelerate tumor growth and initiate metastasis [90, 91]. Dutsch-Wicherek et al. observed that the immunoreactivity levels of MTs in pharyngeal squamous cell carcinoma were statistically higher than those in the reference tissues. In addition, higher MT immunoreactivity levels were detected in tumor patients with lymph node metastasis than in patients without metastasis. The authors concluded that MT expression within the tumor cells was associated with tumor aggressiveness and metastasis via microenvironment remodeling [91]. Canpolat and Lynes found that endogenous MTs are synthesized during the normal immune response or as a consequence of toxicant exposure suppressed in vivo immune function, indicating an immunomodulatory role of MTs [97]. Inhibition of the immune response by MTs may indicate that MTs are involved in the remodeling of the immunosuppressive tumor microenvironment [90].

These findings collectively suggest that MTs act as immunomodulators to interfere with the immune response and participate in tumor microenvironment remodeling to drive tumor immune evasion.

Tumor drug resistance
MTs contribute to the development of drug resistance through a variety of mechanisms in many types of cancers. A previous study has demonstrated that the overexpression of MTs was involved in the acquisition of resistance to anticancer drugs, including cis-diamminedichloroplatinum (II), chlorambucil, and melphalan [98]. Since then, the relationship between MT expression and tumor drug resistance has been examined in different tumor types.

In bladder carcinoma, an enhanced expression of MT2 was identified in the cisplatin-resistant cells, suggesting that cisplatin resistance may be partly mediated by MT2

[99]. This result was recently corroborated by Wülfing et al. If bladder cancer cells expressed MTs, the patients treated with cisplatin chemotherapy had a significantly poor survival rate; in other words, MT overexpression may mediate resistance to cisplatin-based chemotherapy [23]. Matsumoto et al. reported an enhanced expression of MTs following chemotherapy in non-small cell lung cancer, which may be related to drug resistance [100]. Similarly, MT expression was found to be correlated with cisplatin resistance in three human small cell lung cancer lines [101]. Lee et al. confirmed that in contrast to those in cisplatin-sensitive cells, MTs were overexpressed in cisplatin-resistant mouse melanoma cancer cells. Reducible poly(oligo-D-arginine) (rPOA) was used to deliver short hairpin RNAs against MTs (shMT) into cells and resulted in the downregulation of MT expression and enhanced the anticancer effect of cisplatin. Additionally, in vivo tumor models showed synergistically enhanced the tumor-suppressive effects of co-administration of shMT/rPOA oligopeptoplex and cisplatin. These results demonstrated that MT overexpression was at least one of the main reasons for cisplatin resistance [102]. Upregulation of MTs was shown to increase irinotecan resistance in gastric cancer patients [103]. Furthermore, MT3 overexpression increased chemotherapeutic drug resistance in PC-3 prostate cancer cells [53, 104].

Although several studies have investigated MT-mediated resistance mechanisms, the results still need to be further validated. Kondo et al. demonstrated that nuclear MTs were indicative of greater resistance to cisplatin than diffuse MTs in human hormone-independent prostatic cell lines, implying that the nuclear localization of MTs is important for the resistance to chemical drugs [105]. In addition, Surowiak et al. demonstrated that the nuclear expression of MTs increased during the exposure to cisplatin and was indicative of drug resistance in ovarian cancer cells [106]. Thus, nuclear MT expression probably represents a mechanism of drug resistance that protects the DNA of tumor cells from the toxic effects of chemical drugs. However, Gansukh et al. showed a divergent result in which the nuclear and cytoplasmic expression of MTs had no effect on cisplatin resistance in non-small cell lung cancer cells, perhaps because the mechanism of cisplatin resistance in this cancer is independent of MTs [107]. Arriaga et al. showed that the overexpression of the MT1G sensitized colorectal cancer cells to the chemotherapeutic agents' oxaliplatin and 5-fluorouracil, which may have been mediated by the activation of p53 and repression of NF-κB activity [108]. Sun et al. also demonstrated a novel molecular mechanism of drug resistance. Specifically, they showed that enhanced MT1G expression contributed to sorafenib resistance in hepatocellular carcinoma by inhibiting lipid peroxidation-mediated ferroptosis [109]. Habel et al. showed that chemotherapy resistance induced by MT2A

was partially due to zinc chelation [57]. A study by Yap et al. revealed that reduced MT2A gene expression could enhance the chemosensitivity to doxorubicin [59]. Hence, it can be speculated that inhibiting the expression of certain MT isoforms can increase the anticancer activity of drugs, thereby providing a potential therapeutic strategy.

Therefore, as a predictor of chemoresistance, MT expression might be evaluated for the selection of appropriate anticancer agents or be modulated to resensitize chemoresistant tumor cells to improve the efficacy of chemotherapy. Although MTs have an ability to increase the chemoresistance, many studies indicate that MTs can prevent cardiotoxicity induced by anticancer agents by scavenging free radicals and attenuating oxidative stress [110–112]. Hence, strategies to balance cardioprotection and chemoresistance deserve to be investigated. Heger et al. had proposed a possible solution that involved heart-specific overexpression of MTs by transient transfection to help overcome unwanted cardiotoxicity without increasing tumor chemoresistance [111]. Further studies are needed to explore the potential mechanisms of MTs, thus enhancing their cardioprotective effect while inhibiting chemoresistance.

MTs as biomarkers for cancer diagnosis and prognosis

MTs can be readily detected in patient's blood, and the level of serum MTs is positively correlated with the pathological state, disease stage, and degree of cancer progression; thus, MTs act as an enriched source of biomarkers.

Petrlova et al. had described various electroanalytical techniques to detect MTs in human serum [113]. Through electrochemical analysis, MT levels were found to be elevated in most patients with melanoma, breast, and colon cancer [114]. Tariba et al. selected 25 patients with newly diagnosed testicular germ cell tumors (TGCTs) and 22 healthy volunteers in their study and found that serum MT concentration in patients with TGCT was significantly higher than that in control individuals; additionally, in combination with the commonly used markers, MTs could improve the early diagnosis rate [115]. In another study with 46 prostate cancer patients diagnosed by biopsy, total prostate-specific antigen (tPSA) levels and MT levels were examined in serum samples. In the first cohort ($n = 17$) diagnosed with prostate cancer, tPSA levels were within the physiological range of 0–4 ng/mL for over 36.9% of cases, indicating the unreliability of tPSA as a marker of prostate cancer. However, although tPSA levels were normal in the first group, MT levels were significantly elevated ($p = 0.05$), indicating that MTs might be used as an additional prostate cancer marker to increase the reliability of prostate cancer diagnosis [116]. Krizkova et al. also demonstrated that determination of serum MT levels by differential pulse voltammetry could be considered as a promising diagnostic tool for childhood solid tumors [117].

Previous reports had revealed MT overexpression as a valuable prognostic marker for tumor progression and drug resistance in a wide range of cancers, such as ovarian cancer [22, 118], breast cancer [119, 120], small cell lung cancer [121], non-small cell lung cancer [122], renal cell carcinoma [123, 124], melanoma [24, 125], bladder cancer [23, 126], oral squamous cell carcinoma [127], and cholangiocarcinoma [128]. Surowiak et al. indicated that increased expression of MTs represented an unfavorable predictive factor in cisplatin-treated ovarian cancer patients [118]. In primary ovarian cancer, MT-positive patients had shorter survival than MT-negative patients, and this result could be explained by the positive correlation between MT expression and histological grade [22]. In primary invasive ductal breast carcinoma, MT-positive patients had a significantly poorer prognosis than MT-negative patients ($p < 0.01$), which suggested a prognostic value of MT expression [129]. Similarly, MT3 overexpression has been reported to be associated with poor prognosis in breast cancer [130]. The association of high MT expression with short-term survival had been demonstrated in small cell lung cancer [121] and non-small cell lung cancer [122], and enhanced expression of MT1F and MT2A isoforms predicted poor clinical outcomes in non-small cell lung cancer in which upregulated MT1F expression was associated with larger primary tumor size and higher grade of malignancy [131]. In a prospective study on 520 melanoma patients, MT overexpression was related to an increased risk of melanoma progression with poor prognosis and survival rate [125]. In 2006, the authors updated this study with an 11-year prospective cohort comprising 1270 melanoma patients to confirm the previous results [24]. Another study compared the predictive roles of MT overexpression with those of sentinel lymph node biopsy and found that MT overexpression was an excellent prognostic predictor of cancer progression and patient survival [132]. Additionally, a significant correlation was found between MT overexpression and poor overall survival ($p = 0.0005$), disease-specific survival ($p = 0.0004$), disease-free survival ($p = 0.05$), and disease-free progression ($p = 0.0008$) in patients with transitional cell carcinoma of the bladder [126]. Another study also demonstrated that the overexpression of MTs ($p = 0.003$) was an independent risk factor associated with poor survival in bladder cancer patients [23]. Similar results were observed in oral squamous cell carcinoma patients [127] and in cholangiocarcinoma patients suffering from either intrahepatic cholangiocarcinoma or hilar extrahepatic cholangiocarcinoma [128].

However, in other types of cancers such as prostate cancer [10], hepatocellular carcinoma [133, 134], and gastric cancer [135], the downregulation of MT expression was associated with poor prognosis. Demidenko and colleagues attempted to identify the prognostic biomarkers for predicting biochemical recurrence (BCR) of prostate cancer. They identified 455 differentially expressed genes through global gene expression profiling, among which seven genes (*CHI3L2*, *FABP7*, *GHRH*, *GPR52*, *MT1E*, *OLR1*, and *SAA2*) were selected for further validation in two independent prostate cancer cohorts. The results suggested that MT1E downregulation was a potential biomarker of early BCR and poor prognosis in prostate cancer patients [10]. Park and Yu demonstrated that MT1 and MT2 are important prognostic markers in hepatocellular carcinoma. The loss of nuclear expression of MT1 and MT2 was associated with high Edmondson-Steiner grade and microvascular invasion and poor prognosis indicated by recurrence-free survival ($p = 0.029$) and overall survival ($p = 0.007$) [133]. In another study, low MT1M expression was found to be linked to high alpha-fetoprotein (AFP) levels and high tumor recurrence rates following curative resection in patients with hepatocellular carcinoma [134]. In addition, combined MT1M and MT1G promoter methylation in hepatocellular carcinoma patients was associated with a high incidence of vascular invasion and lymph node or extrahepatic metastasis, thereby acting as an effective prognostic marker [136]. Decreased MT2A expression was reported to be associated with advanced TNM stages, tumor differentiation, and poor outcomes in patients with gastric cancer [135].

Taken together, these findings indicate that MTs play critical roles in almost all aspects of cancer, thereby providing opportunities for the development of MTs as novel diagnostic and prognostic biomarkers.

Mechanisms involving MTs in cancer

MTs can act as zinc donors to mediate the activity of zinc-dependent transcription factors such as P53 and NF-κB to regulate cell apoptosis and tumor cell growth. MTs can remove zinc ions from P53 protein molecules, leading to the changes in its spatial structure and loss of function, similar to p53 mutations, and resulting in uncontrolled cell proliferation. Meplan et al. demonstrated that MT overexpression exerted a potent inhibitory effect on the transcriptional activity of P53, consistent with the metal chelation effect of MTs [137]. Interaction of MTs with the tumor suppressor P53 appears to be crucial for the development and progression of tumors [46, 138, 139]. Conversely, the activation of P53 has been shown to be an important factor in the expression and induction of MTs in cancer cells [140]. Positive correlations between MT and p53 expression were found in endometrial carcinoma, implying that MTs can regulate p53 expression [141]. The study by Hengstler et al. also showed a significant correlation between MT expression and mutant p53 in ovarian carcinoma [22]. Furthermore, the antiapoptotic role of MTs may also be related to its modulation of NF-κB activity. Abdel-Mageed and Agrawal revealed that MTs cause the transactivation of NF-κB, which results in the inhibition of apoptosis [47]. In contrast, Sakurai et al. demonstrated MTs as a negative regulator of NF-κB activity by using the MT-null embryonic cell lines [48]. MT2A has been shown to regulate NF-κB pathway activation to participate in tumor progression in gastric cancer [135] and colorectal cancer [49]. Downregulation of MT1M can also contribute to hepatocellular carcinogenesis by increasing the activity of NF-κB [142].

Numerous studies have demonstrated that the elimination of tumor suppressor gene activity by promoter methylation is responsible for carcinogenesis, a mechanism that has been confirmed in many human cancers. Demidenko et al. revealed MT1E promoter methylation as a possible mechanism of gene inactivation, which resulted in the reduced expression of MT1E in prostate cancer [10]. Similar observations were validated in patients with endometrial carcinoma [143] and melanoma [144]. In previous studies, MT1G suppression was reported to contribute to carcinogenesis in papillary thyroid carcinoma, prostate cancer, esophageal squamous cell carcinoma, hepatocellular carcinoma, and hepatoblastoma, and the mechanism of MT1G gene silencing was related to promoter hypermethylation [145–150]. In gastric carcinoma, Deng et al. showed that the reduced expression of MT3 was due to the hypermethylation of CpG islands on intron 1 [151]. DNA methylation of MT3 was detected in esophageal adenocarcinoma, resulting in MT3 gene silencing. Moreover, DNA methylation of MT3 from − 127 to − 8 sites was shown to be significantly correlated with advanced tumor stages and lymph node metastasis, implying that the methylation of promoter regions may be involved in tumor progression [152]. DNA methylation of MT3 was also confirmed in esophageal squamous cell carcinoma, but there was no significant association between the MT3 methylation status and prognosis [153]. Tao et al. observed epigenetic inactivation of MT3 via promoter hypermethylation in pediatric acute myeloid leukemia, and MT3 could act as a tumor suppressor by inhibiting tumor cell proliferation and inducing apoptosis [154]. Han et al. demonstrated that MT1H acts as a tumor suppressor by interacting with euchromatin histone methyltransferase 1 (EHMT1) to increase the methyltransferase activity of EHMT1 on histone 3 [26]. Earlier studies have shown that MT1G inactivation was mediated by promoter methylation in thyroid cancer [7, 149]. Fu et al. revealed in-depth molecular mechanisms of MT1G as a tumor suppressor in thyroid carcinogenesis, which involved the inhibition of cell growth and invasion and induction of cell cycle arrest and apoptosis via the inhibition of the phosphorylation of Akt and Rb, that is, through modulation of the phosphatidylinositol 3-kinase (PI3K)/AKT and Rb/E2F signaling pathways [89].

Beyond DNA methylation, there are other potential mechanisms of MTs in carcinogenesis. The suppression of MT1 and MT2A in human hepatocellular carcinoma was related to the dephosphorylation (inactivation) of the transcription factor CCAAT/enhancer-binding protein (C/EBP) α through the PI3K/AKT signaling pathway rather than the gene hypermethylation [25]. Zheng et al. established stable hepatocellular cancer cell lines with constitutive expression of MT1H to examine the potential role of MT1H in hepatocellular carcinogenesis. They found that MT1H could suppress Wnt/β-catenin signaling to inhibit tumor progression, including hepatocellular cancer cell proliferation, invasion, and migration [8]. In terms of the studies on genomic changes, Chan et al. noted that MT1G downregulation in hepatocellular carcinoma was due to the allelic loss on chromosome 16q12.1-q23.1 [155]. Additionally, Yan et al. demonstrated that the potential mechanism of MT1F downregulation in colon cancer was a loss of heterozygosity (LOH) [52]. Furthermore, Krzeslak et al. found that single nucleotide polymorphism (SNP) (rs28336003) could affect the expression of MT2A in prostate cancer and that this may be associated with metal accumulation, causing the cells to lose protection against heavy metal toxicity and carcinogenicity [14].

As described above, many potential molecular mechanisms of MTs in tumorigenesis have been reported by scholars (Table 3), but countless challenges remain to be overcome. Further studies should be conducted to fully elucidate the exact mechanisms mediating the complex roles of MTs in cancer. In addition to focusing on currently known mechanisms, we need to do a search for potential targets and ultimately provide novel strategies for cancer therapy.

MTs as cancer therapeutic targets

Given the importance of MTs in physiological and pathological processes, accumulating data have exhibited the possible role of MTs as a therapeutic molecular target against human diseases, such as neurodegenerative diseases, cerebral ischemia and retinal diseases, liver diseases, chemical- and radiation-induced carcinogenesis, pulmonary inflammation, and obesity [156–158].

MT overexpression promotes cell growth, angiogenesis, metastasis, and chemoresistance in many kinds of human tumors. Thus, MT gene KO is gaining interest as a therapeutic approach for the treatment of these cancers. RNA interference is widely employed as a strategy to stably inhibit gene expression. Packaging RNA (pRNA) of bacteriophage phi29 has been used to deliver short interfering RNA (siRNA) into the cells for gene therapy [159, 160]. Tarapore et al. constructed pRNA/siRNA chimeras targeting MT2A in ovarian cancer cells and showed that the pRNA/siRNA complex could inhibit the expression of MT2A, resulting in a decreased cell proliferation. This

Table 3 Roles of MTs in carcinogenesis

MT isoforms	Mechanisms	References
MTs	Regulation of P53 activity	[22, 46, 137–139, 141]
MTs	Regulation of NF-κB activity	[47–49, 135, 142]
MTs	Methylation of DNA promoters	[7, 10, 143–152, 154, 204]
MT1H	Increasing the methyltransferase activity of EHMT1 on histone 3	[26]
MT1G	Modulation of the PI3K/AKT and Rb/E2F signaling pathways	[89]
MT1, MT2A	Modulation of the PI3K/AKT signaling pathway	[25]
MT1H	Suppression of the Wnt/β-catenin signaling pathway	[8]
MT1G	Allelic loss on chromosome 16q12.1-q23.1	[155]
MT1F	Loss of heterozygosity	[52]
MT2A	SNP (rs28336003)	[14]

result was also confirmed in breast and prostate cancer cells [161]. Therefore, the pRNA/siMT2A chimera represents a highly potent therapeutic approach against cancer. Lai et al. reported that silencing the MT2A gene by siRNAs induced entosis (the internalization of a cell into another cell) [162] in breast cancer, and this result may provide new insights into strategies to limit tumor cell growth [163]. Similarly, Lee et al. used shMT/rPOA oligo-peptoplexes to downregulate MT expression and reverse the cisplatin resistance and verified enhanced anticancer efficacy in both cisplatin-resistant cell lines and in vivo mouse cancer models [102]. Antisense approaches targeting unique mRNA molecules are intended to reduce the expression of specific proteins, and this strategy is possibly applicable for cancer therapy [164]. The downregulation of MTs by antisense approaches has been shown to induce growth inhibition in breast cancer cells [165], leukemia cells [166], and nasopharyngeal cancer [167].

Sharma et al. highlighted the clinical significance of MTs in cell therapy and nanomedicine [168]. The study and application of nanoparticles (NPs) are increasingly gaining focus in biological systems and nanomedicine. MT expression can be specifically induced by metal nanoparticles and cancer to serve as a defensive mechanism and provide protection by acting as free radical scavengers, anti-inflammatory agents, and antiapoptotic agents and by mediating zinc-dependent gene expression involved in cell apoptosis, proliferation, or differentiation [111, 168, 169]. Hence, MTs could be used as early and sensitive biomarkers to assess the effectiveness and environmental safety of newly developed NPs. Based on these properties, MT-capped semiconductor NPs are now being further developed for their theranostic applications as third-generation NPs.

MT isoforms can be targeted to treat cancer and enhance the efficacy of anticancer therapies. However, not many strategies of targeting MT isoforms have reached the clinical practice as therapeutic agents.

Further work is needed to achieve and update these technologies and to evaluate the clinical safety of these strategies modulating MT expression. Targeting particular MT isoforms in various cancer types indicates a promising future for the biomedical applications of MTs in the field of cancer treatment.

Conclusions

MTs, a unique class of metalloproteins, are emerging as important players in carcinogenesis. MTs play a pivotal role in multiple biological processes by virtue of their unusual metal-binding functions, such as participating in metal ion homeostasis and detoxification, regulating cell growth and proliferation, and protecting the body against DNA damage and oxidative stress. Moreover, currently available experimental evidence suggests vital roles of MTs in tumor growth, differentiation, angiogenesis, metastasis, immune escape, and drug resistance. However, the data on the relationship between MT expression and tumor types are variable, that is, MT expression is not universal in all human cancers not only because the functions of MTs are isoform- and tissue-specific but also because MT expression varies with different environmental stimuli or gene mutations and interactions with other cell signaling pathways or the tumor microenvironment. In addition, contradictory results in the same kind of cancer may be because some studies had only been carried out in a small number of cases. This review provides a comprehensive summary of the complicated roles of MTs in carcinogenesis. The identification of changes in the expression of particular MT isoforms can contribute to tumor diagnosis and targeted therapy. Future studies of MTs will not only reveal their functions in the pathogenesis of cancer but also provide new insights into cancer diagnosis and therapy.

Abbreviations

AFP: Alpha-fetoprotein; ATM: Ataxia telangiectasia mutated; ATRA: All-trans retinoic acid; BCR: Biochemical recurrence; b-FGF: b-fibroblast growth factor; C/EBP: CCAAT/enhancer-binding protein; cdc25A: Cell division cycle 25A; CMM: Cutaneous malignant melanoma; ECM: Extracellular matrix; ECs: Endothelial cells; EHMT1: Euchromatin histone methyltransferase 1; ELFEMFs: Extremely low-frequency electromagnetic fields; ER: Estrogen receptor; FADD: Fas-associated death domain; GIF: Growth inhibitory factor; HIF-1α: Hypoxia-inducible factor-1α; IL: Interleukin; KO: Knockout; LOH: Loss of heterozygosity; MCM-2: Minichromosome maintenance protein 2; MMP: Matrix metalloproteinase; MTs: Metallothioneins; NCBI: National Center of Biotechnology Information; NF-κB: Nuclear factor-κB; NPs: Nanoparticles; PDGF: Platelet-derived growth factor; PI3K: Phosphatidylinositol 3-kinase; pRNA: Packaging RNA; rPOA: Reducible poly(oligo-ᴅ-arginine); shMT: Short hairpin RNAs against MTs; siRNA: Short interfering RNA; SMCs: Smooth muscle cells; SNP: Single nucleotide polymorphism; TGCTs: Testicular germ cell tumors; TGFβ1: Transforming growth factor β1; TNM: Tumor node metastasis; tPSA: Total prostate-specific antigen; VEGF: Vascular endothelial growth factor

Authors' contributions

LJH was responsible for the conception and design of the manuscript. SMF was a major contributor in writing the manuscript. Both authors read and approved the final manuscript.

Authors' information

LJH is an expert on gynecological oncology at the Chinese Academy of Engineering and the head of the Department of Obstetrics and Gynecology, Peking Union Medical College Hospital, Peking Union Medical College, Chinese Academy of Medical Sciences, No. 1 Shuaifuyuan, Dongcheng District, Beijing 100730, China.

Consent for publication

Not applicable.

Competing interests

The authors declare that they have no competing interests.

References

1. Coyle P, Philcox JC, Carey LC, Rofe AM. Metallothionein: the multipurpose protein. Cell Mol Life Sci. 2002;59:627–47.
2. Albrecht AL, Singh RK, Somji S, Sens MA, Sens DA, Garrett SH. Basal and metal-induced expression of metallothionein isoform 1 and 2 genes in the RWPE-1 human prostate epithelial cell line. J Appl Toxicol. 2008;28:283–93.
3. Margoshes M, Vallee BL. A cadmium protein from equine kidney cortex. J Am Chem Soc. 1957;79:4813–4.
4. Klaassen CD, Liu J, Diwan BA. Metallothionein protection of cadmium toxicity. Toxicol Appl Pharmacol. 2009;238:215–20.
5. Kumari MV, Hiramatsu M, Ebadi M. Free radical scavenging actions of metallothionein isoforms I and II. Free Radic Res. 1998;29:93–101.
6. Arriaga JM, Levy EM, Bravo AI, Bayo SM, Amat M, Aris M, Hannois A, Bruno L, Roberti MP, Loria FS, et al. Metallothionein expression in colorectal cancer: relevance of different isoforms for tumor progression and patient survival. Hum Pathol. 2012;43:197–208.
7. Ferrario C, Lavagni P, Gariboldi M, Miranda C, Losa M, Cleris L, Formelli F, Pilotti S, Pierotti MA, Greco A. Metallothionein 1G acts as an oncosupressor in papillary thyroid carcinoma. Lab Investig. 2008;88:474–81.
8. Zheng Y, Jiang L, Hu Y, Xiao C, Xu N, Zhou J, Zhou X. Metallothionein 1H (MT1H) functions as a tumor suppressor in hepatocellular carcinoma through regulating Wnt/beta-catenin signaling pathway. BMC Cancer. 2017;17:161.
9. Pedersen MO, Larsen A, Stoltenberg M, Penkowa M. The role of metallothionein in oncogenesis and cancer prognosis. Prog Histochem Cytochem. 2009;44:29–64.
10. Demidenko R, Daniunaite K, Bakavicius A, Sabaliauskaite R, Skeberdyte A, Petroska D, Laurinavicius A, Jankevicius F, Lazutka JR, Jarmalaite S. Decreased expression of MT1E is a potential biomarker of prostate cancer progression. Oncotarget. 2017;8:61709–18.
11. Vasak M. Advances in metallothionein structure and functions. J Trace Elem Med Biol. 2005;19:13–7.
12. Thirumoorthy N, Manisenthil Kumar KT, Shyam Sundar A, Panayappan L, Chatterjee M. Metallothionein: an overview. World J Gastroenterol. 2007;13:993–6.
13. Moleirinho A, Carneiro J, Matthiesen R, Silva RM, Amorim A, Azevedo L. Gains, losses and changes of function after gene duplication: study of the metallothionein family. PLoS One. 2011;6:e18487.
14. Krzeslak A, Forma E, Chwatko G, Jozwiak P, Szymczyk A, Wilkosz J, Rozanski W, Brys M. Effect of metallothionein 2A gene polymorphism on allele-specific gene expression and metal content in prostate cancer. Toxicol Appl Pharmacol. 2013;268:278–85.
15. Ruttkay-Nedecky B, Nejdl L, Gumulec J, Zitka O, Masarik M, Eckschlager T, Stiborova M, Adam V, Kizek R. The role of metallothionein in oxidative stress. Int J Mol Sci. 2013;14:6044–66.
16. Krezel A, Maret W. The functions of metamorphic metallothioneins in zinc and copper metabolism. Int J Mol Sci. 2017;18(6). https://doi.org/10.3390/ijms18061237.
17. Cherian MG, Jayasurya A, Bay BH. Metallothioneins in human tumors and potential roles in carcinogenesis. Mutat Res. 2003;533:201–9.
18. Shimoda R, Achanzar WE, Qu W, Nagamine T, Takagi H, Mori M, Waalkes MP. Metallothionein is a potential negative regulator of apoptosis. Toxicol Sci. 2003;73:294–300.
19. Dutsch-Wicherek M, Sikora J, Tomaszewska R. The possible biological role of metallothionein in apoptosis. Front Biosci. 2008;13:4029–38.
20. Gomulkiewicz A, Podhorska-Okolow M, Szulc R, Smorag Z, Wojnar A, Zabel M, Dziegiel P. Correlation between metallothionein (MT) expression and selected prognostic factors in ductal breast cancers. Folia Histochem Cytobiol. 2010;48:242–8.
21. Jayasurya A, Bay BH, Yap WM, Tan NG, Tan BK. Proliferative potential in nasopharyngeal carcinoma: correlations with metallothionein expression and tissue zinc levels. Carcinogenesis. 2000;21:1809–12.
22. Hengstler JG, Pilch H, Schmidt M, Dahlenburg H, Sagemuller J, Schiffer I, Oesch F, Knapstein PG, Kaina B, Tanner B. Metallothionein expression in ovarian cancer in relation to histopathological parameters and molecular markers of prognosis. Int J Cancer. 2001;95:121–7.
23. Wulfing C, van Ahlen H, Eltze E, Piechota H, Hertle L, Schmid KW. Metallothionein in bladder cancer: correlation of overexpression with poor outcome after chemotherapy. World J Urol. 2007;25:199–205.
24. Weinlich G, Eisendle K, Hassler E, Baltaci M, Fritsch PO, Zelger B. Metallothionein - overexpression as a highly significant prognostic factor in melanoma: a prospective study on 1270 patients. Br J Cancer. 2006;94:835–41.
25. Datta J, Majumder S, Kutay H, Motiwala T, Frankel W, Costa R, Cha HC, MacDougald OA, Jacob ST, Ghoshal K. Metallothionein expression is suppressed in primary human hepatocellular carcinomas and is mediated through inactivation of CCAAT/enhancer binding protein alpha by phosphatidylinositol 3-kinase signaling cascade. Cancer Res. 2007;67:2736–46.
26. Han YC, Zheng ZL, Zuo ZH, Yu YP, Chen R, Tseng GC, Nelson JB, Luo JH. Metallothionein 1 h tumour suppressor activity in prostate cancer is mediated by euchromatin methyltransferase 1. J Pathol. 2013;230:184–93.
27. Theocharis S, Karkantaris C, Philipides T, Agapitos E, Gika A, Margeli A, Kittas C, Koutselinis A. Expression of metallothionein in lung carcinoma: correlation with histological type and grade. Histopathology. 2002;40:143–51.
28. Lee JD, Wu SM, Lu LY, Yang YT, Jeng SY. Cadmium concentration and metallothionein expression in prostate cancer and benign prostatic hyperplasia of humans. J Formos Med Assoc. 2009;108:554–9.
29. Dziegiel P, Pula B, Kobierzycki C, Stasiolek M, Podhorska-Okolow M: The role of metallothioneins in carcinogenesis. Metallothioneins in Normal and Cancer Cells 2016; 218:29–63.
30. Uchida Y, Takio K, Titani K, Ihara Y, Tomonaga M. The growth inhibitory factor that is deficient in the Alzheimer's disease brain is a 68 amino acid metallothionein-like protein. Neuron. 1991;7:337–47.
31. Palmiter RD, Findley SD, Whitmore TE, Durnam DM. MT-III, a brain-specific member of the metallothionein gene family. Proc Natl Acad Sci U S A. 1992;89:6333–7.

32. Quaife CJ, Findley SD, Erickson JC, Froelick GJ, Kelly EJ, Zambrowicz BP, Palmiter RD. Induction of a new metallothionein isoform (MT-IV) occurs during differentiation of stratified squamous epithelia. Biochemistry. 1994;33:7250–9.

33. Haq F, Mahoney M, Koropatnick J. Signaling events for metallothionein induction. Mutat Res. 2003;533:211–26.

34. Krizkova S, Kepinska M, Emri G, Eckschlager T, Stiborova M, Pokorna P, Heger Z, Adam V. An insight into the complex roles of metallothioneins in malignant diseases with emphasis on (sub)isoforms/isoforms and epigenetics phenomena. Pharmacol Ther. 2018;183:90–117.

35. Cherian MG, Huang PC, Klaassen CD, Liu YP, Longfellow DG, Waalkes MP. National Cancer Institute Workshop on the possible roles of metallothionein in carcinogenesis. Cancer Res. 1993;53:922–5.

36. Nagel WW, Vallee BL. Cell cycle regulation of metallothionein in human colonic cancer cells. Proc Natl Acad Sci U S A. 1995;92:579–83.

37. Chesters JK, Petrie L, Vint H. Specificity and timing of the Zn2+ requirement for DNA synthesis by 3T3 cells. Exp Cell Res. 1989;184:499–508.

38. Chesters JK, Boyne R. Nature of the Zn2+ requirement for DNA synthesis by 3T3 cells. Exp Cell Res. 1991;192:631–4.

39. Lim D, Jocelyn KM, Yip GW, Bay BH. Silencing the metallothionein-2A gene inhibits cell cycle progression from G1- to S-phase involving ATM and cdc25A signaling in breast cancer cells. Cancer Lett. 2009;276:109–17.

40. Werynska B, Pula B, Muszczynska-Bernhard B, Piotrowska A, Jethon A, Podhorska-Okolow M, Dziegiel P, Jankowska R. Correlation between expression of metallothionein and expression of Ki-67 and MCM-2 proliferation markers in non-small cell lung cancer. Anticancer Res. 2011;31:2833–9.

41. Jin RX, Chow VTK, Tan PH, Dheen ST, Duan W, Bay BH. Metallothionein 2A expression is associated with cell proliferation in breast cancer. Carcinogenesis. 2002;23:81–6.

42. Dziegiel P, Forgacz J, Suder E, Surowiak P, Kornafel J, Zabel M. Prognostic significance of metallothionein expression in correlation with Ki-67 expression in adenocarcinomas of large intestine. Histol Histopathol. 2003;18:401–7.

43. Bieniek A, Pula B, Piotrowska A, Podhorska-Okolow M, Salwa A, Koziol M, Dziegiel P. Expression of metallothionein I/II and Ki-67 antigen in various histological types of basal cell carcinoma. Folia Histochem Cytobiol. 2012;50:352–7.

44. Dziegiel P, Salwa-Zurawska W, Zurawski J, Wojnar A, Zabel M. Prognostic significance of augmented metallothionein (MT) expression correlated with Ki-67 antigen expression in selected soft tissue sarcomas. Histol Histopathol. 2005;20:83–9.

45. Alkamal I, Ikromov O, Tolle A, Fuller TF, Magheli A, Miller K, Krause H, Kempkensteffen C. An epigenetic screen unmasks metallothioneins as putative contributors to renal cell carcinogenesis. Urol Int. 2015;94:99–110.

46. Ostrakhovitch EA, Olsson PE, Jiang S, Cherian MG. Interaction of metallothionein with tumor suppressor p53 protein. FEBS Lett. 2006;580:1235–8.

47. Abdel-Mageed AB, Agrawal KC. Activation of nuclear factor kappaB: potential role in metallothionein-mediated mitogenic response. Cancer Res. 1998;58:2335–8.

48. Sakurai A, Hara S, Okano N, Kondo Y, Inoue J, Imura N. Regulatory role of metallothionein in NF-kappaB activation. FEBS Lett. 1999;455:55–8.

49. Marikar FM, Jin G, Sheng W, Ma D, Hua Z. Metallothionein 2A an interactive protein linking phosphorylated FADD to NF-kappaB pathway leads to colorectal cancer formation. Chin Clin Oncol. 2016;5:76.

50. Klaassen CD, Liu J, Choudhuri S. Metallothionein: an intracellular protein to protect against cadmium toxicity. Annu Rev Pharmacol Toxicol. 1999;39:267–94.

51. Wang GW, Klein JB, Kang YJ. Metallothionein inhibits doxorubicin-induced mitochondrial cytochrome c release and caspase-3 activation in cardiomyocytes. J Pharmacol Exp Ther. 2001;298:461–8.

52. Yan DW, Fan JW, Yu ZH, Li MX, Wen YG, Li DW, Zhou CZ, Wang XL, Wang Q, Tang HM, Peng ZH. Downregulation of metallothionein 1F, a putative oncosuppressor, by loss of heterozygosity in colon cancer tissue. Biochim Biophys Acta. 1822;2012:918–26.

53. Dutta R, Sens DA, Somji S, Sens MA, Garrett SH. Metallothionein isoform 3 expression inhibits cell growth and increases drug resistance of PC-3 prostate cancer cells. Prostate. 2002;52:89–97.

54. Aikins AR, Hong SW, Kim HJ, Yoon CH, Chung JH, Kim MJ, Kim CW. Extremely low-frequency electromagnetic field induces neural differentiation of hBM-MSCs through regulation of (Zn)-metallothionein-3. Bioelectromagnetics. 2017;38:364–73.

55. Wu C, Pot C, Apetoh L, Thalhamer T, Zhu B, Murugaiyan G, Xiao S, Lee Y, Rangachari M, Yosef N, Kuchroo VK. Metallothioneins negatively regulate IL-27-induced type 1 regulatory T-cell differentiation. Proc Natl Acad Sci U S A. 2013;110:7802–7.

56. Hirako N, Nakano H, Takahashi S. A PU.1 suppressive target gene, metallothionein 1G, inhibits retinoic acid-induced NB4 cell differentiation. PLoS One. 2014;9:e103282.

57. Habel N, Hamidouche Z, Girault I, Patino-Garcia A, Lecanda F, Marie PJ, Fromigue O. Zinc chelation: a metallothionein 2A's mechanism of action involved in osteosarcoma cell death and chemotherapy resistance. Cell Death Dis. 2013;4:e874.

58. Jin R, Bay BH, Chow VT, Tan PH. Metallothionein 1F mRNA expression correlates with histological grade in breast carcinoma. Breast Cancer Res Treat. 2001;66:265–72.

59. Yap XL, Tan HY, Huang JX, Lai YY, Yip GWC, Tan PH, Bay BH. Over-expression of metallothionein predicts chemoresistance in breast cancer. J Pathol. 2009;217:563–70.

60. Gallicchio LM, Flaws JA, Fowler BA, Ioffe OB. Metallothionein expression in invasive and in situ breast carcinomas. Cancer Detect Prev. 2005;29:332–7.

61. Rezk NA, Zidan HE, Riad M, Mansy W, Mohamad SA. Metallothionein 2A expression and its relation to different clinical stages and grades of breast cancer in Egyptian patients. Gene. 2015;571:17–22.

62. Ohshio G, Imamura T, Okada N, Wang ZH, Yamaki K, Kyogoku T, Suwa H, Yamabe H, Imamura M. Immunohistochemical study of metallothionein in pancreatic carcinomas. J Cancer Res Clin Oncol. 1996;122:351–5.

63. Shukla VK, Aryya NC, Pitale A, Pandey M, Dixit VK, Reddy CD, Gautam A. Metallothionein expression in carcinoma of the gallbladder. Histopathology. 1998;33:154–7.

64. Izawa JI, Moussa M, Cherian MG, Doig G, Chin JL. Metallothionein expression in renal cancer. Urology. 1998;52:767–72.

65. McCluggage WG, Strand K, Abdulkadir A. Immunohistochemical localization of metallothionein in benign and malignant epithelial ovarian tumors. Int J Gynecol Cancer. 2002;12:62–5.

66. McCluggage WG, Maxwell P, Hamilton PW, Jasani B. High metallothionein expression is associated with features predictive of aggressive behaviour in endometrial carcinoma. Histopathology. 1999;34:51–5.

67. Arriaga JM, Bravo AI, Mordoh J, Bianchini M. Metallothionein 1G promotes the differentiation of HT-29 human colorectal cancer cells. Oncol Rep. 2017;37:2633–51.

68. Eichhorn ME, Kleespies A, Angele MK, Jauch KW, Bruns CJ. Angiogenesis in cancer: molecular mechanisms, clinical impact. Langenbecks Arch Surg. 2007;392:371–9.

69. Miyashita H, Sato Y. Metallothionein 1 is a downstream target of vascular endothelial zinc finger 1 (VEZF1) in endothelial cells and participates in the regulation of angiogenesis. Endothelium. 2005;12:163–70.

70. Penkowa M, Carrasco J, Giralt M, Molinero A, Hernandez J, Campbell IL, Hidalgo J. Altered central nervous system cytokine-growth factor expression profiles and angiogenesis in metallothionein-I+II deficient mice. J Cereb Blood Flow Metab. 2000;20:1174–89.

71. Wierzowiecka B, Gomulkiewicz A, Cwynar-Zajac L, Olbromski M, Grzegrzolka J, Kobierzycki C, Podhorska-Okolow M, Dziegiel P. Expression of metallothionein and vascular endothelial growth factor isoforms in breast cancer cells. In Vivo. 2016;30:271–8.

72. Kim HG, Hwang YP, Jeong HG. Metallothionein-III induces HIF-1 alpha-mediated VEGF expression in brain endothelial cells. Biochem Biophys Res Commun. 2008;369:666–71.

73. Schuermann A, Helker CSM, Herzog W. Metallothionein 2 regulates endothelial cell migration through transcriptional regulation of vegfc expression. Angiogenesis. 2015;18:463–75.

74. Farina AR, Mackay AR. Gelatinase B/MMP-9 in tumour pathogenesis and progression. Cancers. 2014;6:240–96.

75. Zalewska M, Trefon J, Milnerowicz H. The role of metallothionein interactions with other proteins. Proteomics. 2014;14:1343–56.

76. Zbinden S, Wang JS, Adenika R, Schmidt M, Tilan JU, Najafi AH, Peng XZ, Lassance-Soares RM, Iantorno M, Morsli H, et al. Metallothionein enhances angiogenesis and arteriogenesis by modulating smooth muscle cell and macrophage function. Arterioscler Thromb Vasc Bio. 2010;30:477–U240.

77. Emri E, Egervari K, Varvolgyi T, Rozsa D, Miko E, Dezso B, Veres I, Mehes G, Emri G, Remenyik E. Correlation among metallothionein expression, intratumoural macrophage infiltration and the risk of metastasis in human cutaneous malignant melanoma. J Eur Acad Dermatol Venereol. 2013;27:e320–7.

78. Hishikawa Y, Kohno H, Ueda S, Kimoto T, Dhar DK, Kubota H, Tachibana M, Koji T, Nagasue N. Expression of metallothionein in colorectal cancers and synchronous liver metastases. Oncology. 2001;61:162–7.

79. Haerslev T, Jacobsen K, Nedergaard L, Zedeler K. Immunohistochemical detection of metallothionein in primary breast carcinomas and their axillary lymph node metastases. Pathol Res Pract. 1994;190:675–81.

80. Hishikawa Y, Koji T, Dhar DK, Kinugasa S, Yamaguchi M, Nagasue N. Metallothionein expression correlates with metastatic and proliferative potential in squamous cell carcinoma of the oesophagus. Br J Cancer. 1999;81:712–20.

81. Galizia G, Ferraraccio F, Lieto E, Orditura M, Castellano P, Imperatore V, La Manna G, Pinto M, Ciardiello F, La Mura A, De Vita F. p27 downregulation and metallothionein overexpression in gastric cancer patients are associated with a poor survival rate. J Surg Oncol. 2006;93:241–52.

82. Kim HG, Kim JY, Han EH, Hwang YP, Choi JH, Park BH, Jeong HG. Metallothionein-2A overexpression increases the expression of matrix metalloproteinase-9 and invasion of breast cancer cells. FEBS Lett. 2011;585:421–8.

83. Kmiecik AM, Pula B, Suchanski J, Olbromski M, Gomulkiewicz A, Owczarek T, Kruczak A, Ambicka A, Rys J, Ugorski M, et al. Metallothionein-3 increases triple-negative breast cancer cell invasiveness via induction of metalloproteinase expression. PLoS One. 2015;10:e0124865.

84. Hur H, Ryu HH, Li CH, Kim IY, Jang WY, Jung S. Metallothinein 1E enhances glioma invasion through modulation matrix metalloproteinases-2 and 9 in U87MG mouse brain tumor model. J Korean Neurosurg Soc. 2016;59:551–8.

85. Ryu HH, Jung S, Jung TY, Moon KS, Kim IY, Jeong YI, Jin SG, Pei J, Wen M, Jang WY. Role of metallothionein 1E in the migration and invasion of human glioma cell lines. Int J Oncol. 2012;41:1305–13.

86. Ramaswamy S, Ross KN, Lander ES, Golub TR. A molecular signature of metastasis in primary solid tumors. Nat Genet. 2003;33:49–54.

87. Giorgi RR, Correa-Giannella MLC, Casarini APM, Machado MC, Bronstein MD, Cescato VA, Giannella-Neto D. Metallothionein isoform 3 gene is differentially expressed in corticotropin-producing pituitary adenomas. Neuroendocrinology. 2005;82:208–14.

88. Gomulkiewicz A, Jablonska K, Pula B, Grzegrzolka J, Borska S, Podhorska-Okolow M, Wojnar A, Rys J, Ambicka A, Ugorski M, et al. Expression of metallothionein 3 in ductal breast cancer. Int J Oncol. 2016;49:2487–97.

89. Fu J, Lv H, Guan H, Ma X, Ji M, He N, Shi B, Hou P. Metallothionein 1G functions as a tumor suppressor in thyroid cancer through modulating the PI3K/Akt signaling pathway. BMC Cancer. 2013;13:462.

90. Dutsch-Wicherek M, Lazar A, Tomaszewska R. The potential role of MT and vimentin immunoreactivity in the remodeling of the microenvironment of parotid adenocarcinoma. Cancer Microenviron. 2010;4:105–13.

91. Dutsch-Wicherek M, Lazar A, Tomaszewska R, Kazmierczak W, Wicherek L. Analysis of metallothionein and vimentin immunoreactivity in pharyngeal squamous cell carcinoma and its microenvironment. Cell Tissue Res. 2013;352:341–9.

92. Dutsch-Wicherek M. RCAS1, MT, and vimentin as potential markers of tumor microenvironment remodeling. Am J Reprod Immunol. 2010;63:181–8.

93. Subramanian Vignesh K, Deepe GS Jr. Metallothioneins: emerging modulators in immunity and infection. Int J Mol Sci. 2017;18(10). https://doi.org/10.3390/ijms18102197.

94. Popiela TJ, Rudnicka-Sosin L, Dutsch-Wicherek M, Klimek M, Basta P, Galazka K, Wicherek L. The metallothionein and RCAS1 expression analysis in breast cancer and adjacent tissue regarding the immune cells presence and their activity. Neuroendocrinol Lett. 2006;27:786–94.

95. Borghesi LA, Youn J, Olson EA, Lynes MA. Interactions of metallothionein with murine lymphocytes: plasma membrane binding and proliferation. Toxicology. 1996;108:129–40.

96. Youn J, Lynes MA. Metallothionein-induced suppression of cytotoxic T lymphocyte function: an important immunoregulatory control. Toxicol Sci. 1999;52:199–208.

97. Canpolat E, Lynes MA. In vivo manipulation of endogenous metallothionein with a monoclonal antibody enhances a T-dependent humoral immune response. Toxicol Sci. 2001;62:61–70.

98. Kelley SL, Basu A, Teicher BA, Hacker MP, Hamer DH, Lazo JS. Overexpression of metallothionein confers resistance to anticancer drugs. Science. 1988;241:1813–5.

99. Siegsmund MJ, Marx C, Seemann O, Schummer B, Steidler A, Toktomambetova L, Kohrmann KU, Rassweiler J, Alken P. Cisplatin-resistant bladder carcinoma cells: enhanced expression of metallothioneins. Urol Res. 1999;27:157–63.

100. Matsumoto Y, Oka M, Sakamoto A, Narasaki F, Fukuda M, Takatani H, Terashi K, Ikeda K, Tsurutani J, Nagashima S, et al. Enhanced expression of

101. Kasahara K, Fujiwara Y, Nishio K, Ohmori T, Sugimoto Y, Komiya K, Matsuda T, Saijo N. Metallothionein content correlates with the sensitivity of human small cell lung cancer cell lines to cisplatin. Cancer Res. 1991;51:3237–42.

102. Lee JH, Chae JW, Kim JK, Kim HJ, Chung JY, Kim YH. Inhibition of cisplatin-resistance by RNA interference targeting metallothionein using reducible oligo-peptoplex. J Control Release. 2015;215:82–90.

103. Chun JH, Kim HK, Kim E, Kim IH, Kim JH, Chang HJ, Choi IJ, Lim HS, Kim IJ, Kang HC, et al. Increased expression of metallothionein is associated with irinotecan resistance in gastric cancer. Cancer Res. 2004;64:4703–6.

104. Juang HH, Chung LC, Sung HC, Feng TH, Lee YH, Chang PL, Tsui KH. Metallothionein 3: an androgen-upregulated gene enhances cell invasion and tumorigenesis of prostate carcinoma cells. Prostate. 2013;73:1495–506.

105. Kondo Y, Kuo SM, Watkins SC, Lazo JS. Metallothionein localization and cisplatin resistance in human hormone-independent prostatic tumor cell lines. Cancer Res. 1995;55:474–7.

106. Surowiak P, Materna V, Maciejczyk A, Pudelko M, Markwitz E, Spaczynski M, Dietel M, Zabel M, Lage H. Nuclear metallothionein expression correlates with cisplatin resistance of ovarian cancer cells and poor clinical outcome. Virchows Arch. 2007;450:279–85.

107. Gansukh T, Donizy P, Halon A, Lage H, Surowiak P. In vitro analysis of the relationships between metallothionein expression and cisplatin sensitivity of non-small cellular lung cancer cells. Anticancer Res. 2013;33:5255–60.

108. Arriaga JM, Greco A, Mordoh J, Bianchini M. Metallothionein 1G and zinc sensitize human colorectal cancer cells to chemotherapy. Mol Cancer Ther. 2014;13:1369–81.

109. Sun XF, Niu XH, Chen RC, He WY, Chen D, Kang R, Tang DL. Metallothionein-1G facilitates sorafenib resistance through inhibition of ferroptosis. Hepatology. 2016;64:488–500.

110. Shuai Y, Guo JB, Peng SQ, Zhang LS, Guo J, Han G, Dong YS. Metallothionein protects against doxorubicin-induced cardiomyopathy through inhibition of superoxide generation and related nitrosative impairment. Toxicol Lett. 2007;170:66–74.

111. Heger Z, Rodrigo MAM, Krizkova S, Ruttkay-Nedecky B, Zalewska M, del Pozo EMP, Pelfrene A, Pourrut B, Stiborova M, Eckschlager T, et al. Metallothionein as a scavenger of free radicals - new cardioprotective therapeutic agent or initiator of tumor chemoresistance? Curr Drug Targets. 2016;17:1438–51.

112. Jing L, Yang M, Li Y, Yu Y, Liang BL, Cao LG, Zhou XQ, Peng SQ, Sun ZW. Metallothionein prevents doxorubicin cardiac toxicity by indirectly regulating the uncoupling proteins 2. Food Chem Toxicol. 2017;110:204–13.

113. Petrlova J, Potesil D, Mikelova R, Blastik O, Adam V, Trnkova L, Jelen F, Prusa R, Kukacka J, Kizek R. Attomole voltammetric determination of metallothionein. Electrochim Acta. 2006;51:5112–9.

114. Eckschlager T, Adam V, Hrabeta J, Figova K, Kizek R. Metallothioneins and cancer. Curr Protein Pept Sci. 2009;10:360–75.

115. Tariba B, Zivkovic T, Krasnici N, Marijic VF, Erk M, Gamulin M, Grgic M, Pizent A. Serum metallothionein in patients with testicular cancer. Cancer Chemother Pharmacol. 2015;75:813–20.

116. Krizkova S, Ryvolova M, Gumulec J, Masarik M, Adam V, Majzlik P, Hubalek J, Provaznik I, Kizek R. Electrophoretic fingerprint metallothionein analysis as a potential prostate cancer biomarker. Electrophoresis. 2011;32:1952–61.

117. Krizkova S, Masarik M, Majzlik P, Kukacka J, Kruseova J, Adam V, Prusa R, Eckschlager T, Stiborova M, Kizek R. Serum metallothionein in newly diagnosed patients with childhood solid tumours. Acta Biochim Pol. 2010;57:561–6.

118. Surowiak P, Materna V, Kaplenko I, Spaczynski M, Dietel M, Lage H, Zabel M. Augmented expression of metallothionein and glutathione S-transferase pi as unfavourable prognostic factors in cisplatin-treated ovarian cancer patients. Virchows Arch. 2005;447:626–33.

119. Jin RX, Huang JX, Tan PH, Bay BH. Clinicopathological significance of metallothioneins in breast cancer. Pathol Oncol Res. 2004;10:74–9.

120. Goulding H, Jasani B, Pereira H, Reid A, Galea M, Bell JA, Elston CW, Robertson JF, Blamey RW, Nicholson RA, et al. Metallothionein expression in human breast cancer. Br J Cancer. 1995;72:968–72.

121. Joseph MG, Banerjee D, Kocha W, Feld R, Stitt LW, Cherian MG. Metallothionein expression in patients with small cell carcinoma of the lung: correlation with other molecular markers and clinical outcome. Cancer. 2001;92:836–42.

122. Dziegiel P, Jelen M, Muszczynska B, Maciejczyk A, Szulc A, Podhorska-Okolow M, Cegielski M, Zabel M. Role of metallothionein expression in non-small cell lung carcinomas. Rocz Akad Med Bialymst. 2004;49(Suppl 1):43–5.

metallothionein in human non-small-cell lung carcinomas following chemotherapy. Anticancer Res. 1997;17:3777–80.

123. Tuzel E, Kirkali Z, Yorukoglu K, Mungan MU, Sade M. Metallothionein expression in renal cell carcinoma: subcellular localization and prognostic significance. J Urol. 2001;165:1710–3.

124. Mitropoulos D, Kyroudi-Voulgari A, Theocharis S, Serafetinides E, Moraitis E, Zervas A, Kittas C. Prognostic significance of metallothionein expression in renal cell carcinoma. World J Surg Oncol. 2005;3:5.

125. Weinlich G, Bitterlich W, Mayr V, Fritsch PO, Zelger B. Metallothionein-overexpression as a prognostic factor for progression and survival in melanoma. A prospective study on 520 patients. Br J Dermatol. 2003;149:535–41.

126. Yamasaki Y, Smith C, Weisz D, van Huizen I, Xuan J, Moussa M, Stitt L, Hideki S, Cherian MG, Izawa JI. Metallothionein expression as prognostic factor for transitional cell carcinoma of bladder. Urology. 2006;67:530–5.

127. Cardoso SV, Barbosa HM, Candellori IM, Loyola AM, Aguiar MC. Prognostic impact of metallothionein on oral squamous cell carcinoma. Virchows Arch. 2002;441:174–8.

128. Schmitz KJ, Lang H, Kaiser G, Wohlschlaeger J, Sotiropoulos GC, Baba HA, Jasani B, Schmid KW. Metallothionein overexpression and its prognostic relevance in intrahepatic cholangiocarcinoma and extrahepatic hilar cholangiocarcinoma (Klatskin tumors). Hum Pathol. 2009;40:1706–14.

129. Zhang R, Zhang H, Wei H, Luo X. Expression of metallothionein in invasive ductal breast cancer in relation to prognosis. J Environ Pathol Toxicol Oncol. 2000;19:95–7.

130. Sens MA, Somji S, Garrett SH, Beall CL, Sens DA. Metallothionein isoform 3 overexpression is associated with breast cancers having a poor prognosis. Am J Pathol. 2001;159:21–6.

131. Werynska B, Pula B, Muszczynska-Bernhard B, Gomulkiewicz A, Piotrowska A, Prus R, Podhorska-Okolow M, Jankowska R, Dziegiel P. Metallothionein 1F and 2A overexpression predicts poor outcome of non-small cell lung cancer patients. Exp Mol Pathol. 2013;94:301–8.

132. Weinlich G, Topar G, Eisendle K, Fritsch PO, Zelger B. Comparison of metallothionein-overexpression with sentinel lymph node biopsy as prognostic factors in melanoma. J Eur Acad Dermatol Venereol. 2007;21:669–77.

133. Park Y, Yu E. Expression of metallothionein-1 and metallothionein-2 as a prognostic marker in hepatocellular carcinoma. J Gastroenterol Hepatol. 2013;28:1565–72.

134. Ding J, Lu SC. Low metallothionein 1M expression association with poor hepatocellular carcinoma prognosis after curative resection. Genet Mol Res. 2016;15(4). https://doi.org/10.4238/gmr.15048735.

135. Pan Y, Huang J, Xing R, Yin X, Cui J, Li W, Yu J, Lu Y. Metallothionein 2A inhibits NF-kappaB pathway activation and predicts clinical outcome segregated with TNM stage in gastric cancer patients following radical resection. J Transl Med. 2013;11:173.

136. Ji XF, Fan YC, Gao S, Yang Y, Zhang JJ, Wang K. MT1M and MT1G promoter methylation as biomarkers for hepatocellular carcinoma. World J Gastroenterol. 2014;20:4723–9.

137. Meplan C, Richard MJ, Hainaut P. Metalloregulation of the tumor suppressor protein p53: zinc mediates the renaturation of p53 after exposure to metal chelators in vitro and in intact cells. Oncogene. 2000;19:5227–36.

138. Ostrakhovitch EA, Olsson PE, von Hofsten J, Cherian MG. P53 mediated regulation of metallothionein transcription in breast cancer cells. J Cell Biochem. 2007;102:1571–83.

139. Cardoso SV, Silveira-Junior JB, De Carvalho MV, De-Paula AM, Loyola AM, De Aguiar MC. Expression of metallothionein and p53 antigens are correlated in oral squamous cell carcinoma. Anticancer Res. 2009;29:1189–93.

140. Fan LZ, Cherian MG. Potential role of p53 on metallothionein induction in human epithelial breast cancer cells. Br J Cancer. 2002;87:1019–26.

141. Ioachim EE, Kitsiou E, Carassavoglou C, Stefanaki S, Agnantis NJ. Immunohistochemical localization of metallothionein in endometrial lesions. J Pathol. 2000;191:269–73.

142. Mao J, Yu HX, Wang CJ, Sun LH, Jiang W, Zhang PZ, Xiao QY, Han DB, Saiyin H, Zhu JD, et al. Metallothionein MT1M is a tumor suppressor of human hepatocellular carcinomas. Carcinogenesis. 2012;33:2568–77.

143. Tse KY, Liu VW, Chan DW, Chiu PM, Tam KF, Chan KK, Liao XY, Cheung AN, Ngan HY. Epigenetic alteration of the metallothionein 1E gene in human endometrial carcinomas. Tumour Biol. 2009;30:93–9.

144. Faller WJ, Rafferty M, Hegarty S, Gremel G, Ryan D, Fraga MF, Esteller M, Dervan PA, Gallagher WM. Metallothionein 1E is methylated in malignant melanoma and increases sensitivity to cisplatin-induced apoptosis. Melanoma Res. 2010;20:392–400.

145. Roth MJ, Abnet CC, Hu N, Wang QH, Wei WQ, Green L, D'Alelio M, Qiao YL, Dawsey SM, Taylor PR, Woodson K. p16, MGMT, RARbeta2, CLDN3, CRBP

146. and MT1G gene methylation in esophageal squamous cell carcinoma and its precursor lesions. Oncol Rep. 2006;15:1591–7.

146. Kumar A, Chatopadhyay T, Raziuddin M, Ralhan R. Discovery of deregulation of zinc homeostasis and its associated genes in esophageal squamous cell carcinoma using cDNA microarray. Int J Cancer. 2007;120:230–42.

147. Sakamoto LH, DEC B, Cajaiba M, Soares FA, Vettore AL. MT1G hypermethylation: a potential prognostic marker for hepatoblastoma. Pediatr Res. 2010;67:387–93.

148. Kanda M, Nomoto S, Okamura Y, Nishikawa Y, Sugimoto H, Kanazumi N, Takeda S, Nakao A. Detection of metallothionein 1G as a methylated tumor suppressor gene in human hepatocellular carcinoma using a novel method of double combination array analysis. Int J Oncol. 2009;35:477–83.

149. Huang Y, de la Chapelle A, Pellegata NS. Hypermethylation, but not LOH, is associated with the low expression of MT1G and CRABP1 in papillary thyroid carcinoma. Int J Cancer. 2003;104:735–44.

150. Henrique R, Jeronimo C, Hoque MO, Nomoto S, Carvalho AL, Costa VL, Oliveira J, Teixeira MR, Lopes C, Sidransky D. MT1G hypermethylation is associated with higher tumor stage in prostate cancer. Cancer Epidemiol Biomark Prev. 2005;14:1274–8.

151. Deng D, El-Rifai W, Ji J, Zhu B, Trampont P, Li J, Smith MF, Powel SM. Hypermethylation of metallothionein-3 CpG island in gastric carcinoma. Carcinogenesis. 2003;24:25–9.

152. Peng DF, Hu TL, Jiang AX, Washington MK, Moskaluk CA, Schneider-Stock R, El-Rifai W. Location-specific epigenetic regulation of the metallothionein 3 gene in esophageal adenocarcinomas. PLoS One. 2011;6(7):e22009.

153. Smith E, Drew PA, Tian ZQ, De Young NJ, Liu JF, Mayne GC, Ruszkiewicz AR, Watson DI, Jamieson GG. Metallothionein 3 expression is frequently down-regulated in oesophageal squamous cell carcinoma by DNA methylation. Mol Cancer. 2005;4. https://doi.org/10.1186/1476-4598-4-42.

154. Tao YF, Xu LX, Lu J, Cao L, Li ZH, Hu SY, Wang NN, Du XJ, Sun LC, Zhao WL, et al. Metallothionein III (MT3) is a putative tumor suppressor gene that is frequently inactivated in pediatric acute myeloid leukemia by promoter hypermethylation. J Transl Med. 2014;12:182.

155. Chan KYY, Lai PBS, Squire JA, Beheshti B, Wong NLY, Sy SMH, Wong N. Positional expression profiling indicates candidate genes in deletion hotspots of hepatocellular carcinoma. Mod Pathol. 2006;19:1546–54.

156. Inoue K, Satoh M. Metallothionein as a therapeutic molecular target against human diseases. Curr Pharm Biotechnol. 2013;14:391–3.

157. Ito Y, Tanaka H, Hara H. The potential roles of metallothionein as a therapeutic target for cerebral ischemia and retinal diseases. Curr Pharm Biotechnol. 2013;14:400–7.

158. Fujiwara Y, Satoh M. Protective role of metallothionein in chemical and radiation carcinogenesis. Curr Pharm Biotechnol. 2013;14:394–9.

159. Guo S, Huang F, Guo P. Construction of folate-conjugated pRNA of bacteriophage phi29 DNA packaging motor for delivery of chimeric siRNA to nasopharyngeal carcinoma cells. Gene Ther. 2006;13:814–20.

160. Guo S, Tschammer N, Mohammed S, Guo P. Specific delivery of therapeutic RNAs to cancer cells via the dimerization mechanism of phi29 motor pRNA. Hum Gene Ther. 2005;16:1097–109.

161. Tarapore P, Shu Y, Guo P, Ho SM. Application of phi29 motor pRNA for targeted therapeutic delivery of siRNA silencing metallothionein-IIA and survivin in ovarian cancers. Mol Ther. 2011;19:386–94.

162. Overholtzer M, Mailleux AA, Mouneimne G, Normand G, Schnitt SJ, King RW, Cibas ES, Brugge JS. A nonapoptotic cell death process, entosis, that occurs by cell-in-cell invasion. Cell. 2007;131:966–79.

163. Lai Y, Lim D, Tan PH, Leung TK, Yip GW, Bay BH. Silencing the metallothionein-2A gene induces entosis in adherent MCF-7 breast cancer cells. Anat Rec (Hoboken). 2010;293:1685–91.

164. Krizkova S, Ryvolova M, Hrabeta J, Adam V, Stiborova M, Eckschlager T, Kizek R. Metallothioneins and zinc in cancer diagnosis and therapy. Drug Metab Rev. 2012;44:287–301.

165. Abdel-Mageed A, Agrawal KC. Antisense down-regulation of metallothionein induces growth arrest and apoptosis in human breast carcinoma cells. Cancer Gene Ther. 1997;4:199–207.

166. Takeda A, Hisada H, Okada S, Mata JE, Ebadi M, Iversen PL. Tumor cell growth is inhibited by suppressing metallothionein-I synthesis. Cancer Lett. 1997;116:145–9.

167. Tan OJ, Bay BH, Chow VT. Differential expression of metallothionein isoforms in nasopharyngeal cancer and inhibition of cell growth by antisense down-regulation of metallothionein-2A. Oncol Rep. 2005;13:127–31.

168. Sharma S, Rais A, Sandhu R, Nel W, Ebadi M. Clinical significance of metallothioneins in cell therapy and nanomedicine. Int J Nanomedicine. 2013;8:1477–88.

169. Penkowa M. Metallothioneins are multipurpose neuroprotectants during brain pathology. FEBS J. 2006;273:1857–70.

170. Levadoux-Martin M, Hesketh JE, Beattie JH, Wallace HM. Influence of metallothionein-1 localization on its function. Biochem J. 2001;355:473–9.

171. Karin M, Eddy RL, Henry WM, Haley LL, Byers MG, Shows TB. Human metallothionein genes are clustered on chromosome 16. Proc Natl Acad Sci U S A. 1984;81:5494–8.

172. West AK, Stallings R, Hildebrand CE, Chiu R, Karin M, Richards RI. Human metallothionein genes: structure of the functional locus at 16q13. Genomics. 1990;8:513–8.

173. Heguy A, West A, Richards RI, Karin M. Structure and tissue-specific expression of the human metallothionein IB gene. Mol Cell Biol. 1986;6:2149–57.

174. Varshney U, Jahroudi N, Foster R, Gedamu L. Structure, organization, and regulation of human metallothionein IF gene: differential and cell-type-specific expression in response to heavy metals and glucocorticoids. Mol Cell Biol. 1986;6:26–37.

175. Foster R, Jahroudi N, Varshney U, Gedamu L. Structure and expression of the human metallothionein-IG gene. Differential promoter activity of two linked metallothionein-I genes in response to heavy metals. J Biol Chem. 1988;263:11528–35.

176. Stennard FA, Holloway AF, Hamilton J, West AK. Characterisation of six additional human metallothionein genes. Biochim Biophys Acta. 1994;1218:357–65.

177. Cai X, Wang J, Huang X, Fu W, Xia W, Zou M, Wang Y, Wang J, Xu D. Identification and characterization of MT-1X as a novel FHL3-binding partner. PLoS ONE [Electronic Resource]. 2014;9:e93723.

178. Karin M, Richards RI. Human metallothionein genes–primary structure of the metallothionein-II gene and a related processed gene. Nature. 1982;299:797–802.

179. Yamazaki S, Nakanishi M, Hamamoto T, Hirata H, Ebihara A, Tokue A, Kagawa Y. Expression of human metallothionein-II fusion protein in Escherichia coli. Biochem Int. 1992;28:451–60.

180. Vasak M, Meloni G. Mammalian metallothionein-3: new functional and structural insights. Int J Mol Sci. 2017;18(6):1117. https://doi.org/10.3390/ijms18061117.

181. Chen HI, Chiu YW, Hsu YK, Li WF, Chen YC, Chuang HY. The association of metallothionein-4 gene polymorphism and renal function in long-term lead-exposed workers. Biol Trace Elem Res. 2010;137:55–62.

182. Sauerbrey A, Zintl F, Hermann J, Volm M. Multiple resistance mechanisms in acute nonlymphoblastic leukemia (ANLL). Anticancer Res. 1998;18:1231–6.

183. Imoto A, Okada M, Okazaki T, Kitasato H, Harigae H, Takahashi S. Metallothionein-1 isoforms and vimentin are direct PU.1 downstream target genes in leukemia cells. J Biol Chem. 2010;285:10300–9.

184. Alves SM, Cardoso SV, de Fatima BV, Machado VC, Mesquita RA, Vieira do Carmo MA, Ferreira Aguiar MC. Metallothionein immunostaining in adenoid cystic carcinomas of the salivary glands. Oral Oncol. 2007;43:252–6.

185. Rossen K, Haerslev T, Hou-Jensen K, Jacobsen GK. Metallothionein expression in basaloid proliferations overlying dermatofibromas and in basal cell carcinomas. Br J Dermatol. 1997;136:30–4.

186. Pula B, Tazbierski T, Zamirska A, Werynska B, Bieniek A, Szepietowski J, Rys J, Dziegiel P, Podhorska-Okolow M. Metallothionein 3 expression in normal skin and malignant skin lesions. Pathol Oncol Res. 2015;21:187–93.

187. Slusser A, Zheng Y, Zhou XD, Somji S, Sens DA, Sens MA, Garrett SH. Metallothionein isoform 3 expression in human skin, related cancers and human skin derived cell cultures. Toxicol Lett. 2015;232:141–8.

188. Saika T, Tsushima T, Ochi J, Akebi N, Nasu Y, Matsumura Y, Ohmori H. Over-expression of metallothionein and drug-resistance in bladder cancer. Int J Urol. 1994;1:135–9.

189. Sens MA, Somji S, Lamm DL, Garrett SH, Slovinsky F, Todd JH, Sens DA. Metallothionein isoform 3 as a potential biomarker for human bladder cancer. Environ Health Perspect. 2000;108:413–8.

190. Somji S, Sens MA, Lamm DL, Garrett SH, Sens DA. Metallothionein isoform 1 and 2 gene expression in the human bladder: evidence for upregulation of MT-1X mRNA in bladder cancer. Cancer Detect Prev. 2001;25:62–75.

191. Tai SK, Tan OJ, Chow VT, Jin R, Jones JL, Tan PH, Jayasurya A, Bay BH. Differential expression of metallothionein 1 and 2 isoforms in breast cancer lines with different invasive potential: identification of a novel nonsilent metallothionein-1H mutant variant. Am J Pathol. 2003;163:2009–19.

192. Jansova E, Koutna I, Krontorad P, Svoboda Z, Krivankova S, Zaloudik J, Kozubek M, Kozubek S. Comparative transcriptome maps: a new approach to the diagnosis of colorectal carcinoma patients using cDNA microarrays. Clin Genet. 2006;69:218–27.

193. Jin R, Bay BH, Chow VTK, Tan PH, Lin VCL. Metallothionein 1E mRNA is highly expressed in oestrogen receptor-negative human invasive ductal breast cancer. Br J Cancer. 2000;83:319–23.

194. Hishikawa Y, Abe S, Kinugasa S, Yoshimura H, Monden N, Igarashi M, Tachibana M, Nagasue N. Overexpression of metallothionein correlates with chemoresistance to cisplatin and prognosis in esophageal cancer. Oncology. 1997;54:342–7.

195. Oka D, Yamashita S, Tomioka T, Nakanishi Y, Kato H, Kaminishi M, Ushijima T. The presence of aberrant DNA methylation in noncancerous esophageal mucosae in association with smoking history a target for risk diagnosis and prevention of esophageal cancers. Cancer. 2009;115:3412–26.

196. Suganuma K, Kubota T, Saikawa Y, Abe S, Otani Y, Furukawa T, Kumai K, Hasegawa H, Watanabe M, Kitajima M, et al. Possible chemoresistance-related genes for gastric cancer detected by cDNA microarray. Cancer Sci. 2003;94:355–9.

197. An J, Pan Y, Yan Z, Li W, Cui J, Yuan J, Tian L, Xing R, Lu Y. MiR-23a in amplified 19p13.13 loci targets metallothionein 2A and promotes growth in gastric cancer cells. J Cell Biochem. 2013;114:2160–9.

198. Lin ZH, Lai SC, Zhuo W, Chen SJ, Si JM, Wang L. Gastric cancer related lncRNA-MTM involved in cell migration and invasion by interacting with MT1F. Gastroenterology. 2016;150:S359.

199. Yang J, Zhang YB, Liu P, Yan HL, Ma JC, Da MX. Decreased expression of long noncoding RNA MT1JP may be a novel diagnostic and predictive biomarker in gastric cancer. Int J Clin Exp Pathol. 2017;10:432–8.

200. Lu DD, Chen YC, Zhang XR, Cao XR, Jiang HY, Yao L. The relationship between metallothionein-1F (MT1F) gene and hepatocellular carcinoma. Yale J Biol Med. 2003;76:55–62.

201. Tao X, Zheng JM, Xu AM, Chen XF, Zhang SH. Downregulated expression of metallothionein and its clinicopathological significance in hepatocellular carcinoma. Hepatol Res. 2007;37:820–7.

202. Li H, Lu YF, Chen H, Liu J. Dysregulation of metallothionein and circadian genes in human hepatocellular carcinoma. Chronobiol Int. 2017;34:192–202.

203. Fu CL, Pan B, Pan JH, Gan MF. Metallothionein 1M suppresses tumorigenesis in hepatocellular carcinoma. Oncotarget. 2017;8:33037–46.

204. Subrungruang I, Thawornkuno C, Chawalitchewinkoon-Petmitr P, Pairojkul C, Wongkham S, Petmitr S. Gene expression profiling of intrahepatic cholangiocarcinoma. Asian Pac J Cancer Prev. 2013;14:557–63.

205. Liang GY, Lu SX, Xu G, Liu XD, Li J, Zhang DS. Expression of metallothionein and Nrf2 pathway genes in lung cancer and cancer-surrounding tissues. World J Surg Oncol. 2013;11:199.

206. da Motta LL, De Bastiani MA, Stapenhorst F, Klamt F. Oxidative stress associates with aggressiveness in lung large-cell carcinoma. Tumour Biol. 2015;36:4681–8.

207. Hou XF, Fan QX, Wang LX, Lu SX. Role of metallothionein1h in cisplatin resistance of non-small cell lung cancer cells. Chin J Cancer Res. 2009;21:247–54.

208. Werynska B, Pula B, Muszczynska-Bernhard B, Gomulkiewicz A, Jethon A, Podhorska-Okolow M, Jankowska R, Dziegiel P. Expression of metallothionein-III in patients with non-small cell lung cancer. Anticancer Res. 2013;33:965–74.

209. Brazao-Silva MT, Rodrigues MF, Eisenberg AL, Dias FL, de Castro LM, Nunes FD, Faria PR, Cardoso SV, Loyola AM, de Sousa SC. Metallothionein gene expression is altered in oral cancer and may predict metastasis and patient outcomes. Histopathology. 2015;67:358–67.

210. Endo-Munoz L, Cumming A, Sommerville S, Dickinson I, Saunders NA. Osteosarcoma is characterised by reduced expression of markers of osteoclastogenesis and antigen presentation compared with normal bone. Br J Cancer. 2010;103:73–81.

211. Tekur S, Ho SM. Ribozyme-mediated downregulation of human metallothionein II(a) induces apoptosis in human prostate and ovarian cancer cell lines. Mol Carcinog. 2002;33:44–55.

212. Mougeot JLC, Bahrani-Mostafavi Z, Vachris JC, McKinney KQ, Gurlov S, Zhang J, Naumann RW, Higgins RV, Hall JB. Gene expression profiling of ovarian tissues for determination of molecular pathways reflective of tumorigenesis. J Mol Biol. 2006;358:310–29.

213. Garrett SH, Sens MA, Shukla D, Nestor S, Somji S, Todd JH, Sens DA. Metallothionein isoform 3 expression in the human prostate and cancer-derived cell lines. Prostate. 1999;41:196–202.

214. Garrett SH, Sens MA, Shukla D, Flores L, Somji S, Todd JH, Sens DA. Metallothionein isoform 1 and 2 gene expression in the human prostate: downregulation of MT-1X in advanced prostate cancer. Prostate. 2000;43:125–35.

215. Prueitt RL, Yi M, Hudson RS, Wallace TA, Howe TM, Yfantis HG, Lee DH, Stephens RM, Liu CG, Calin GA, et al. Expression of microRNAs and protein-coding genes associated with perineural invasion in prostate cancer. Prostate. 2008;68:1152–64.

216. Nguyen A, Jing Z, Mahoney PS, Davis R, Sikka SC, Agrawal KC, Abdel-Mageed AB. In vivo gene expression profile analysis of metallothionein in renal cell carcinoma. Cancer Lett. 2000;160:133–40.

217. Takahashi M, Rhodes DR, Furge KA, Kanayama H, Kagawa S, Haab BB, Teh BT. Gene expression profiling of clear cell renal cell carcinoma: gene identification and prognostic classification. Proc Natl Acad Sci U S A. 2001;98:9754–9.

218. Tan Y, Sinniah R, Bay BH, Singh G. Metallothionein expression and nuclear size in benign, borderline, and malignant serous ovarian tumours. J Pathol. 1999;189:60–5.

219. Skubitz KM, Francis P, Skubitz APN, Luo XH, Nilbert M. Gene expression identifies heterogeneity of metastatic propensity in high-grade soft tissue sarcomas. Cancer. 2012;118:4235–43.

220. Sundelin K, Jadner M, Norberg-Spaak L, Davidsson A, Hellquist HB. Metallothionein and Fas (CD95) are expressed in squamous cell carcinoma of the tongue. Eur J Cancer. 1997;33:1860–4.

221. Theocharis S, Klijanienko J, Giaginis C, Rodriguez J, Jouffroy T, Girod A, Point D, Tsirouflis G, Sastre-Garau X. Metallothionein expression in mobile tongue squamous cell carcinoma: associations with clinicopathological parameters and patient survival. Histopathology. 2011;59:514–25.

222. Chin JL, Banerjee D, Kadhim SA, Kontozoglou TE, Chauvin PJ, Cherian MG. Metallothionein in testicular germ cell tumors and drug resistance. Clinical correlation. Cancer. 1993;72:3029–35.

14

Insulin-like growth factor 2 mRNA-binding protein 1 (IGF2BP1) in cancer

Xinwei Huang[1,2†], Hong Zhang[3†], Xiaoran Guo[2], Zongxin Zhu[2], Haibo Cai[4*] and Xiangyang Kong[2*]

Abstract

The insulin-like growth factor-2 mRNA-binding protein 1 (IGF2BP1) plays essential roles in embryogenesis and carcinogenesis. IGF2BP1 serves as a post-transcriptional fine-tuner regulating the expression of some essential mRNA targets required for the control of tumor cell proliferation and growth, invasion, and chemo-resistance, associating with a poor overall survival and metastasis in various types of human cancers. Therefore, IGF2BP1 has been traditionally regarded as an oncogene and potential therapeutic target for cancers. Nevertheless, a few studies have also demonstrated its tumor-suppressive role. However, the details about the contradictory functions of IGF2BP1 are unclear. The growing numbers of microRNAs (miRNAs) and long non-coding RNAs (lncRNAs) have been identified as its direct regulators, during tumor cell proliferation, growth, and invasion in multiple cancers. Thus, the mechanisms of post-transcriptional modulation of gene expression mediated by IGF2BP1, miRNAs, and lncRNAs in determining the fate of the development of tissues and organs, as well as tumorigenesis, need to be elucidated. In this review, we summarized the tissue distribution, expression, and roles of IGF2BP1 in embryogenesis and tumorigenesis, and focused on modulation of the interconnectivity between IGF2BP1 and its targeted mRNAs or non-coding RNAs (ncRNAs). The potential use of inhibitors of IGF2BP1 and its related pathways in cancer therapy was also discussed.

Keywords: IGF2BP, IGF2 mRNA-binding protein, IMP, CRD-BP, VICKZ, Cancer

Background

The insulin-like growth factor-2 mRNA-binding protein 1 (IGF2BP1), a member of a conserved family of single-stranded RNA-binding proteins (IGF2BP1-3), expresses in a broad range of fetal tissues and more than 16 cancers but only in a limited number of normal adult tissues. This gene is required for the transport of certain mRNAs that play essential roles in embryogenesis, carcinogenesis, and chemo-resistance [1, 2], by affecting their stability, translatability, or localization [1, 3, 4]. IGF2BP1 consists of six canonical RNA-binding domains, including four K homology (KH) domains and two RNA recognition motifs (RRMs) (Fig. 1a) [5]. Even though the RRM domains of IGF2BP1 can potentially contribute to the stabilization of IGF2BP-RNA complexes in a target-dependent manner [6], in vitro studies indicated that RNA binding was majorly facilitated by the KH domains [7]. The KH1/2 domain is significant for the stabilization of IGF2BP-RNA complexes. For example, the KH1/2 domain could regulate binding of IGF2BP1 to cis-determinants in the ACTB 3′-UTR as well as, more strikingly, the MYC-CRD (coding region stability determinant) RNA in vitro [8]. However, recent structural analyses of KH3/4 domain of human IGF2BP1 showed the formation of an antiparallel pseudo-dimer conformation where KH3 and KH4 each contacts the targeted RNA [9]. As far as we know, the KH domains, particularly the KH3−4 di-domain, are essential for the binding of IGF2BP1 to targeted mRNAs in a N6-methyladenosine (m6A)-dependent manner in which KH domains recognize the consensus GG (m6A) C sequence of mRNAs [10]. IGF2BP1 is considered as a m6A-binding protein, with > 3000 mRNA transcript targets [11]. Importantly, as shown in Fig. 1b, the m6A alterations of those mRNAs are required for the targeting of IGF2BP1 with mRNAs such as MYC, as well as for

* Correspondence: XP8557@163com; 3517826707@qq.com
†Xinwei Huang and Hong Zhang contributed equally to this work.
⁴Department of Oncology, Yunfeng Hospital, Xuanwei City 655400, Yunnan Province, China
²Medical School, Kunming University of Science and Technology, Kunming City 650504, Yunnan Province, China
Full list of author information is available at the end of the article

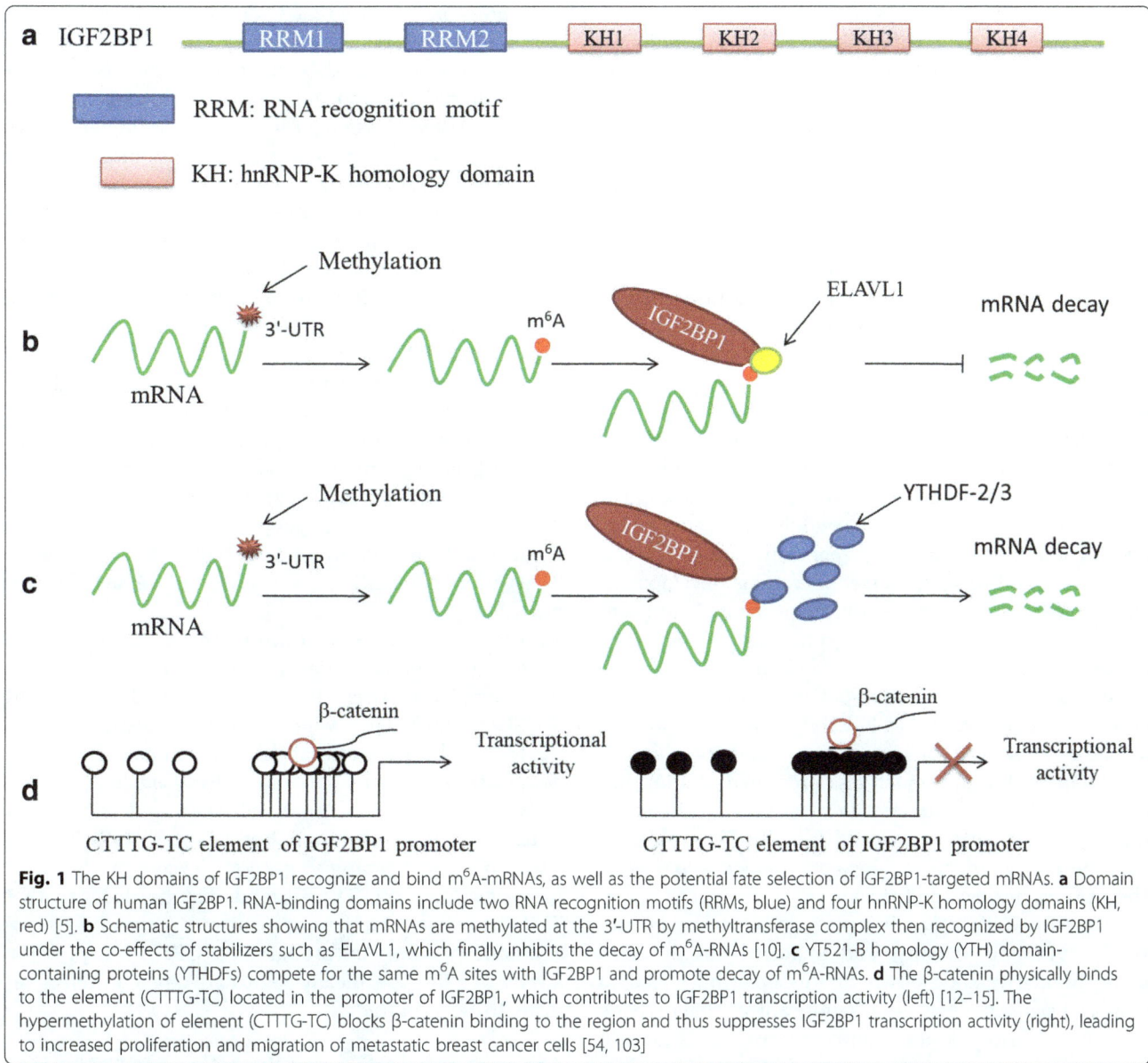

Fig. 1 The KH domains of IGF2BP1 recognize and bind m6A-mRNAs, as well as the potential fate selection of IGF2BP1-targeted mRNAs. **a** Domain structure of human IGF2BP1. RNA-binding domains include two RNA recognition motifs (RRMs, blue) and four hnRNP-K homology domains (KH, red) [5]. **b** Schematic structures showing that mRNAs are methylated at the 3′-UTR by methyltransferase complex then recognized by IGF2BP1 under the co-effects of stabilizers such as ELAVL1, which finally inhibits the decay of m6A-RNAs [10]. **c** YT521-B homology (YTH) domain-containing proteins (YTHDFs) compete for the same m6A sites with IGF2BP1 and promote decay of m6A-RNAs. **d** The β-catenin physically binds to the element (CTTTG-TC) located in the promoter of IGF2BP1, which contributes to IGF2BP1 transcription activity (left) [12–15]. The hypermethylation of element (CTTTG-TC) blocks β-catenin binding to the region and thus suppresses IGF2BP1 transcription activity (right), leading to increased proliferation and migration of metastatic breast cancer cells [54, 103]

IGF2BP1-mediated control of mRNA expression. In addition, some co-factors of IGF2BP1, such as ELAV-like RNA binding protein 1 (ELAVL1), which may be recruited by IGF2BP1, protect m6A-containing mRNAs from degradation and subsequently promote their translation [10]. However, other m6A-binding proteins may be also the readers of the m6A-containing mRNAs that are also recognized by IGF2BP1, whereas result in different effects on those mRNAs from that of IGF2BP1 does. A set of YT521-B homology (YTH) domain-containing proteins (YTHDFs), for instance, can read and control the fate of m6A-containing mRNAs via modulating pre-mRNA splicing, promoting translation, or facilitating mRNA decay (Fig. 1c) [12–15].

In numerous studies in vivo and in vitro, the emerging cancer-related mRNAs have been found, including PTEN, ACTB, MAPK4, MKI67, c-MYC, and CD44. By regulating those mRNAs, IGF2BP1 has been identified to play important roles in cell proliferation and growth of normal tissues and tumor tissues, as well as tumor cell adhesion, apoptosis, migration, and invasion [8]. Thus, IGF2BP1 is considered to be one of the most promising therapeutic targets for treating cancers, as well as the use of inhibitors of IGF2BP1-mediated cell signaling would emerge as a potential strategy for cancer treatment. However, a few recent studies have found its suppressive role in tumor growth and metastasis [16, 17]. Therefore, mechanisms resulting in the paradoxical findings need to be elucidated. Additionally, the emerging non-coding RNAs (ncRNAs) including micro-RNAs (miRNAs) and long non-coding RNAs (lncRNAs) have been demonstrated to be involved in the mediation of cancer onset and progression by targeting IGFBP1 and thus could become novel therapeutic targets of cancers. In this review, we provided a new overview of the roles of IGF2BP1 in embryo development and in multiple cancers. We focused on the interconnectivity between IGF2BP1 and its targeted mRNAs or ncRNAs involved in the biological processes of embryogenesis and tumorigenesis, as well as aid in the identification of potential targets for cancer therapy and contribute to the cancer drug-discovery research.

IGF2BP1's role in modulating embryogenesis

The essential role of IGF2BP1 in embryo development has been established. IGF2BP1 is highly expressed during the stages between zygote and embryo phases, and nearly abolished in the normal adult organism [8]. In embryo studies of Xenopus, zebrafish, and mice, this gene was found to be expressed in various developmental cell types, including the migrating neural crest and branchial arches, and cranial neural crest (CNC) [18]. Notably, its modest expression was observed in the lung, spleen, and brain of 16-week-old male mice [8]. However, one report found that IGF2BP1 is not only ubiquitously expressed in organs during human embryonic development, but also much less presented in adult human prostate, testis, kidneys, and ovaries [19]. Therefore, the expression pattern observed for IGF2BP1 could indeed be characterized as "oncofetal," since it is largely absent from normal adult tissues.

Mice with IGF2BP1 deficiency exhibit dwarfism, severely decreased viability, and impaired gut development. Similarly, knockdown of this gene may lead to 60% of perinatal death and significantly smaller body with hypoplastic tissues among almost all organs in mice [20]. The SNP rs9674544 in IGF2BP1 was identified to be significantly associated with primary tooth development in infancy [21]. Furthermore, in the neuronal development, IGF2BP1 regulates the neurite outgrowth, neuronal cell migration, and axonal guidance partially by controlling the spatiotemporal activation of protein synthesis such as ACTB mRNA [22, 23]. IGF2BP1 controls the subcellular sorting of the ACTB in primary fibroblasts and neurons by binding to the cis-acting zipcode in the ACTB's 3-UTR [24]. Moreover, IGF2BP1 was also involved in determining cell fate in testis stem cells and controlling neuronal differentiation and matured neuronal system during regeneration [25–27]. One study showed that downregulation of IGF2BP1 expression in the dorsal neural tube was both necessary and sufficient for the delamination and emigration of CNC, whereas inhibition of its expression enhanced CNC delamination and induced epithelial dissociation. Furthermore, IGF2BP1 expression is negatively associated with epithelial-to-mesenchymal transition and plays an important role in sustaining epithelial integrity. Those regulation processes might involve partly the mechanism of which IGF2BP1 interacts with ITGA6 mRNA, either directly or indirectly, to control its expression [28]. In another study on the role of IGF2BP1 in amphibian neural crest migration, the reduced IGF2BP1 expression by antisense morpholino oligonucleotides (AMO), throughout the entire embryo, was showed to increase CNC migration, suggesting the reduction in CNC migration originally observed in the AMO-injected Xenopus embryos is a result of a global, non-cell autonomous reduction in IGF2BP1 expression [18]. Those findings reveal the essential roles of IGF2BP1 in regulating cell growth and differentiation during development of organisms and suggest that aberrant expression of this gene could cause dysplasia of tissues and organs by dysregulating the expression levels of its targets such as ACTB mRNA and ITGA6 mRNA.

So far, the regulatory networks that IGF2BP1 participates in embryonic development are little known. Interestingly, a novel ultra-conserved lncRNA, THOR (ENSG00000226856), which is testis-specific in adult tissues of human, zebrafish, and mouse, has been demonstrated to be broadly expressed during the early development of both zebrafish and mouse. By IGF2BP1 binding to exons 2 and 3 of THOR, it regulates IGF2BP1's target mRNA levels to promote tumorigenesis [29]. Therefore, it may be deduced that THOR involves the development of organs and tissues and tumorigenesis by modulating IGF2BP1 expression levels, but the specifically regulated target mRNAs remain to be explored.

Aberrant expression and the roles of IGF2BP1 in cancers

IGF2BP1 and 3 have an amino acid sequence identity of 73% with each other and many the same or similar functions in cytosol. The main IGF2BP family member described in the context of cancers is IGF2BP3 [30, 31]. The comprehensive description in the regulative mechanisms of IGF2BP1 in human cancers is little, although this gene has been demonstrated to play important roles in tumorigenesis and drug-resistance of cancer therapy in vitro and in vivo studies. Even though most of the presently found cancer-related mRNA targets of IGF2BP1 have been identified to promote tumor proliferation and growth, migration, and invasion, some mRNAs have been indicated to at least indirectly suppress tumor growth and metastasis. Additionally, some ncRNAs were found to involve the regulation of tumor events by targeting IGF2BP1. Thus, bearing in mind the described limitation of post-transcriptional modulation of gene expression mediated by RNA-binding proteins (RBPs), miRNAs, and lncRNAs in determining fate of tumorigenesis, we in the following review recent findings on the expression of IGF2BP1 in cancers and focus on the interconnectivity of IGF2BP1 with its targeted mRNAs or ncRNAs.

Lung and esophageal cancer

The in vitro and in vivo studies, and TCGA data indicated that IGF2BP1 is significantly overexpressed in non-small cell lung cancer (NSCLC), especially both lung squamous cell carcinoma (LUSC) and lung adenocarcinoma (LUAD), and that its high expression correlates with the disease progression [32, 33]. IGF2BP1 overexpression was showed to significantly associate with younger onset age in LUSC and bigger tumor size and poor overall survival in LUAD [32]. Notably, another analysis from TCGA data indicated that the higher expression of IGF2BP1 is associated with poorer survival in esophageal adenocarcinomas (EAC), LUAD, and the pooled several other adenocarcinomas (ADCs) including cancers of the endometrium, prostate, endocervix, ovary, pancreas, kidney, endometrium, rectum, colon, breast, and thyroid. However, the same trend was not found in a pooled squamous cell carcinoma (SCC) dataset [34], suggesting the gene is a potential driver of ADs and may act as a therapeutic target for cancers, particularly ADCs.

At present, at least two miRNAs have been identified to inhibit lung cancer development partly by targeting 3′-UTR of IGF2BP1. MiR-494 was found to be significantly enhanced in cell lines and serum of NSCLC patients as well as closely associated with poor clinical outcome [35, 36]. However, the upregulation of miR-494 was demonstrated to suppress colony-forming activity and cell proliferation, as well as induce senescence in A549 cells via directly downregulating IGF2BP1 levels and increasing the levels of IGF2BP1's target IGF2 mRNA [37]. This means that the tumor-suppressive role of miR-494 by downregulating IGF2BP1 in lung cancer might be covered by other carcinogenic effects from elevating IGF2BP1 levels. MiR-491-5p, which may suppress the growth and metastasis of multiple types of tumors by targeting some cancer-related genes, was observed to be downregulated in NSCLC tissues and cell lines. In a mouse model, upregulation of miR-491-5p was observed to enhance the tumor cell cycle arrest at the G1/G0 stage and promote tumor cell apoptosis, as well as repress tumor cell proliferation, migration, and invasion, and growth by inhibiting IGF2BP1 [24].

Liver cancer

IGF2BP1 expression has been reported in gallbladder cancer (GC), hepatocellular carcinoma (HCC), and fibrolamellar hepatocellular carcinoma (FL-HCC). In GC tissues, the positive expression of IGF2BP1 was 72.4%, with the lower expression levels compared to control tissues. Furthermore, IGF2BP1 expression was observed to be related to longer survival and better prognosis [38]. However, IGF2BP1 expression was found to promote HCC cell proliferation, migration, and invasion [39, 40], and correlate with poor survival and prognosis [41–43]. Those observations indicated the different roles of IGF2BP1 in survival and prognosis for distinct liver cancers.

In vitro, SOX12 upregulation was found to promote HCC cell growth and apoptosis, invasion, and metastasis partly via enhancing IGF2BP1 expression that elevates the expression of c-MYC and the proliferation marker MKI67 [3, 41, 44]. Some lncRNAs function in HCC progression by various mechanisms, such as splicing regulation and lncRNA-miRNA/protein interaction [45–47]. In previous reports, lncRNA HCG11 was showed to be a tumor suppressor in prostate cancer (PCa) [48] and may serve as prognostic markers in both breast and gastric cancers [49, 50]. However, in HCC development, HCG11 was demonstrated to be highly expressed and unregulated in the activity of IGF2BP1, by which it modulated the downstream signaling of IGF2BP1, including p21/capase-3 and MAPK, and subsequently affected the growth and metastasis of HCC. Nevertheless, knockdown of HCG11 was showed to lead to IGF2BP1 suppression and inhibition of cell viability and proliferation, cell migration and invasion, and colony formation ability of HepG2 cells, as well as induce cell apoptosis and cell cycle arrest at G1 stage, which is similar to the effects of IGF2BP1 suppression by shRNA [40]. Another lncRNA HULC was also found to be overexpressed in HCC tissues and correlate with low-grade and low-stage HCC, indicating a functional role of HULC in the early stages of tumor development. Interestingly, IGF2BP1 served as a trans-acting factor to inhibit HULC expression by recruiting CNOT1 and bringing HULC into close proximity to the CCR4-NOT deadenylase complex [51]. Significantly, in HCC samples, both IGF2BP1 and HULC were upregulated [51], suggesting that other modulation may antagonize the suppressive effects of IGF2BP1 on HULC.

Presently, some miRNAs including miR-625, miR-98-5p, miR-9, miR-1275, and miRNA-196b were showed to be frequently downregulated in HCC samples, and their upregulation may hinder HCC development [39, 42, 43, 52, 53]. miR-625 was found to bind to IGF2BP1 and inhibit tumor migration and invasion, which may have partly resulted from the speculated

IGF2BP1/PTEN/HSP27 pathway in which the re-expression of miR-625 might indirectly reduce PTEN expression through depressing IGF2BP1, subsequently contributing to the Akt-mediated phosphorylation of HSP27 and suppressing F-actin polymerization [42]. miR-98-5p was reported to associate with poor survival of HCC patients and could depress HCC cell proliferation and induce cell apoptosis by targeting and inhibiting IGF2BP1 [39]. Another potential prognostic marker for HCC, miR-9, was observed to promote HCC cell proliferation and migration by hypermethylation-mediated downregulation of it and inhibit HCC development via suppressing AKT and ERK phosphorylation that are well known for their oncogenic properties after targeting IGF2BP1 [43]. miR-1275, prevalent frequently in various cancers, could hinder HCC cell growth partially by simultaneously regulating the oncogenic IGF2BP1–3 and IGF1R [52]. Furthermore, IGF2BP1 was found to be targeted by miRNA-196b and suppress cell proliferation and induce apoptosis in HepG2 cell [53].

Breast cancer

IGF2BP1 was found to ubiquitously express in normal adult breast epithelial cells, and mouse and human breast tumor cell [1]. However, the suppression of invasion and metastasis by IGF2BP1 was seen in breast carcinoma cells of human and rat. IGF2BP1 activation may depress chemotaxis and metastasis of breast cancer cells through sustaining cell polarity and directional movement by modulating the localization of β-actin mRNA [54–56]. The high promoter methylation and significant downregulation of IGF2BP1 was observed in all metastatic cell lines including MTLn3, MDA435, MDA231, and 4T1 but slightly in non-metastatic cell lines including MTC in T47D, and the promoter demethylation of IGF2BP1 induced its endogenous expression in metastatic MTLn3 cells, indicating epigenetic modifications could act a role in silencing the IGF2BP1 in metastatic breast tumor cells [54, 57]. Furthermore, IGF2BP1 can depress metastatic breast tumor cell proliferation and invasion by targeting and regulating localized expression of multiple adhesion- and motility-related mRNAs. Repression of IGF2BP1 expression may reduce the accumulation of E-cadherin, a crucial cell adhesion protein, at cell–cell contacts, as well as impair the dynamics of focal adhesions, subsequently converting the polarized adherent phenotype into an unpolarized morphological one with invasive behavior [57]. Notably, promoter methylation of IGF2BP1 was not detected in normal tissues including the breast, liver, and brain of adult rat. Taken together, it seems possible to draw a conclusion from these in vitro and in vivo studies that methylation events of IGF2BP1 are becoming more frequent with the higher breast cancer grade, and this leads to more

silence and downregulation events of IGF2BP1, resulting in dysregulated effects on IGF2BP1-target mRNAs. Significantly, in addition to methylation, other factors also cause silence event of IGF2BP1 [54]. However, in another observation of metastatic human breast tumor-driving cell and xenograft mouse model, the gain expression of IGF2BP1 inhibited tumor growth and metastases, which may be through the function of the KH3/4 domain of IGF2BP1 on its targeted mRNAs [17], suggesting other tumor-related inhibition paths for IGF2BP1 exist in addition to methylation-induced effects. For example, IGF2BP1 expression might upregulate RGS4 mRNA and inhibit tumor cell proliferation and invasion, while downregulate GDF15, IGF2, and PTG2 mRNAs and lead to suppression of tumor cell proliferation and invasion [17].

However, inconsistent with the suppressive role in the breast tumor cell-derived cell and xenograft mouse models, some in vivo studies revealed that IGF2BP1 plays an enhancive role in tumorigenesis and metastasis in breast cancer cells [57]. The probable explanations for contradictive function of IGF2BP1 might result from the cell-specific differences and the endogenous difference between non-metastatic cells and metastatic cells, for example, the significantly high promoter methylation of IGF2BP1 in metastatic breast tumor cells compared with that in non-metastatic breast tumor cells results in the more common silence events of IGF2BP1. In addition, in cancer cells advance to metastasis, crucial genes have incensed changes in the pattern of expression including both the gain and loss of gene function [58].

Gynecologic cancers

IGF2BP1 was reported to be significantly elevated in cervical cancer (CC) tissues and cell lines and in ovarian cancer tissues [59–61]. Two miRNAs including miR-140-5p and miR-124-3p were significantly downregulated in CC tissues compared with that in normal cervical tissues and cell lines. In addition, CC patients with higher miR-140-5p levels had significantly longer survival, ectopic expression of miR-124-3p, and inhibited tumor cell growth and metastasis. Therefore, miR-140-5p and miR-124-3p might act as an inhibitor of cell proliferation, migration and invasion, growth, and metastasis in CC by targeting and downregulating IGF2BP1 levels [60].

In ovarian carcinoma (OC) cells, IGF2BP1 was showed to act as an oncogenic factor that contributes to enhanced proliferation by stabilizing the c-MYC mRNA. Furthermore, elevated IGF2BP1 expression was observed preferentially in high-grade and high-stage cases [61], indicating its prognostic role for decreased recurrence-free and overall survival. Additionally, IGF2BP1 was demonstrated to sustain tumor cell survival upon binding eIF5A and suppressing eIF5A-mediated apoptotic effects that depends on the cytoplasmic IGF2BP1 levels in ovarian and breast cancer of mouse [62], indicating their important role in the therapeutic trials using inhibitors of exportin1 (XPO1) that is the key nuclear export protein and essential for transporting cargo proteins with leucine-rich nuclear export sequences from the nucleus to the cytoplasm, such as leptomycin B [62, 63]. The let-7 miRNA family was dysregulated in various cancers, including OC, and had a tumor-suppressive role by interfering in the expression of multiple oncogenic factors, including IGF2BP1 [64, 65]. let-7 was demonstrated to inhibit tumor cell growth and migration, and self-renewal via depressing the oncogenic "triangle" composed of HMGA2-IGF2BP1-LIN28B [65]. Interestingly, another underexpressed miR-708 was observed to enhance the susceptibility of OC cells to cisplatin through targeting IGF2BP1 and inducing an inhibition of Akt signaling that plays a critical role in cisplatin resistance in OC. However, the upregulated expression of IGF2BP1 might restore resistance of miR-708-overexpressing OC cells to cisplatin [66].

Gastrointestinal cancers

IGF2BP1 was demonstrated to play tumor-suppressive or tumorigenic roles in gastrointestinal cancers. Stromal IGF2BP1 is a contributor to normal intestinal development and homeostasis. Mongroo et al. have identified the tumorigenic role of IGF2BP1 in colon cancer cell. IGF2BP1 loss was found to inhibit the expression of K-Ras and Cdc34, the let-7 repressor Lin-28B, and c-Myc, concomitantly depress anchorage-independent growth and colon cancer cell proliferation, and trigger caspase-mediated cell death [67]. During the process, c-Myc and IGF2BP1 constitute a potential feedback mechanism to reciprocally regulate expression of each other in colon cancer. In the study, IGF2BP1 was established to promote colon cancer cell survival and regulate K-Ras expression via targeting 3′-UTR of K-Ras mRNA that frequently mutates in human cancers and regulates distinct cellular pathways important for the growth, differentiation, and survival of cell [68], in part by suppressing CYFIP2, which is a p53-inducible gene and may depress cell proliferation and caspase activation, and induce apoptosis in colon cancer [69]. However, different from the oncogenic role in previous colorectal tumors and cells, and other cancers [67, 70], IGF2BP1 was demonstrated to have tumor-suppressive roles. Under the stromal knockdown of IGF2BP1 in the mouse model of colitis-associated cancer, the mice showed elevated tumor burden such as enhanced tumor initiation and progression, which is partly explained by the effects of chronic inflammatory damage caused by IGF2BP1 detection [16]. Additionally, IGF2BP1 loss

enhanced the levels of HGF, which is produced by stromal fibroblasts and contributes to epithelial cell proliferation and invasive growth of CRC cells by the interaction with β-catenin signaling, and conferred resistance to EGFR inhibitors in colon tumor-initiating cells in fibroblasts in vitro, and increased fibroblast cell growth [16, 71–74], indicating a potentially tumor-suppressive role of IGF2BP1 via modulating HGF in fibroblasts. The contradictory function of IGF2BP1 in colon cancer cells and mouse models of colitis-associated cancer may result from use of different tumor models or the complexity of colon cancer tumorigenesis, suggesting that tumor cells arrived from different origins or conditions might have different responses to IGF2BP1 expression.

LncRNA GHET1 was found to be upregulated in gastric carcinoma tissues and correlate with poor prognosis, with a positive relationship with tumor size and invasion, and the shorter survival. Enhanced GHET1 expression can contribute to gastric carcinoma cell proliferation and tumor growth in vitro and in vivo by physically associating with IGF2BP1 and increasing the physical interaction of IGF2BP1 with c-Myc mRNA, consequently enhancing c-Myc mRNA stability and expression [75].

Sarcoma

Although the study of IGF2BP1 in osteosarcoma (OS) is little, the observation of the restoration of miR-150 expression in OS cells could suppress the proliferation, migration and invasion, and growth of tumor cell and induce apoptosis by targeting it was reported [76]. MiR-150, which has been demonstrated to play important roles in various human cancers, was showed to be downregulated in OS tissues and cell lines in contrast to the matched adjacent tissues as well as human normal osteoblast cells.

IGF2BP1 is a critical modulator of cellular inhibitor of apoptosis 1 (cIAP1) expression and of apoptotic resistance in rhabdomyosarcoma (RMS), controlling cell death and drug resistance by medicating translation of cIAP1. In rhabdomyosarcoma tissues and cell lines, IGF2BP1 was found to be overexpressed and drive the expression of cIAP1 that is a key modulator of apoptosis and contributes to tumor cell survival through controlling the nuclear factor-κB signalling and extrinsic cell death pathways, as well as promote disease progression and chemo-resistance by increasing IRES-mediated translation of cIAP1 [77, 78]. Decreasing levels of cIAP1 in RMS cell lines upon IGF2BP1 knockdown sensitize RMS cells to tumor necrosis factor-α (TNFα)-mediated cell death, similar to the result by Smac mimetic compound (SMC) treatment. Moreover, targeting cIAP1 by SMC suppresses the formation and growth of RMS xeno-graft tumors in mice [78].

Central nervous system cancer

The important roles of IGF2BP1 in neuroblastoma, meningiomas, and glioblastoma were reported [79]. IGF2BP1 was showed to highly express in neuroblastoma tissues and identified as a significantly important gene in this disease because of its clear negative prognostic effect at the DNA, mRNA, and protein levels, and its positive correlation with MYCN, a most prominent oncogene in neuroblastoma and other aggressive tumors. In the 69 neuroblastoma tissues, IGF2BP1 DNA copy number, mRNA, and protein abundance were strikingly higher in stage 4 than stage 1 tumor. Additionally, IGF2BP1 mRNA and protein levels were correlated with poor overall survival. IGF2BP1 clearly influenced MYCN expression and neuroblastoma cell survival [80].

The significantly frequent promoter methylation of IGF2BP1 in recurrent meningioma cases was found [81]. IGF2BP1 increased the malignant potential of meningiomas, with significantly higher methylation levels in atypical (grade II/III) than benign (grade I), indicating its prognostic role. Notably, the median production of protein of this gene for both of the two-set atypical meningiomas was reduced, though without statistically significant difference [82]. Those findings show that methylation of IGF2BP1 involves tumor development and regulates its expression and thus modulates the downstream biological pathway.

Glioblastoma multiforme (GBM) is known as the most highly malignant and active primary brain tumor with a poor prognosis [44]. Some miRNAs including miR-506 and miR-873 were showed to be lowly expressed in GBM tissues or cells and play a tumor-suppressive role in this disease by targeting and modulating IGF2BP1. However, their overexpression was observed to repress the cell proliferation and migration, and invasion of GBM through downregulating the IGF2BP1 levels, which reduces the level of c-MYC, CD44, MKI67, and PTEN mRNA in GBM cells or blocks G1/S transition in glioblastoma cell [44, 83]. C-MYC and MKI67 act as effective modulators of cell proliferation and apoptosis with the stability by IGF2BP1 [41]. Furthermore, suppression of CD44 mRNA degradation may promote invadopodia formation under the IGF2BP1 upregulation [84]. PTEN has a cell-migration role in early neural precursors, and IGF2BP1 can enhance the directionality of cell migration with the functional PTEN-dependent manner [85, 86]. Those studies support a hypothesis that reduced levels of miR-506 and miR-873 or other miR-NAs contribute to carcinogenesis and metastasis via upregulating IGF2BP1 expression and subsequently modulating its target RNA transcripts.

Melanoma

Upregulation of IGF2BP1 expression in human melanoma or mouse model was observed [87, 88]. Its overexpression influences various proto-oncogenes and oncogenic signaling pathways that involve tumor development, survival, and drug resistance [88]. In metastatic melanoma, IGF2BP1 expression was observed to confer a resistance to chemotherapeutic agents, whereas its inhibition or knockdown enhanced the effects of chemotherapy and reduced tumorigenic characteristics [88]. Moreover, IGF2BP1 knockdown was found to reduce levels of c-MYC, which contributes to the suppression of NF-kB activity and of anchorage-independent growth of melanoma cells and proliferation, as well as induces apoptosis [89]. Thus, IGF2BP1 could be a reduce-chemoresistance target for melanoma.

Leukemia

The role of IGF2BP1 in hematological malignancies, including acute myeloid leukemia (AML) and B acute lymphoblastic leukemia (ALL) was found [4], although its expression and exact function is little known. LIN28B, a stem cell reprogramming factor, may down-regulate the let-7 family to promote stem cell differentiation [90, 91]. The overexpression of this gene is common in advance leukemias [92] and could depress cancer stem cell (CSC) differentiation [93–96], while its inhibition might induce G2/M cell-cycle arrest which regulates cell proliferation and colony formation in AML. Importantly, IGF2BP1 has been identified as a downstream effector of LIN28B by let-7 miRNA. By this mechanism, overexpression of LIN28B may inhibit let-7 miRNAs, thus elevating IGF2BP1 expression in AML cells [4]. Additionally, the loss of IGF2BP1 was indicated to increase tumor cell proliferation related to increased IGF-II protein levels in K562 leukemia cells [97] and promote PARP- and caspase-3 mediated apoptosis in colorectal cancer cells [67]. However, whether LIN28B also induces PARP- and caspase-3-mediated apoptosis in AML and other cancers by downregulating IGF2BP1 is unknown. In t(12;21) (p13;q22)-positive ALL, IGF2BP1 was found as a potent regulator of ETV6/RUNX1 mRNA stability and potentially linked this evolutionary highly conserved protein to cell transformation events [98].

Other cancers

IGF2BP1 was showed to be overexpressed in both retinoblastoma and choriocarcinoma. In retinoblastoma, the gene promotes tumor cell proliferation and migration [99]. In choriocarcinoma cell lines, the depletion of ribosomal protein S6 kinase (RSK2) or protein phosphatase methylesterase 1 (PPME1) inhibits cell migration and invasion, which is similar to that after knockdown of IGF2BP1 that controls RSK2 and PPME expression,

Table 1 The expression and roles of IGF2BP1 in human cancer

Cancer type	Incidence	Method	The status of expression in tissues	The roles of IGF2BP1 expression in cancers	Reference
Lung cancer and esophageal adenocarcinomas					
Non-small cell lung cancer	27% (4/11)–52% (139/267)	Microarray, qRT-PCR, Western blot	Overexpressed	Promoting lung cancer development and progression	[8, 33]
Lung adenocarcinoma	17% (1/6)	IHC, TCGA datasets	Significantly upregulated	Poor overall survival; bigger primary tumor size	[32, 34, 79]
Lung squamous cell carcinoma	37.5% (3/8)	IHC, TCGA datasets	Significantly upregulated	Younger age at diagnosis	[32, 79]
Esophageal adenocarcinomas	Unknown	TCGA datasets	Significantly upregulated	Poor survival	[34]
Breast cancer					
Breast cancer	59% (59/118)	IHC, immunofluorescence, Western Blotting, RNASeq	High and ubiquitously expressed	Tumorigenic activity, clonogenic growth	[1, 8]
Breast cancer		qRT-PCR	Wildly expressed	Inhibiting tumor growth and metastasis	[17, 54–57]
Liver cancer					
Gallbladder carcinoma	72.4%	IHC	Ubiquitously expressed but lower expressed than controls	Longer survival	[38]
Hepatocellular carcinoma	Unknown	TCGA, IHC, qRT-PCR, Western blot		Poor survival	[3]
Hepatocellular carcinoma		qRT-PCR, Western blot	Overexpressed	Positively correlated with tumor size, advanced stages and grading of poor differentiation	[41]
Hepatocellular carcinoma		IHC	Significantly upregulated	Promoting progression; migration and invasion	[40]
Hepatocellular carcinoma		IHC	Significantly upregulated	Poor prognosis	[42]
Hepatocellular carcinoma		qRT-PCR, Western blot	Significantly upregulated	Promoting tumor cell proliferation, migration, and invasion	[39]
Hepatocellular carcinoma		ELISA, qRT-PCR, Western blot	Significantly upregulated	Poor post-surgery prognosis	[43]
Hepatocellular carcinoma		qRT-PCR	Significantly upregulated		[52]
Fibrolamellar hepatocellular carcinoma (FL-HCC)	Unknown	ACGH, RNA-seq	Significantly upregulated		[50]
Leukemia					
Chronic myelogenous leukemia (CML)	Unknown	qRT-PCR	Significantly upregulated	Promoting cell proliferation	[97]
Acute lymphoblastic leukemia (ALL)	Unknown		Overexpressed		[98]
Melanoma					
Melanoma	34% (13/38)	RT-PCR	Upregulated	Promoting tumor growth and drug resistance	[8, 87–89]
Osteosarcoma (OS)					
Osteosarcoma (OS)	Unknown	Western blot	High expression	Promoting the proliferation, migration and invasion,	[76]

Table 1 The expression and roles of IGF2BP1 in human cancer *(Continued)*

Cancer type	Incidence	Method	The status of expression in tissues	The roles of IGF2BP1 expression in cancers	Reference
				and growth of tumor cell, and inhibiting apoptosis	
Gastrointestinal cancer					
Colon	50% (36/79)– 59% (46/78)	IHC		Tumor-suppressive role	[8, 16]
Colon		qRT-PCR, immunofluorescence, IHC, Western Blotting	Upregulated	Promoting cell proliferation, growth, and survival	[67]
CNS cancer					
Neuroblastoma	Unknown	Microarray data	High expression	Poor survival, advanced stages	[80]
Glioblastoma multiforme (GBM)	54.5% (6/11)	qRT-PCR, Western blotting	Significantly upregulated	Inducing carcinogenesis and metastasis	[44, 79]
Meningiomas	63.6% (14/22)	Western blotting	Reduced expression	Promoting tumor development and the malignant potential	[81, 79]
Rhabdomyosarcomas (RMS)	Unknown	IHC	Overexpressed tumors and cell lines	Regulating cell death and drug resistance	[78]
Gynecologic cancers					
Cervical cancer (CC)	Unknown	Western blotting, qRT-PCR	Significantly upregulated	Promoting cell viability, migration, and invasion	[59, 60]
Ovarian cancer	69% (73/106)	IHC	High expression	Poor prognosis and poor overall survival	[8, 61]
Other cancers					
Choriocarcinoma (CC)	Unknown	IHC, Western blotting, qRT-PCR	Overexpressed	Promoting cell migration and invasion	[100]
Retinoblastoma	Unknown	LC–MS/MS,IHC	Overexpressed	Promoting cell proliferation and migration	[99]

whereas it did not influence cellular proliferation and morphology [100], indicating that IGF2BP1 promotes choriocarcinoma cell migration and invasion partly via the effect of RSK2 and PPME1.

The interconnectivity of IGF2BP1 with its targeted RNAs in cancers

IGF2BP1 was found to be commonly and significantly up-regulated in almost all tumor cell lines and tumor tissues with a range from 17 to 72.4% of incidence (Table 1) and act as an essential oncogene that promotes the stability, localization, and translation of cancer-related mRNA targets by the regulation of some lncRNAs and miRNAs (Table 2). Almost all of the reported miRNAs including miR-491-5p, miR-625, miR-98-5p, miR-9, miR-196b, miR-1275, miR-708, let-7 miRNA family, miR-150, miR-506, miR-873, miR-140-5p, and miR-124-3p are downregulated in corresponding cancer samples, whereas all of the three lncRNAs including HCG11, GHET1, and THOR are highly expressed in corresponding solid tumors. As shown in Fig. 2, upregulation of the three lncRNAs can elevate IGF2BP1 level, while upregulation of

the miRNAs could repress IGF2BP1 expression. HCG11 can upregulate the activity of IGF2BP1 and thus leads to activation of MAPK signaling [40]. GHET1 may enhance he stability of c-Myc mRNA and expression by physically associating with IGF2BP1 and elevating the physical interaction between c-Myc mRNA and IGF2BP1 [75]. However, THOR indirectly controls the levels of IGF2BP1-target mRNAs including KRAS, IGF2, CD44, PABPC1, ACTB, GLI1, MYC, CTNNB1, MAPT, PPP1R9B, PTEN, BTRC, and H19. Nearly the levels of all those targets are reduced in both MM603 and H1299 cells with THOR knock down similar to that with IGF2BP1 knockdown, whereas elevates with overexpression of THOR in SKMEL5 and H1437 cells [29]. Taken together, those findings show that lncRNAs HCG11, GHET1, and THOR dysregulate the expression of IGF2BP1-downstream targets by modulating IGF2BP1. Similarly, the miRNAs in tumors target the 3′-UTR of IGF2BP1, by which they regulate the expression of IGF2BP1-downstream targets and affect tumor cell proliferation, migration and invasion, and growth.

Table 2 Target mRNAs of IGF2BP1

Identified/putative target mRNAs	Cis-element on RNA	Regulation of IGF2BP1 for target mRNA	The biological roles of those target mRNAs (http://www.genecards.org/)	Ref.
eEF2		Increasing basal protein translation rates	Enhancing basal proliferation rates	[102]
CD44	3'-UTR	Stabilization of the transcript	Involving in invadopodia formation, cell migration, tumor growth and progression.	[83]
c-Myc	CDS	Inhibition of CRD-dependent mRNA decay	Promoting the tumor cell proliferation	[40]
ACTB	3'-UTR	Inhibition of mRNA translation;	Involving in various types of cell motility	[101]
IGF2	5'-UTR	Inhibition of mRNA translation	Promoting cell growth and proliferation	[8]
PTEN	CDS	Inhibition of CRD-dependent mRNA decay	Modulation of actin dynamics and cell migration; modulating cell cycle progression and cell survival; promoting cell polarization and directed movement.	[100]
MDR1	CDS	Inhibition of CRD-dependent mRNA decay	NA	[8]
MAPK4	3'-UTR	Inhibition of mRNA translation	Modulating actin dynamics and cell migration; promoting entry in the cell cycle	[100]
PPP1R9B	3'-UTR	mRNA transport	Involving in linking the actin cytoskeleton to the plasma membrane at the synaptic junction	[8]
BTRC	CDS	Inhibition of betaTrCP1 mRNA degradation	Mediating the ubiquitination and subsequent proteasomal degradation of target proteins	[102]
CTNNB1	3'-UTR	Inhibition of mRNA decay	Regulating cell adhesion; promoting neurogenesis	[8]
KRAS	CDS, 3'-UTR	Inhibition of mRNA decay	Modulating cell proliferation; promoting oncogenic events	[66, 67]
PABPC1	5'-UTR	mRNA translation	Regulating mRNA metabolism, and translationally coupled mRNA turnover	[29]
H19	3'-UTR	mRNA localization	Involving in migration and invasion	[29]
GLI1	CDS	Inhibition of mRNA decay	Regulating cell proliferation and differentiation; promoting cancer cell migration	[29]
cIAP1	5'-UTR IRES	Enhancing IRES-mediated translation	Modulating cell proliferation, as well as cell invasion and metastasis, and cell cycle	[77]
RAPGEF2			Inhibiting cell proliferation of melanoma cells and promotes their apoptosis; regulating embryonic blood vessel formation; establishment of basal junction integrity and endothelial barrier function	[100]
RPS6KA5			Involving in neuronal cell death; limiting the production of pro-inflammatory cytokines	[100]
RSK2		Stabilization of the transcript	Promoting cell migration and invasion	[99]
PPME1		Stabilization of the transcript	Promoting cell migration and invasion	[99]
ITGA6	NA	NA	Mediating cell adhesion to extra cellular matrix or to other cells, and fertilization of ova and embryonic development	[28]
ETV6/RUNX1 mRNA (potential)		Stability of this transcript	NA	[97]
GDF15	3'-UTR	Inhibition of this transcript	Inhibiting breast cancer cell migration and invasion	[17]
RGS4			Inhibiting signal transduction and breast cancer cell migration and invasion	[17]
PTGS2			Modulating production of inflammatory prostaglandins, and motility, proliferation, and resistance to apoptosis.	[17]
CDH1		Localization of the mRNAs	Regulating cell–cell adhesions, mobility, and proliferation of epithelial cells; downregulation of cell growth	[53]
β-actin		Localization of the mRNAs	Involving in establishment of cell polarity and cell motility	[53]
α-actinin		Localization of the mRNAs	Regulating focal adhesion metabolism	[53]
Arp2/3		Localization of the mRNAs		[53]

Table 2 Target mRNAs of IGF2BP1 *(Continued)*

Identified/putative target mRNAs	Cis-element on RNA	Regulation of IGF2BP1 for target mRNA	The biological roles of those target mRNAs (http://www.genecards.org/)	Ref.
			Regulating focal adhesion metabolism, actin polymerization, and the formation of branched actin networks	
TAU	3'-UTR	Localization of the mRNAs	Promoting microtubule assembly and stability; establishment and maintenance of neuronal polarity	[53]
MKI67		Stability of this transcript	Promoting the tumor cell proliferation	[40]

In the context of modulation by miRNAs/lncRNAs (Fig. 2), aberrant upregulation of IGF2BP1 promotes the expression of c-MYC and MKI67, as well as CD44 and PTEN [41, 44, 84, 101]. By stabilizing c-MYC and MKI67 transcripts, IGF2BP1 enhances tumor cell proliferation and growth. Interestingly, c-Myc and IGF2BP1 each constitutes a potential feedback mechanism to reciprocally regulate expression of the other. Additionally, IGF2BP1 prevents CD44 and PTEN mRNA turnover, consequently enhances CD44 expression, and induces the formation of invadopodia and therefore may promote tumor cell migration and invasiveness [84]. The elevation of PTEN inhibits PIP3/PIP2 ratios and then interferes with the activation of RAC1, which enhances cell polarization, and thus, this contributes to directed tumor cell migration as well as tumor invasion. However, the increased RGS4 expression enhanced by IGF2BP1 depresses tumor cell migration and invasion [17]. Although the expression levels of PTGS2, ACTB, and MAPK4 are reduced by IGF2BP1 interfering with their mRNA translation, there are different results on tumor events. Reduced PTGS2 decreases the suppression of tumor cell apoptosis and the promotion of tumor cell invasion [17]. The inhibition of MAPK4 antagonizes MK5-directed phosphorylation of HSP27. PHSP27 at both residues induces the degradation of oligomers and increases the sequestering of actin monomers by the phosphorylated protein [101]. The reduced ACTB also decreases G-actin levels. This shift in the cellular G-/F-actin equilibrium contributes to cell adhesion and actin dynamics, and finally promotes cell migration velocity [102]. In addition, promoter methylation of IGF2BP1 may silence its expression and subsequently modulates the downstream biological pathways [81, 82]. Taken together, we can deduce a conclusion that IGF2BP1 plays an important role in the occurrence of tumor events and shows a degree of tumor suppressor effect. However, determining whether the occurrence of tumor events or not partly depends on IGF2BP1 targeting different cancer-related mRNAs, although the driving factors that contribute to this gene to choose different mRNA targets are unclear. It is worth noting that the methylation events of the promoter in IGF2BP1 at least involve the selected process because high promoter methylation of IGF2BP1 was demonstrated to

block β-catenin binding to the IGF2BP promoter, leading to inactivation of the gene and enhancing proliferation and migration of metastatic breast cancer cells (Fig. 1d) [54, 103]. Additionally, the selective manner may partially result from the competitive combination on m^6A-containing mRNAs between IGF2BP1 and other m^6A-binding proteins such as YTHDFs, since they could read the same m^6A regions of mRNAs while determining a totally different fate of m^6A-containing mRNAs (Fig. 1c).

As per the tumor-promotion role of IGF2BP1 in most of cancers, it seems that IGF2BP1 and its targeted transcripts could be attractive anticancer drug targets; however, small molecule inhibitors of IGF2BP1 and other cancer-related mRNA stabilizing proteins, as well as the upstream ncRNAs, are little known [8]. Note worthily, a small molecule, BTYNB, might function as a potential therapeutics by inhibiting cell proliferation of IGF2BP1-positive cancer cells without effect in IGF2BP1-negative cells. BTYNB may restrain binding of IGF2BP1 to the coding region stability determinant of c-Myc mRNA and downregulate several mRNA transcripts including c-Myc, β-TrCP1, and eEF2 both in IGROV-1 and SK-MEL2 cancer cells, as well as decrease activation of nuclear transcriptional factors-kappa B (NF-κB). Moreover, it also selectively reduces the levels of other cancer-related IGF2BP1 mRNA targets including CALM1, CDC34, COL5A, and BTRC, similar to the effect by RNAi knockdown of IGF2BP1 both in IGROV-1 and SK-MEL2 cancer cells [104].

Conclusions

IGF2BP1 is broadly and highly expressed in embryonic and tumor tissues. The bulk of correlative studies describing enhanced expression or de novo synthesis of IGF2BP1 in human cancer and animal model provide strong evidence that IGF2BP1 serves important roles in controlling embryonic development, as well as functions as an oncogenic factor in most of cancers. In most of the cancers, IGF2BP1 enhances tumor cell proliferation, survival, adhesion-independent growth and invasion, and chemo-resistance. The upregulated expression of IGF2BP1 is associated with poor overall survival and metastasis in multiple cancers. However, the tumor-suppressive role of IGF2BP1 has been observed

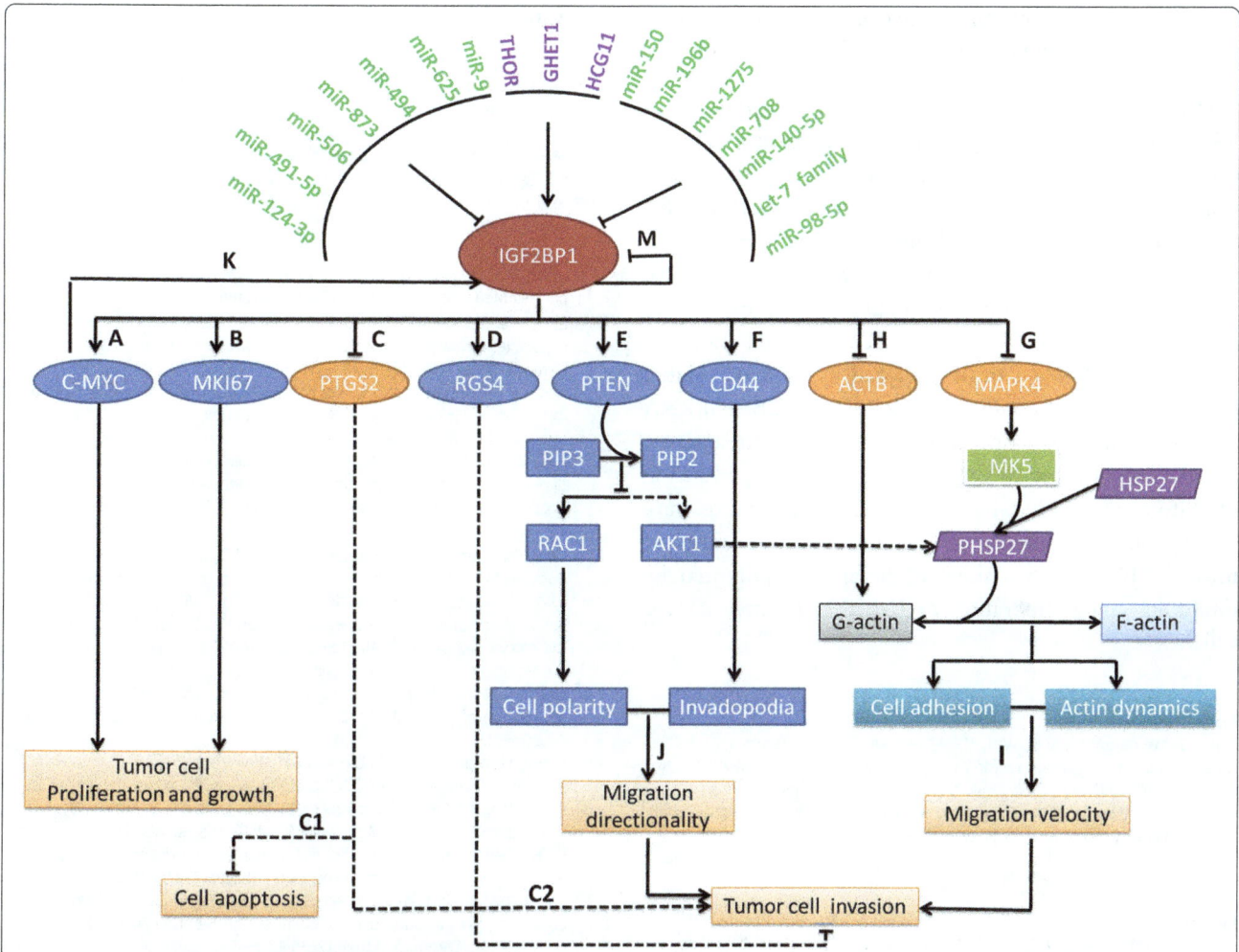

Fig. 2 The roles of IGF2BP1 in promoting and suppressing tumor growth and invasion via regulating different mRNA targets, under the modulation of upstream non-coding RNAs. (1) Some miRNAs/lncRNAs upregulate or downregulate IGF2BP1 expression levels. (2) IGF2BP1 promotes the expression of c-MYC and MKI67 by stabilizing their transcripts and promotes tumor cell proliferation and growth (**a**, **b**). In addition, IGF2BP1 elevates CD44 and PTEN expression via preventing mRNA turnover. The enhancement of CD44 expression induces the formation of invadopodia and therefore may promote the tumor cell migration and invasiveness (**f**, **j**). Elevation of PTEN inhibits PIP3/PIP2 ratios and then interferes with the activation of RAC1, which enhances cell polarization and thus contributes to directed tumor cell migration as well as tumor invasion (**e**, **j**). IGF2BP1 suppresses the expression of MAPK4 and ACTB through interfering with mRNA translation (**g**, **h**). The inhibition of MAPK4 antagonizes MK5-directed phosphorylation of HSP27. PHSP27 at both residues induces the degradation of oligomers and increases the sequestering of actin monomers by the phosphorylated protein. The reduced ACTB also decreases G-actin levels. This shifts the cellular G-/F-actin equilibrium contributes to cell adhesion and actin dynamics and finally promotes cell migration velocity (I) [41, 84–86, 101, 102]. Furthermore, IGF2BP1 promotes RGS4 expression and thus indirectly depresses tumor cell invasion (**d**). IGF2BP1 inhibits PTGS2 expression (**c**). The reduction of PTGS2 indirectly promotes tumor cell invasion and releases the suppression for cell apoptosis (C1, C2) [17]. C-Myc and IGF2BP1 constitute a potential feedback mechanism to reciprocally regulate expression of each other (**k**) [68]. The hypermethylation of promoter in IGF2BP1 leads to its expression silencing (**m**) [81, 82].The gray dotted lines show that the interaction of the depicted pathways needs to be explored. The part of Fig. 2 including pathway from (**e**, **f**, **h**, and **g** to **i** and **j** is adapted from the Figure 3 of the paper by Stohr et al. [102]

in breast cancer and colon stromal cells. At least in breast cancer, it is confirmed that IGF2BP1 inhibits tumor cell growth and invasion. IGF2BP1 has both tumor-driving and tumor-suppressive roles in cancers in a context-based manner.

Although the origin of difference between oncogenic and tumor-suppressive roles is unclear, the apparently contradictory functions of IGF2BP1 may result from tumor cells arrived from different origins or conditions with different responses to IGF2BP1 expression. In this context, it seems that some undefined driver factors contribute to IGF2BP1 selectively binding and regulating its mRNA targets and lead to either development or suppression for tumors. Though the mechanism of IGF2BP1 selectively binding to its mRNA targets is unclear, epigenetic modifications of IGF2BP1 at least are involved in the process. In addition, the selective manner may partially result from the competitive combination on m^{6}A-containing mRNAs between IGF2BP1 and other m^{6}A-binding proteins such as YTHDFs.

The reasonable inferences about the functions of IGF2BP1 in cancer biology can be confirmed in the future by in vivo and in vitro studies, according to specific origins or conditions of the tumor cells. Additionally, the emerging miRNAs and lncRNAs that target and regulate IGF2BP1 have been ascertained to involve IGF2BP1-mediated mRNA modulation. Therefore, more interconnectivity between IGF2BP1 and its targeted mRNAs or ncRNAs can be explored in contexts related to specific cancer conditions. NcRNA-IGF2BP1-mRNA target-axes may be worth of more studies as their target potential for cancer therapy. Though currently available inhibitors of ncRNA-IGF2BP1-mRNA target-axes are limited, an inhibitor of IGF2BP1 binding to targeted mRNAs, BTYNB, has showed therapeutic potential by inhibiting cell proliferation of IGF2BP1-positive cancer cells.

Abbreviations
CNC: Cranial neural crest; ELAVL1: ELAV-like RNA binding protein 1; IGF2BP1: Insulin-like growth factor 2 mRNA-binding protein 1 (IGF2BP1), also known as IMP/CRD-BP/VICKZ; lncRNA: Long non-coding RNA; miRNA: MicroRNA; ncRNAs: Non-coding RNA; RRMs: RNA recognition motifs; YTHDFs: YT521-B homology (YTH) domain-containing proteins

Funding
This work was supported by The National Natural Science Foundation of China (81460007), the Cooperative Innovation Center for Old-age Care and Geriatric Health of Sichuan Province of China (YLZBZ1515), and the Natural Science Foundation of Sichuan provincial department of education of China (17A0130).

Authors' contributions
XH and HZ drafted the manuscript. XK and HC read and approved the final manuscript. XG and ZZ participated in planning. All authors read and approved the final manuscript.

Consent for publication
Not applicable.

Competing interests
The authors declare that they have no competing interests.

Author details
[1]Faculty of Environmental Science and Engineering, Kunming University of Science and Technology, Kunming City 650504, Yunnan Province, China. [2]Medical School, Kunming University of Science and Technology, Kunming City 650504, Yunnan Province, China. [3]Department of Rehabilitation Medicine, The First Affiliated Hospital of Chengdu Medical College, Chengdu City 610500, Sichuan Province, China. [4]Department of Oncology, Yunfeng Hospital, Xuanwei City 655400, Yunnan Province, China.

References
1. Fakhraldeen SA, Clark RJ, Roopra A, Chin EN, Huang W, Castorino J, et al. Two isoforms of the RNA binding protein, coding region determinant-binding protein (CRD-BP/IGF2BP1), are expressed in breast epithelium and support clonogenic growth of breast tumor cells. J Biol Chem. 2015;290(21): 13386–400.
2. Mahaira LG, Katsara O, Pappou E, Iliopoulou EG, Fortis S, Antsaklis A, et al. IGF2BP1 expression in human mesenchymal stem cells significantly affects their proliferation and is under the epigenetic control of TET1/2 demethylases. Stem Cells Dev. 2014;23(20):2501–12.
3. Yuan P, Meng L, Wang N. SOX12 upregulation is associated with metastasis of hepatocellular carcinoma and increases CDK4 and IGF2BP1 expression. Eur Rev Med Pharmacol Sci. 2017;21(17):3821–6.
4. Zhou J, Bi C, Ching YQ, Chooi JY, Lu X, Quah JY, et al. Inhibition of LIN28B impairs leukemia cell growth and metabolism in acute myeloid leukemia. J Hematol Oncol. 2017;10(1):138.
5. Wachter K, Kohn M, Stohr N, Huttelmaier S. Subcellular localization and RNP formation of IGF2BPs (IGF2 mRNA-binding proteins) is modulated by distinct RNA-binding domains. Biol Chem. 2013;394(8):1077–90.
6. Nielsen J, Kristensen MA, Willemoes M, Nielsen FC, Christiansen J. Sequential dimerization of human zipcode-binding protein IMP1 on RNA: a cooperative mechanism providing RNP stability. Nucleic Acids Res. 2004; 32(14):4368–76.
7. Farina KL, Huttelmaier S, Musunuru K, Darnell R, Singer RH. Two ZBP1 KH domains facilitate beta-actin mRNA localization, granule formation, and cytoskeletal attachment. J Cell Biol. 2003;160(1):77–87.
8. Bell JL, Wachter K, Muhleck B, Pazaitis N, Kohn M, Lederer M, et al. Insulin-like growth factor 2 mRNA-binding proteins (IGF2BPs): post-transcriptional drivers of cancer progression? Cell Mol Life Sci. 2013;70(15):2657–75.
9. Chao JA, Patskovsky Y, Patel V, Levy M, Almo SC, Singer RH. ZBP1 recognition of beta-actin zipcode induces RNA looping. Genes Dev. 2010; 24(2):148–58.
10. Huang H, Weng H, Sun W, Qin X, Shi H, Wu H, et al. Recognition of RNA N(6)-methyladenosine by IGF2BP proteins enhances mRNA stability and translation. Nat Cell Biol. 2018;20(3):285–95.
11. Dominissini D, Moshitch-Moshkovitz S, Schwartz S, Salmon-Divon M, Ungar L, Osenberg S, et al. Topology of the human and mouse m6A RNA methylomes revealed by m6A-seq. Nat. 2012;485(7397):201–6.
12. Du H, Zhao Y, He J, Zhang Y, Xi H, Liu M, et al. YTHDF2 destabilizes m(6)A-containing RNA through direct recruitment of the CCR4-NOT deadenylase complex. Nat Commun. 2016;7:12626.
13. Xiao W, Adhikari S, Dahal U, Chen YS, Hao YJ, Sun BF, et al. Nuclear m(6)a reader YTHDC1 regulates mRNA splicing. Mol Cell. 2016;61(4):507–19.
14. Wang X, Zhao BS, Roundtree IA, Lu Z, Han D, Ma H, et al. N(6)-methyladenosine modulates messenger RNA translation efficiency. Cell. 2015;161(6):1388–99.
15. Wang X, Lu Z, Gomez A, Hon GC, Yue Y, Han D, et al. N6-methyladenosine-dependent regulation of messenger RNA stability. Nat. 2014;505(7481):117–20.
16. Hamilton KE, Chatterji P, Lundsmith ET, Andres SF, Giroux V, Hicks PD, et al. Loss of stromal IMP1 promotes a tumorigenic microenvironment in the colon. Mol Cancer Res. 2015;13(11):1478–86.
17. Wang G, Huang Z, Liu X, Huang W, Chen S, Zhou Y, et al. IMP1 suppresses breast tumor growth and metastasis through the regulation of its target mRNAs. Oncotarget. 2016;7(13):15690–702.
18. Yaniv K, Fainsod A, Kalcheim C, Yisraeli JK. The RNA-binding protein Vg1 RBP is required for cell migration during early neural development. Dev. 2003;130(23):5649–61.
19. Hammer NA, Hansen T, Byskov AG, Rajpert-De Meyts E, Grondahl ML, Bredkjaer HE, et al. Expression of IGF-II mRNA-binding proteins (IMPs) in gonads and testicular cancer. Reprod. 2005;130(2):203–12.
20. Hansen TV, Hammer NA, Nielsen J, Madsen M, Dalbaeck C, Wewer UM, et al. Dwarfism and impaired gut development in insulin-like growth factor II mRNA-binding protein 1-deficient mice. Mol Cell Biol. 2004;24(10):4448–64.
21. Pillas D, Hoggart CJ, Evans DM, O'Reilly PF, Sipila K, Lahdesmaki R, et al. Genome-wide association study reveals multiple loci associated with primary tooth development during infancy. PLoS Genet. 2010;6(2): e1000856.
22. Perycz M, Urbanska AS, Krawczyk PS, Parobczak K, Jaworski J. Zipcode binding protein 1 regulates the development of dendritic arbors in hippocampal neurons. J Neurosci. 2011;31(14):5271–85.

23. Fabrizio JJ, Hickey CA, Stabrawa C, Meytes V, Hutter JA, Talbert C, et al. Imp (IGF-II mRNA-binding protein) is expressed during spermatogenesis in Drosophila melanogaster. Fly (Austin). 2008;2(1):47–52.

24. Gong F, Ren P, Zhang Y, Jiang J, Zhang H. MicroRNAs-491-5p suppresses cell proliferation and invasion by inhibiting IGF2BP1 in non-small cell lung cancer. Am J Transl Res. 2016;8(2):485–95.

25. Boylan KL, Mische S, Li M, Marques G, Morin X, Chia W, et al. Motility screen identifies Drosophila IGF-II mRNA-binding protein—zipcode-binding protein acting in oogenesis and synaptogenesis. PLoS Genet. 2008;4(2):e36.

26. Toledano H, D'Alterio C, Czech B, Levine E, Jones DL. The let-7-Imp axis regulates ageing of the Drosophila testis stem-cell niche. Nat. 2012; 485(7400):605–10.

27. Donnelly CJ, Willis DE, Xu M, Tep C, Jiang C, Yoo S, et al. Limited availability of ZBP1 restricts axonal mRNA localization and nerve regeneration capacity. EMBO J. 2011;30(22):4665–77.

28. Carmel MS, Kahane N, Oberman F, Miloslavski R, Sela-Donenfeld D, Kalcheim C, et al. A novel role for VICKZ proteins in maintaining epithelial integrity during embryogenesis. PLoS One. 2015;10(8):e0136408.

29. Hosono Y, Niknafs YS, Prensner JR, Iyer MK, Dhanasekaran SM, Mehra R, et al. Oncogenic role of THOR, a conserved cancer/testis long non-coding RNA. Cell. 2017;171(7):1559–1572.e20.

30. Findeis-Hosey JJ, Xu H. The use of insulin like-growth factor II messenger RNA binding protein-3 in diagnostic pathology. Hum Pathol. 2011;42(3): 303–14.

31. Lederer M, Bley N, Schleifer C, Huttelmaier S. The role of the oncofetal IGF2 mRNA-binding protein 3 (IGF2BP3) in cancer. Semin Cancer Biol. 2014;29:3–12.

32. Shi R, Yu X, Wang Y, Sun J, Sun Q, Xia W, et al. Expression profile, clinical significance, and biological function of insulin-like growth factor 2 messenger RNA-binding proteins in non-small cell lung cancer. Tumour Biol. 2017;39(4):1010428317695928.

33. Kato T, Hayama S, Yamabuki T, Ishikawa N, Miyamoto M, Ito T, et al. Increased expression of insulin-like growth factor-II messenger RNA-binding protein 1 is associated with tumor progression in patients with lung cancer. Clin Cancer Res. 2007;13(2 Pt 1):434–42.

34. Lin EW, Karakasheva TA. Comparative transcriptomes of adenocarcinomas and squamous cell carcinomas reveal molecular similarities that span classical anatomic boundaries. PLoS Genet. 2017;13(8):e1006938. https://doi. org/10.1371/journal.pgen.1006938. eCollection 2017 Aug.

35. Zhang J, Wang T, Zhang Y, Wang H, Wu Y, Liu K, et al. Upregulation of serum miR-494 predicts poor prognosis in non-small cell lung cancer patients. Cancer Biomark. 2018;21(4):763-8. https://doi.org/10.3233/CBM-170337.

36. Xiang Z, Sun M, Yuan Z, Zhang C, Jiang J, Huang S, et al. Prognostic and clinicopathological significance of microRNA-494 overexpression in cancers: a meta-analysis. Oncotarget. 2018;9(1):1279–90.

37. Ohdaira H, Sekiguchi M, Miyata K, Yoshida K. MicroRNA-494 suppresses cell proliferation and induces senescence in A549 lung cancer cells. Cell Prolif. 2012;45(1):32–8.

38. Kessler SM, Lederer E, Laggai S, Golob-Schwarzl N, Hosseini K, Petzold J, et al. IMP2/IGF2BP2 expression, but not IMP1 and IMP3, predicts poor outcome in patients and high tumor growth rate in xenograft models of gallbladder cancer. Oncotarget. 2017;8(52):89736–45.

39. Jiang T, Li M, Li Q, Guo Z, Sun X, Zhang X, et al. MicroRNA-98-5p inhibits cell proliferation and induces cell apoptosis in hepatocellular carcinoma via targeting IGF2BP1. Oncol Res. 2017;25(7):1117–27.

40. Xu Y, Zheng Y, Liu H, Li T. Modulation of IGF2BP1 by long non-coding RNA HCG11 suppresses apoptosis of hepatocellular carcinoma cells via MAPK signaling transduction. Int J Oncol. 2017;51(3):791–800.

41. Gutschner T, Hammerle M, Pazaitis N, Bley N, Fiskin E, Uckelmann H, et al. Insulin-like growth factor 2 mRNA-binding protein 1 (IGF2BP1) is an important protumorigenic factor in hepatocellular carcinoma. Hepatology. 2014;59(5):1900–11.

42. Zhou X, Zhang CZ, Lu SX, Chen GG, Li LZ, Liu LL, et al. miR-625 suppresses tumour migration and invasion by targeting IGF2BP1 in hepatocellular carcinoma. Oncogene. 2015;34(8):965–77.

43. Zhang J, Cheng J, Zeng Z, Wang Y, Li X, Xie Q, et al. Comprehensive profiling of novel microRNA-9 targets and a tumor suppressor role of microRNA-9 via targeting IGF2BP1 in hepatocellular carcinoma. Oncotarget. 2015;6(39):42040–52.

44. Wang RJ, Li JW, Bao BH, Wu HC, Du ZH, Su JL, et al. MicroRNA-873

(miRNA-873) inhibits glioblastoma tumorigenesis and metastasis by suppressing the expression of IGF2BP1. J Biol Chem. 2015;290(14) :8938–48.

45. Huang JL, Zheng L, Hu YW, Wang Q. Characteristics of long non-coding RNA and its relation to hepatocellular carcinoma. Carcinogenesis. 2014;35(3): 507–14.

46. Yang X, Xie X, Xiao YF, Xie R, Hu CJ, Tang B, et al. The emergence of long non-coding RNAs in the tumorigenesis of hepatocellular carcinoma. Cancer Lett. 2015;360(2):119–24.

47. He Y, Meng XM, Huang C, Wu BM, Zhang L, Lv XW, et al. Long noncoding RNAs: novel insights into hepatocelluar carcinoma. Cancer Lett. 2014;344(1):20–7.

48. Zhang Y, Zhang P, Wan X, Su X, Kong Z, Zhai Q, et al. Downregulation of long non-coding RNA HCG11 predicts a poor prognosis in prostate cancer. Biomed Pharmacother. 2016;83:936–41.

49. Liu H, Li J, Koirala P, Ding X, Chen B, Wang Y, et al. Long non-coding RNAs as prognostic markers in human breast cancer. Oncotarget. 2016;7(15): 20584–96.

50. Gu Y, Chen T, Li G, Yu X, Lu Y, Wang H, et al. LncRNAs: emerging biomarkers in gastric cancer. Future Oncol. 2015;11(17):2427–41.

51. Hammerle M, Gutschner T, Uckelmann H, Ozgur S, Fiskin E, Gross M, et al. Posttranscriptional destabilization of the liver-specific long noncoding RNA HULC by the IGF2 mRNA-binding protein 1 (IGF2BP1). Hepatol. 2013;58(5): 1703–12.

52. Fawzy IO, Hamza MT, Hosny KA, Esmat G, El Tayebi HM, Abdelaziz AI. miR-1275: a single microRNA that targets the three IGF2-mRNA-binding proteins hindering tumor growth in hepatocellular carcinoma. FEBS Lett. 2015; 589(17):2257–65.

53. Rebucci M, Sermeus A, Leonard E, Delaive E, Dieu M, Fransolet M, et al. miRNA-196b inhibits cell proliferation and induces apoptosis in HepG2 cells by targeting IGF2BP1. Mol Cancer. 2015;14:79.

54. Gu W, Pan F, Singer RH. Blocking beta-catenin binding to the ZBP1 promoter represses ZBP1 expression, leading to increased proliferation and migration of metastatic breast-cancer cells. J Cell Sci. 2009;122(Pt 11):1895–905.

55. Lapidus K, Wyckoff J, Mouneimne G, Lorenz M, Soon L, Condeelis JS, et al. ZBP1 enhances cell polarity and reduces chemotaxis. J Cell Sci. 2007;120(Pt 18):3173–8.

56. Wang W, Goswami S, Lapidus K, Wells AL, Wyckoff JB, Sahai E, et al. Identification and testing of a gene expression signature of invasive carcinoma cells within primary mammary tumors. Cancer Res. 2004;64(23): 8585–94.

57. Gu W, Katz Z, Wu B, Park HY, Li D, Lin S, et al. Regulation of local expression of cell adhesion and motility-related mRNAs in breast cancer cells by IMP1/ ZBP1. J Cell Sci. 2012;125(Pt 1):81–91.

58. Wang W, Wyckoff JB, Frohlich VC, Oleynikov Y, Huttelmaier S, Zavadil J, et al. Single cell behavior in metastatic primary mammary tumors correlated with gene expression patterns revealed by molecular profiling. Cancer Res. 2002; 62(21):6278–88.

59. Wang P, Zhang L, Zhang J, Xu G. MicroRNA-124-3p inhibits cell growth and metastasis in cervical cancer by targeting IGF2BP1. Exp Ther Med. 2018; 15(2):1385–93.

60. Su Y, Xiong J, Hu J, Wei X, Zhang X, Rao L. MicroRNA-140-5p targets insulin like growth factor 2 mRNA binding protein 1 (IGF2BP1) to suppress cervical cancer growth and metastasis. Oncotarget. 2016;7(42):68397–411.

61. Kobel M, Weidensdorfer D, Reinke C, Lederer M, Schmitt WD, Zeng K, et al. Expression of the RNA-binding protein IMP1 correlates with poor prognosis in ovarian carcinoma. Oncogene. 2007;26(54):7584–9.

62. Miyake T, Pradeep S, Wu SY, Rupaimoole R, Zand B, Wen Y, et al. XPO1/CRM1 inhibition causes antitumor effects by mitochondrial accumulation of eIF5A. Clin Cancer Res. 2015;21(14):3286–97.

63. Xu D, Grishin NV, Chook YM. NESdb: a database of NES-containing CRM1 cargoes. Mol Biol Cell. 2012;23(18):3673–6.

64. van Jaarsveld MT, Helleman J, Berns EM, Wiemer EA. MicroRNAs in ovarian cancer biology and therapy resistance. Int J Biochem Cell Biol. 2010;42(8):1282–90.

65. Busch B, Bley N, Muller S, Glass M, Misiak D, Lederer M, et al. The oncogenic triangle of HMGA2, LIN28B and IGF2BP1 antagonizes tumor-suppressive actions of the let-7 family. Nucleic Acids Res. 2016;44(8): 3845–64.

66. Qin X, Sun L, Wang J. Restoration of microRNA-708 sensitizes ovarian cancer cells to cisplatin via IGF2BP1/Akt pathway. Cell Biol Int. 2017;41(10):1110–8.

67. Mongroo PS, Noubissi FK, Cuatrecasas M, Kalabis J, King CE, Johnstone CN, et al. IMP-1 displays cross-talk with K-Ras and modulates colon cancer cell survival through the novel proapoptotic protein CYFIP2. Cancer Res. 2011; 71(6):2172–82.

68. Friday BB, Adjei AA. K-ras as a target for cancer therapy. Biochim Biophys Acta. 2005;1756(2):127–44.

69. Jackson RS 2nd, Cho YJ, Stein S, Liang P. CYFIP2, a direct p53 target, is leptomycin-B sensitive. Cell Cycle. 2007;6(1):95–103.

70. Hamilton KE, Noubissi FK, Katti PS, Hahn CM, Davey SR, Lundsmith ET, et al. IMP1 promotes tumor growth, dissemination and a tumor-initiating cell phenotype in colorectal cancer cell xenografts. Carcinogenesis. 2013;34(11): 2647–54.

71. Goke M, Kanai M, Podolsky DK. Intestinal fibroblasts regulate intestinal epithelial cell proliferation via hepatocyte growth factor. Am J Phys. 1998; 274(5 Pt 1):G809–18.

72. Rasola A, Fassetta M, De Bacco F, D'Alessandro L, Gramaglia D, Di Renzo MF, et al. A positive feedback loop between hepatocyte growth factor receptor and beta-catenin sustains colorectal cancer cell invasive growth. Oncogene. 2007;26(7):1078–87.

73. Luraghi P, Reato G, Cipriano E, Sassi F, Orzan F, Bigatto V, et al. MET signaling in colon cancer stem-like cells blunts the therapeutic response to EGFR inhibitors. Cancer Res. 2014;74(6):1857–69.

74. Takahashi N, Yamada Y, Furuta K, Honma Y, Iwasa S, Takashima A, et al. Serum levels of hepatocyte growth factor and epiregulin are associated with the prognosis on anti-EGFR antibody treatment in KRAS wild-type metastatic colorectal cancer. Br J Cancer. 2014;110(11):2716–27.

75. Yang F, Xue X, Zheng L, Bi J, Zhou Y, Zhi K, et al. Long non-coding RNA GHET1 promotes gastric carcinoma cell proliferation by increasing c-Myc mRNA stability. FEBS J. 2014;281(3):802–13.

76. Qu Y, Pan S, Kang M, Dong R, Zhao J. MicroRNA-150 functions as a tumor suppressor in osteosarcoma by targeting IGF2BP1. Tumour Biol. 2016;37(4): 5275–84.

77. Silke J, Meier P. Inhibitor of apoptosis (IAP) proteins-modulators of cell death and inflammation. Cold Spring Harb Perspect Biol. 2013;5(2) https:// doi.org/10.1101/cshperspect.a008730.

78. Faye MD, Beug ST, Graber TE, Earl N, Xiang X, Wild B, et al. IGF2BP1 controls cell death and drug resistance in rhabdomyosarcomas by regulating translation of cIAP1. Oncogene. 2015;34(12):1532–41.

79. Ioannidis P, Kottaridi C, Dimitriadis E, Courtis N, Mahaira L, Talieri M, et al. Expression of the RNA-binding protein CRD-BP in brain and non-small cell lung tumors. Cancer Lett. 2004;209(2):245–50.

80. Bell JL, Turlapati R, Liu T, Schulte JH, Huttelmaier S. IGF2BP1 harbors prognostic significance by gene gain and diverse expression in neuroblastoma. J Clin Oncol. 2015;33(11):1285–93.

81. Kishida Y, Natsume A, Kondo Y, Takeuchi I, An B, Okamoto Y, et al. Epigenetic subclassification of meningiomas based on genome-wide DNA methylation analyses. Carcinogenesis. 2012;33(2):436–41.

82. Vengoechea J, Sloan AE, Chen Y, Guan X, Ostrom QT, Kerstetter A, et al. Methylation markers of malignant potential in meningiomas. J Neurosurg. 2013;119(4):899–906.

83. Luo Y, Sun R, Zhang J, Sun T, Liu X, Yang B. miR-506 inhibits the proliferation and invasion by targeting IGF2BP1 in glioblastoma. Am J Transl Res. 2015;7(10):2007–14.

84. Vikesaa J, Hansen TV, Jonson L, Borup R, Wewer UM, Christiansen J, et al. RNA-binding IMPs promote cell adhesion and invadopodia formation. EMBO J. 2006;25(7):1456–68.

85. Fraser MM, Zhu X, Kwon CH, Uhlmann EJ, Gutmann DH, Baker SJ. Pten loss causes hypertrophy and increased proliferation of astrocytes in vivo. Cancer Res. 2004;64(21):7773–9.

86. Yue Q, Groszer M, Gil JS, Berk AJ, Messing A, Wu H, et al. PTEN deletion in Bergmann glia leads to premature differentiation and affects laminar organization. Development. 2005;132(14):3281–91.

87. Fortis SP, Anastasopoulou EA, Voutsas IF, Baxevanis CN, Perez SA, Mahaira LG. Potential prognostic molecular signatures in a preclinical model of melanoma. Anticancer Res. 2017;37(1):143–8.

88. Kim T, Havighurst T, Kim K, Albertini M, Xu YG, Spiegelman VS. Targeting insulin-like growth factor 2 mRNA-binding protein 1 (IGF2BP1) in metastatic melanoma to increase efficacy of BRAF(V600E) inhibitors. Mol Carcinog. 2018; https://doi.org/10.1002/mc.22786

89. Elcheva I, Tarapore RS, Bhatia N, Spiegelman VS. Overexpression of mRNA-binding protein CRD-BP in malignant melanomas. Oncogene. 2008;27(37): 5069–74.

90. Zhou J, Ng SB, Chng WJ. LIN28/LIN28B: an emerging oncogenic driver in cancer stem cells. Int J Biochem Cell Biol. 2013;45(5):973–8.

91. Su JL, Chen PS, Johansson G, Kuo ML. Function and regulation of let-7 family microRNAs. Microrna. 2012;1(1):34–9.

92. Alam M, Ahmad R, Rajabi H, Kufe D. MUC1-C induces the LIN28B–>LET-7– >HMGA2 axis to regulate self-renewal in NSCLC. Mol Cancer Res. 2015;13(3): 449–60.

93. Ali Hosseini Rad SM, Bavarsad MS, Arefian E, Jaseb K, Shahjahani M, Saki N. The role of microRNAs in stemness of cancer stem cells. Oncol Rev. 2013; 7(1):e8.

94. Viswanathan SR, Powers JT, Einhorn W, Hoshida Y, Ng TL, Toffanin S, et al. Lin28 promotes transformation and is associated with advanced human malignancies. Nat Genet. 2009;41(7):843–8.

95. Viswanathan SR, Daley GQ. Lin28: a microRNA regulator with a macro role. Cell. 2010;140(4):445–9.

96. Yang X, Lin X, Zhong X, Kaur S, Li N, Liang S, et al. Double-negative feedback loop between reprogramming factor LIN28 and microRNA let-7 regulates aldehyde dehydrogenase 1-positive cancer stem cells. Cancer Res. 2010;70(22):9463–72.

97. Liao B, Patel M, Hu Y, Charles S, Herrick DJ, Brewer G. Targeted knockdown of the RNA-binding protein CRD-BP promotes cell proliferation via an insulin-like growth factor II-dependent pathway in human K562 leukemia cells. J Biol Chem. 2004;279(47):48716–24.

98. Stoskus M, Vaitkeviciene G, Eidukaite A, Griskevicius L. ETV6/RUNX1 transcript is a target of RNA-binding protein IGF2BP1 in t(12;21) (p13;q22)-positive acute lymphoblastic leukemia. Blood Cells Mol Dis. 2016;57:30–4.

99. Danda R, Ganapathy K, Sathe G, Madugundu AK, Ramachandran S, Krishnan UM, et al. Proteomic profiling of retinoblastoma by high resolution mass spectrometry. Clin Proteomics. 2016;13:29.

100. Hsieh YT, Chou MM, Chen HC, Tseng JJ. IMP1 promotes choriocarcinoma cell migration and invasion through the novel effectors RSK2 and PPME1. Gynecol Oncol. 2013;131(1):182–90.

101. Stohr N, Kohn M, Lederer M, Glass M, Reinke C, Singer RH, et al. IGF2BP1 promotes cell migration by regulating MK5 and PTEN signaling. Genes Dev. 2012;26(2):176–89.

102. Stohr N, Huttelmaier S. IGF2BP1: a post-transcriptional "driver" of tumor cell migration. Cell Adh Migr. 2012;6(4):312–8.

103. Gu W, Wells AL, Pan F, Singer RH. Feedback regulation between zipcode binding protein 1 and beta-catenin mRNAs in breast cancer cells. Mol Cell Biol. 2008;28(16):4963–74.

104. Mahapatra L, Andruska N, Mao C, Le J, Shapiro DJ. A novel IMP1 inhibitor, BTYNB, targets c-Myc and inhibits melanoma and ovarian cancer cell proliferation. Transl Oncol. 2017;10(5):818–27.

15

Cyclin D1-CDK4 activity drives sensitivity to bortezomib in mantle cell lymphoma by blocking autophagy-mediated proteolysis of NOXA

Simon Heine[1,6]* (iD), Markus Kleih[1,6], Neus Giménez[2], Kathrin Böpple[1,6], German Ott[3], Dolors Colomer[2], Walter E. Aulitzky[4], Heiko van der Kuip[1,6]^ and Elisabeth Silkenstedt[1,4,5,6]

Abstract

Background: Mantle cell lymphoma (MCL) is an aggressive B-non-Hodgkin lymphoma with generally poor outcome. MCL is characterized by an aberrantly high cyclin D1-driven CDK4 activity. New molecular targeted therapies such as inhibitors of the ubiquitin-proteasome system (UPS) have shown promising results in preclinical studies and MCL patients. Our previous research revealed stabilization of the short-lived pro-apoptotic NOXA as a critical determinant for sensitivity to these inhibitors. It is currently unclear how cyclin D1 overexpression and aberrant CDK4 activity affect NOXA stabilization and treatment efficacy of UPS inhibitors in MCL.

Methods: The effect of cyclin D1-driven CDK4 activity on response of MCL cell lines and primary cells to proteasome inhibitor treatment was investigated using survival assays (Flow cytometry, AnnexinV/PI) and Western blot analysis of NOXA protein. Half-life of NOXA protein was determined by cycloheximide treatment and subsequent Western blot analysis. The role of autophagy was analyzed by LC3-II protein expression and autophagolysosome detection. Furthermore, silencing of autophagy-related genes was performed using siRNA and MCL cells were treated with autophagy inhibitors in combination with proteasome and CDK4 inhibition.

Results: In this study, we show that proteasome inhibitor-mediated cell death in MCL depends on cyclin D1-driven CDK4 activity. Inhibition of cyclin D1/CDK4 activity significantly reduced proteasome inhibitor-mediated stabilization of NOXA protein, mainly driven by an autophagy-mediated proteolysis. Bortezomib-induced cell death was significantly potentiated by compounds that interfere with autophagosomal function. Combined treatment with bortezomib and autophagy inhibitors enhanced NOXA stability leading to super-induction of NOXA protein. In addition to established autophagy modulators, we identified the fatty acid synthase inhibitor orlistat to be an efficient autophagy inhibitor when used in combination with bortezomib. Accordingly, this combination synergistically induced apoptosis both in MCL cell lines and in patient samples.

Conclusion: Our data demonstrate that CDK4 activity in MCL is critical for NOXA stabilization upon treatment with UPS inhibitors allowing preferential induction of cell death in cyclin D transformed cells. Under UPS blocked conditions, autophagy appears as the critical regulator of NOXA induction. Therefore, inhibitors of autophagy are promising candidates to increase the activity of proteasome inhibitors in MCL.

Keywords: Mantle cell lymphoma, Bortezomib, NOXA, CDK4, Autophagy

* Correspondence: simon.heine@ikp-stuttgart.de
^Deceased
[1]Dr. Margarete Fischer-Bosch-Institute of Clinical Pharmacology, Stuttgart, Germany
[6]University of Tübingen, Tübingen, Germany
Full list of author information is available at the end of the article

Background

Mantle cell lymphoma (MCL) is a rare B cell neoplasia often characterized by an aggressive clinical course, relatively short response to conventional chemotherapy and frequent relapses [1]. The initial molecular pathogenic event of this malignancy is the t(11;14)(q13;q32) translocation leading to juxtaposition of the *CCND1* gene (coding for cyclin D1) to the immunoglobulin heavy chain complex (IgH) gene [2]. Normally, the G1 phase regulator cyclin D1 is not expressed at high levels in normal B cells but gets overexpressed as a result of this translocation [3]. As a binding partner and activator of the cyclin-dependent kinases CDK4 and CDK6, cyclin D1 plays a crucial role in G1-S transition and promotes proliferation by phosphorylating RB1 and preventing its inhibitory interaction with the E2Fs [4]. As CDK6 is hardly expressed in MCL cells, cyclin D1 mainly exerts its functions via CDK4 [5]. In addition to its role in cell cycle progression, cyclin D1 affects different cellular processes via both CDK4-dependent and CDK4-independent mechanisms [6]. Cyclin D1/CDK4 activity has also been shown to suppress the autophagic degradation machinery [7–11].

The proteasome inhibitor bortezomib which was approved for treatment of relapsed or refractory MCL was recently included in the first-line treatment of MCL [12, 13]. As there are still many patients who are poorly responding to bortezomib treatment, there is urgent need to elucidate the basis for bortezomib sensitivity and resistance [12]. Different resistance mechanisms to bortezomib have been proposed including accumulation of Bcl-2 protein in lymphoma cells, mutation as well as overexpression of proteasomal subunits in THP1 cells and plasmacytic differentiation, elevated nuclear factor-κB activity, or increased autophagy in MCL cells [14–18]. Combination of bortezomib with substances that target the DNA methyltransferase, histone acetylation, prosurvival chaperones, PI3K/AKT signaling, or the anti-apoptotic protein MCL1 have been shown to enhance the efficacy of bortezomib in MCL [19–23]. Work from our group revealed that extensive proteasomal degradation of the pro-apoptotic Bcl-2 family protein NOXA and corresponding low protein levels is crucial for sensitivity of MCL to the proteasome inhibitor bortezomib [24].

The aim of the present work is to investigate how cyclin D1 overexpression and aberrant CDK4 activity affect treatment efficacy of bortezomib in MCL. Furthermore, we seek to elucidate underlying molecular mechanisms and identify novel combinations to enhance bortezomib treatment in MCL.

Methods

Cell culture

The MCL cell lines Mino, Jeko-1, Rec-1, Jvm2, and Granta-519 were obtained from the German Collection of Microorganisms and Cell Cultures GmbH (Germany). NIH3T3 cells stably transfected with human CD40 ligand were a kind gift from Dr. Martina Seiffert from the German Cancer Research Center, DKFZ (Germany). All cell lines were tested for mycoplasma contamination and recently authenticated by short tandem repeat profiling. Cell lines as well as the primary MCL cells were cultivated in RPMI-1640 (Biochrom, Germany) supplemented with 20% fetal calf serum, 0.1 g/l penicillin-streptomycin (Gibco, Germany), and 2 mM L-glutamine (Biochrom, Germany).

Reagents

Cycloheximide, 3-methyladenine, hydroxychloroquine, Spautin-1, orlistat, BEZ235, Cerulenin, and hydrogen peroxide were purchased from Sigma-Aldrich Chemie GmbH (Germany). Liensinine was obtained from ChemFaces (China) and bortezomib, carfilzomib, and palbociclib from Selleck Chemicals (USA).

Protein expression analysis

Cells were lysed, sonicated, and boiled to obtain cellular proteins according to standard protocols. Western blots were performed using a SDS-PAGE Gel Electrophoresis system. Proteins were blotted on Amersham Protran 0.1 NC nitrocellulose membranes, except for LC3 which was blotted on Amersham Hybond P 0.2 PVDF membranes (GE Healthcare, USA). The primary antibodies used were anti-NOXA antibody (Calbiochem, USA), anti-cyclin D1 antibody (Santa Cruz Biotechnology, USA), anti-MCL1, RB1, β-actin, α-tubulin, ATG5, ATG7, LC3, CDK4, PUMA, BAX, BAK, and GAPDH (Cell Signaling, USA).

Autophagolysosome detection

After treatment, samples containing 5×10^5 to 1×10^6 cells were stained with Cyto-ID Green Detection Reagent (Enzo Life Sciences, USA) according to manufacturer's instructions for 30 min at 37 °C in the dark. Afterwards, cells were stained with AnnexinV-APC (BD Pharmingen, Germany) and subsequently analyzed by flow cytometry. The Cyto-ID fluorescence intensity of AnnexinV-APC negative cells was detected and compared by histogram overlays for the different treatments.

mRNA expression analysis

RNA was extracted using RNeasy Mini Kit (QIAGEN N.V., Netherlands) and transcribed to cDNA according to standard protocols. *NOXA* (*PMAIP1*) expression was analyzed using TaqMan Gene Expression Assay Hs00560402_m1 (Applied Biosystems, USA) on 7900 HT Fast Real-Time PCR System (Applied Biosystems) according to the manufacturer's instructions. TBP (Hs00427620_m1) was used for normalization of *NOXA* mRNA expression.

Gene silencing

For gene silencing, we used siGENOME siRNA Reagents - Human SMARTpool siRNA (Dharmacon, UK). Sequences targeted by the siRNAs are shown in Additional file 1: Table S1. As control, siRNA (cosi) non-targeting siRNA#1 (Dharmacon, UK) was used. For electroporation, the Nucleofector™ II/2B, the Cell Line Nucleofector® Kit V, and the program X-001 (Lonza Group Ltd., Basel, Switzerland) were used. Knockdown efficacy was analyzed by Western blot.

Cell death detection

Cell death was assessed by staining the cells with AnnexinV-FITC (BD Pharmingen, Heidelberg, Germany) and propidium iodide (PI) (Sigma-Aldrich, Steinheim, Germany) and subsequent analysis by flow cytometry. Combination index (CI) values were determined with the CalcuSyn Software (Biosoft, UK), whose algorithm is based on the Chou and Talalay's method [25]. A combination index smaller than 0.9 indicates a synergistic effect between two substances.

Measurement of cell cycle distribution

Analysis of cell cycle distribution was carried out using BrdU staining as previously described [26].

Determination of protein half-life

The half-life of NOXA protein was determined by treating the cells with 20 µg/ml cycloheximide and harvesting cell pellets at different time points for subsequent analysis by Western blot.

Statistics

Data are obtained from at least three independent experiments and expressed as standard deviation (SD) of the mean. Statistics were calculated using GraphPadPrism 4.0 software (GraphPad Software, La Jolla, CA, USA). Changes in paired samples were analyzed using two-sided paired t test, and results were considered statistically significant when $p < 0.05$ (*$p < 0.05$; **$p < 0.01$; ***$p < 0.001$).

Results

Cyclin D1-driven CDK4 activity is required for cell death and induction of NOXA protein upon proteasome inhibitor treatment

Sensitivity of MCL cells to inhibitors of the ubiquitin-proteasome pathway (UPS), such as bortezomib, has been associated with the BH3 only protein NOXA [24, 27, 28]. A recently published preclinical study also demonstrated a link between cyclin D1 expression and bortezomib sensitivity in multiple myeloma cell lines [29]. However, it is not well established if bortezomib sensitivity is dependent on the kinase activity of the cyclin D1/CDK4 complex and if NOXA is affected by this activity in MCL cells. To address this issue, we first incubated MCL cell lines Mino, Jeko-1, and Granta-519 with or without palbociclib, a potent and selective CDK4/6 inhibitor and co-treated the cell lines with bortezomib. In all three MCL cell lines investigated, co-treatment with palbociclib partially rescued cells from bortezomib-induced cell death (Fig. 1a, left). Co-treatment of bortezomib with palbociclib led to a reduced induction of NOXA protein in the MCL cell lines and in patient-derived primary MCL cells (Fig. 1a, right). Importantly, palbociclib treatment inhibited CDK4-dependent phosphorylation of RB1 in Mino, Jeko-1, and Granta-519 (Additional file 2: Figure S1). In order to prevent excessive cell death caused by the extended cultivation duration during the co-treatment schedule, we co-cultivated the primary MCL cells with CD40 ligand-expressing fibroblasts and different cytokines. This resulted in an acquired therapy resistance of the primary MCL cells which did not exhibit cell death after bortezomib treatment with or without palbociclib co-treatment (data not shown). The development of therapy resistance mechanisms after co-culturing primary MCL cells is known and involves the activation of survival pathways and the increased expression of anti-apoptotic Bcl-2 family proteins [30, 31]. In order to analyze if the antagonism on the bortezomib effect after palbociclib treatment was dependent on inhibition of cyclin D1-driven CDK4 activity, we performed siRNA-mediated knockdown of either cyclin D1 or CDK4. We observed a comparable reduction in bortezomib sensitivity in MCL cell lines Mino and Jeko-1 after knockdown of cyclin D1 or CDK4 (Fig. 1b, left and Additional file 3: Figure S2). In addition, NOXA induction after bortezomib treatment was also antagonized by knockdown of cyclin D1 or CDK4 (Fig. 1b, right). Double knockdown of cyclin D1 and CDK4 did not increase the antagonism on bortezomib-induced cell death (Additional file 4: Figure S3), indicating that in this context, both of these proteins exert their function through the same pathways.

Collectively, these data demonstrate that cyclin D1/CDK4 activity is required for effective accumulation of NOXA protein and thus also for complete execution of bortezomib-induced cell death in MCL.

We next asked if inhibition of CDK4 activity might also reduce sensitivity to other clinically relevant proteasome inhibitors such as carfilzomib. In contrast to bortezomib, which not only reversibly blocks the chymotrypsin- and caspase-like activity of the proteasome but also binds different serine proteases, carfilzomib is more specific and irreversibly binds the N-terminal threonine active sites of the proteasome [32, 33]. As shown in Fig. 1c, the effect of palbociclib on carfilzomib-induced cell death and NOXA accumulation in MCL cell line Mino was identical to that observed with bortezomib. Importantly, this could also be shown for other compounds which have been identified to

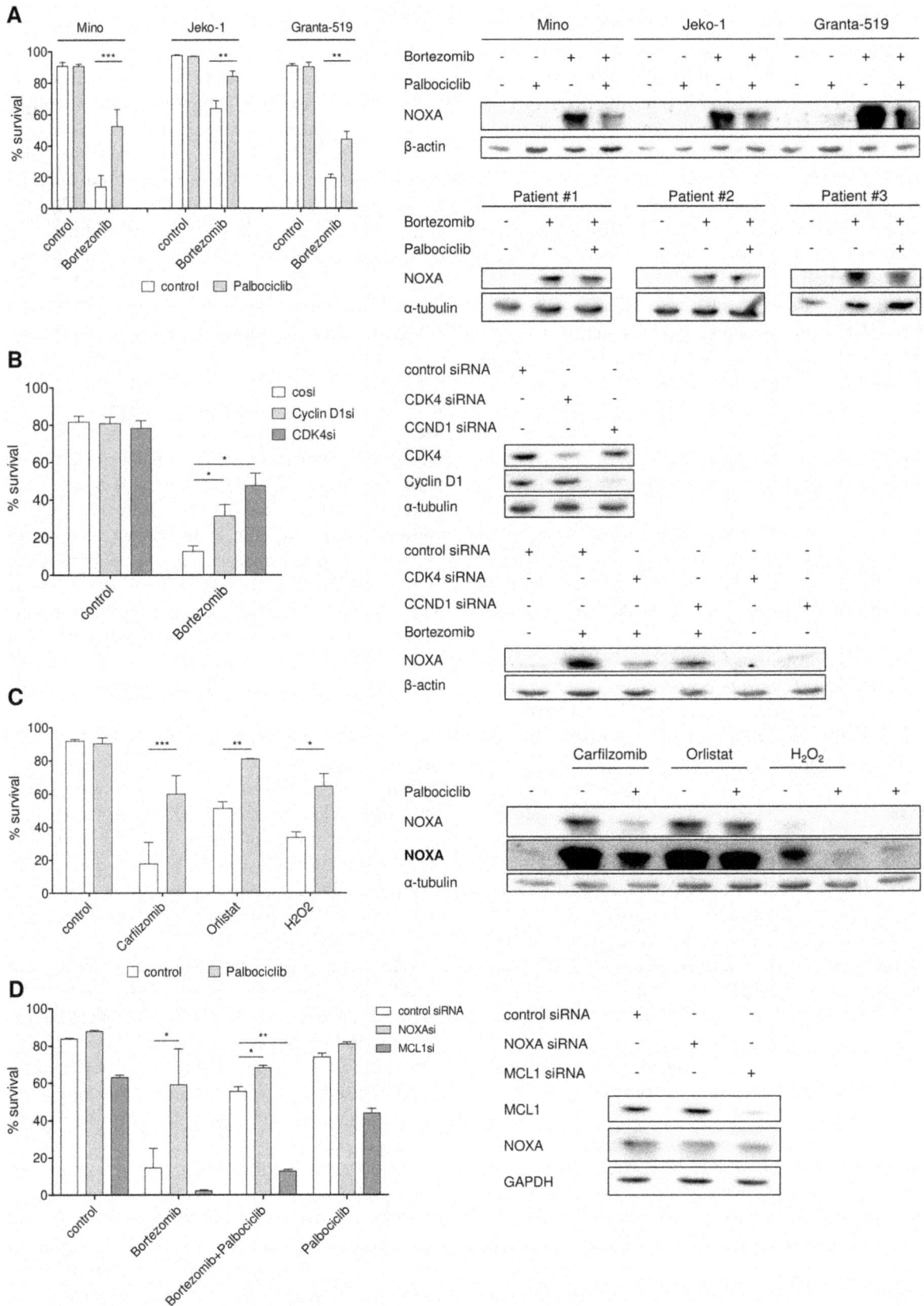

Fig. 1 (See legend on next page.)

be effective in MCL cells via upregulation of NOXA, such as the fatty acid synthase inhibitor orlistat (Fig. 1c; [24]) as well as for hydrogen peroxide (Fig. 1c; [34]). Similar results were also observed in the MCL cell line Jeko-1 (Additional file 5: Figure S4). In order to confirm that the inability to induce cell death after co-treatment of bortezomib with palbociclib is dependent on NOXA, we performed knockdowns of NOXA and its anti-apoptotic binding partner MCL1. NOXA knockdown rescued bortezomib-induced cell death (Fig. 1d). Furthermore, knockdown of MCL1 reversed the palbociclib-mediated antagonism on bortezomib-induced cell death, whereas NOXA knockdown further increased the antagonism on cell death induction (Fig. 1d).

Together, these observations indicate that cyclin D1-driven CDK4 activity is required for effective upregulation of NOXA and concomitant induction of cell death not only upon treatment with proteasome inhibitors but also other NOXA protein inducing agents.

Inhibition of CDK4 activity antagonizes proteasome inhibitor-mediated stabilization of NOXA by autophagy-driven proteolysis

Previous studies have shown that inhibition of the proteasome leads to induction of *NOXA* transcript [28, 35]. However, the predominant mechanism by which NOXA protein is enhanced seems to be protein stabilization by targeting the rapid NOXA protein turnover both in MCL and in melanoma cells [24, 36]. To uncover the mechanism by which CDK4 inhibition diminishes NOXA protein in bortezomib-treated cells, we first quantified *NOXA* RNA levels. We found only minor differences of *NOXA* transcript induction upon bortezomib in cells pre-incubated with or without palbociclib, indicating that transcriptional regulation of *NOXA* upon bortezomib is not the predominant effect of CDK4 inhibition on *NOXA* regulation (Additional file 6: Figure S5). Palbociclib

antagonism on bortezomib-induced cell death might also be mediated by alterations in cell cycle distribution. We therefore performed a knockdown of RB1 to allow cells to progress to s-phase while CDK4 is inhibited. Even though cells progressed to s-phase (Additional file 7: Figure S6, left panel), palbociclib antagonized bortezomib-induced cell death in RB1 knockdown cells in the same extent as cells transfected with control siRNA (Additional file 7: Figure S6, middle panel). Furthermore, bortezomib treatment led to a similar decrease of s-phase cells as palbociclib treatment (Additional file 7: Figure S6, left panel). Consequently, we conclude that it is unlikely that cell cycle distribution does mediate palbociclib effects on bortezomib-induced cell death.

We therefore studied NOXA protein stability using cycloheximide pulse-chase experiments. In accordance with previous studies [24, 37], bortezomib significantly prolonged NOXA half-life in MCL cell line Mino (Fig. 2a), whereas palbociclib alone had no effect on NOXA protein stability. Interestingly, the stabilizing effect of bortezomib was almost completely antagonized when co-treated with palbociclib indicating that CDK4 inhibition activates a proteasome-independent degradation of NOXA.

Several groups have shown that CDK4 activity [7–11] can suppress autophagy, which represents another central degradation mechanism delivering cytosolic proteins, aggregates, or organelles to lysosomes [38]. In line with this, we observed an increase of the autophagy marker LC3-II in MCL cell line Mino upon co-treatment of bortezomib with palbociclib or after treatment with palbociclib alone (Fig. 2b, upper panel). LC3-II protein levels can be elevated either because the completion of autophagy is impaired which leads to an accumulation of autophagosomes or because there is an actual increase of the autophagic flux [39]. To differentiate this, we treated the MCL cell line Mino with palbociclib and the downstream autophagy inhibitor hydroxychloroquine which

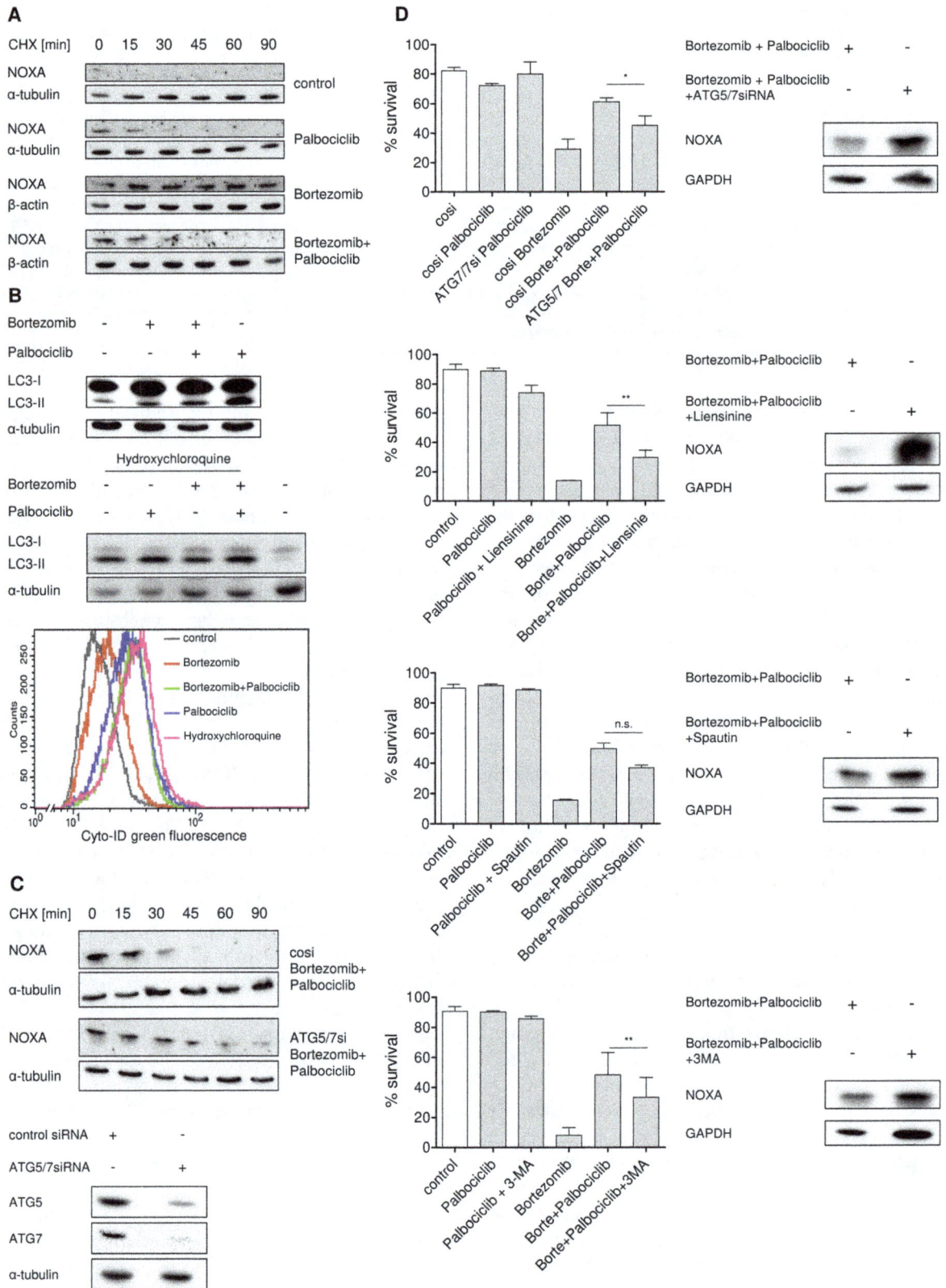

Fig. 2 (See legend on next page.)

(See figure on previous page.)
Fig. 2 Proteasome inhibitor-mediated stabilization of NOXA is abrogated through an autophagy-driven proteolysis. **a** Increased half-life of Noxa protein after bortezomib treatment is diminished after palbociclib co-treatment. MCL cell line Mino was treated with 100 nM palbociclib for 16 h and subsequently co-treated with 8 nM bortezomib. After 8 h co-treatment, 20 µg/ml cycloheximide was added to the cells and samples were harvested 0, 15, 30, 45, 60, and 90 min after cycloheximide exposition for Western blot analysis. **b** Palbociclib treatment induces autophagy. MCL cell line Mino was treated with 100 nM palbociclib for 16 h and subsequently co-treated with 8 nM bortezomib. After 8 h, protein expression was analyzed (upper panel). MCL cell line Mino was treated with 40 µM hydroxychloroquine and 100 nM palbociclib for 16 h and subsequently co-treated with 8 nM bortezomib. After 8 h, protein expression was analyzed (middle panel). MCL cell line Mino was treated with 40 µM hydroxychloroquine for 24 h or treated with 100 nM palbociclib for 16 h and subsequently co-treated with 8 nM bortezomib for 24 h. After treatment, autophagic vesicles were measured by Cyto-ID staining (lower panel). **c** Knockdown of autophagy-related genes reverses the palbociclib-mediated antagonism on bortezomib-mediated stabilization of NOXA. MCL cell line Mino was transfected with siRNA targeting ATG5 and ATG7. Twenty-four hours after transfection, cells were treated with 100 nM palbociclib for 16 h and subsequently co-treated with 8 nM bortezomib. After 8 h, cells were exposed to 20 µg/ml cycloheximide and samples were harvested 0, 15, 30, 45, 60, and 90 min after cycloheximide addition and analyzed by Western blot. **d** Knockdown of autophagy-related genes as well as autophagy inhibitors counteract palbociclib-mediated antagonism on bortezomib-induced cell death and NOXA induction. MCL cell line Mino was transfected with siRNA targeting ATG5 and ATG7. Twenty-four hours after transfection, cells were treated with 100 nM palbociclib for 16 h and subsequently co-treated with 8 nM bortezomib. After 8 h, protein expression was analyzed (upper right) and cell death was assessed by AnnexinV-PI staining 24 h post-treatment (upper left). MCL cell line Mino was treated with 100 nM palbociclib and 20 µM liensinine (upper middle panel), 5 µM Spautin-1 (lower middle panel), or 2 mM 3-MA (lower panel) for 16 h and subsequently co-treated with 8 nM bortezomib. After 8 h, protein expression was analyzed (right) and cell death was assessed by AnnexinV-PI staining 24 h post-treatment (left). Data represent means ± S.D. from three independent experiments

inhibits the acidification of lysosomes, completely blocks autophagy in its final step and therefore leads to the accumulation of autophagosomes [40]. Hydroxychloroquine treatment induced LC3-II protein levels which, importantly, were further increased by co-treatment with palbociclib (Fig. 2b, middle panel). We can thereby conclude that inhibition of CDK4 activity results in increased autophagic flux. In addition, direct staining of autophagic vacuoles with the autophagy Cyto-ID Green dye and subsequent cytometric analysis corroborated our results that we obtained by analyzing LC3-II protein expression. CDK4 inhibition with palbociclib alone or after co-treatment with bortezomib induced an increase in green fluorescence, indicative of elevated levels of autophagic vesicles (Fig. 2b, lower panel). Similar results were observed in MCL cell line Jeko-1, where palbociclib treatment led to an increase in green fluorescence (Additional file 8: Figure S7A). Furthermore, co-treatment of palbociclib with hydroxychloroquine showed higher green fluorescence than hydroxychloroquine alone (Additional file 8: Figure S7A), corroborating our result that CDK4 inhibition results in increased autophagic flux (Fig. 2b, middle panel). Short-term treatment of MCL cell line Mino with Palbociclib, however, did not led to an increase in autophagic vacuoles (Additional file 8: Figure S7B), indicating that it requires more time to activate intermediate signals that induce autophagy.

To test whether the antagonizing effect of palbociclib on bortezomib-induced NOXA stability is mediated by activating an autophagy-lysosome pathway (ALP)-dependent degradation of NOXA, we performed RNAi-mediated knockdowns of autophagy-related proteins (ATG5/7) and investigated NOXA protein stability. Indeed, compared to control siRNA genetic blockade of autophagy by pre-incubation with ATG5/7 siRNA prolonged

NOXA half-life in the MCL cell line Mino co-treated with palbociclib (Fig. 2c), reaching a protein stability comparable to that observed in cells treated with bortezomib alone (Fig. 2a). Importantly, in cells co-treated with palbociclib, genetic or pharmacologic inhibition of autophagy with Spautin-1, liensinine, or 3-methyladenine (3-MA) also restored the effect of bortezomib on cell death induction in MCL cell lines Mino and Jeko-1 (Fig. 2d, left and Additional file 9: Figure S8) and on NOXA induction in MCL cell line Mino (Fig. 2d, right). These results indicate that inhibition of CDK4 antagonizes bortezomib efficacy via an autophagy-mediated degradation of NOXA.

Inhibition of autophagy synergizes with bortezomib-induced cell death and NOXA stabilization in MCL

If NOXA stability is targeted by UPS and ALP-mediated proteolysis, we would expect an enhanced half-life of NOXA upon inhibition of both the proteasome and the autophagy pathway as well as an increase of cell death as compared to proteasome inhibition alone. To address this issue, we used a cell line with reduced sensitivity to proteasome inhibitors, namely Jeko-1 (Fig. 1), and performed cycloheximide pulse-chase experiments. For evaluation of NOXA protein stability, cells were incubated in presence or absence of the UPS inhibitor bortezomib, the autophagy inhibitor 3-MA, and the combination of both. Interestingly, inhibition of autophagy alone had no effect on NOXA protein half-life (Fig. 3a) indicating that ALP has a minor role for NOXA degradation in cells with active UPS. However, compared to inhibition of the proteasome alone, combined inhibition of the ubiquitin-proteasome and the autophagy-lysosome pathways led to a significant

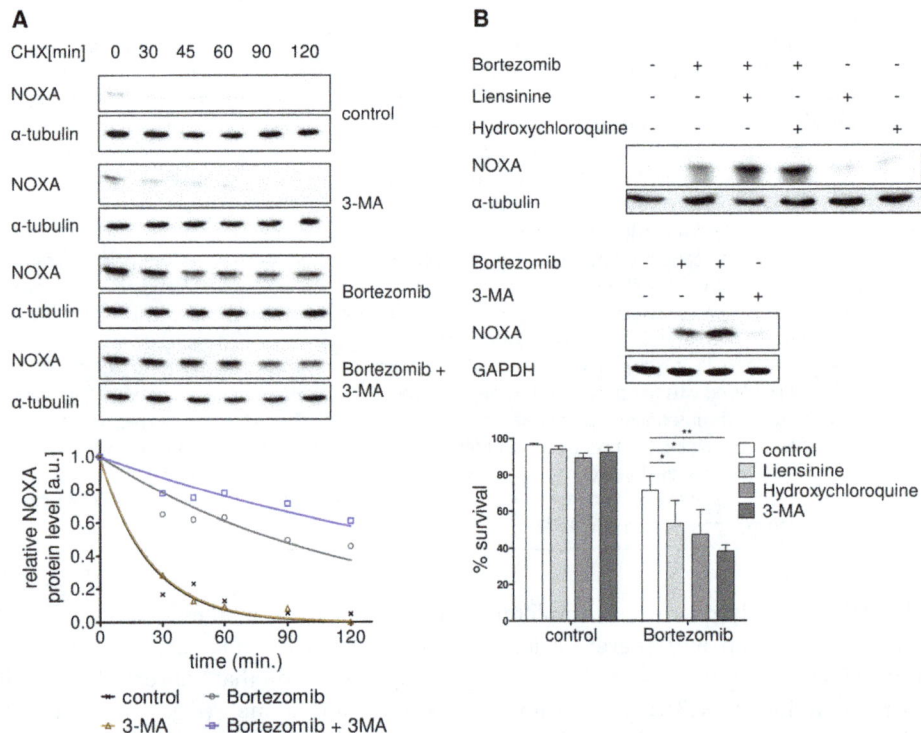

Fig. 3 Autophagy inhibitors potentiate bortezomib-induced cell death through NOXA stabilization. **a** Co-treatment of bortezomib with an autophagy inhibitor potentiates half-life increase of NOXA protein. MCL cell line Jeko-1 was treated with 2 mM 3-MA for 16 h and subsequently co-treated with 7 nM bortezomib. After 14 h, 20 μg/ml cycloheximide was added to the cells and samples were harvested 0, 30, 45, 60, 90, and 120 min after cycloheximide exposition for Western blot analysis (upper panel) and corresponding densitometric analysis of NOXA protein stability (lower panel). **b** Co-treatment of Bortezomib with autophagy inhibitors potentiates cell death induction as well as NOXA protein accumulation. MCL cell line Jeko-1 was treated with 20 μM liensinine, 40 μM hydroxychloroquine, or 2 mM 3-MA for 16 h and subsequently co-treated with 8 nM bortezomib. After 8 h, protein expression was analyzed (upper panel), and after 24 h treatment, cell death was assessed by AnnexinV-PI staining (lower panel). Data represent means ± S.D. from three independent experiments

increase of NOXA stability as shown by Western blot analysis (Fig. 3a, upper panel) and corresponding densitometric quantification (Fig. 3a, lower panel). Importantly, this elevated NOXA accumulation upon combined inhibition of autophagy and proteasome was accompanied by a significantly enhanced cell death as compared to proteasome inhibition alone (Fig. 3b, lower panel). Analogous to the results obtained with 3-MA, combination of bortezomib with the autophagy inhibitors liensinine or hydroxychloroquine also resulted in an elevated NOXA accumulation as well as enhanced cell death compared to proteasome inhibition alone (Fig. 3b). In line with this, autophagy inhibitors also potentiated bortezomib-induced cell death in another bortezomib-resistant cell line, namely Rec-1 (Additional file 10: Figure S9).

Together, these results indicate that bortezomib-mediated accumulation of NOXA is partially hampered by a parallel degradation of NOXA via autophagy. Therefore, combined inhibition of both UPS and autophagy potentiates both stabilization of NOXA protein and induction of cell death in MCL cells.

Orlistat acts synergistically with bortezomib to accumulate NOXA and induce potent cell death in MCL cells

Previous work of our group showed that MCL cells can be efficiently treated using the fatty acid synthase inhibitor (FASNi) orlistat [24, 41]. This cell death relies on the efficient stabilization of NOXA protein. The FASNi orlistat has been shown to block palmitate synthesis [42]. Interestingly, many studies have shown that palmitate levels are linked to ER stress and autophagy regulation [43–45]. Therefore, we investigated if bortezomib effects could be potentiated by orlistat co-treatment in analogy to the observation with autophagy inhibitors (Fig. 3).

Co-treatment of bortezomib with the fatty acid inhibitor orlistat led to a blockade of autophagic degradation in MCL cell line Mino (Fig. 4a), which is characterized by an elevated LC-3 II protein expression and a concomitant accumulation of the P62 protein which is exclusively degraded by autophagy [46]. Consequentially, orlistat prolonged bortezomib-mediated NOXA half-life in bortezomib-resistant cell line Jeko-1 as shown by Western blot analysis (Fig. 4b, upper panel) and corresponding

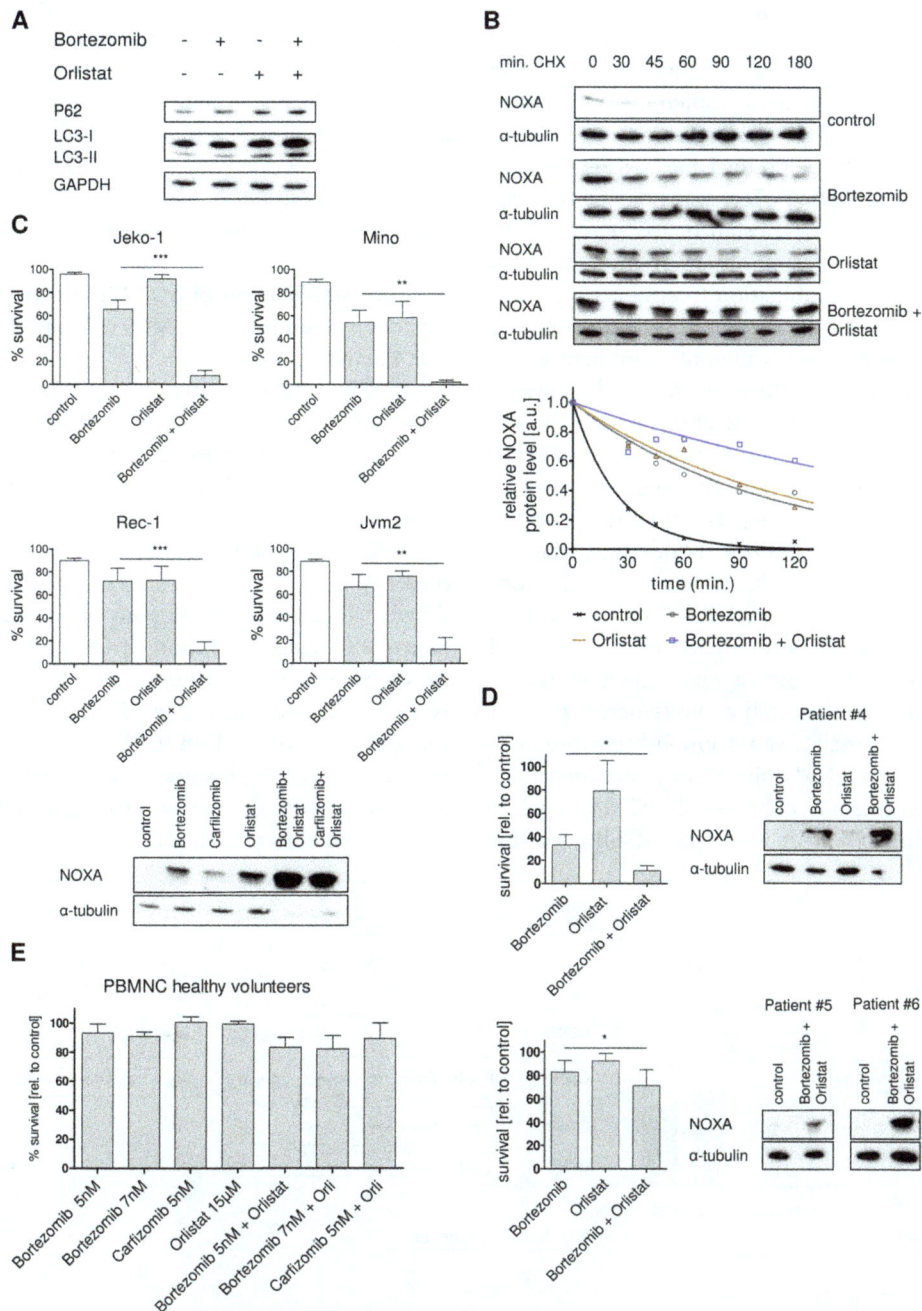

Fig. 4 FASNi modulates autophagy upon proteasome inhibition and leads to synergistic cell death in MCL cells. **a** Co-treatment of bortezomib with the fatty acid synthase inhibitor orlistat blocks autophagy. MCL cell line Mino was treated with 15 μM orlistat and 7 nM bortezomib. After 8 h, samples were harvested for Western blot analysis. **b** Inhibition of proteasome and fatty acid synthase further increases NOXA half-life. MCL cell line Jeko-1 was treated with 15 μM orlistat and 7 nM bortezomib. After 14 h, 20 μg/ml cycloheximide was added to the cells and samples were harvested 0, 30, 45, 60, 90, 120, and 180 min after cycloheximide exposition for Western blot analysis (upper panel) and quantification of NOXA protein stability (lower panel). **c** Co-treatment of bortezomib with orlistat induces cell death in MCL cell lines. MCL cell lines were treated with 15 μM orlistat and 7 nM (Jeko-1 and Rec-1) or 5 nM (Mino and Jvm2) bortezomib. After 14 h, protein expression was analyzed (Jeko-1), and after 24 h, cell death was assessed by AnnexinV-PI staining. **d** Co-treatment of bortezomib with orlistat induces cell death in primary MCL cells. Primary MCL cells were treated with 15 μM orlistat and 7 nM (four patients, upper panel) or 5 nM (six patients, lower panel) bortezomib. After 24 h, samples were taken for Western blot analysis (left) and cell death was assessed by AnnexinV-PI staining (right). **e** Healthy lymphocytes and monocytes are hardly affected by co-treatment of proteasome inhibitors with orlistat. Peripheral blood mononuclear cells were treated with 15 μM orlistat and 5 nM or 7 nM bortezomib. After 24 h, cell death was assessed by AnnexinV-PI staining. Data represent means ± S.D. from three independent experiments

densitometric quantification (Fig. 4b, lower panel). This enhanced protein stability resulted in super-induction of NOXA protein and an almost complete loss of viability in four MCL cell lines characterized by different sensitivity to bortezomib monotherapy (Fig. 4c). The same results were obtained with carfilzomib (Additional file 11: Figure S10) indicating that the potentiating effect was not due to a differential bortezomib uptake or substance cross-interaction.

Changes in expression levels of other apoptotic proteins apart from NOXA after combination treatments were not observed (Additional file 12: Figure S11). Treatment of the MCL cell line Jeko-1 with different combinations of orlistat and bortezomib or carfilzomib resulted in synergistic cell death even at low concentrations of bortezomib and carfilzomib (Additional file 13: Figure S12). Cell death induced by these combinations was dependent on caspase activity and could be blocked by pre-incubation with the pan-caspase inhibitor Z-VAD-FMK (Additional file 11: Figure S10). Importantly, similar effects were also observed in patient-derived primary MCL cells. Combination of orlistat together with bortezomib led to an enhanced NOXA protein expression and significantly potentiated the cytotoxic effect of bortezomib alone (when applied at 7 nM; Fig. 4d upper panel). Even a low bortezomib concentration of 5 nM which had only minor effects in monotherapy led to a significant increase of cell death when combined with orlistat (Fig. 4d, lower panel). Of note, this combinatory treatment had only minor effects on peripheral blood mononuclear cells (PBMNC) from healthy donors (Fig. 4e).

Collectively, these data demonstrate that the combination of bortezomib with a FASNi provides a potent tool to effectively induce MCL cell death via super-induction of NOXA presumably by parallel inhibition of the proteasome as well as the autophagic degradation machinery.

Effective stabilization of NOXA and concomitant induction of apoptosis in MCL cells requires cyclin D1-CDK4 activity

After demonstrating that cyclin D1-CDK4 activity is important for response to bortezomib in MCL cells (Fig. 1), we next asked if this also holds true for the more effective combination of bortezomib with orlistat. Indeed, knockdown of cyclin D1 or CDK4 in MCL cell line Jeko-1 blocked accumulation of NOXA upon combinatory treatment as effective as direct NOXA knockdown (Fig. 5a). Analogous to bortezomib alone, pharmacological inhibition of CDK4 by palbociclib prior to combination treatment was sufficient to abrogate NOXA accumulation (Fig. 5b). Again, consistent with the effects observed in cells treated with bortezomib alone, genetic or pharmacologic blockade of cyclin D1/CDK4 also partially rescued the more effective apoptosis upon co-treatment with orlistat.

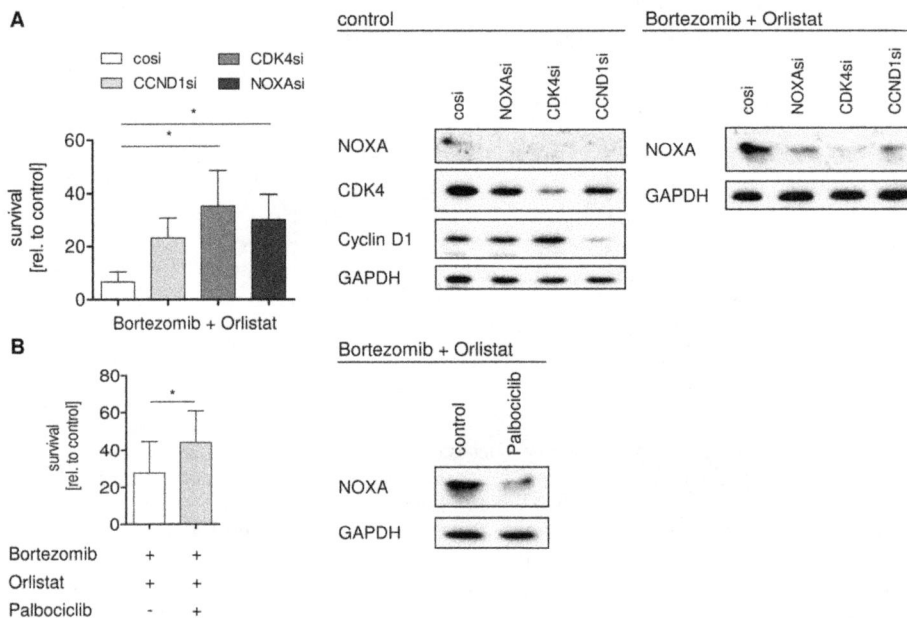

Fig. 5 CDK4 activity is required for cell death induction after combined fatty acid synthase and proteasome inhibition. a Knockdown of either cyclin D1 or CDK4 antagonizes cell death as well as NOXA protein induction as efficient as knockdown of NOXA. MCL cell line Jeko-1 was transfected with siRNA targeting NOXA, CCND1, and CDK4. Twenty-four hours after transfection, cells were treated with 15 μM orlistat and 7 nM bortezomib. After 14 h, protein expression was analyzed (right) and cell death was assessed by AnnexinV-PI staining (left) 24 h post-treatment. b Co-treatment of bortezomib with orlistat is antagonized by palbociclib treatment. MCL cell line Jeko-1 was treated with 300 nM palbociclib and subsequently co-treated with 15 μM orlistat and 7 nM bortezomib. After 14 h, protein expression was analyzed (right) and cell death was assessed by AnnexinV-PI staining (left). Data represent means ± S.D. from three independent experiments

Together, these results demonstrate that effective NOXA accumulation and induction of cell death after combined proteasome and fatty acid synthase inhibition is dependent on cyclin D1/CDK4 activity in MCL cells.

Discussion

In MCL stabilization of the short-lived pro-apoptotic BH3-only protein, NOXA is a major determinant for its sensitivity to bortezomib and other therapeutics [24, 28]. Our results show that the aberrant cyclin D1/CDK4 activity in MCL is critical for NOXA protein induction and thereby directly contributes to cell death triggered by proteasome inhibition. Similar to MCL, in multiple myeloma, cyclin D1 overexpression is also frequently observed and the disease is responding well to proteasomal inhibition [47, 48]. Interestingly, the susceptibility to bortezomib was also shown to be dependent both on cyclin D1 and on NOXA protein expression [29, 49]. In addition, a correlation between cyclin D1 overexpression and response to bortezomib treatment was also shown in breast cancer [50]. We show that in MCL, both induction of NOXA protein and cell death by bortezomib are largely abolished when CDK4 activity is blocked by pharmacologic inhibition or genetic manipulation. Furthermore, our experiments clarify that autophagy is the biological mechanism underlying the interaction between proteasome inhibition and CDK4 activity in the regulation of cell death in MCL cells. When MCL cells are exposed to bortezomib, NOXA can only be efficiently induced if the aberrant cyclin D1/CDK4 activity inhibits autophagy. This allows the very efficient induction of NOXA protein and explains the preferential sensitivity of cyclin D1 transformed cells to bortezomib.

The autophagy-lysosomal degradation pathway is known to be suppressed by cyclin D1/CDK4 activity [8–10]. The exact mechanism of how autophagy and CDK4 activity is linked in MCL remains to be determined. It has recently been reported that autophagy triggered by CDK4 inhibition relies on the induction of reactive oxygen species (ROS) [9]. Other reports identified AMPK signaling as a link between CDK4 activity and autophagy, as AMPK can directly phosphorylate the autophagy activating kinase ULK1 or inhibit the mTOR pathway which again blocks autophagy by inhibiting ULK1 [51–53]. Of note, the mTOR inhibitor Everolimus has been shown to induce autophagy in MCL [54]. In line with these data, we also observed an antagonism on bortezomib-induced cell death by the dual PI3K/mTOR inhibitor BEZ235 as well as by the AMPK activator metformin (data not shown).

We show for the first time that in the absence of proteasomal activity, NOXA can be degraded by the autophagy-lysosome pathway. Many proteins are degraded by both autophagosome and the proteasome [55]. Proteasomal degradation of NOXA has been extensively studied [56]. It is known that proteasome inhibition may reveal a crosstalk between the ubiquitin-proteasome system and the autophagy-lysosomal pathway enabling a so-called compensatory autophagy [57]. Whether NOXA can be directed to the autophagosomal degradation machinery has never been described. Chaperone-mediated autophagy (CMA) is a selective catabolic pathway that mediates proteins to lysosomes. This pathway involves specific chaperones, the lysosome-associated membrane protein type 2A (LAMP-2A) and the presence of a peptide motif biochemically related to KFERQ [58]. As this motif is mandatory for CMA and as it is not present in the NOXA protein sequence, it is unlikely that NOXA is a target for CMA. Macroautophagy (generally referred to as autophagy), however, involves proteins of the ATG8 family which promote the entry of cargo receptors into the autophagy pathway through interaction with the LC3-interacting regions (LIR) [59]. Interestingly, a LIR motif can be found in the NOXA protein sequence (Additional file 14: Figure S13) and might therefore target NOXA for ALP-dependent proteolysis.

Our findings have important implications for further development of combinatorial strategies with proteasomal inhibitors. Co-treatment of bortezomib with agents that either induce autophagy or abrogate its inhibition such as palbociclib reduces the efficacy of proteasome inhibitors. In contrast, combined treatment with agents that inhibit autophagy and/or lysosomal degradation might act synergistically with proteasome inhibitors. The clinical consequences are therefore twofold: When combining proteasome inhibitors with other chemotherapeutics, particular care must be taken. Co-treatment with a chemotherapeutic agent might cause nutrient starvation, inhibit the PI3K/AKT/mTOR pathway, activate AMPK signaling pathway, and induce ROS or ER stress which could eventually lead to prosurvival autophagy induction. Furthermore, co-treatment could impair CDK4 activity which, as we have shown, prevents prosurvival autophagy upon proteasome inhibition in MCL. On the other hand, proteasome inhibitors can be combined with approved therapeutics that block autophagy. Chloroquine and its derivative hydroxychloroquine, which have been initially FDA approved as antimalarial drug, are currently repurposed to inhibit autophagy and are well tolerated in clinical use [60]. Interestingly, a phase 1 clinical trial including patients with relapsed/refractory myeloma showed promising results for the combination of bortezomib with the autophagy inhibitor hydroxychloroquine corroborating our results [61]. More importantly, there are several more potent and specific autophagy inhibitors under preclinical investigation [62].

As we have shown here with the fatty acid synthase inhibitor orlistat, it is a highly interesting approach to investigate established compounds for their potential to regulate autophagy. This approach of re-positioning conventional drugs to target autophagy and induce cancer cell death was already shown for several therapeutics [63]. Orlistat might impair the autophagic machinery due to a reduction in palmitate levels [43–45]. Our group has previously shown that orlistat-induced cell death in MCL is indeed palmitate-dependent [24]. Alternatively, there are recent reports showing that lipid droplets and their components triglycerides are linked to endoplasmic reticulum homeostasis and autophagy regulation [64]. In line with this, another fatty acid synthase inhibitor Cerulenin has also been shown to inhibit autophagy due to lipid droplet downregulation [65]. Furthermore, we observed that co-treatment of bortezomib with Cerulenin potentiates cell death in a similar manner as orlistat does (data not shown).

NOXA contains six lysine sites and is substrate for polyubiquitination [56]. The only reported polyubiquitin chains for NOXA are K11 or K48 linkages [36, 66]. Although the K63 linkage has been shown to direct proteins preferentially towards autophagy instead of proteasomal degradation, all ubiquitin linkages including K11 and K48 have been shown to be involved in autophagosomal trafficking [67, 68]. Interestingly, our results show that orlistat is more effective in potentiating proteasomal inhibitor-mediated cell death and NOXA accumulation as compared to autophagy inhibitors. Our group previously demonstrated that orlistat interferes with NOXA ubiquitination [24]. Polyubiquitination is important for substrate selectivity of UPS as well as ALP [57, 69]. Therefore, in addition to orlistat blocking the late steps of ALP process (Fig. 4a), orlistat potentially impairs proteasomal degradation as well as trafficking of NOXA protein to autophagy in parallel and thus subsequently causing hyper-accumulation of NOXA protein.

In addition to the aforementioned mechanisms, many chemotherapeutics have shown to cause oxidative stress [70]. Therefore, it might be a promising approach investigating concomitant autophagy induction as oxidative stress regulates autophagy [71]. There is also growing insight into the interaction between DNA damage response and autophagy regulation [72]. It will be highly interesting to investigate if standard therapy regimes like R-CHOP could benefit from autophagy inhibitors.

Conclusion

Our data demonstrate for the first time that the high CDK4 activity in MCL is a prerequisite for the response to bortezomib therapy as well as for other compounds that require stabilization of NOXA for efficient cell death induction. We found out that the underlying molecular mechanism is a mitigated autophagy due to high CDK4

activity, offering novel combination treatment strategies in MCL and bortezomib-resistant cells. We show that NOXA can be degraded by the autophagosome and that blocking the residual autophagic activity combined with proteasome inhibition leads to highly efficient cell death in MCL due to super induction of NOXA protein.

Additional files

Additional file 1: Table S1. Sequences targeted by the siRNAs used for gene silencing. (TIFF 883 kb)

Additional file 2: Figure S1. CDK4 inhibition by palbociclib treatment inhibits RB1 phosphorylation. MCL cell lines Jeko-1 and Granta-519 were treated with 300 nM and MCL cell line Mino with 100 nM palbociclib. After 16 h, proteins were analyzed by Western blot. (TIFF 360 kb)

Additional file 3: Figure S2. Knockdown of cyclin D1 and CDK4 antagonizes bortezomib-induced cell death. MCL cell line Jeko-1 was transfected with siRNA targeting *CCND1* and *CDK4*. Twenty-four hours after transfection, protein expression was analyzed (right) and cells were treated with 8 nM bortezomib. Cell death was assessed by AnnexinV-PI staining 24 h post-treatment (left). Data represent means ± S.D. from three independent experiments. (TIFF 833 kb)

Additional file 4: Figure S3. Double knockdown of cyclin D1 and CDK4 antagonizes bortezomib-induced cell death similar to single knockdown of CDK4. MCL cell line Mino was transfected with siRNA targeting CCND1, CDK4, or both. Twenty-four hours after transfection, protein expression was analyzed (right) and cells were treated with 8 nM bortezomib. Cell death was assessed by AnnexinV-PI staining 24 h post-treatment (left). Data represent means ± S.D. from three independent experiments. (TIFF 903 kb)

Additional file 5: Figure S4. CDK4 inhibition antagonizes cell death of NOXA inducing substances. MCL cell line Jeko-1 was pretreated with 300 nM palbociclib for 16 h and subsequently co-treated with either 8 nM carfilzomib, 40 μM orlistat, or 500 μM hydrogen peroxide. After 24 h treatment, cell death was assessed by AnnexinV-PI staining. Data represent means ± S.D. from three independent experiments. (TIFF 950 kb)

Additional file 6: Figure S5. Inhibition CDK4 activity hardly alters *NOXA* mRNA levels after proteasome inhibition. MCL cell line Mino was treated with 100 nM and Granta-519 with 300 nM Palbociclib for 16 h and subsequently co-treated with 8 nM bortezomib. After 8 h co-treatment samples were taken and analyzed by real-time PCR. *NOXA* mRNA expression was normalized to TBP. Data represent means ± SD from three experiments. (TIFF 569 kb)

Additional file 7: Figure S6. Palbociclib-mediated antagonism on bortezomib-induced cell death is not caused by alterations in cell cycle distribution. MCL cell line Mino was transfected with siRNA targeting RB1 and treated with 100 nM palbociclib 24 h post-transfection. After 16 h, cells were treated with 8 nM bortezomib. Twenty-four hours after treatment, cell cycle distribution was measured by BrdU staining (left), cell death was assessed by AnnexinV-PI staining (middle panel), and proteins were analyzed by Western blot (right). Data represent means ± S.D. from three independent experiments. (TIFF 802 kb)

Additional file 8: Figure S7. Palbociclib treatment induces autophagy but not after a short treatment period. (A) MCL cell line Jeko-1 was treated with 300 nM palbociclib for 24 h with or without 40 μM hydroxychloroquine. After treatment, autophagic vesicles were measured with Cyto-ID staining. (B) MCL cell line Mino was treated with 100 nM palbociclib for 6 h. After treatment autophagic vesicles were measured with Cyto-ID staining. (TIFF 1187 kb)

Additional file 9: Figure S8. Autophagy inhibitors counteract palbociclib-mediated antagonism on bortezomib-induced cell death. MCL cell line Jeko-1 was treated with 20 μM liensinine (left), 2 mM 3-MA (left), or 10 μM Spautin-1 (right) with or without 300 nM palbociclib. After 16 h, cells were treated with 8 nM bortezomib for 24 h and analyzed by

AnnexinV-PI staining to assess cell death. Data represent means ± S.D. from three independent experiments. (TIFF 690 kb)

Additional file 10: Figure S9. Co-treatment of bortezomib with autophagy inhibitors potentiates cell death induction. MCL cell line Rec-1 was pretreated with 20 μM liensinine, 120 μM hydroxychloroquine, or 5 mM 3-MA for 16 h and subsequently co-treated with 8 nM bortezomib. After 24 h treatment, cell death was assessed by AnnexinV-PI staining. Data represent means ± S.D. from three independent experiments. (TIFF 725 kb)

Additional file 11: Figure S10. Synergistic cell death after proteasome inhibition and simultaneous fatty acid inhibition is caspase dependent. MCL cell line Jeko-1 was treated with 50 μM of the pan-caspase inhibitor Z-VAD-FMK for 2 h subsequently treated with 7 nM bortezomib or carfilzomib and co-treated with 15 μM orlistat. After 24 h, cell death was assessed by AnnexinV-PI staining. Data represent means ± S.D. from three experiments. (TIFF 774 kb)

Additional file 12: Figure S11. Combination of proteasome inhibition and simultaneous fatty acid inhibition regulates mainly NOXA protein levels and not PUMA, BAX, BAK, or MCL1. MCL cell line Jeko-1 was treated with 7 nM bortezomib or carfilzomib and co-treated with 15 μM orlistat. After 14 h, protein expression was analyzed by Western blot. (TIFF 1502 kb)

Additional file 13: Figure S12. Proteasome inhibitors combined with fatty acid inhibition induce synergistic cell death. MCL cell line Jeko-1 was treated with either five concentrations of carfilzomib or four concentrations of bortezomib and co-treated with four concentrations of orlistat (concentrations in the table). After 24 h, cell death was assessed by AnnexinV-PI staining. Induced cell death was used as fractional effect for determining the combination index (CI). (TIFF 1773 kb)

Additional file 14: Figure S13. NOXA protein contains a potential LIR motif. The amino acid sequence DGFRRL at the position 29-34 in the NOXA protein represents a potential LIR motif with the core consensus sequence ((W/F/Y) XX (L/I/V)). The acidic amino acid is highlighted in red. (TIFF 829 kb)

Abbreviations
3-MA: 3-Methyladenine; ALP: Autophagy lysosome pathway; CDK4: Cyclin-dependent kinase 4; CI: Combination index; CMA: Chaperone-mediated autophagy; cosi: Control siRNA; FASNi: Fatty acid synthase inhibitor; MCL: Mantle cell lymphoma; PBMNC: Peripheral blood mononuclear cells; ROS: Reactive oxygen species; SD: Standard deviation; UPS: Ubiquitin proteasome

Acknowledgements
We thank Dr. Martina Seiffert for kindly providing the NIH3T3 cell line (German Cancer Research Center DKFZ, Germany). We are grateful to Kerstin Willecke for excellent technical assistance.

Funding
This study was supported by the Robert Bosch Stiftung (project O2).

Authors' contributions
HvdK, WEA, SH, ES, GO, and DC designed the study. SH, ES, HvdK, and NG performed the experimental work. SH, HvdK, ES, MK, and KB analyzed the data. SH and HvdK wrote the manuscript. All authors read and approved the final manuscript.

Consent for publication
Not applicable.

Competing interests
The authors declare that they have no competing interests.

Author details
[1]Dr. Margarete Fischer-Bosch-Institute of Clinical Pharmacology, Stuttgart, Germany. [2]Hematopathology Unit, Hospital Clínic – Institut d'Investigacions Biomèdiques August Pi i Sunyer (IDIBAPS), CIBERONC, Barcelona, Spain. [3]Department of Clinical Pathology, Robert-Bosch-Hospital, Stuttgart, Germany. [4]Department of Hematology and Oncology, Robert-Bosch-Hospital, Stuttgart, Germany. [5]LMU Klinikum der Universität München, Med. Klinik und Poliklinik III, Munich, Germany. [6]University of Tübingen, Tübingen, Germany.

References
1. Dreyling M, Campo E, Hermine O, Jerkeman M, Le Gouill S, Rule S, et al. Newly diagnosed and relapsed mantle cell lymphoma: ESMO Clinical Practice Guidelines for diagnosis, treatment and follow-up. Ann Oncol. 2017; 28:iv62–71. https://doi.org/10.1093/annonc/mdx223.
2. Jares P, Colomer D, Campo E. Molecular pathogenesis of mantle cell lymphoma. J Clin Invest. 2012;122:3416–23. https://doi.org/10.1172/JCI61272.
3. Fernàndez V, Hartmann E, Ott G, Campo E, Rosenwald A. Pathogenesis of mantle-cell lymphoma: all oncogenic roads lead to dysregulation of cell cycle and DNA damage response pathways. J Clin Oncol. 2005;23:6364–9. https://doi.org/10.1200/JCO.2005.05.019.
4. Sherr CJ. G1 phase progression: cycling on cue. Cell. 1994;79:551–5.
5. Marzec M, Kasprzycka M, Lai R, Gladden AB, Wlodarski P, Tomczak E, et al. Mantle cell lymphoma cells express predominantly cyclin D1a isoform and are highly sensitive to selective inhibition of CDK4 kinase activity. Blood. 2006;108:1744–50. https://doi.org/10.1182/blood-2006-04-016634.
6. Qie S, Diehl JA. Cyclin D1, cancer progression, and opportunities in cancer treatment. J Mol Med. 2016;94:1313–26. https://doi.org/10.1007/s00109-016-1475-3.
7. Valenzuela CA, Vargas L, Martinez V, Bravo S, Brown NE. Palbociclib-induced autophagy and senescence in gastric cancer cells. Exp Cell Res. 2017;360: 390–6. https://doi.org/10.1016/j.yexcr.2017.09.031.
8. Acevedo M, Vernier M, Mignacca L, Lessard F, Huot G, Moiseeva O, et al. A CDK4/6-dependent epigenetic mechanism protects cancer cells from PML-induced senescence. Cancer Res. 2016;76:3252–64. https://doi.org/10.1158/0008-5472.CAN-15-2347.
9. Vijayaraghavan S, Karakas C, Doostan I, Chen X, Bui T, Yi M, et al. CDK4/6 and autophagy inhibitors synergistically induce senescence in Rb positive cytoplasmic cyclin E negative cancers. Nat Commun. 2017;8:15916. https://doi.org/10.1038/ncomms15916.
10. Brown NE, Jeselsohn R, Bihani T, Hu MG, Foltopoulou P, Kuperwasser C, Hinds PW. Cyclin D1 activity regulates autophagy and senescence in the mammary epithelium. Cancer Res. 2012;72:6477–89. https://doi.org/10.1158/0008-5472.CAN-11-4139.
11. Okada Y, Kato S, Sakamoto Y, Oishi T, Ishioka C. Synthetic lethal interaction of CDK inhibition and autophagy inhibition in human solid cancer cell lines. Oncol Rep. 2017;38:31–42. https://doi.org/10.3892/or.2017.5684.
12. Doorduijn JK, Minnema MC, Kersten MJ, Lugtenburg PJ, Schipperus MR, van Marwijk Kooy M, et al. Bortezomib maintenance therapy after induction with R-CHOP, ARA-C and autologous stem cell transplantation in newly diagnosed MCL patients, results of a multicenter phase II HOVON study. Blood. 2015;23:339.
13. Robak T, Huang H, Jin J, Zhu J, Liu T, Samoilova O, et al. Bortezomib-based therapy for newly diagnosed mantle-cell lymphoma. N Engl J Med. 2015; 372:944–53. https://doi.org/10.1056/NEJMoa1412096.
14. Smith AJ, Dai H, Correia C, Takahashi R, Lee S-H, Schmitz I, Kaufmann SH. Noxa/Bcl-2 protein interactions contribute to bortezomib resistance in human lymphoid cells. J Biol Chem. 2011;286:17682–92. https://doi.org/10.1074/jbc.M110.189092.
15. Oerlemans R, Franke NE, Assaraf YG, Cloos J, van Zantwijk I, Berkers CR, et al. Molecular basis of bortezomib resistance: proteasome subunit beta5 (PSMB5) gene mutation and overexpression of PSMB5 protein. Blood. 2008; 112:2489–99. https://doi.org/10.1182/blood-2007-08-104950.
16. Pérez-Galán P, Mora-Jensen H, Weniger MA, Shaffer AL, Rizzatti EG, Chapman CM, et al. Bortezomib resistance in mantle cell lymphoma is

associated with plasmacytic differentiation. Blood. 2011;117:542–52. https://doi.org/10.1182/blood-2010-02-269514.

17. Yang DT, Young KH, Kahl BS, Markovina S, Miyamoto S. Prevalence of bortezomib-resistant constitutive NF-kappaB activity in mantle cell lymphoma. Mol Cancer. 2008;7:40. https://doi.org/10.1186/1476-4598-7-40.

18. Chen Z, Teo AE, McCarty N. ROS-induced CXCR4 signaling regulates mantle cell lymphoma (MCL) cell survival and drug resistance in the bone marrow microenvironment via autophagy. Clin Cancer Res. 2016;22:187–99. https://doi.org/10.1158/1078-0432.CCR-15-0987.

19. Heider U, von Metzler I, Kaiser M, Rosche M, Sterz J, Rötzer S, et al. Synergistic interaction of the histone deacetylase inhibitor SAHA with the proteasome inhibitor bortezomib in mantle cell lymphoma. Eur J Haematol. 2008;80:133–42. https://doi.org/10.1111/j.1600-0609.2007.00995.x.

20. Roué G, Pérez-Galán P, Mozos A, López-Guerra M, Xargay-Torrent S, Rosich L, et al. The Hsp90 inhibitor IPI-504 overcomes bortezomib resistance in mantle cell lymphoma in vitro and in vivo by down-regulation of the prosurvival ER chaperone BiP/Grp78. Blood. 2011;117:1270–9. https://doi.org/10.1182/blood-2010-04-278853.

21. Qu F-L, Xia B, Li S-X, Tian C, Yang H-L, Li Q, et al. Synergistic suppression of the PI3K inhibitor CAL-101 with bortezomib on mantle cell lymphoma growth. Cancer Biol Med. 2015;12:401–8. https://doi.org/10.7497/j.issn.2095-3941.2015.0013.

22. Zhao L-L, Liu Y-F, Peng L-J, Fei A-M, Cui W, Miao S-C, et al. Arsenic trioxide rewires mantle cell lymphoma response to bortezomib. Cancer Med. 2015;4:1754–66. https://doi.org/10.1002/cam4.511.

23. Leshchenko VV, Kuo P-Y, Jiang Z, Weniger MA, Overbey J, Dunleavy K, et al. Harnessing Noxa demethylation to overcome Bortezomib resistance in mantle cell lymphoma. Oncotarget. 2015;6:27332–42. https://doi.org/10.18632/oncotarget.2903.

24. Dengler MA, Weilbacher A, Gutekunst M, Staiger AM, Vöhringer MC, Horn H, et al. Discrepant NOXA (PMAIP1) transcript and NOXA protein levels: a potential Achilles' heel in mantle cell lymphoma. Cell Death Dis. 2014;5:e1013. https://doi.org/10.1038/cddis.2013.552.

25. Chou T-C, Talalay P. Quantitative analysis of dose-effect relationships: the combined effects of multiple drugs or enzyme inhibitors. Adv Enzym Regul. 1984;22:27–55. https://doi.org/10.1016/0065-2571(84)90007-4.

26. Haubeiss S, Schmid JO, Mürdter TE, Sonnenberg M, Friedel G, van der Kuip H, Aulitzky WE. Dasatinib reverses cancer-associated fibroblasts (CAFs) from primary lung carcinomas to a phenotype comparable to that of normal fibroblasts. Mol Cancer. 2010;9:168. https://doi.org/10.1186/1476-4598-9-168.

27. Weniger MA, Rizzatti EG, Pérez-Galán P, Liu D, Wang Q, Munson PJ, et al. Treatment-induced oxidative stress and cellular antioxidant capacity determine response to bortezomib in mantle cell lymphoma. Clin Cancer Res. 2011;17:5101–12. https://doi.org/10.1158/1078-0432.CCR-10-3367.

28. Pérez-Galán P, Roué G, Villamor N, Montserrat E, Campo E, Colomer D. The proteasome inhibitor bortezomib induces apoptosis in mantle-cell lymphoma through generation of ROS and Noxa activation independent of p53 status. Blood. 2006;107:257–64. https://doi.org/10.1182/blood-2005-05-2091.

29. Bustany S, Cahu J, Guardiola P, Sola B. Cyclin D1 sensitizes myeloma cells to endoplasmic reticulum stress-mediated apoptosis by activating the unfolded protein response pathway. BMC Cancer. 2015;15:262. https://doi.org/10.1186/s12885-015-1240-y.

30. Medina DJ, Goodell L, Glod J, Gélinas C, Rabson AB, Strair RK. Mesenchymal stromal cells protect mantle cell lymphoma cells from spontaneous and drug-induced apoptosis through secretion of B-cell activating factor and activation of the canonical and non-canonical nuclear factor κB pathways. Haematologica. 2012;97:1255–63. https://doi.org/10.3324/haematol.2011.040659.

31. Chiron D, Dousset C, Brosseau C, Touzeau C, Maïga S, Moreau P, et al. Biological rational for sequential targeting of Bruton tyrosine kinase and Bcl-2 to overcome CD40-induced ABT-199 resistance in mantle cell lymphoma. Oncotarget. 2015;6:8750–9. https://doi.org/10.18632/oncotarget.3275.

32. Demo SD, Kirk CJ, Aujay MA, Buchholz TJ, Dajee M, Ho MN, et al. Antitumor activity of PR-171, a novel irreversible inhibitor of the proteasome. Cancer Res. 2007;67:6383–91. https://doi.org/10.1158/0008-5472.CAN-06-4086.

33. Arastu-Kapur S, Anderl JL, Kraus M, Parlati F, Shenk KD, Lee SJ, et al. Nonproteasomal targets of the proteasome inhibitors bortezomib and carfilzomib: a link to clinical adverse events. Clin Cancer Res. 2011;17:2734–43. https://doi.org/10.1158/1078-0432.CCR-10-1950.

34. Aikawa T, Shinzawa K, Tanaka N, Tsujimoto Y. Noxa is necessary for hydrogen peroxide-induced caspase-dependent cell death. FEBS Lett. 2010;584:681–8. https://doi.org/10.1016/j.febslet.2010.01.026.

35. Qin J-Z, Ziffra J, Stennett L, Bodner B, Bonish BK, Chaturvedi V, et al. Proteasome inhibitors trigger NOXA-mediated apoptosis in melanoma and myeloma cells. Cancer Res. 2005;65:6282–93. https://doi.org/10.1158/0008-5472.CAN-05-0676.

36. Brinkmann K, Zigrino P, Witt A, Schell M, Ackermann L, Broxtermann P, et al. Ubiquitin C-terminal hydrolase-L1 potentiates cancer chemosensitivity by stabilizing NOXA. Cell Rep. 2013;3:881–91. https://doi.org/10.1016/j.celrep.2013.02.014.

37. Baou M, Kohlhaas SL, Butterworth M, Vogler M, Dinsdale D, Walewska R, et al. Role of NOXA and its ubiquitination in proteasome inhibitor-induced apoptosis in chronic lymphocytic leukemia cells. Haematologica. 2010;95:1510–8. https://doi.org/10.3324/haematol.2010.022368.

38. Yu L, Chen Y, Tooze SA. Autophagy pathway: cellular and molecular mechanisms. Autophagy. 2017:1–9. https://doi.org/10.1080/15548627.2017.1378838.

39. Klionsky DJ, Abdelmohsen K, Abe A, Abedin MJ, Abeliovich H, Acevedo Arozena A, et al. Guidelines for the use and interpretation of assays for monitoring autophagy (3rd edition). Autophagy. 2016;12:1–222. https://doi.org/10.1080/15548627.2015.1100356.

40. Amaravadi RK, Lippincott-Schwartz J, Yin X-M, Weiss WA, Takebe N, Timmer W, et al. Principles and current strategies for targeting autophagy for cancer treatment. Clin Cancer Res. 2011;17:654–66. https://doi.org/10.1158/1078-0432.CCR-10-2634.

41. Höring E, Montraveta A, Heine S, Kleih M, Schaaf L, Vöhringer MC, et al. Dual targeting of MCL1 and NOXA as effective strategy for treatment of mantle cell lymphoma. Br J Haematol. 2017;177:557–61. https://doi.org/10.1111/bjh.14571.

42. Kridel SJ, Axelrod F, Rozenkrantz N, Smith JW. Orlistat is a novel inhibitor of fatty acid synthase with antitumor activity. Cancer Res. 2004;64:2070–5. https://doi.org/10.1158/0008-5472.CAN-03-3645.

43. Liu J, Chang F, Li F, Fu H, Wang J, Zhang S, et al. Palmitate promotes autophagy and apoptosis through ROS-dependent JNK and p38 MAPK. Biochem Biophys Res Commun. 2015;463:262–7. https://doi.org/10.1016/j.bbrc.2015.05.042.

44. Chen Y-Y, Sun L-Q, Wang B-A, Zou X-M, Mu Y-M, Lu J-M. Palmitate induces autophagy in pancreatic β-cells via endoplasmic reticulum stress and its downstream JNK pathway. Int J Mol Med. 2013;32:1401–6. https://doi.org/10.3892/ijmm.2013.1530.

45. Park M, Sabetski A, Kwan Chan Y, Turdi S, Sweeney G. Palmitate induces ER stress and autophagy in H9c2 cells: implications for apoptosis and adiponectin resistance. J Cell Physiol. 2015;230:630–9. https://doi.org/10.1002/jcp.24781.

46. Komatsu M, Ichimura Y. Physiological significance of selective degradation of p62 by autophagy. FEBS Lett. 2010;584:1374–8. https://doi.org/10.1016/j.febslet.2010.02.017.

47. Specht K, Haralambieva E, Bink K, Kremer M, Mandl-Weber S, Koch I, et al. Different mechanisms of cyclin D1 overexpression in multiple myeloma revealed by fluorescence in situ hybridization and quantitative analysis of mRNA levels. Blood. 2004;104:1120–6. https://doi.org/10.1182/blood-2003-11-3837.

48. Rajkumar SV, Kumar S. Multiple myeloma: diagnosis and treatment. Mayo Clin Proc. 2016;91:101–19. https://doi.org/10.1016/j.mayocp.2015.11.007.

49. Gomez-Bougie P, Wuillème-Toumi S, Ménoret E, Trichet V, Robillard N, Philippe M, et al. Noxa up-regulation and Mcl-1 cleavage are associated to apoptosis induction by bortezomib in multiple myeloma. Cancer Res. 2007;67:5418–24. https://doi.org/10.1158/0008-5472.CAN-06-4322.

50. Ishii Y, Pirkmaier A, Alvarez JV, Frank DA, Keselman I, Logothetis D, et al. Cyclin D1 overexpression and response to bortezomib treatment in a breast cancer model. J Natl Cancer Inst. 2006;98:1238–47. https://doi.org/10.1093/jnci/djj334.

51. Hsieh F-S, Chen Y-L, Hung M-H, Chu P-Y, Tsai M-H, Chen L-J, et al. Palbociclib induces activation of AMPK and inhibits hepatocellular carcinoma in a CDK4/6-independent manner. Mol Oncol. 2017;11:1035–49. https://doi.org/10.1002/1878-0261.12072.

52. Kim J, Kundu M, Viollet B, Guan K-L. AMPK and mTOR regulate autophagy through direct phosphorylation of Ulk1. Nat Cell Biol. 2011;13:132–41. https://doi.org/10.1038/ncb2152.

53. Drakos E, Atsaves V, Li J, Leventaki V, Andreeff M, Medeiros LJ, Rassidakis GZ. Stabilization and activation of p53 downregulates mTOR signaling through AMPK in mantle cell lymphoma. Leukemia. 2009;23:784–90. https://doi.org/10.1038/leu.2008.348.

54. Rosich L, Xargay-Torrent S, López-Guerra M, Campo E, Colomer D, Roué G. Counteracting autophagy overcomes resistance to everolimus in mantle cell lymphoma. Clin Cancer Res. 2012;18:5278–89. https://doi.org/10.1158/1078-0432.CCR-12-0351.

55. Liu WJ, Ye L, Huang WF, Guo LJ, Xu ZG, Wu HL, et al. p62 links the autophagy pathway and the ubiquitin-proteasome system upon ubiquitinated protein degradation. Cell Mol Biol Lett. 2016;21:29. https://doi.org/10.1186/s11658-016-0031-z.

56. Craxton A, Butterworth M, Harper N, Fairall L, Schwabe J, Ciechanover A, Cohen GM. NOXA, a sensor of proteasome integrity, is degraded by 26S proteasomes by an ubiquitin-independent pathway that is blocked by MCL-1. Cell Death Differ. 2012;19:1424–34. https://doi.org/10.1038/cdd.2012.16.

57. Ji CH, Kwon YT. Crosstalk and interplay between the ubiquitin-proteasome system and autophagy. Mol Cells. 2017;40:441–9. https://doi.org/10.14348/molcells.2017.0115.

58. Kaushik S, Bandyopadhyay U, Sridhar S, Kiffin R, Martinez-Vicente M, Kon M, et al. Chaperone-mediated autophagy at a glance. J Cell Sci. 2011;124:495–9. https://doi.org/10.1242/jcs.073874.

59. D-w W, Z-j P, G-f R, G-x W. The different roles of selective autophagic protein degradation in mammalian cells. Oncotarget. 2015;6:37098–116. https://doi.org/10.18632/oncotarget.5776.

60. Morgan MJ, Gamez G, Menke C, Hernandez A, Thorburn J, Gidan F, et al. Regulation of autophagy and chloroquine sensitivity by oncogenic RAS in vitro is context-dependent. Autophagy. 2014;10:1814–26. https://doi.org/10.4161/auto.32135.

61. Vogl DT, Stadtmauer EA, Tan K-S, Heitjan DF, Davis LE, Pontiggia L, et al. Combined autophagy and proteasome inhibition: a phase 1 trial of hydroxychloroquine and bortezomib in patients with relapsed/refractory myeloma. Autophagy. 2014;10:1380–90. https://doi.org/10.4161/auto.29264.

62. Chude CI, Amaravadi RK. Targeting autophagy in cancer: update on clinical trials and novel inhibitors. Int J Mol Sci. 2017; https://doi.org/10.3390/ijms18061279.

63. Yoshida GJ. Therapeutic strategies of drug repositioning targeting autophagy to induce cancer cell death: from pathophysiology to treatment. J Hematol Oncol. 2017;10:67. https://doi.org/10.1186/s13045-017-0436-9.

64. Velázquez AP, Tatsuta T, Ghillebert R, Drescher I, Graef M. Lipid droplet-mediated ER homeostasis regulates autophagy and cell survival during starvation. J Cell Biol. 2016;212:621–31. https://doi.org/10.1083/jcb.201508102.

65. Shpilka T, Welter E, Borovsky N, Amar N, Mari M, Reggiori F, Elazar Z. Lipid droplets and their component triglycerides and steryl esters regulate autophagosome biogenesis. EMBO J. 2015;34:2117–31. https://doi.org/10.15252/embj.201490315.

66. Zhou W, Xu J, Li H, Xu M, Chen ZJ, Wei W, et al. Neddylation E2 UBE2F promotes the survival of lung cancer cells by activating CRL5 to degrade NOXA via the K11 linkage. Clin Cancer Res. 2017;23:1104–16. https://doi.org/10.1158/1078-0432.CCR-16-1585.

67. Tan JMM, Wong ESP, Kirkpatrick DS, Pletnikova O, Ko HS, Tay S-P, et al. Lysine 63-linked ubiquitination promotes the formation and autophagic clearance of protein inclusions associated with neurodegenerative diseases. Hum Mol Genet. 2008;17:431–9. https://doi.org/10.1093/hmg/ddm320.

68. Riley BE, Kaiser SE, Shaler TA, Ng ACY, Hara T, Hipp MS, et al. Ubiquitin accumulation in autophagy-deficient mice is dependent on the Nrf2-mediated stress response pathway: a potential role for protein aggregation in autophagic substrate selection. J Cell Biol. 2010;191:537–52. https://doi.org/10.1083/jcb.201005012.

69. Deng Z, Purtell K, Lachance V, Wold MS, Chen S, Yue Z. Autophagy receptors and neurodegenerative diseases. Trends Cell Biol. 2017;27:491–504. https://doi.org/10.1016/j.tcb.2017.01.001.

70. Conklin KA. Dietary antioxidants during cancer chemotherapy: impact on chemotherapeutic effectiveness and development of side effects. Nutr Cancer. 2000;37:1–18. https://doi.org/10.1207/S15327914NC3701_1.

71. Szumiel I. Autophagy, reactive oxygen species and the fate of mammalian cells. Free Radic Res. 2011;45:253–65. https://doi.org/10.3109/10715762.2010.525233.

72. Eliopoulos AG, Havaki S, Gorgoulis VG. DNA damage response and autophagy: a meaningful partnership. Front Genet. 2016;7:204. https://doi.org/10.3389/fgene.2016.00204.

16

Ube2v1-mediated ubiquitination and degradation of Sirt1 promotes metastasis of colorectal cancer by epigenetically suppressing autophagy

Tong Shen[1†], Ling-Dong Cai[1†], Yu-Hong Liu[2†], Shi Li[1], Wen-Juan Gan[1], Xiu-Ming Li[1], Jing-Ru Wang[1], Peng-Da Guo[1], Qun Zhou[1], Xing-Xing Lu[1], Li-Na Sun[1] and Jian-Ming Li[1*]

Abstract

Background: Ubiquitination is a basic post-translational modification for cellular homeostasis, and members of the conjugating enzyme (E2) family are the key components of the ubiquitin–proteasome system. However, the role of E2 family in colorectal cancer (CRC) is largely unknown. Our study aimed to investigate the role of Ube2v1, one of the ubiquitin-conjugating E2 enzyme variant proteins (Ube2v) but without the conserved cysteine residue required for the catalytic activity of E2s, in CRC.

Methods: Immunohistochemistry and real-time RT-PCR were used to study the expressions of Ube2v1 at protein and mRNA levels in CRC, respectively. Western blotting and immunofluorescence, transmission electron microscopy, and in vivo rescue experiments were used to study the functional effects of Ube2v1 on autophagy and EMT program. Quantitative mass spectrometry, immunoprecipitation, ubiquitination assay, western blotting, and real-time RT-PCR were used to analyze the effects of Ube2v1 on histone H4 lysine 16 acetylation, interaction with Sirt1, ubiquitination of Sirt1, and autophagy-related gene expression.

Results: Ube2v1 was elevated in CRC samples, and its increased expression was correlated with poorer survival of CRC patients. Ube2v1 promoted migration and invasion of CRC cells in vitro and tumor growth and metastasis of CRC cells in vivo. Interestingly, Ube2v1suppressed autophagy program and promoted epithelial mesenchymal transition (EMT) and metastasis of CRC cells in an autophagy-dependent pattern in vitro and in vivo. Moreover, both rapamycin and trehalose attenuated the enhanced Ube2v1-mediated lung metastasis by inducing the autophagy pathway in an orthotropic mouse xenograft model of lung metastasis. Mechanistically, Ube2v1 promoted Ubc13-mediated ubiquitination and degradation of Sirt1 and inhibited histone H4 lysine 16 acetylation, and finally epigenetically suppressed autophagy gene expression in CRC.

Conclusions: Our study functionally links Ube2v1, an E2 member in the ubiquitin–proteasome system, to autophagy program, thereby shedding light on developing Ube2v1 targeted therapy for CRC patients.

Keywords: Ubiquitin-conjugating E2 enzyme, Autophagy, Epithelial mesenchymal transition, Metastasis, Colorectal cancer

* Correspondence: jianmingli@suda.edu.cn
†Tong Shen, Ling-Dong Cai and Yu-Hong Liu contributed equally to this work.
[1]Department of Pathology, Soochow University Medical School, Suzhou 215123, People's Republic of China
Full list of author information is available at the end of the article

Background

Ubiquitination mediated by the ubiquitin–proteasome system is basically required for the protein homeostasis in the cells [1]. The conjugation of ubiquitin to substrates usually involves three key steps, an activation step initiated by E1, an intermediate step covalently linking ubiquitin to a conjugating enzyme (E2), and a final step usually facilitated by a ligase enzyme (E3) which catalyzes the transfer of ubiquitin from the E2 to the protein substrate [2]. Members of the E2 family are key components for the ubiquitin–proteasome system. However, the role of the E2 family in autophagy and colorectal cancer (CRC) progression remains poorly defined.

Autophagy is an alternative mechanism to maintain cellular homeostasis, which is characterized by an autophagosome-dependent lysosomal degradation of long-lived proteins and unneeded organelles [3]. Although autophagy and proteasomal mediated lysosomal degradation use distinct components, they may also have some shared specific mechanisms [4–7]. Recently, the roles of autophagy in malignant transformation and cancer progression are concerned [8–18]. However, the roles of autophagy in tumorigenesis and progression are still not well characterized.

Ubiquitin-conjugating E2 enzyme variant proteins constitute a distinct subfamily within the E2 protein family, which lack the conserved cysteine residue needed for the catalytic activity of E2s [19, 20]. The functions of ubiquitin-conjugating E2 enzyme variant proteins are not well understood. Ubiquitin-conjugating E2 enzyme variant 1 (Ube2v1), one member of ubiquitin-conjugating E2 enzyme variant proteins, has been controversially suggested as both a candidate oncogene or a tumor suppressor [19, 21–23]. In addition, Ube2v1 has been found as one of the key components of TRAF6 to control NF-κB activation [20, 24–28]. Nevertheless, the role of Ube2v1 in autophagy and cancer including CRC and the mechanisms involved are still largely unknown.

Here, we reported that Ube2v1 promoted ubiquitination and degradation of Sirt1 by the help of Ubc13, inhibited histone H4 lysine 16 acetylation, and finally epigenetically suppressed gene expression of autophagy genes. Importantly, Ube2v1 promoted epithelial mesenchymal transition (EMT) and metastasis using an autophagy-related mechanism. Ube2v1 is employed as a new effective therapeutic target for CRC.

Methods

Cell lines and reagents

The human CRC cell lines DLD-1, SW480, and HCT116 (Additional file 1) were obtained from the Cell Bank at the Chinese Academy of Sciences (Shanghai, People's Republic of China) and cultured in RPMI-1640 or DMEM containing 10% fetal bovine serum. Human Ube2v1 cDNA were cloned into the GV218 expression vector (Genechem) and GV248 expression vector (Genechem), respectively. Stable overexpression and low expression Ube2v1 cell lines were selected by puromycin (1 mg/ml) and confirmed by RT-qPCR and western blots. Cells were transfected using the Lipofectamine 2000 (Invitrogen, CA, USA). siRNAs (RiboBio silencer siRNA: negative control, Ube2v1 [ID#siG1463152832 and siG1463152844]), Ubc13 (ID#stB000527A and ID#stB0005287B), Sirt1 (ID#siB09 917110134 and ID#siB09917110218), ATG5 (ID#siB071 03014081), ATG7 (ID#siB101210103531) were transfected at a final concentration of 10 nM using Lipofectamine™R-NAiMAX (Invitrogen). 3-MA (SigmaAldrich) was dissolved in DMSO (50 mM stock solution) and always used at a final concentration of 5 mM unless otherwise indicated. BafA1 was diluted in dimethylsulfoxide (DMSO) and used at a final working concentration of 1 μmol/l for 6 and 12 h, respectively. NSC697923 (Selleckchem), specifically inhibiting the activity of Ubc13-Uev1A, was dissolved in DMSO and used at 0.5 and 1 μM for 5 min. The proteasome inhibitor MG132 (Sigma Aldrich) was dissolved in DMSO and added in media at a final concentration of 10 μM for 4 h. Cycloheximide (CHX, Cell Signaling Technology) was added in the culture medium at concentrations of 100 μg/ml for 3, 6, and 9 h, respectively. Sirt1 expression construct has been described previously [29]. The constructs for GFP-LC3, pCMV-myc-Ube2v1, GFP-Ubc13, pCMV-myc-Ubc13, hemagglutinin (HA)-tagged ubiquitin gene (HA-Ub), and mCherry-GFP-LC3B were generated by PCR and confirmed by sequencing.

Lung metastases in vivo

To analyze lung metastases, CRC cells ($1 \times 10^7/0.2$ ml) were injected into the lateral tail vein of 6-week-old BALB/C-nu mice. Ten weeks after tail vein injection, mice were sacrificed, and the lungs were weighed. The lung metastases were examined using H&E staining. The number of surface metastases per lung was determined under a dissecting microscope. For comparison, we also prepared rapamycin for IP injection. Rapamycin (Tokyo Chemical Industry) was dissolved in ethanol, which was then diluted with PBS to a final concentration of 1 mg/ml directly before use. Mice were administered daily via intraperitoneal injections of 5 mg/kg rapamycin for 3 days per week following injection of SW480/Ube2v1 into the lateral tail vein for 2 weeks. Lung pairs were prepared for immunohistochemistry. All animal protocols were performed with the approval of the ethics committee of the Soochow University.

The wound-healing assay

The cancer cells were cultured in 6-well plates and grown in medium containing 10% FBS to nearly confluent cell monolayer, then carefully scratched using a

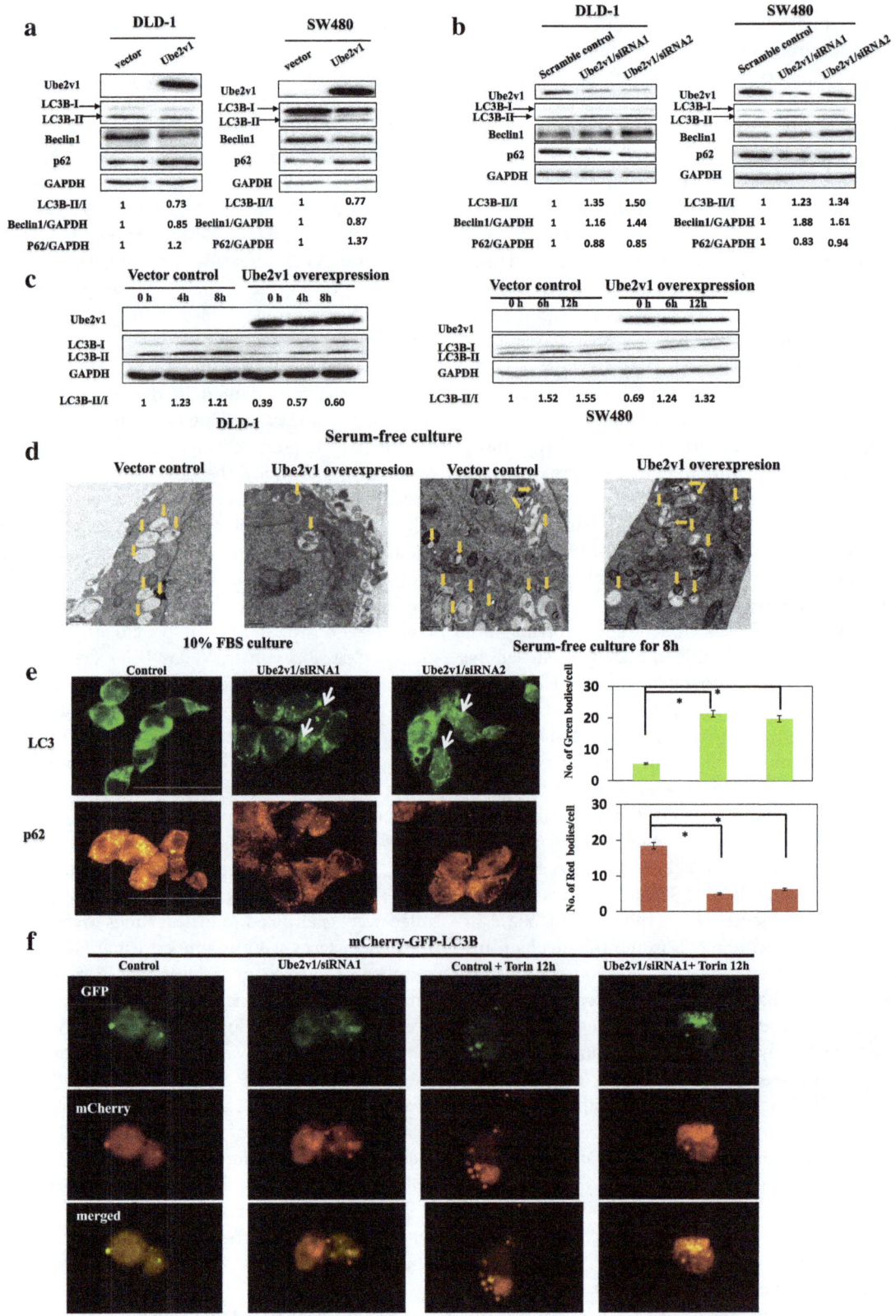

Fig. 1 (See legend on next page.)

(See figure on previous page.)
Fig. 1 The effects of Ube2v1 on autophagy program in colorectal cancer. **a, b** Protein expressions of LC3-II, Beclin1, and P62 level were examined by western blots when Ube2v1was overexpressed (**a**) or knocked down (**b**) in DLD-1 and SW480 cells under normal medium culture condition. **c** Protein expression of LC3-II was examined by western blots when Ube2v1was overexpressed in DLD-1 and SW480 cells under starvation in Hank's buffered saline solution (HBSS). **d** Enlarged multivesicular structures corresponding to autophagic vacuole in cells with stable Ube2v1 overexpression under normal condition or starvation condition were observed by transmission electron microscope (TEM). **e** Immunofluorescence staining of endogenous LC3 or P62 puncta was analyzed in SW480 cells after Ube2v1 expression was knocked down. **f** A mCherry-GFP-LC3B reporter was transfected into the cells to monitor the autophagy progression from the autophagosome characterized with green fluorescent protein (GFP) to autolysosome characterized with red fluorescent protein (RFP) after Ube2v1 knockdown or and Torin (concentration) treatment for 12 h

plastic pipette tip to draw a linear "wound" in the cell monolayer of each well. The monolayer was washed twice with PBS to remove debris or the detached cells from the monolayer. The cells were incubated at 37 °C and monitored by time lapse (photographed per 20 min for 12 h) in the Nikon microscope Ti-S (Japan). Under the microscope, the number of cells that migrated into the cell-free zone, base on the zero line of the linear "wound," was evaluated. The experiments were performed thrice in triplicate and were counted double blind by at least two investigators.

Transwell migration assay

For transwell migration assays, 5×10^5 cells were plated in the top chamber (serum-free medium) onto the non-coated membrane (24-well insert; pore size, 8 μm; Corning Costar) and allowed to migrate toward 10% serum-containing medium in the lower chamber. Cells were fixed after 36 h of incubation with methanol and stained with Giemsa solution. The number of cells invading through the membrane was counted under a light microscope (× 40, three random fields per well).

Transwell invasion assay

For invasion assay, 5×10^5 cells were plated in the top chamber onto the Matrigel-coated membrane (24-well insert; pore size, 8 μm; Corning Costar). Each well was coated freshly with Matrigel (60 μg; BD Bioscience) before the invasion assay. Cells were plated in medium without serum or growth factors, and medium supplemented with serum was used as a chemoattractant in the lower chamber. The cells were incubated for 48 h, and cells that did invade through the pores were removed by a cotton swab. Cells on the lower surface of the membrane were fixed with methanol and stained with Giemsa solution. The number of cells invading through the membrane was counted under a light microscope (× 40, three random fields per well).

Human CRC samples

Surgically resected CRC specimens with paired normal mucosal counterparts were obtained from The First Affiliated Hospital of Soochow University. All procedures involving human tumor biopsies were performed with the approval of the ethics committee of the Soochow University. The patients had given written informed consent.

RNA isolation and qPCR

Total RNA was isolated using the Trizol (Invitrogen) according to the manufacturer's instructions. For mRNA, cDNA was generated from 1 μg total RNA per sample using the Transcriptor First Strand cDNA Synthesis Kit (Roche). qPCR was performed by using the ABI StepOne Plus and the SYBR® Select Master Mix (ABI). mRNA expression was normalized using detection of 18S ribosomal RNA. Results are represented as fold induction using the $\Delta\Delta Ct$ method with the control set to 1. The sequences of qPCR primers are listed in Additional file 2: Table S1.

Western blot analysis and antibodies

Cell lysates were collected in RIPA lysis buffer (1% Triton-X-100, 20 mM Tris, pH 7.5, 137 mM NaCl, 1 mM EGTA, 10% glycerol, 1.5 mM $MgCl_2$, and protease inhibitor mixture and phosphatase inhibitors; latter 2 were from Roche). Lysates were sonicated and centrifuged at 4 °C. Per lane, whole-cell lysate was separated on 12% SDS-acrylamide gels and transferred on Immobilon PVDF membranes (Millipore). The membranes were probed with primary antibodies overnight at 4 °C and incubated for 1 h with secondary peroxidase-conjugated antibodies (CST). Chemiluminescent signals were then developed with Lumiglo reagent (Cell Signaling Technology) and detected by the ChemiDoc XRS gel documentation system (Bio-rad). Antibodies include anti-Ube2v1 (Abcam, monoclonal ab151725), anti-E-cadherin (Santa Cruz, monoclonal sc-21791), anti-N-cadherin (Boster, polyclonal BA0673), anti-Fibronectin (Boster, polyclonal BA1771), anti-Vimentin (Abcam, monoclonal, ab8978), anti-β-Catenin (Cell Signaling Technology, monoclonal #8480), anti-Twist1 (Proteintech, 25465), anti-Snai1 (Bioss, bs-2441R), anti-LC3B (CST, monoclonal 3868), anti-SQSTM1/p62 (CST, polyclonal 5114), anti-H4K16ac (Immunoway, polyclonal YM3317), anti-Beclin1 (Boster, polyclonal PB0014), anti-histone H3 (Abcam, polyclonal ab1791), and anti-Sirt1 (Santa Cruz, monoclonal sc-74504).

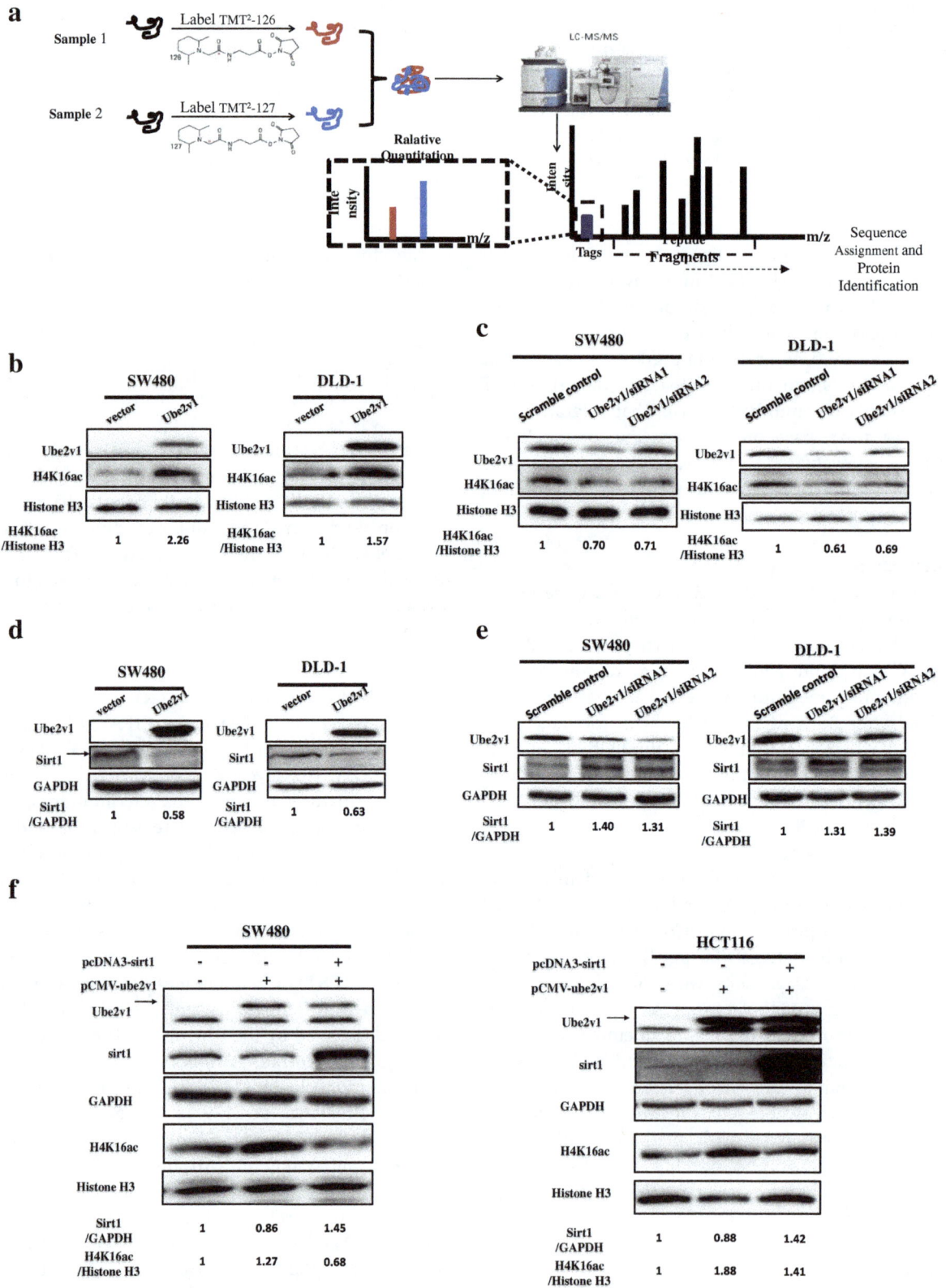

a

Sample 1 — Label TMT²-126

Sample 2 — Label TMT²-127

LC-MS/MS

Relative Quantitation

Intensity / m/z

Intensity

Tags / Peptide Fragments / m/z

Sequence Assignment and Protein Identification

b

	SW480			DLD-1	
	vector	Ube2v1		vector	Ube2v1
Ube2v1			Ube2v1		
H4K16ac			H4K16ac		
Histone H3			Histone H3		
H4K16ac /Histone H3	1	2.26	H4K16ac /Histone H3	1	1.57

c

	SW480			DLD-1		
	Scramble control	Ube2v1/siRNA1	Ube2v1/siRNA2	Scramble control	Ube2v1/siRNA1	Ube2v1/siRNA2
Ube2v1				Ube2v1		
H4K16ac				H4K16ac		
Histone H3				Histone H3		
H4K16ac /Histone H3	1	0.70	0.71	1	0.61	0.69

d

	SW480			DLD-1	
	vector	Ube2v1		vector	Ube2v1
Ube2v1			Ube2v1		
Sirt1			Sirt1		
GAPDH			GAPDH		
Sirt1 /GAPDH	1	0.58	Sirt1 /GAPDH	1	0.63

e

	SW480			DLD-1		
	Scramble control	Ube2v1/siRNA1	Ube2v1/siRNA2	Scramble control	Ube2v1/siRNA1	Ube2v1/siRNA2
Ube2v1				Ube2v1		
Sirt1				Sirt1		
GAPDH				GAPDH		
Sirt1 /GAPDH	1	1.40	1.31	1	1.31	1.39

f

	SW480		
pcDNA3-sirt1	-	-	+
pCMV-ube2v1	-	+	+
Ube2v1			
sirt1			
GAPDH			
H4K16ac			
Histone H3			
Sirt1 /GAPDH	1	0.86	1.45
H4K16ac /Histone H3	1	1.27	0.68

	HCT116		
pcDNA3-sirt1	-	-	+
pCMV-ube2v1	-	+	+
Ube2v1			
sirt1			
GAPDH			
H4K16ac			
Histone H3			
Sirt1 /GAPDH	1	0.88	1.42
H4K16ac /Histone H3	1	1.88	1.41

Fig. 2 (See legend on next page.)

(See figure on previous page.)
Fig. 2 The effects of Ube2v1 on histone H4 lysine 16 acetylation and expression of Sirt1. **a** Quantitative mass spectrometry was used to analyze differential proteins between control cells and cells with Ube2v1 stable overexpression. **b, c** Expression of histone H4 lysine 16 acetylation (H4K16ac) in histone extracts was examined after Ube2v1 was overexpressed (**b**) or knocked down (**c**) in SW480 and DLD-1 cells. **d, e** Sirt1 expression was detected after Ube2v1 was overexpressed (**d**) or knocked down (**e**) in SW480 and DLD-1 cells. **f** The effects of Ube2v1 overexpression on H4K16ac with or without Sirt1 overexpression

Co-immunoprecipitation and ubiquitination assays

Antibodies include anti-Sirt1 (Santa Cruz, polyclonal sc-15404), anti-HA-probe (Santa Cruz, polyclonal sc-805), anti-Myc (Proteintech Group, Inc., 10828-1-AP), anti-GFP (GeneTex, Inc., Monoclonal GT859), anti-Ubc13 (Cell Signaling Technology, Monoclonal #6999), and anti-IgG (Santa Cruz, polyclonal sc-66931). SW480 cells were lysed in Tris/HCl, pH 7.5, buffered with 1% Triton containing protease inhibitors as described above. Supernatant was incubated with appropriate antibody (2 µg) for at least 90 min at 4 °C followed by incubation overnight with Protein A/G-Sepharose beads (GE Healthcare). After overnight incubation, the agarose beads were washed four times with cold lysis buffer, incubated for 10 min at 108 °C with loading buffer, and subjected to SDS-PAGE and western blot analysis. To detect Sirt1 ubiquitination, 10 mM N-ethylmaleimide was included in the lysis buffer containing a protease inhibitor cocktail (Roche, Hongkong, China).

Immunohistochemistry

Paraffin-embedded slides were incubated with primary antibodies: anti-Ube2v1 (Abcam, polyclonal ab88679), anti-E-cadherin (Dako, monoclonal M3612), anti-Fibronectin (Boster, polyclonal BA1771), anti-Vimentin (Abcam, monoclonal, ab8978), anti-β-catenin (Cell Signaling Technology, monoclonal #8480), anti-SQSTM1/p62 (CST, polyclonal 5114), and anti-Beclin1 (Boster, polyclonal PB0014). Staining was done on a SPlink Detection Kit (SP-9000). We quantified staining intensity and percentage of stained cells. Positive tumor cells were quantified by two independent observers. The staining intensity was scored on a scale of 0–3 as negative (0), weak (1), medium (2), or strong (3). The extent of the staining, defined as the percentage of positive staining areas of tumor cells in relation to the whole tumor area, was scored on a scale of 0 (0%), 1 (1–25%), 2 (26–50%), 3 (51–75%), and 4 (76–100%). An overall protein expression score (overall score range, 0–12) was calculated by multiplying the intensity and extent positively scores.

Immunofluorescence microscopy

Cells were permeabilized with 0.3% Triton X-100 for 10 min followed by fixation with 2–4% Methanal for 15 min, and blocked with 3% sheep serum at room temperature for 60 min. Then, probed with primary antibodies anti-LC3B, anti-E-cadherin, anti-β-catenin, anti-Vimentine, and anti-SQSTM1/p62 were described before overnight at room temperature, and cells were washed three times with PBS. Stained with anti-rabbit IgG H&L (FITC) (abcam #ab6717) and anti-mouse IgG H&L (FITC) (abcam #ab6785) for 1 h at room temperature, and then the cells were washed three times with PBS. SW480 cells expressing GFP-RFP-LC3 were treated with Torin (Cayman Chemical) 250 nM for 6 h. Nuclei were visualized by staining with DAPI (Sigma Aldrich, USA) for 2 min. The stained cells were observed with an inverted fluorescence microscope (Nikon Ni-U). Autophagy was measured by quantitation of GFP-LC3 puncta per cell using fluorescence microscopy. All GFP-LC3 puncta quantitation was performed by an observer blinded to experimental condition.

Electron microscopy

Cells plated at 2×10^6 cells/mL were treated. In a primary case, each sample was fixed with 2% glutaraldehyde–paraformaldehyde in 0.1 M phosphate buffer (PB), pH 7.4 for 2 h and washed three times for 30 min each in 0.1 M PB. Samples were then postfixed with 1% OsO4 dissolved in 0.1 M PB for 2 h and dehydrated in an ascending gradual series (50–100%) of ethanol and infiltrated with propylene oxide. After sectioning and staining with uranyl acetate and lead citrate, they were observed under an electron microscope (JEM 1200EX; JEOL).

Quantitative mass spectrometry

Proteins were extracted from SW480cell lines with stable overexpressioning Ube2v1 and its control. Total protein concentrations were estimated with the bicinchoninic acid assay (Pierce BCA Protein Assay Kit; Thermo Fisher Scientific Inc. #23227, Waltham, MA, USA). A quantity of 50 mg of protein from each sample was used following the manufacturer's protocol (Expedeon, San Diego, CA, USA) with a minor modification by substituting urea with triethylammonium bicarbonate (TEAB) buffer for sample washes to avoid the primary amine group containing chemical that would interfere with TMT labeling. Each sample was digested with sequencing-grade trypsin (Promega, Fitchburg, WI, USA) in 500 mM TEAB buffer overnight in an enzyme to substrate ratio of 1:100 (wt:wt) at room temperature with gentle shaking, followed by a second digestion for

4 h with the same amount of trypsin. The digested peptide from different samples were labeled with tandem mass tags (TMT) reagents (Thermo, Pierce Biotechnology) according to the manufacturer's instruction (TMT 127, 126 for the samples). Briefly, the TMT label reagents were dissolved by anhydrous acetonitrile and carefully added to each digestion products. The reaction was performed for 1 h at room temperature, and hydroxylamine was used to quench the reaction. The TMT-labeled peptides were desalted using the stage tips. For LC-MS/MS analysis, the MS/MS spectra from each LC-MS/MS run were searched against the selected database using an in-house Mascot or Proteome Discovery searching algorithm. Peptides that have 127/126 scores > 1.2 and 126/127 scores < 0.8 were used for protein identification, and MS/MS spectra for all matched peptides were manually interpreted and confirmed. The QMS experiments were repeated for three times, and similar results were obtained.

Statistical analysis

Data were expressed as mean ± SD. Each experiment was performed in at least three repetitions. Student's t test (unpaired, two-tailed) was used to compare two groups of independent samples. One-way ANOVA was used for multiple comparisons. For analyses of associations of Ube2v1 expression with clinical parameters of CRC patients, the chi-square test was performed. P values of 0.05 or less were considered statistically significant.

Results

Ube2v1 suppresses autophagy in colorectal cancer

The role of autophagy in cancer progression is recently suggested [18]. However, the role of E2 family in autophagy is largely unclear. In our experiments, changes of LC3-II, Beclin1, and p62 protein levels were used as indicators of autophagy program. Surprisingly, decreased LC3-II and Beclin1 levels and increased P62 expression were observed when Ube2v1was overexpressed in DLD-1 and SW480 cells (Fig. 1a). Moreover, Ube2v1 knockdown in DLD-1 and SW480 cells led to increased LC3-II and Beclin1 levels and decreased P62 level (Fig. 1b). Given that starvation will initiate the autophagy program, we further evaluated the effects of Ube2v1 on starvation-mediated autophagy program. Cells were cultured under starvation in Hank's buffered saline solution (HBSS) for different interval, and we found that Ube2v1 overexpression attenuated the starvation initiated autophagy program (Fig. 1c). Moreover, even when the cells were treated with bafilomycin A1 (BafA1), an autophagy inhibitor which blocks autophagosome–lysosome fusion and leads to accumulation of autophosome characterized with increased expression of LC3-II, Ube2v1 overexpression still had suppressive effect on

autophagy under both normal culture and starvation conditions (Additional file 3: Figure S1). Ultrastructurally, the number of enlarged multivesicular structures corresponding to autophagic vacuoles was significantly decreased in SW480 cells with stable Ube2v1 overexpression under both normal condition or starvation condition by transmission electron microscope (TEM) and (Fig. 1d). To further quantify the changes of autophagy flux affected by Ube2v1, immunofluorescence staining of endogenous LC3 or P62 puncta were analyzed in SW480 cells after Ube2v1 expression was knocked down. Our results showed that Ube2v1 knockdown increased autophagy flux in SW480 cells (Fig. 1e). To further study the role of Ube2v1 on autophagy flux, A mCherry-GFP-LC3 assay were used to monitor the autophagy progression from the autophagosome labeled with green fluorescent protein (GFP) to autolysosome labeled with red fluorescent protein (RFP). We found that Ube2v1 knockdown led to increased autophagy flux, indicating as increasing expression of both green and red puncta within the cells (Fig. 1f). Torin, an inhibitor for mTOR pathway, was used to induce the autophagy program as a positive control in our experiment. Interestingly, Ube2v1 knockdown and Torin treatment had synergistic effect on autophagy (Fig. 1f). Together, these data demonstrate that Ube2v1 suppresses the autophagy program in CRC cells.

Ube2v1 inhibits histone H4 lysine 16 acetylation by downregulating expression of Sirt1 and epigenetically suppresses gene expression of autophagy-related genes in CRC

To delineate how Ube2v1 interferes with autophagy program, quantitative mass spectrometry was used to analyze differentially expressed proteins between control cells and cells with Ube2v1 stable overexpression (Fig. 2a). Interestingly, histones were enriched in these differentially expressed proteins (Additional file 2: Table S2), suggesting Ube2v1 may play a role in chromatin modification. It was suggested that reduction of histone H4 lysine 16 acetylation (H4K16ac) could lead to induction of autophagy [30, 31]. Based on our results from quantitative mass spectrometry, we speculated that histone H4 lysine 16 acetylation (H4K16ac) might be affected by Ube2v1. Surprisingly, we observed that H4K16acin histone extracts was significantly increased in Ube2v1 overexpressed SW480 and DLD-1 cells (Fig. 2b). Accordingly, H4K16ac in histone extracts was significantly decreased after Ube2v1 was knocked down in SW480 and DLD-1 cells (Fig. 2c). As we know, H4K16ac is one of the primary histone targets of Sirtuin 1 (Sirt1) [32]. Therefore, we postulated that the regulatory effects of Ube2v1 on H4K16ac are related to the effects of Ube2v1 on Sirt1. Interestingly, we found that Sirt1 expression was significantly decreased

Ube2v1-mediated ubiquitination and degradation of Sirt1 promotes metastasis of colorectal cancer...

223

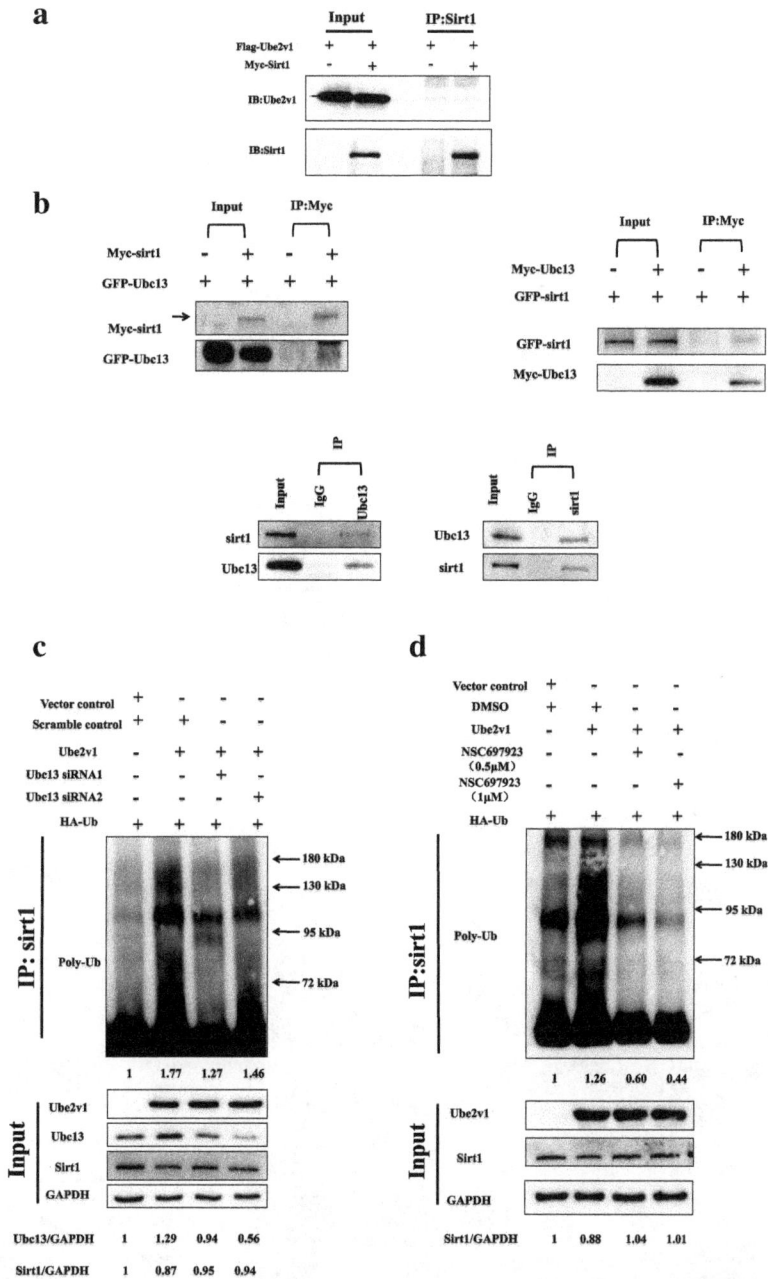

Fig. 3 The role of Ubc13 in Ube2v1 mediates Sirt1 ubiquitination in CRC cells. **a** Immunoprecipitation assay for the exogenous interaction between Ube2v1 and Sirt1in SW480 cells transfected with Flag-Ube2v1 and Myc-Sirt1. **b** Immunoprecipitation assay for the exogenous and endogenous interaction between Ubc13 and Sirt1 in SW480 cells. **c** Ubiquitination assays of endogenousSirt1 in the lysates from SW480 cells cotransfected with GFP-Ube2v1, HA-Ub, two siRNAs targeting Ubc13, or vector control. The cells were treated with or without MG132 (20 μM) before harvest and then immunoprecipitated them with anti-Sirt1 antibody. **d** Ubiquitination assays of endogenous Sirt1 in the lysates from SW480 cells cotransfected with GFP-Ube2v1, HA-Ub, NSC697923 (a small-molecule inhibitor targeting Ubc13), or DMSO control. The cells were treated with or without MG132 (20 μM) before harvest and then immunoprecipitated them with anti-Sirt1 antibody

in Ube2v1 overexpressed SW480 and DLD-1 cells (Fig. 2d), while Sirt1 expression was significantly increased after Ube2v1was knocked down in SW480 and DLD-1 cells (Fig. 2e). Moreover, the suppressive effects of Ube2v1 overexpression on H4K16ac can be successfully rescued by Sirt1 overexpression (Fig. 2f), suggesting that the role of Ube2v1 in autophagy program is at least partly depending on Sirt1 function.

Sirt1 is a key epigenetic player for gene regulation of autophagy genes. Thus, the regulatory effects of Ube2v1

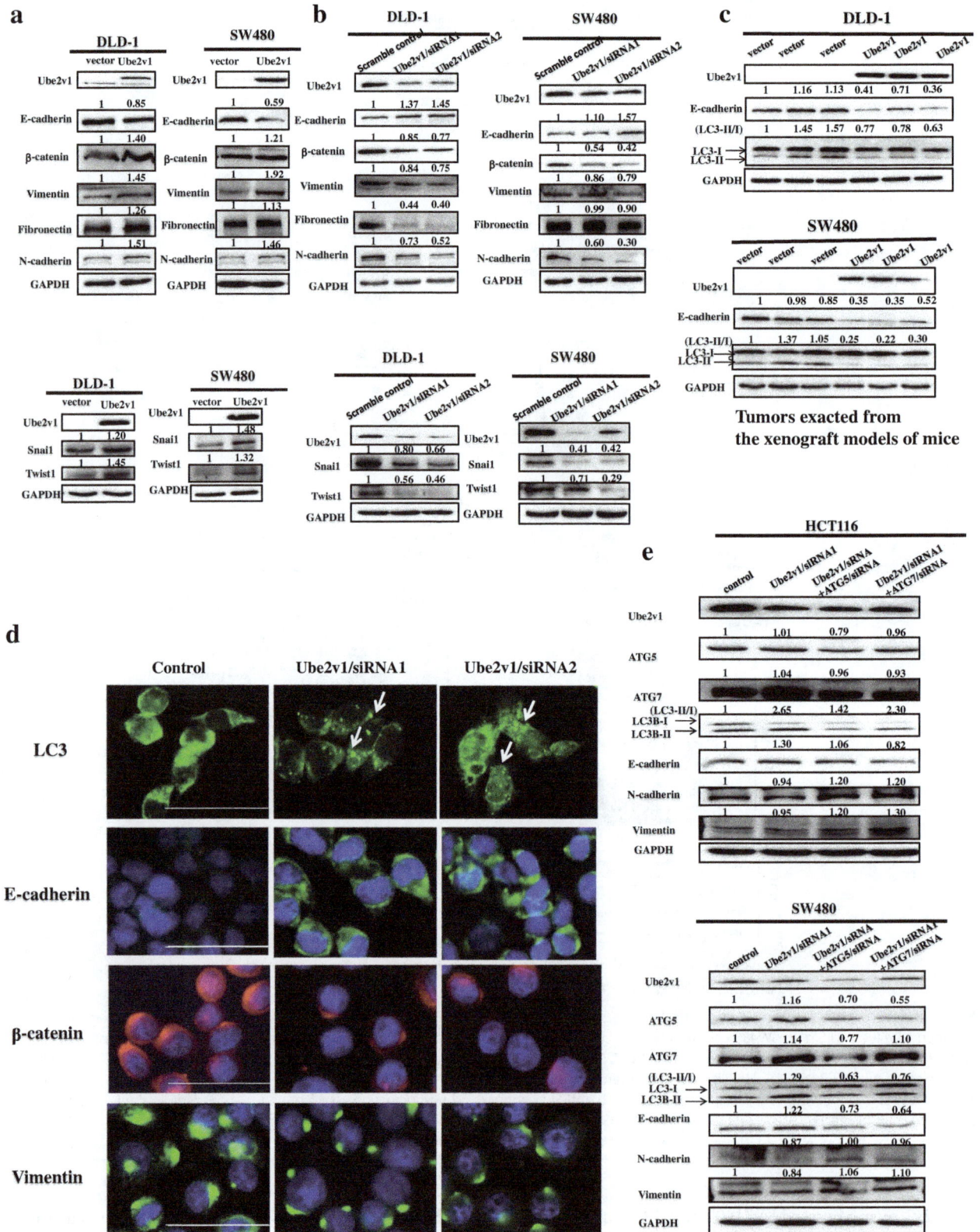

Fig. 4 (See legend on next page.)

on Sirt1 and H4K16ac might involve the epigenetic suppression of autophagy gene expression in CRC. qRT-PCR analysis showed that mRNA levels of many autophagy-related genes (LC3, Beclin1, ATG16L1, ATG3, ATG5, ATG7, ATG12, ATG10, ATG4a, ATG4b, ATG4c, and ATG4d) were significantly elevated when Ube2v1 expression was knocked down in SW480 cells (Additional file 3: Figure S2A), which were similar to gene expression patterns of autophagy genes induced by Sirt1 overexpression (Additional file 3: Figure S2D). In con7trast, Ube2v1 overexpression in SW480 cells significantly inhibited autophagy gene expression (Additional file 3: Figure S2B), which were similar to those induced by Sirt1 knockdown (Additional file 3: Figure S2C).

Generally, our study shows Ube2v1 as an epigenetic regulator for autophagy gene expression.

Ube2v1 destabilizes Sirt1 and promotes Sirt1 ubiquitination by the help of Ubc13

To determine the mechanism by which Ube2v1 regulates Sirt1 expression, we examined whether Ube2v1 affects the turnover of Sirt1 protein. CRC cells were treated with cycloheximide (CHX), an inhibitor of protein synthesis, and Sirt1 expression was determined by western blotting at various intervals. We found that silencing of Ube2v1 in SW480 cells significantly increased the half-life of Sirt1 (Additional file 3: Figure S3A), while overexpression of Ube2v1 in SW480 cells significantly decreased the half-life of Sirt1 (Additional file 3: Figure S3B), indicating that Ube2v1 promotes the turnover of Sirt1 protein.

Furthermore, we determine whether Ube2v1 affects Sirt1 ubiquitination. Ube2v1 overexpressed SW480 cells were treated with MG132 to block the degradation of Sirt1. Interestingly, overexpression of Ube2v1 significantly increased the ubiquitination of Sirt1 (Additional file 3: Figure S3C). Consistent with this finding, knockdown of Ube2v1 expression led to the dramatic decrease of Sirt1 ubiquitination in the presence or absence of MG132 (Additional file 3: Figure S3D).

To study the underlying mechanisms by which Ube2v1 mediates Sirt1 ubiquitination, we examined whether there is an interaction between Ube2v1 and Sirt1. Co-immunoprecipitation assay showed that there was no direct interaction between Ube2v1 and Sirt1 in CRC

cells (Fig. 3a). As Ube2v1 is a ubiquitin-conjugating E2 enzyme variant proteins without the conserved cysteine residue essential for the catalytic activity of E2s, the functions of Ube2v1 might be mediated by Ubc13 [33]. Interestingly, we found that Ubc13 can directly interact with Sirt1 in both exogenous and endogenous cell systems by co-immunoprecipitation (Fig. 3b). Functionally, knockdown of Ubc13 (Fig. 3c) or NSC697923 treatment (Fig. 3d), a small molecular inhibitor targeting interaction between Ubc13 and Ube2v1, can effectively attenuate the Sirt1 ubiquitination, demonstrating that Ubc13 is required for the regulatory effects of Ube2v1 on Sirt1 ubiquitination.

Ube2v1 promotes epithelial mesenchymal transition by suppressing autophagy program in CRC cells

The role of autophagy in cancer is very complex, depending on context and types of cancers [34, 35]. Epithelial mesenchymal transition (EMT) has been implicated to play a key role in tumor progression and metastasis [36]. Whether Ube2v1 is involved in EMT through autophagy program is unknown.

We found that Ube2v1 promotes EMT of CRC cells as demonstrated by decreased expression of E-cadherin, as well as increased expressions of β-catenin, Vimentin, Fibronectin, N-cadherin, Snai1, and Twist1 following Ube2v1 overexpression in DLD-1 and SW480 cells (Fig. 4a). Consistently, increased expression of E-cadherin and decreased expressions of β-catenin, Vimentin, Fibronectin, N-cadherin, Snai1, and Twist1 were found after Ube2v1was knocked down in DLD-1 and SW480 cells (Fig. 4b).

To explore the potential link between EMT and autophagy program, we used tumor samples from mouse xenograft model for western blotting and immunohistochemical staining. Western blots showed that decreased expression of E-cadherin and LC3-II was found in both DLD-1 and SW480 cells with Ube2v1 stable overexpression (Fig. 4c). In addition, immunofluorescence results indicated that increased endogenous LC3 puncta and E-cadherin was found after Ube2v1 was knocked down in SW480 cells (Fig. 4d), suggesting the link between EMT and autophagy program.

To further establish the regulatory effects of autophagy program mediated by Ube2v1 on EMT, inhibition of autophagy program by silencing expression of ATG5 or

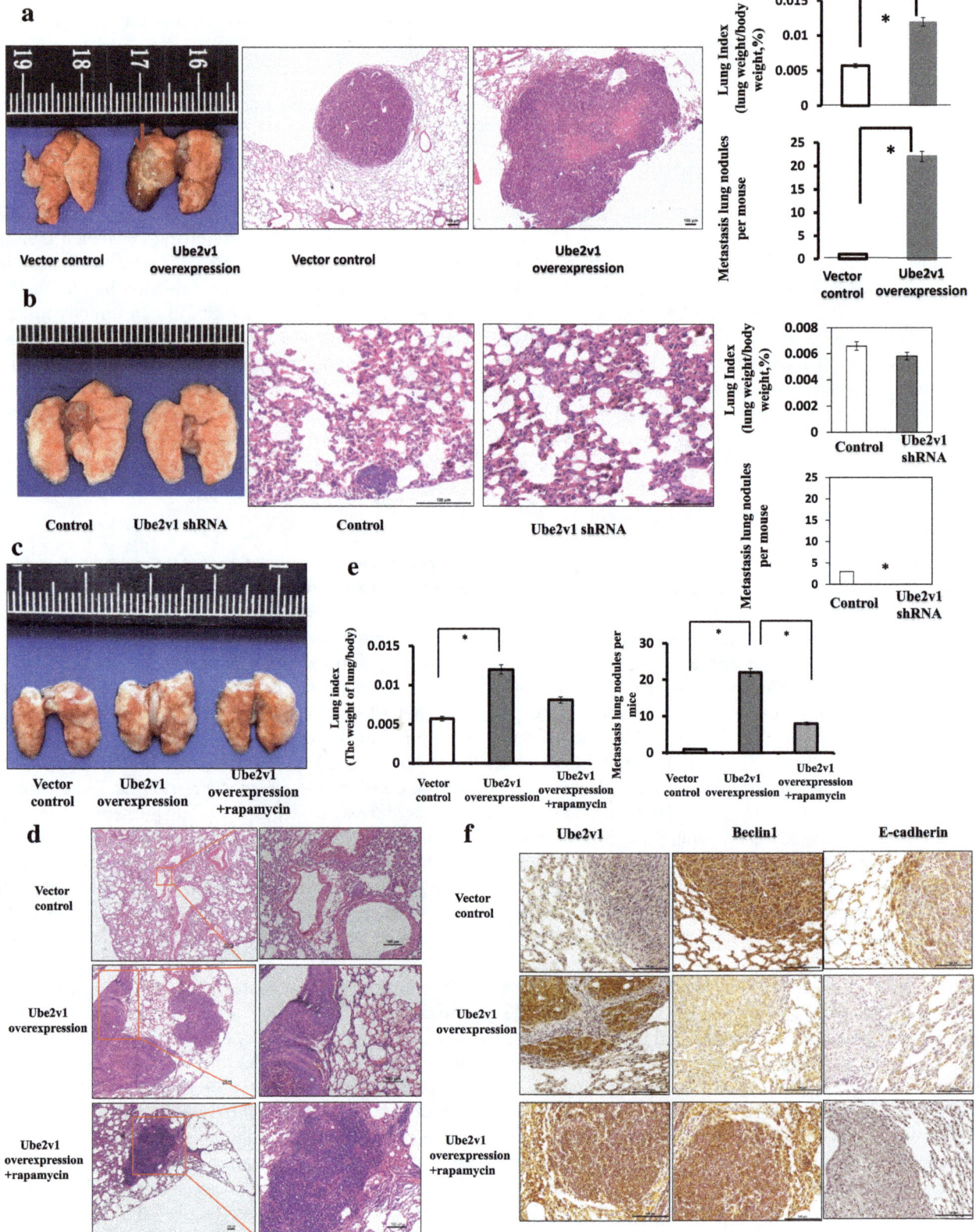

Fig. 5 (See legend on next page.)

(See figure on previous page.)
Fig. 5 Effects of rapamycin on Ube2v1-mediated lung metastasis in the orthotropic mouse xenograft models of CRC. **a** Lung index and numbers of metastatic lung nodules of mice administrated intravenously with SW480 cells stably overexpressing Ube2v1 (2×10^6 cells) were determined ($n = 6$ per group). **b** Lung index and numbers of metastatic lung nodules of mice administrated intravenously with SW480 cells stably knocked down expression of Ube2v1 (2×10^6 cells) were determined ($n = 6$ per group). Representative photographs of the lung with metastatic nodules are shown (arrow heads). Representative micrographs of the lung with metastatic cells are shown by H&E staining at a magnification of $\times 200$. M metastatic lesion, N adjacent normal lung tissue. Expressions of E-cadherin and LC3-II were detected after Ube2v1 was overexpressed with or without rapamycin (final concentration 10 ng/ml) stimulation. **c** Representative photographs of the lung with metastatic nodules are shown. **d** Representative micrographs of the lung with metastatic cells are shown by H&E staining at a magnification of $\times 100$ (left) and $\times 200$ (right). **e** Lung index and numbers of metastatic lung nodules of mice were determined ($n = 6$ per group). M metastatic lesion, N adjacent normal lung tissue. Error bars represent mean $\pm$ s.d. Statistical significance was determined by a two-tailed, unpaired Student's t test. $*p < 0.05$, $**p < 0.01$. **f** Expressions of Ube2v1, Beclin1, and E-cadherin were analyzed by immunohistochemical staining. Error bars represent mean $\pm$ s.d. Statistical significance was determined by a two-tailed, unpaired Student's t test. $*p < 0.05$

ATG7 can successfully rescued the suppressive effects on EMT initiated by Ube2v1 knockdown in HCT116 and SW480 cells (Fig. 4e). Additionally, 3-methyladenine (3-MA), an autophagy inhibitor, can effectively abolish the enhanced expression of E-cadherin induced by Ube2v1 knockdown (Additional file 3: Figure S4).

Rapamycin attenuates the Ube2v1-mediated migration and invasion in vitro and lung metastasis of CRC cells in an orthotropic mouse xenograft model by restoring autophagy program

To further study the functional role of Ube2v1 in CRC, the expression levels of Ube2v1 in CRC cell lines were inspected at first and we found that SW480 and DLD-1 expressed low levels of Ube2v1. Therefore, Ube2v1 was stably overexpressed in SW480 and DLD-1 cells using a lentiviral system. The expression efficiency was confirmed at both mRNA and protein levels by Western blotting and qRT-PCR (data not showed). Scratch-wound healing assays showed that overexpression of Ube2v1 significantly enhanced CRC cell migration (Additional file 3: Figure S5A), consistent with the observations in the migration assay after Ube2v1 was overexpressed (Additional file 3: Figure S5B). Similarly, invasion assays indicated enhanced invasion ability for cells with Ube2v1 stable overexpression (Additional file 3: Figure S5C). Furthermore, we found that treatment with rapamycin, an agonist of autophagy, can successfully alleviate the increased migration and invasion abilities of CRC cells after Ube2v1 overexpression (Additional file 3: Figure S6).

Lung metastasis models were used to monitor the effects of Ube2v1 overexpression or knockdown on metastasis of CRC in vivo. SW480 cells with Ube2v1 stable overexpression or knockdown were respectively injected into the lateral vein in the tails of the nude BALB/c mice. Five weeks after implantation, the lung metastatic index in mice administrated with SW480 cells with Ube2v1 stable overexpression increased significantly compared with those mice administrated with control SW480 cells (Fig. 5a). Histological examination showed SW480 cells with Ube2v1 stable overexpression were

found to develop more and larger micrometastases in the lung of mice than control cells (Fig. 5a). In accordance with these results, knockdown of Ube2v1 resulted in less and smaller micrometastases in the lung (Fig. 5b). More importantly, rapamycin, an agonist of autophagy, can rescue the enhanced effects of lung metastasis induced by Ube2v1 overexpression in vivo (Fig. 5c–e). Immunohistochemical staining indicated that Beclin1 expression was significantly restored, accompanied by increased expressions of E-cadherin after administration of rapamycin (Fig. 5f).

Collectively, Ube2v1 promotes EMT and metastasis of CRC in an autophagy-dependent mechanism in vitro and in vivo.

High Ube2v1 expression in CRC samples is correlated with poorer survival of CRC patients

Finally, the clinical significance of Ube2v1 in CRC was determined by analyzing the mRNA and protein levels of Ube2v1 in CRC patient samples. At both mRNA and protein levels, Ube2v1 expression was significantly increased in primary CRC tissue samples compared with that in their normal counterparts (Fig. 6a, b). More interestingly, Ube2v1 expression was markedly increased in CRC patients with distant metastases (Fig. 6c) or advanced clinical stage such as TNM stage IV when compared with that in patients without distant metastases or early clinical stage such as TNM stage I (Fig. 6d). Thus, the Ube2v1 exhibits a stage-specific expression which is correlated with CRC progression. Using data from Public Gene Expression Profile (GSE17537), meta-analysis of the prognostic value of Ube2v1 mRNA by PrognoScan showed that CRC patients with high levels of Ube2v1 mRNA might have shorter disease-free survival (Fig. 6e).

Discussion

Ube2v1 (also named as Uev1A), one of ubiquitin-conjugating E2 enzyme variant proteins, belongs to a distinct subfamily of the E2 protein family [20, 37]. Based on its structure characteristics, Ube2v1 may have unknown functions different from those classic E2s.

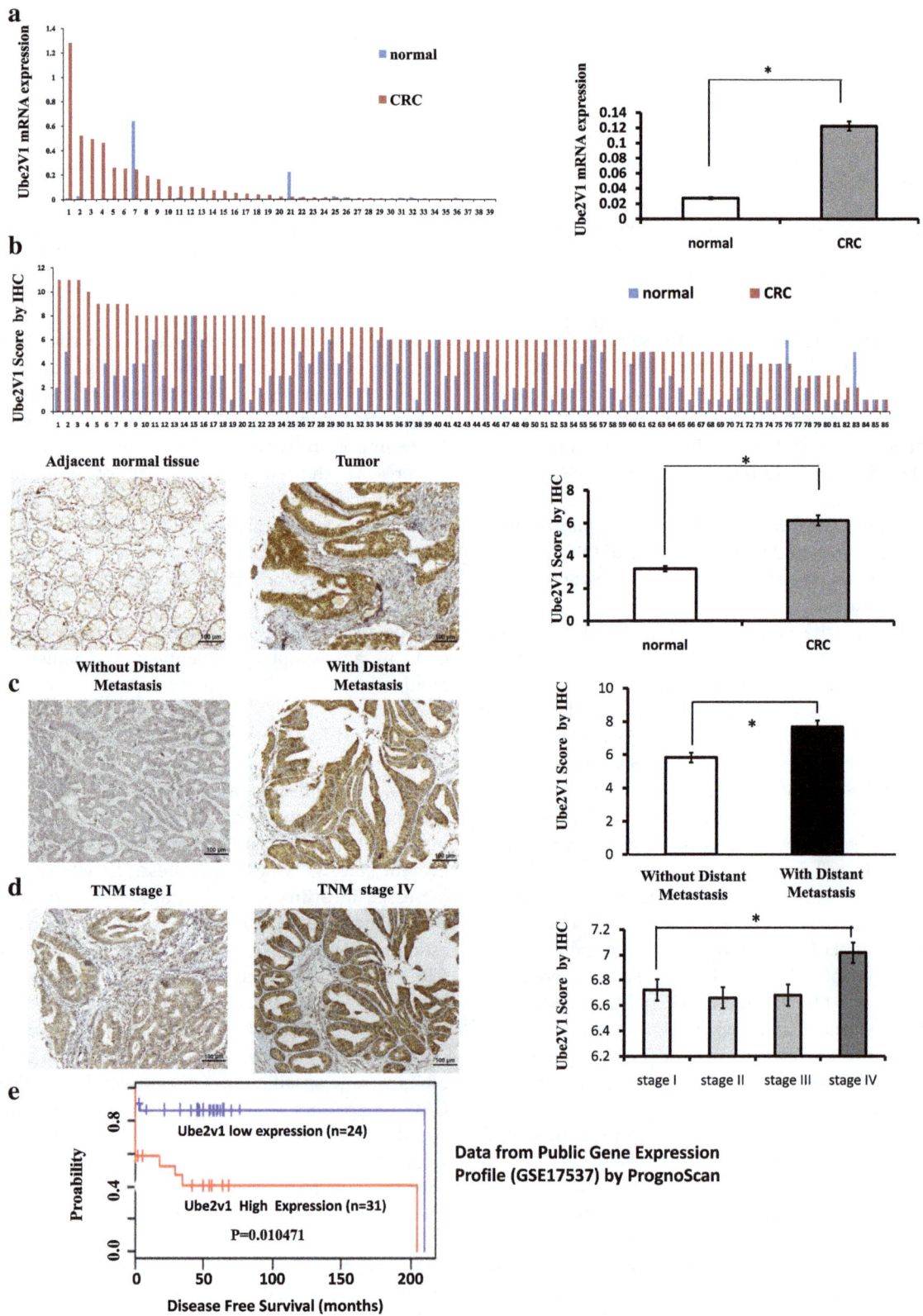

Fig. 6 (See legend on next page.)

Ube2v1-mediated ubiquitination and degradation of Sirt1 promotes metastasis of colorectal cancer...

229

(See figure on previous page.)
Fig. 6 Ube2v1 expression in clinical samples of colorectal cancer. **a** mRNA levels of Ube2v1 in a tumor and its adjacent tissue from a CRC patient using qPCR. **b** Scores for Ube2v1 staining in paired, adjacent normal and tumor tissue samples from CRC patients by immunohistochemical staining. Typical staining for Ube2v1 in paired, adjacent normal and tumor tissue sample from a CRC patient. **c** Scores for Ube2v1 staining in tumor samples from CRC patients with or without distant metastasis by immunohistochemical staining. **d** Scores for Ube2v1 staining in tumor samples from CRC patients with different TNM stages by immunohistochemical staining. Typical staining for Ube2v1 in tumor samples from CRC patients in TNM stage I and stage IV was shown. **e** Disease-free survival of CRC patients according to the expression levels of Ube2v1 mRNA by PrognoScan using data from Public Gene Expression Profile (GSE17537). Statistical significance was determined by using a two-tailed, unpaired Student's t test. *$p < 0.05$

Here, we present a critical role of Ube2v1 in autophagy program. We found Ube2v1 can epigenetically regulate autophagy genes. Ube2v1 can globally suppress gene expression of autophagy-related genes. Mechanistically, Ube2v1 promotes ubiquitination and degradation of Sirt1 through Ubc13, subsequently reduces H4K16ac, and suppresses gene expression of autophagy genes epigenetically. It has been shown that H4K16ac is one of the primary histone target of Sirt1 which is a key epigenetic player involved in autophagy. Our study provided a novel mechanistic understanding about the functional regulation of Sirt1 by Ube2v1-Ubc13-mediated ubiquitination. Noteworthily, our study link the classic ubiquitin-proteasome system especially the E2 member with autophagy machine in CRC, suggesting cooperative interaction between these two systems to control cellular homeostasis in CRC. For a long time, Ube2v1-UBC13, as a key components working with TRAF6, controls NF-κB signaling pathways. Recent reports showed that TAK1 kinase and OTUB1 controls NF-κB activation using similar Ube2v1-UBC13/TRAF6 signaling axis. The understanding of Ube2v1-UBC13 in autophagy discovered a new regulatory pathway for autophagy.

Moreover, we also uncovered a key mechanism by which Ube2v1 promotes metastasis of CRC cells. Accumulating evidences demonstrated that cancer cells usually undergo EMT program to facilitate invasion and metastasis [36, 38–40]. Ube2v1 promotes an autophagy-dependent EMT of CRC cells in vitro and in vivo. Our study functionally links the EMT with autophagy program in CRC. Nevertheless, the role of autophagy in cancer is very complex, depending on cell types and specific process involved [10, 18, 41–44]. In general, tumor cell autophagy has evolved to deal with intracellular and environmental stress, thus favoring tumor growth and progression [43]. This implies that autophagy may have differential impact in distinct phases of tumorigenesis including metastasis. For example, the role of autophagy in EMT processes is also diverse. Autophagy induction impairs migration and invasion by reversing EMT in glioblastoma cells [45]. On the contrary, Beclin1 overexpression promoted EMT process through Wnt/β-catenin pathway under starvation [46]. Moreover, the pan-inhibitor of Aurora kinases danusertib

induces autophagy and suppresses EMT in human breast cancer cells [47]. Autophagy deficiency stabilizes Twist1 to promote EMT [48]. DEDD interacts with PI3KC3 to activate autophagy and attenuate EMT in human breast cancer [49, 50]. In liver-specific autophagy-deficient mice (Alb-Cre; ATG7(fl/fl)), autophagy deficiency in vivo reduces epithelial markers' expression and increases the levels of mesenchymal markers [51]. In this study, we found that the tumor cells survived and metastasized to distant organs by a suppressive autophagy program.

Our study presented here has illuminated pro-metastatic function of Ube2v1 in CRC. We present a critical role of Ube2v1 in tumor growth and metastasis of CRC in vivo and in vitro. In CRC patients, Ube2v1 expression is elevated in tumor samples especially in advanced TNM staging and correlated with poorer survival of patients. In vivo studies using orthotopic mouse xenograft models of CRC showed that Ube2v1 promotes tumor growth and metastasis. To our knowledge, the role of Ube2v1 in CRC progression and metastasis has not been established. Only several papers have reported its controversial roles in cancer. Ube2v1, first named as CROC-1, was suggesting as a candidate oncogene by transcriptionally activating FOS proto-oncogene [19]. Inconsistently, Ube2v1 can also function as a tumor suppressor by protecting cells from DNA damage [21]. And Ube2v1 expression is increased significantly in the early stage for the acquisition of immortality of tumor cells [22]. Recently, Ube2v1 was reported to mediate matrix metalloproteinase-1 gene regulation through nuclear factor-κB and promote breast cancer metastasis [23]. Although concrete evidence for the role of Ube2v1 in cancer remains, some inhibitors targeting Ube2v1 pathway have been developed to treat some type of cancers, such as diffuse large B cell lymphoma cells [33]. Our study presented here has paved the path forward to develop small-molecule inhibitor targeting Ube2v1 for CRC treatment.

Conclusion

Ube2v1 suppresses autophagy program and promotes metastasis of CRC by an autophagy-related EMT mechanism (Additional file 3: Figure S7), shedding light on developing Ube2v1 as a potential target for CRC treatment.

Additional files

Additional file 1: Identification information of cell lines. (PDF 2605 kb)

Additional file 2: Table S1. Primers for qPCR or DNA sequencing. **Table S2.** Differential proteins between control cells and cells with Ube2v1 stable overexpression by quantitative mass spectrometry. (PDF 107 kb)

Additional file 3: Figure S1. Protein expressions of LC3-II and Beclin1 were examined by western blots when Ube2v1 was overexpressed in DLD-1 and SW480 cells under both normal medium culture condition (a) and starvation in Hank's buffered saline solution (HBSS) (b). The cells were treated with Bafilomycin A1(BafA1), an autophagy inhibitor which blocks autophagosome–lysosome fusion. **Figure S2.** The effects of Ube2v1 on gene expressions of autophagy genes. A-B. mRNA levels of autophagy genes (LC3, Beclin1, ATG16L1, ATG3, ATG5, ATG7, ATG12, ATG10, ATG4a, ATG4b, ATG4c and ATG4d) were detected by qPCR analysis when Ube2v1 expression was knocked down (a) or overexpressed (b) in SW480 cells. C-D. mRNA levels of autophagy genes (LC3, Beclin1, ATG16L1, ATG3, ATG5, ATG7, ATG12, ATG10, ATG4a, ATG4b, ATG4c and ATG4d) were detected by qPCR analysis when Sirt1 expression was knocked down (c) or overexpressed (d) in SW480 cells. **Figure S3.** The effects of Ube2v1 on stabilization and ubiquitination of Sirt1 in CRC cells. The expression of Sirt1 was detected by western blotting in shRNA-transduced cells (a) or Ube2v1 overexpressed (b) SW480 cells treated with cyclohexamide (CHX) (100 μg/ml) for the indicated time intervals. The intensity of endogenous Sirt1 expression for each time point was quantified by densitometry. c Ubiquitination assays of exogenous Sirt1 in the lysates from SW480 cells cotransfected with GFP-Ube2v1, HA-Ub, Myc-Sirt1 or vector control. The cells were treated with or without MG132 (20 μM) before harvest and then immunoprecipitated them with anti-myc antibody. d Ubiquitination assays of exogenous Sirt1 in the lysates from SW480 cells cotransfected with HA-Ub, Myc-Sirt1 in the lysates from SW480 cells stably expressing Ube2v1 shRNA(shRNA/Ube2v1) or shRNA (shRNA/Control). **Figure S4.** Expressions of E-cadherin after Ube2v1 knockdown with stimulation of Autophagy inhibitor, 3-Methyladenine (3-MA) (5 mM) for 24 h. **Figure S5.** The effects of Ube2v1overexpression on wound-healing, migration and invasion of CRC cells. Wound healing (a), migration (b) and invasion (c) of SW480 and DLD-1 cells after Ube2v1 expression was stably overexpressed. Statistical significance was determined by using a two-tailed, unpaired student's t-test.*$p < 0.05$. **Figure S6.**The effects of rapamycin on Ube2v1 mediated in vitro migration and invasion of CRC cells. a Expressions of E-cadherin and LC3-II, were detected after Ube2v1 was overexpressed with or without rapamycin (final concentration:10 ng/ml) stimulation. B-C. In vitro migration (b) and invasion (c) assays of CRC cells after Ube2v1 overexpression with or without rapamycin (final concentration:10 ng/ml) stimulation for 36 h. **Figure S7.** A proposed model for the role of Ube2v1 in CRC metastasis. Ube2v1 promotes ubiquitination and degradation of Sirt1 by the help of Ubc13, reduces H4K16ac, and finally epigenetically suppresses gene expression of autophagy genes. Then, Ube2v1 promotes autophagy-dependent EMT and metastasis in CRC. (PDF 2486 kb)

Abbreviations
3-MA: 3-Methyladenine; CHX: Cycloheximide; CRC: Colorectal cancer; EMT: Epithelial mesenchymal transition; H4K16ac: Histone H4 lysine 16 acetylation; Sirt1: Sirtuin 1; Ube2v1: Ubiquitin-conjugating E2 enzyme variant 1

Funding
This work was supported by the National Nature Science Foundation of China (Grants81525020, 81502033, 81272300, and 31570753), the Postdoctoral Science Foundation (1302029B) of Jiangsu Province, and Science and Technology Foundation of Suzhou (SYS201412).

Authors' contributions
TS and JML contributed to the study concept and design; TS, LDC, and YHL contributed to the acquisition of data; TS, LDC, YHL, and JML contributed to the analysis and interpretation of data; TS and JML contributed to the drafting of the manuscript for important intellectual content; TS and LDC contributed to the statistical analysis; TS and JML obtained the funding; WJG, XML, JLW, PDG, QZ, XXL, and LNS contributed to the technical for material support; and JML contributed to the study supervision. All authors read and approved the final manuscript.

Consent for publication
Not applicable.

Competing interests
The authors declare that they have no competing interests.

Author details
[1]Department of Pathology, Soochow University Medical School, Suzhou 215123, People's Republic of China. [2]Department of Pathology, Baoan Hospital, Southern Medical University, Shenzhen 518101, People's Republic of China.

References
1. Burger AM, Seth AK. The ubiquitin-mediated protein degradation pathway in cancer: therapeutic implications. Eur J Cancer. 2004;40:2217–29.
2. Hershko A, Heller H, Elias S, Ciechanover A. Components of ubiquitin-protein ligase system. Resolution, affinity purification, and role in protein breakdown. J Biol Chem. 1983;258:8206–14.
3. He C, Klionsky DJ. Regulation mechanisms and signaling pathways of autophagy. Annu Rev Genet. 2009;43:67–93.
4. Kraft C, Peter M, Hofmann K. Selective autophagy: ubiquitin-mediated recognition and beyond. Nat Cell Biol. 2010;12:836–41.
5. Kirkin V, McEwan DG, Novak I, Dikic I. A role for ubiquitin in selective autophagy. Mol Cell. 2009;34:259–69.
6. Rogov V, Dotsch V, Johansen T, Kirkin V. Interactions between autophagy receptors and ubiquitin-like proteins form the molecular basis for selective autophagy. Mol Cell. 2014;53:167–78.
7. Lu K, Psakhye I, Jentsch S. A new class of ubiquitin-Atg8 receptors involved in selective autophagy and polyQ protein clearance. Autophagy. 2014;10:2381–2.
8. Perera RM, Stoykova S, Nicolay BN, Ross KN, Fitamant J, Boukhali M, et al. Transcriptional control of autophagy-lysosome function drives pancreatic cancer metabolism. Nature. 2015;524:361–5.
9. Moscat J, Diaz-Meco MT. p62 at the crossroads of autophagy, apoptosis, and cancer. Cell. 2009;137:1001–4.
10. Edinger AL, Thompson CB. Defective autophagy leads to cancer. Cancer Cell. 2003;4:422–4.
11. Liu Z, Chen P, Gao H, Gu Y, Yang J, Peng H, et al. Ubiquitylation of autophagy receptor Optineurin by HACE1 activates selective autophagy for tumor suppression. Cancer Cell. 2014;26:106–20.
12. Sheen JH, Zoncu R, Kim D, Sabatini M. Defective regulation of autophagy upon leucine deprivation reveals a targetable liability of human melanoma cells in vitro and in vivo. Cancer Cell. 2011;19:613–28.
13. Liang XH, Jackson S, Seaman M, Brown K, Kempkes B, Hibshoosh H, et al. Induction of autophagy and inhibition of tumorigenesis by beclin 1. Nature. 1999;402:672–6.
14. Degenhardt K, Mathew R, Beaudoin B, Bray K, Anderson D, Chen G, et al. Autophagy promotes tumor cell survival and restricts necrosis, inflammation, and tumorigenesis. Cancer Cell. 2006;10:51–64.
15. Mathew R, Karp CM, Beaudoin B, Vuong N, Chen G, Chen HY, et al. Autophagy suppresses tumorigenesis through elimination of p62. Cell. 2009;137:1062–75.
16. Liu H, He Z, Simon HU. Autophagy suppresses melanoma tumorigenesis by inducing senescence. Autophagy. 2014;10:372–3.
17. Yang S, Wang X, Contino G, Liesa M, Sahin E, Ying H, et al. Pancreatic cancers require autophagy for tumor growth. Genes Dev. 2011;25:717–29.
18. Galluzzi L, Pietrocola F, Bravo-San Pedro JM, Amaravadi RK, Baehrecke EH, Cecconi F, et al. Autophagy in malignant transformation and cancer progression. EMBO J. 2015;34:856–80.
19. Rothofsky ML, Lin SL. CROC-1 encodes a protein which mediates transcriptional activation of the human FOS promoter. Gene. 1997;195:141–9.

20. Deng L, Wang C, Spencer E, Yang L, Braun A, You J, et al. Activation of the IkappaB kinase complex by TRAF6 requires a dimeric ubiquitin-conjugating enzyme complex and a unique polyubiquitin chain. Cell. 2000;103:351–61.

21. Thomson TM, Khalid H, Lozano JJ, Sancho E, Arino J. Role of UEV-1A, a homologue of the tumor suppressor protein TSG101, in protection from DNA damage. FEBS Lett. 1998;423:49–52.

22. Ma L, Broomfield S, Lavery C, Lin SL, Xiao W, Bacchetti S. Up-regulation of CIR1/CROC1 expression upon cell immortalization and in tumor-derived human cell lines. Oncogene. 1998;17:1321–6.

23. Wu Z, Shen S, Zhang Z, Zhang W, Xiao W. Ubiquitin-conjugating enzyme complex Uev1A-Ubc13 promotes breast cancer metastasis through nuclear factor-small ka, CyrillicB mediated matrix metalloproteinase-1 gene regulation. Breast Cancer Res. 2014;16:R75.

24. Wang C, Deng L, Hong M, Akkaraju GR, Inoue J, Chen ZJ. TAK1 is a ubiquitin-dependent kinase of MKK and IKK. Nature. 2001;412:346–51.

25. Sun L, Deng L, Ea CK, Xia ZP, Chen ZJ. The TRAF6 ubiquitin ligase and TAK1 kinase mediate IKK activation by BCL10 and MALT1 in T lymphocytes. Mol Cell. 2004;14:289–301.

26. Lamothe B, Besse A, Campos AD, Webster WK, Wu H, Darnay BG. Site-specific Lys-63-linked tumor necrosis factor receptor-associated factor 6 auto-ubiquitination is a critical determinant of I kappa B kinase activation. J Biol Chem. 2007;282:4102–12.

27. Petroski MD, Zhou X, Dong G, Daniel-Issakani S, Payan DG, Huang J. Substrate modification with lysine 63-linked ubiquitin chains through the UBC13-UEV1A ubiquitin-conjugating enzyme. J Biol Chem. 2007;282:29936–45.

28. Xia ZP, Sun L, Chen X, Pineda G, Jiang X, Adhikari A, et al. Direct activation of protein kinases by unanchored polyubiquitin chains. Nature. 2009;461:114–9.

29. Sun L, Li H, Chen J, Dehennaut V, Zhao Y, Yang Y, et al. A SUMOylation-dependent pathway regulates SIRT1 transcription and lung cancer metastasis. J Natl Cancer Inst. 2013;105:887–98.

30. Fullgrabe J, Klionsky DJ, Joseph B. Histone post-translational modifications regulate autophagy flux and outcome. Autophagy. 2013;9:1621–3.

31. Fullgrabe J, Lynch-Day MA, Heldring N, Li W, Struijk RB, Ma Q. The histone H4 lysine 16 acetyltransferase hMOF regulates the outcome of autophagy. Nature. 2013;500:468–71.

32. Ryall JG, Dell'Orso S, Derfoul A, Juan A, Zare H, Feng XS, et al. The NAD(+)-dependent SIRT1 deacetylase translates a metabolic switch into regulatory epigenetics in skeletal muscle stem cells. Cell Stem Cell. 2015;16:171–83.

33. Pulvino M, Liang Y, Oleksyn D, DeRan M, Van Pelt E, Shapiro J, et al. Inhibition of proliferation and survival of diffuse large B-cell lymphoma cells by a small-molecule inhibitor of the ubiquitin-conjugating enzyme Ubc13-Uev1A. Blood. 2012;120:1668–77.

34. Mathew R, Karantza-Wadsworth V, White E. Role of autophagy in cancer. Nat Rev Cancer. 2007;7:961–7.

35. White E, Karp C, Strohecker AM, Guo Y, Mathew R. Role of autophagy in suppression of inflammation and cancer. Curr Opin Cell Biol. 2010;22:212–7.

36. Kalluri R, Weinberg RA. The basics of epithelial-mesenchymal transition. J Clin Invest. 2009;119:1420–8.

37. Wiener R, Zhang X, Wang T, Wolberger C. The mechanism of OTUB1-mediated inhibition of ubiquitination. Nature. 2012;483:618–22.

38. Qi J, Yu Y, Akilli Ozturk O, Holland JD, Besser D, Fritzmann J, et al. New Wnt/beta-catenin target genes promote experimental metastasis and migration of colorectal cancer cells through different signals. Gut. 2015; 65:1690–1701.

39. Hur K, Toiyama Y, Takahashi M, Balaguer F, Nagasaka T, Koike J, et al. MicroRNA-200c modulates epithelial-to-mesenchymal transition (EMT) in human colorectal cancer metastasis. Gut. 2013;62:1315–1326.

40. Bronsert P, Enderle-Ammour K, Bader M, Timme S, Kuehs M, Csanadi A, et al. Cancer cell invasion and EMT marker expression: a three-dimensional study of the human cancer-host interface. J Pathol. 2014;234:410–22.

41. Guo JY, Xia B, White E. Autophagy-mediated tumor promotion. Cell. 2013; 155:1216–9.

42. Grimm WA, Messer JS, Murphy SF, Nero T, Lodolce JP, Weber CR, et al. The Thr300Ala variant in ATG16L1 is associated with improved survival in human colorectal cancer and enhanced production of type I interferon. Gut. 2016;65:456–64.

43. White E. The role for autophagy in cancer. J Clin Invest. 2015;125:42–6.

44. White E. Deconvoluting the context-dependent role for autophagy in cancer. Nat Rev Cancer. 2012;12:401–10.

45. Catalano M, D'Alessandro G, Lepore F, Corazzari M, Caldarola S, Valacca C, et al. Autophagy induction impairs migration and invasion by reversing EMT in glioblastoma cells. Mol Oncol. 2015;9:1612–25.

46. Cicchini M, Chakrabarti R, Kongara S, Price S, Nahar R, Lozy F, et al. Autophagy regulator BECN1 suppresses mammary tumorigenesis driven by WNT1 activation and following parity. Autophagy. 2014;10:2036–52.

47. Li JP, Yang YX, Liu QL, Zhou ZW, Pan ST, He ZX, et al. The pan-inhibitor of Aurora kinases danusertib induces apoptosis and autophagy and suppresses epithelial-to-mesenchymal transition in human breast cancer cells. Drug Des Devel Ther. 2015;9:1027–62.

48. Qiang L, He YY. Autophagy deficiency stabilizes TWIST1 to promote epithelial-mesenchymal transition. Autophagy. 2014;10:1864–5.

49. Lv Q, Hua F, Hu ZW. DEDD, a novel tumor repressor, reverses epithelial-mesenchymal transition by activating selective autophagy. Autophagy. 2012;8:1675–6.

50. Lv Q, Wang W, Xue J, Hua F, Mu R, Lin H, et al. DEDD interacts with PI3KC3 to activate autophagy and attenuate epithelial-mesenchymal transition in human breast cancer. Cancer Res. 2012;72:3238–50.

51. Grassi G, Di Caprio G, Santangelo L, Fimia GM, Cozzolino AM, Komatsu M, et al. Autophagy regulates hepatocyte identity and epithelial-to-mesenchymal and mesenchymal-to-epithelial transitions promoting Snail degradation. Cell Death Dis. 2015;6:e1880.

Permissions

The contributors of this book come from diverse backgrounds, making this book a truly international effort. This book will bring forth new frontiers with its revolutionizing research information and detailed analysis of the nascent developments around the world.

We would like to thank all the contributing authors for lending their expertise to make the book truly unique. They have played a crucial role in the development of this book. Without their invaluable contributions this book wouldn't have been possible. They have made vital efforts to compile up to date information on the varied aspects of this subject to make this book a valuable addition to the collection of many professionals and students.

This book was conceptualized with the vision of imparting up-to-date information and advanced data in this field. To ensure the same, a matchless editorial board was set up. Every individual on the board went through rigorous rounds of assessment to prove their worth. After which they invested a large part of their time researching and compiling the most relevant data for our readers.

The editorial board has been involved in producing this book since its inception. They have spent rigorous hours researching and exploring the diverse topics which have resulted in the successful publishing of this book. They have passed on their knowledge of decades through this book. To expedite this challenging task, the publisher supported the team at every step. A small team of assistant editors was also appointed to further simplify the editing procedure and attain best results for the readers.

Apart from the editorial board, the designing team has also invested a significant amount of their time in understanding the subject and creating the most relevant covers. They scrutinized every image to scout for the most suitable representation of the subject and create an appropriate cover for the book.

The publishing team has been an ardent support to the editorial, designing and production team. Their endless efforts to recruit the best for this project, has resulted in the accomplishment of this book. They are a veteran in the field of academics and their pool of knowledge is as vast as their experience in printing. Their expertise and guidance has proved useful at every step. Their uncompromising quality standards have made this book an exceptional effort. Their encouragement from time to time has been an inspiration for everyone.

The publisher and the editorial board hope that this book will prove to be a valuable piece of knowledge for researchers, students, practitioners and scholars across the globe.

List of Contributors

Swathi Balaji, Makhdum Ahmed, Elizabeth Lorence, Fangfang Yan, Krystle Nomie and Michael Wang
Department of Lymphoma/Myeloma, University of Texas MD Anderson Cancer Center, 1515 Holcombe Blvd. Unit 0429, Houston, TX 77030-4009, USA

Yingxue Qi, Xinyu Liang, Xiangyu Gu, Jianwen Liu and Xin Liang
State Key Laboratory of Bioreactor Engineering and Shanghai Key Laboratory of New Drug Design, School of Pharmacy, East China University of Science and Technology, 130 Meilong Rd, Shanghai 200237, People's Republic of China

Wenchun Chen and Renhao Li
Aflac Cancer and Blood Disorders Center, Children's Healthcare of Atlanta, Department of Pediatrics, Emory University School of Medicine, Atlanta, GA 30322, USA

Ke Xu
Central laboratory, General Surgery, Putuo Hospital, and Interventional Cancer Institute of Chinese Integrative Medicine, Shanghai University of Traditional Chinese Medicine, 164 Lanxi Rd, Shanghai 200062, People's Republic of China

Fengying Wu and Shengxiang Ren
Department of Medical Oncology, Shanghai Pulmonary Hospital, Thoracic Cancer Institute, Tongji University School of Medicine, Shanghai, People's Republic of China

Xuemei Fan and Junling Liu
Department of Biochemistry and Molecular Cell Biology, Shanghai Key Laboratory of Tumor Microenvironment and Inflammation, Shanghai Jiao Tong University School of Medicine, Shanghai 200025, People's Republic of China

Jun Zhang
Division of Hematology, Oncology and Blood and Marrow Transplantation, Department of Internal Medicine, Holden Comprehensive Cancer Center, University of Iowa Carver College of Medicine, Iowa City, IA 52242, USA

Yiting Geng
Department of Oncology, The Third Affiliated Hospital of Soochow University, 185 Juqian Street, Changzhou 213003, Jiangsu, China

Changping Wu
Department of Oncology, The Third Affiliated Hospital of Soochow University, 185 Juqian Street, Changzhou 213003, Jiangsu, China
Department of Tumor Biological Treatment, The Third Affiliated Hospital of Soochow University, 185 Juqian Street, Changzhou 213003, Jiangsu, China

Jingting Jiang
Department of Tumor Biological Treatment, The Third Affiliated Hospital of Soochow University, 185 Juqian Street, Changzhou 213003, Jiangsu, China

Yang Liu and Yinping Dong
School of Medicine and Life Sciences, University of Jinan-Shandong Academy of Medical Sciences, Jinan, Shandong, China
Department of Radiation Oncology, Shandong Cancer Hospital affiliated to Shandong University, Shandong Academy of Medical Sciences, 440 Jiyan Road, Jinan 250117, Shandong, China

Li Kong and Fang Shi
Department of Radiation Oncology, Shandong Cancer Hospital affiliated to Shandong University, Shandong Academy of Medical Sciences, 440 Jiyan Road, Jinan 250117, Shandong, China

Jinming Yu
Department of Radiation Oncology, Shandong Cancer Hospital affiliated to Shandong University, Shandong Academy of Medical Sciences, 440 Jiyan Road, Jinan 250117, Shandong, China
School of Medicine and Life Sciences, University of Jinan-Shandong Academy of Medical Sciences, Jinan, Shandong, China

Federica Giannotti
Department of Hematology and Cell Therapy, Saint-Antoine Hospital, Paris, France

William Arcese
Rome Transplant Network, Tör Vergatä University of Rome, Stem Cell Transplant Unit, Policlinico Universitario Tor Vergata, Rome, Italy

Emanuele Angelucci
Hematology and transplant Unit, Ospedale Policlinico San Martino, Genoa, Italy

Josep-Maria Ribera Santasusana
ICO-Hospital Universitari Germans Trias i Pujol, Josep Carreras Research Institute, Badalona, Spain.

Stella Santarone
Ospedale Civile, Dipartimento di Ematologia, Medicina Trasfusionale e Biotecnologie, Pescara, Italy

Bruno Benedetto
S. S. C. V. D Trapianto di Cellule Staminali A. O. U Citta della Salute e della Scienza di Torino, Torino, Italy

Frederic Baron
GIGA-I3, University of Liege, Liege, Belgium

Shihua Wang, Meiqian Xu, Xiaodong Su, Xian Xiao and Robert Chunhua Zhao
Center of Excellence in Tissue Engineering, Institute of Basic Medical Sciences, Peking Union Medical College Hospital, Chinese Academy of Medical Sciences, School of Basic Medicine Peking Union Medical College, Beijing 100005, China

Xiaoxia Li
Department of Genetics and Cell Biology, Basic Medical College, Qingdao University, 308 Ningxia Road, Qingdao 266071, China

Armand Keating
Cell Therapy Translational Research Laboratory, Princess Margaret Cancer Centre, Toronto, Ontario M5G 2M9, Canada
Institute of Biomaterials and Biomedical Engineering, University of Toronto, Toronto, Ontario M5G 2M9, Canada
Institute of Medical Science, University of Toronto, Toronto, Ontario M5G 2M9, Canada

Hanxiao Xu, Ming Yi, Weiheng Zhao and Kongming Wu
Department of Oncology, Tongji Hospital of Tongji Medical College, Huazhong University of Science and Technology, 1095 Jiefang Avenue, Wuhan 430030, Hubei, China

Xiaodong Lyu
Central Laboratory, the Affiliated Cancer Hospital of Zhengzhou University, Henan Cancer Hospital, Zhengzhou 450000, Henan, China

Yongping Song
Department of Hematology, the Affiliated Cancer Hospital of Zhengzhou University, Henan Cancer
Federica Giannotti

Shuhua Cheng, Giorgio Inghirami and Wayne Tam
Department of Pathology and Laboratory Medicine, Weill Cornell Medicine, New York, NY 10021, USA

Shuo Cheng
Department of Computer Science, School of Engineering, Cornell University, Ithaca, New York, NY 14853, USA

Junliang Ma, Deliang Cao, Yong Zhou and Wenxiang Wang
Department of the 2nd Department of Thoracic Surgery, Hunan Cance Hospital and The Affiliated Cancer Hospital of Xiangya School of Medicine, Central South University, Changsha 410013, Hunan, People's Republic of China

Min Su
Department of the 2nd Department of Thoracic Surgery, Hunan Cance Hospital and The Affiliated Cancer Hospital of Xiangya School of Medicine, Central South University, Changsha 410013, Hunan, People's Republic of China
Department of the Central Laboratory, Hunan Cancer Hospital and The Affiliated Cancer Hospital of Xiangya School of Medicine, Central South University, Changsha 410013, Hunan, People's Republic of China

Qianjin Liao
Department of the Central Laboratory, Hunan Cancer Hospital and The Affiliated Cancer Hospital of Xiangya School of Medicine, Central South University, Changsha 410013, Hunan, People's Republic of China

Yuhang Xiao
Department of Pharmacy, Xiangya Hospital of Xiangya School of Medicine, Central South University, Changsha 410001, Hunan, People's Republic of China

Hui Wang
Department of Thoracic Radiotherapy, Key laboratory of Translational Radiation Oncology, Department of Radiation Oncology, Hunan Cancer Hospital and The Affiliated Cancer Hospital of Xiangya School of Medicine, Central South University, Changsha 410013, Hunan, People's Republic of China

Ming Liu
State Key Laboratory of Respiratory Diseases, Guangzhou Institute of Respiratory Diseases, The First Affiliated Hospital of Guangzhou Medical University, Guangzhou Medical University, Guangzhou, China
Department of Cancer Biology, Lerner Research Institute, Cleveland Clinic, Cleveland, OH, USA

Xu Wang and Yong Li
Department of Cancer Biology, Lerner Research Institute, Cleveland Clinic, Cleveland, OH, USA

Lei Wang
Department of Cancer Biology, Lerner Research Institute, Cleveland Clinic, Cleveland, OH, USA
Institute for Brain Research and Rehabilitation, South China Normal University, Guangzhou, China

Zhaojian Gong
Department of Cancer Biology, Lerner Research Institute, Cleveland Clinic, Cleveland, OH, USA
Department of Stomatology, The Second Xiangya Hospital, Central South University, Changsha, China

Shanshan Zhang
Department of Cancer Biology, Lerner Research Institute, Cleveland Clinic, Cleveland, OH, USA
Department of Stomatology, Xiangya Hospital, Central South University, Changsha, China

Xiaodong Ma
Institute for Brain Research and Rehabilitation, South China Normal University, Guangzhou, China

Liwei Lang and Yuanping Xiong
Department of Oral Biology, Dental College of Georgia, Augusta University, Augusta, GA, USA

Yong Teng
Department of Oral Biology, Dental College of Georgia, Augusta University, Augusta, GA, USA
Georgia Cancer Center, Department of Biochemistry and Molecular Biology, Medical College of Georgia, Augusta University, Augusta, GA, USA

Department of Medical Laboratory, Imaging and Radiologic Sciences, College of Allied Health, Augusta University, 1120 15th Street, Augusta, GA 30912, USA

Chloe Shay
Department of Pediatrics, Emory Children's Center, Emory University, Atlanta, GA, USA

Parth Thakkar and Ron Chemmalakuzhy
Department of Biology, College of Science and Mathematics, Augusta University, Augusta, GA, USA

Xuli Wang
Department of Radiology and Imaging Sciences, School of Medicine, University of Utah, 201 Presidents Cir, Salt Lake City, UT 84112, USA

Marcia Bellon, Ramona Moles, Hassiba Chaib-Mezrag, Joanna Pancewicz and Christophe Nicot
Department of Pathology and Laboratory Medicine, Center for Viral Pathogenesis, University of Kansas Medical Center, 3901 Rainbow Boulevard, MS 3046, Kansas City, KS 66160, USA

Manfei Si and Jinghe Lang
Department of Obstetrics and Gynecology, Peking Union Medical College Hospital, Peking Union Medical College, Chinese Academy of Medical Sciences, No. 1 Shuaifuyuan, Dongcheng District, Beijing 100730, China

Xinwei Huang
Faculty of Environmental Science and Engineering, Kunming University of Science and Technology, Kunming City 650504, Yunnan Province, China
Medical School, Kunming University of Science and Technology, Kunming City 650504, Yunnan Province, China

Xiaoran Guo, Zongxin Zhu and Xiangyang Kong
Medical School, Kunming University of Science and Technology, Kunming City 650504, Yunnan Province, China

Hong Zhang
Department of Rehabilitation Medicine, The First Affiliated Hospital of Chengdu Medical College, Chengdu City 610500, Sichuan Province, China

Haibo Cai
Department of Oncology, Yunfeng Hospital, Xuanwei City 655400, Yunnan Province, China

Elisabeth Silkenstedt
Dr. Margarete Fischer-Bosch-Institute of Clinical Pharmacology, Stuttgart, Germany
Department of Hematology and Oncology, Robert-Bosch-Hospital, Stuttgart, Germany
LMU Klinikum der Universität München, Med. Klinik und Poliklinik III, Munich, Germany
University of Tübingen, Tübingen, Germany

Simon Heine, Markus Kleih, Kathrin Böpple and Heiko van der Kuip
Dr.Margarete Fischer-Bosch-Institute of Clinical Pharmacology, Stuttgart, Germany
University of Tübingen, Tübingen, Germany

Neus Giménez and Dolors Colomer
Hematopathology Unit, Hospital Clínic – Institut d'Investigacions Biomèdiques August Pi i Sunyer (IDIBAPS), CIBERONC, Barcelona, Spain

German Ott
Department of Clinical Pathology, Robert-Bosch-Hospital, Stuttgart, Germany

Walter E. Aulitzky
Department of Hematology and Oncology, Robert-Bosch-Hospital, Stuttgart, Germany

Tong Shen, Ling-Dong Cai, Shi Li, Wen-Juan Gan, Xiu-Ming Li, Jing-Ru Wang, Peng-Da Guo, Qun Zhou, Xing-Xing Lu, Li-Na Sun and Jian-Ming Li
Department of Pathology, Soochow University Medical School, Suzhou 215123, People's Republic of China

Index

www.ingramcontent.com/pod-product-compliance
Lightning Source LLC
Chambersburg PA
CBHW061256190326

41458CB00011B/3687